IMITATION AND THE SOCIAL MIND

Imitation and the Social Mind

AUTISM AND TYPICAL DEVELOPMENT

Edited by
Sally J. Rogers
Justin H. G. Williams

THE GUILFORD PRESS
New York   London

MT

© 2006 The Guilford Press
A Division of Guilford Publications, Inc.
72 Spring Street, New York, NY 10012
www.guilford.com

Printed in the United States of America

This book is printed on acid-free paper.

Last digit is print number: 9   8   7   6   5   4   3   2   1

Library of Congress Cataloging-in-Publication Data

Imitation and the social mind: autism and typical development / edited by Sally J.
Rogers, Justin H. G. Williams.
      p. cm.
   Includes bibliographical references and index.
   ISBN-10: 1-59385-311-4   ISBN-13: 978-1-59385-311-2
   1. Autism.   2. Child development.   3. Developmental psychology.
4. Imitation.   I. Rogers, Sally J.   II. Williams, Justin H. G.
   RC553.A88I45 2006
   616.85′882—dc22

                                                              2006000653

2/8/07

About the Editors

Sally J. Rogers, PhD, is Professor of Psychiatry and Behavioral Sciences at the M.I.N.D. Institute at the University of California, Davis, Medical Center. Her work in autism represents a lifetime interest in developmental disabilities. Dr. Rogers's first position after graduate school at Ohio State University, as an affiliated clinical faculty member at the University of Michigan, involved one of the earliest university-based early intervention projects for infants and families with developmental disorders. This experience focused her career on early developmental trajectories, infant–parent relations, and the development of early intervention practices, especially for children with autism. Dr. Rogers's research on imitation in autism grew out of her clinical and research experiences with children and adults while Professor of Psychiatry at JFK Partners at the University of Colorado Health Sciences Center. She was intrigued by the puzzling lack of normal mirroring and coordination with others' movements, gestures, and emotional displays that she experienced during social interactions with children and adults with autism. This set in motion a line of studies focused on understanding imitation problems in autism, and creation of clinical interventions designed to promote social responsivity and communication development.

Justin H. G. Williams, MRCPsych, commenced his scientific career in 1993, when he took time out to study ecology and evolutionary biology before returning to clinical practice to pursue postgraduate training in psychiatry. He then specialized in child psychiatry and moved to Scotland, where he established working relationships with Andrew Whiten and David Perrett from the University of St. Andrews. Together, they considered the relationship of imitation to autism at a time when "mirror neurons" were a new phenomenon. In 2000 Dr. Williams took up the post of Senior Lecturer in Child Psychiatry at the University of Aberdeen, where he has been developing a research program to better understand the neural substrate of autism. At the same time, he has served as Honorary Consultant in Child Psychiatry at Royal Aberdeen Children's Hospital, where he has been providing psychiatric input to the Intensive Therapy Team of the Department of Child and Family Mental Health.

Contributors

Shauna Bottos, BA, Behavioral Research Unit, Alberta Children's Hospital, Calgary, Alberta, Canada

Malinda Carpenter, PhD, Department of Developmental and Comparative Psychology, Max Planck Institute for Evolutionary Anthropology, Leipzig, Germany

Tony Charman, PhD, Behavioral and Brain Sciences Unit, Institute of Child Health, University College London, London, United Kingdom

Jean Decety, PhD, Department of Psychology, University of Chicago, Chicago, Illinois

Deborah Dewey, PhD, Department of Pediatrics, University of Calgary, Calgary, Alberta, Canada; Behavioral Research Unit, Alberta Children's Hospital, Calgary, Alberta, Canada

Cheryl Dissanayake, PhD, School of Psychological Science, LaTrobe University, Melbourne, Victoria, Australia

Juan Carlos Gómez, PhD, School of Psychology, University of St. Andrews, Fife, Scotland

Susan L. Hepburn, PhD, Center for Autism and Developmental Disorders Research, Department of Psychiatry, University of Colorado Health Sciences Center, Denver, Colorado

Peter Hobson, PhD, FRCPsych, Developmental Psychopathology Research Unit, Tavistock Clinic, London, United Kingdom; Institute of Child Health, University College London, London, United Kingdom

Eva Loth, PhD, Social, Genetic and Developmental Psychiatry Centre, Institute of Psychiatry, King's College London, London, United Kingdom

Crystal Lowe-Pearce, MA, Department of Psychology, Dalhousie University, Halifax, Nova Scotia, Canada

Elise Frank Masur, PhD, Department of Psychology, Northern Illinois University, DeKalb, Illinois

Daniel N. McIntosh, PhD, Department of Psychology, University of Denver, Denver, Colorado

Jessica Meyer, PhD, Developmental Psychopathology Research Unit, Tavistock Clinic, London, United Kingdom; Institute of Child Health, University College London, London, United Kingdom

Mark Mon-Williams, PhD, School of Psychology, University of Aberdeen, Aberdeen, Scotland

Eric J. Moody, MA, Department of Psychology, University of Denver, Denver, Colorado

Jacqueline Nadel, PhD, Laboratory of Vulnerability, Adaptation, and Psychopathology, Pierre and Marie Curie University, Paris, France; Hôpital de La Salpêtrière, Paris, France

Shana L. Nichols, PhD, North Shore–Long Island Jewish Health System, Bethpage, New York

Mark Nielsen, PhD, School of Psychology, University of Queensland, St. Lucia, Queensland, Australia

Bruce F. Pennington, PhD, Department of Psychology, University of Denver, Denver, Colorado

Sally J. Rogers, PhD, M.I.N.D. Institute and Department of Psychiatry and Behavioral Sciences, University of California, Davis, Medical Center, Sacramento, California

Isabel M. Smith, PhD, Department of Pediatrics and Psychology, Dalhousie University, Halifax, Nova Scotia, Canada; IWK Health Centre, Halifax, Nova Scotia, Canada

Wendy L. Stone, PhD, Treatment and Research Institute for Autism Spectrum Disorders, Center for Child Development, Vanderbilt Children's Hospital, Nashville, Tennessee

Thomas Suddendorf, PhD, School of Psychology, University of Queensland, St. Lucia, Queensland, Australia

James R. Tresilian, PhD, Perception and Motor Systems Laboratory, School of Human Movement Studies, University of Queensland, St. Lucia, Queensland, Australia

Gordon D. Waiter, PhD, Department of Radiology, University of Aberdeen Medical School, Aberdeen, Scotland

Andrew Whiten, PhD, FrSE, FBA, School of Psychology, University of St. Andrews, Fife, Scotland

Justin H. G. Williams, MRCPsych, Department of Child Health, University of Aberdeen Medical School, Aberdeen, Scotland

Preface

When people think about the workings of the human brain and the underpinnings of intelligence, they often think about its symbolic capacity, computational functions, or enormous capacity for memory. However, no less important, and perhaps even more pivotal, is the human ability to represent our own experiences and share these with others. One benefit of this capacity is the ability to learn about the world indirectly, from others, and thus to profit from each other's experiences. We call such a capacity "social cognition," and it has possibly been the most important adaptation of the human brain during its recent evolutionary history. It is a complex and multifaceted affair that involves thinking and communicating about one's own and other people's thoughts and mental states.

For most people, such a capacity comes so naturally and automatically that to even recognize its existence is an effort. However, for people with autism, life is very different. Autism is characterized by a collection of symptoms including impairments in social communication and social cognition, in social responsivity and reciprocity with others, and in the development of symbolic play and other imaginative abilities, as well as the tendency to engage in patterns of repetitive thoughts, language, movements, and behaviors. Both clinicians and researchers want to understand why these symptoms cluster together; whether there is some core ability, or abilities, that, when disrupted, result in this symptom pattern. If so, it would indicate a focus for elucidating the underlying biology of autism, as well as a focus for remedial therapy.

Autism is a compelling disorder because it affects capacities that seem so fundamental to our functioning. It is almost impossible for those without autism to imagine life without emotional contagion, without awareness of others' nonverbal signals, without intuiting others' thoughts and feelings and considering their perspectives in every interaction. Autism brings the type of intelligence we call social cognition into sharp relief. However, while the unusual features of older children and adults with autism capture the public mind, the early impairments are most compelling and captivating to developmental researchers, because the early symptoms give us indicators of the course of development of social cognition in typical human ontogeny. Autism researchers are examining early social developmental processes as if under a microscope—behaviors that occur so early and so universally that we might not even have noticed them if it were not for autism.

Imitation is one of these behaviors. It involves the ability to learn socially from others and to incorporate behaviors seen in others into the behavioral repertoire. It involves the connections between the behavior we observe and the behavior we enact. It can concern simple actions such as opening a container, or it can be as advanced as incorporating other people's ideas when writing a book. It is the means by which we absorb, repeat, and so become integrated with human culture. On the face of it, it is a process with irreducible simplicity, and yet the most sophisticated robotics experts still struggle to produce any machine that can perform the function. Furthermore, the apparently simple connections between the observed behavior (or mental state) and the enacted one seem to be core to other social-cognitive capacities, including the ability to share experiences and attribute mental states.

Developmental psychologists as distinguished as Piaget and Bruner, and more recently Nadel, Užgiris, Meltzoff, and Stern, have championed the possible fundamental role of imitation in interpersonal development. Meltzoff's finding that newborns can imitate suggests that at least the beginnings of imitation are biologically prepared and hard-wired. Such biological preparedness suggests an evolutionary perspective. The ability to take advantage of knowledge acquired by others may have conferred crucial adaptive advantages to evolving humans. Finally, imitation is a gift to researchers as it involves easily observed and manipulated behaviors, an ideal experimental tool for exploring the elemental processes of social-cognitive development.

Imitation is one of the social skills that are markedly impaired by autism. The imitation deficit is a relatively quiet problem in autism, though, easily overshadowed by the prominence of striking language and behavioral abnormalities. It would be easy to overlook this as a possibly crucial variable in the development of autism were it not for its evident importance in human social development. It has taken autism researchers over 25 years to appreciate the possible significance of the imitation problem in autism in terms of its possible significance in the evolution of the disorder. The purpose of this book is to bring together work on this topic into a single volume.

Because imitation and autism are crucial to understanding the development of social cognition and social communication, the topic of this book is of core interest to a broad audience of developmentalists, neuropsychologists, and neuroscientists—clinicians and researchers—from many different disciplines. Thus, such a volume needs to cater to readers from many backgrounds and levels, from graduate students to expert scientists. The book represents these varied disciplines and perspectives, for the authors represent the researchers at the leading edge of imitation research as it relates to autism and social cognition across the globe.

Consistent with the traditions of developmental psychopathology, research involving imitation and autism uses the mirrored approaches of examining atypical development to elucidate normal developmental processes and, conversely, looking deeply into patterns and mechanisms of typical development in order to understand the meaning, nature, and course of atypical patterns when they arise. The typical developmental skills of interest here are those of infants—that earliest capacity to imitate and mirror the behavior of someone else. The infant mirrors not only actions observed in others but also their facial expressions, postures and gestures, and emotional behavior. How do these elementary processes form the foundations for the development of more advanced abilities to communicate socially, including the ability to attribute mental states to others?

At a neural level, we are concerned with the irreducible problem of imitation. How do we map enacted behaviors onto observed ones? How can such a property be laid down in patterns of neural connectivity before birth, before any experience with visual stimuli, as Meltzoff's findings suggest to be the case? The recent discovery of "mirror neurons" has given fresh impetus to this line of research, as they are direct evidence that neurons exist that do in fact fire both to observed behavior and to enacted behavior, and thus react as if these two stimuli are equivalent. In previous papers, each of the contributors to this text has drawn on studies of the psychopathology of autism to suggest that this ability to map one's behavior onto a social partner's behavior is crucial to the development of imitation, and may be equally crucial to the development of emotional contagion, joint attention, and mental state attribution.

This volume highlights the common ground and language between these two research perspectives: those who begin with autism and its associated clinical features, and those who begin with action–perception links and neural connectivity. A developmental context is the setting. A number of issues are addressed. One concerns methodology. Methodology can differ between two disciplines apparently studying the same phenomenon. While imitation has been thoroughly and carefully classified and defined among evolutionary psychologists, the same methods have not been utilized among developmental psychologists. As the primatologists have already done, we need to consider the relationships between different types of social learning such as imitation, emulation, and emotional contagion. We need to ask how they differ, and how they are similar, in their paths of development and their cognitive dependencies.

Another compelling issue concerns the meaning of imitative differences among people with autism. While clinicians have devoted much work to issues of heterogeneity in autism (e.g., classification of variations in autistic disorder and related comorbid conditions), autism tends to be seen as a much more homogeneous entity by the basic scientists who approach the disorder and are sometimes inclined to define it as an absence of some rather specific cognitive ability that is of particular interest to the individual researcher. We need to understand variability of imitative ability in autism, addressing issues of universality, persistence throughout the lifespan, point of emergence in the course of the developing disorder, and specificity as it concerns related neuro-developmental disorders involving speech impairment, language disorder, global delay, and developmental coordination disorder.

Since we started work on this book, the field has moved quickly. The "motor theory" of social cognition is becoming a central topic of debate in cognitive psychology. As we go to press, papers are appearing in high-ranking journals discussing the role of mirror neurons in autism. We hope that this work will provide a solid foundation on which to build and develop what promises to be a strong and lasting perspective.

This volume is the result of the efforts of many people over the past 3 years. Rochelle Serwator, at The Guilford Press, provided the initial impetus and was incredibly helpful and supportive throughout the process. Laura Specht Patchkofsky has marched the production end of the book along in record time. The chapter authors were responsive and professional through-out; their ideas and efforts made the initial imaginings of the book come alive.

From Sally Rogers: Justin Williams was an amazing coeditor—so percep-tive, knowledgeable, and productive. The man must never sleep! My family has put up with many nights with no supper on the table, without complain-ing and with consistent enthusiasm for the book-to-be. My assistant, Debra Galik, provided steady support in her cheerful, calm, and very capable way with all the drafts, formatting, paper gathering, and a thousand other tasks. Bruce F. Pennington deserves a very special acknowledgment for the hours and years of shared discussions, papers, and ideas, and the collaborative for-mulation of many of the questions and thoughts that are addressed in this book. Two very gifted colleagues have been invaluable in conceptualizing and actualizing the research underlying my ideas about autism: Susan Hepburn in Denver and Greg Young in Sacramento. And I particularly want to acknowl-edge my friend and colleague Jacqueline Nadel, who has so steadily modeled for me a creative and enthusiastic approach to thinking about science, devel-opment, and autism. It was Jacqueline who told me that editing books was very rewarding.

From Justin Williams: How can one follow those words (that escaped coeditorial scrutiny until the last moment)? They speak for themselves in showing what good fortune I have had to coedit this book with Sally. The journey has been fun and creative, as I have benefited so much from Sally's immeasurable wisdom, insight, and more than generous spirit. And then, to work with so many great writers has been another honor. This book, for me also, is a staging post in a bigger journey studying developmental psychopath-ology. I wish to acknowledge my mentors and traveling companions, who especially include Andy Whiten, Dave Perrett, and Mark Mon-Williams. Also, my family, of course: my wife, Nina, and children, Brodie, Alexander, and Torben. All keep me on track, and their ideas, reflections, and perspective are all invaluable in helping me to try and maintain a steady course in the right direction.

Contents

PART II. EVOLUTIONARY AND NEURAL BASES OF IMITATION

PART III. IMITATION IN AUTISM AND OTHER CLINICAL GROUPS
Biobehavioral Findings and Clinical Implications

PART I

IMITATION IN TYPICAL DEVELOPMENT

CHAPTER 1

Studies of Imitation in Early Infancy
Findings and Theories

SALLY J. ROGERS

The study of imitative development is currently a "hot" and very fertile area of research, demonstrated by an amazingly broad range of disciplinary sciences. The field of robotics is building computer models of this surprisingly complex skill (Alissandrakis, Nehaniv, & Dautenhahn, 2004). Comparative psychology offers new papers on matching phenomena in birds (Zentall, 2004) and primates (Myowa-Yamakoshi, 2000), as well as thoughtful discussions between comparative and developmental psychologists (Want & Harris, 2002). Neuroimagers are examining the neural mechanisms involved in imitation (see Decety, Chapter 11, this volume) and providing exciting new data in support of embodiment theories of psychological processes (Dapretto et al., 2006; Rizzolatti & Craighero, 2004). Neurology, neuropsychology, and cognitive neuroscience describe brain activation patterns and behavioral patterns of imitation gone awry in persons with atypical patterns of development or those with brain injuries (De Renzi, Motti, & Nichelli, 1980; Heilman, 1979; Maher & Ochipa, 1997). Developmental psychologists document the ways in which this extraordinary ability develops, and the interactional effects of the imitating child and the imitating human models on the child's learning history and patterns of social relations (Meltzoff & Moore, 1999; Nadel, Guérini, Pezé, & Rivet, 1999; Užgiris, 1999).

The current interest and energy in this line of inquiry can be traced back to several main sources. Certainly Piaget's (1962) detailed models of imitative development had a powerful effect on the thinking of all developmental psychologists for the past 50 years. His theories stimulated a series of longitudinal studies on imitation in the 1970s and 1980s that sought to test his suggested sequences of abilities and ages, developed instrumentation and coding systems, and moved imitation into psychology laboratories.

A second powerful line of interest in imitative difficulties can be traced back to Leipmann and Maas's (1907) clinical report of a patient with an apraxia who had lost the ability to imitate and carry out gestures on command with his left arm (as reviewed in Heilman & Rothi, 1997). The neurological research on apraxia led to the development of testing paradigms for adults and drew our attention to the movement, or motoric aspects of imitation, and the possibility that focal neural mechanisms were involved in gestural imitation in autism also.

Meltzoff and Moore's publications concerning neonatal imitation have added considerable fuel to the current wildfire of interest in imitation. Following earlier doctoral dissertation work by Maratos (1973, as described in Maratos, 1982), Meltzoff and Moore published a series of papers beginning in 1977 and spanning the next 15 years in which they demonstrated imitation of multiple gestures by newborns. The importance of imitation to typical social–emotional development was considered in these studies and the flurry of work that followed. A slowly accumulating body of research documenting imitative deficits in autism (see reviews by Rogers & Pennington, 1991; Smith & Bryson, 1994; Williams, Whiten, & Singh, 2004) added clinical significance to the potential importance of early imitation for interpersonal social–emotional development.

The findings and theories generated by the phenomenon of neonatal imitation have had a tremendous impact on theorizing about typical and atypical social development. Given the focus of this entire volume on imitation and social development, the purpose of this first chapter is to begin at the beginning: to review the evidence, and to consider the controversies, concerning research in early infant imitation—imitation occurring before the age of 6 months—and its contributions to social development. For the purposes of this chapter, Butterworth's (1999) definition of the term *imitation* will be used: "[behavior displays in which] one individual voluntarily reproduces behaviour as observed in another who acts as the model for the form of a behaviour" (p. 65). Beginning with the first publications on the phenomenon, the replications, nonreplications, and methodological challenges concerning neonatal imitation will be reviewed. Then data from longitudinal studies concerning consistency and stability of imitation over the first year of life will be provided. Finally, theories and evidence concerning the role of imitation in other aspects of social–communicative development will be covered, ending with research needs and priorities.

THE INITIAL FINDINGS: THE WORK OF MELTZOFF AND MOORE

In their initial paper, Meltzoff and Moore (1977) reported two experiments. The first involved six infants, ages 12–17 days, who were shown one of four movements in randomly assigned order: tongue protrusion (TP), mouth opening (MO), lip protrusion (LP), or hand opening (HO). Following a 90-second still face baseline, the experimenter demonstrated each gesture four times in a 15-second period, followed by a 20-second still period. If the experimenter felt that the infant had not seen the display, it was repeated for up to three total presentation-response blocks. Untrained coders blind to the experimental condition rank-ordered each video segment according to which of the four stimuli the infant's behavior most resembled. Then the four ranks were collapsed into two, yielding dichotomous scores. Analysis revealed significant differences in coder judgments based on the stimulus behavior being modeled. For each behavior, the rate of occurrence in the target condition was significantly elevated over its rate in the other conditions. Potential methodological problems identified by the authors—especially the inconsistent number of presentations according to experimenter judgments—were corrected in the second experiment, which involved 12 infants from 16 to 21 days old. They saw TP and MO counterbalanced, and during the display the infants sucked on a pacifier, so that no infant mouth movements occurred that might have influenced the experimenter. (It probably also helped keep the infants alert and content during the procedure.) The stimulus was delivered "until the experimenter judged that the infant had watched it for 15 seconds." Then the pacifier was removed for 150 seconds for a response, then returned; the second behavior was displayed in the same way. One coder, blind to the experiment, coded behavior in the response periods for all TPs and MOs. In each condition, the target behavior occurred significantly more often in the target condition than the other condition.

Two papers followed (Meltzoff & Moore, 1983, 1989) that described a much more elaborated and standardized method. The 1983 paper described in detail the precise lab setup involved, including a specially prepared, dark, sound dampened chamber; infrared lighting; and spotlight on the face of the experimenter, who was clothed in black. Even the size of the video image was specified. The stimuli were now delivered in a tightly timed and controlled fashion with exactly equal number and length of presentations, and the experimenter's behavior was now rigidly controlled by the method. Coding criteria for the modeled behaviors, TP and MO, are carefully described, as are intra- and interrater reliability data. Newborn infants, all less than 72 hours old, produced both target behaviors significantly more often in the target condition than the alternative condition. The 1989 paper replicated this elaborated method to test a new, nonoral behavior—head turning, as well as TP, again with significant increases of both target behaviors in the target compared to the contrast condition.

With the increasing standardization of the method, and increasingly younger infants, came significant subject attrition. In the 1983 paper, 40 subjects provided data and an additional 62 were dropped. In the 1989 paper 40 infants contributed data and 53 others were dropped. The attrition rate may be an unavoidable by-product of extremely standardized stimulus delivery, even in a paradigm designed to maximize infant attention, given the characteristics of very young infants in terms of state regulation and the brevity of alert attentional states. In studies using methods that provided more support for infant attention or alertness, whether by coordinating stimulus delivery with infant attention (Meltzoff & Moore, 1977), or by use of handling techniques that optimize attention (Field, Woodson, Greenberg, & Cohen, 1982; Kaitz, Meschulach-Sarfaty, Auerbach, & Eidelman, 1988), a higher proportion of infants participate. Examination of infant visual attention is quite helpful in determining the validity of the data (Anisfeld et al., 2001). It is difficult to assess the validity of infant response, even to auditory stimuli, when their eyes are closed (see Chen, Striano, & Rakoczy, 2004).

Topics of the research papers from these scientists in the 1990s moved beyond the question of immediate imitation to explore the phenomenon in greater depth, and to respond to questions and criticisms in the field. In a 1992 paper reporting two experiments, Meltzoff and Moore demonstrated production of imitative TP to both static and dynamic movements in 6- and 12-week-olds. In 1994, they demonstrated deferred imitation in 6-week-old infants, who as a group selectively produced tongue protrusion after a 24-hour delay. In this paper as well, they demonstrated infants' gradually increasing accuracy of response over time. In both of these papers, the MO response did not occur significantly more frequently in the target condition, though the duration was significantly longer. A 1996 paper by Kuhl and Meltzoff examined vocal imitation of three vowel sounds in 12-, 16-, and 20-week-old infants using both spectrograph analysis and phonetically trained coders. The group as a whole demonstrated significantly more matching vowels in the target than the contrast conditions, but when the data were analyzed by age groups, only the 20-week-old group demonstrated significant amounts of imitation of the target. Thus, over a 20-year period, a number of carefully designed experiments from this lab demonstrated, replicated, and extended the findings while generating exciting new hypotheses concerning the nature of the behavior and its role in development.

Replication Efforts

Given the provocative nature of these findings, a large number of attempted replication studies ensued. While a comprehensive literature review will not be attempted here, a number of researchers replicated Meltzoff and Moore's findings, with varying degrees of experimental rigor, with infants in the first 2 months of life (Anisfeld et al., 2001; Heimann, Nelson, & Schaller, 1989; Kaitz et al., 1988; among others, reported TP; imitation of movements other than TP have been reported by Field et al., 1982; Kugiumutzakis, 1999; Maratos, 1982; Reissland, 1988; Vinter, 1986).

However, some investigators reported a complete absence of imitative responses at these very early ages (Abravanel & Sigafoos, 1984; Lewis & Sullivan, 1985). More often, the nonreplications involved behaviors other than TP. Kaitz and colleagues (1988) failed to replicate Field and colleagues'

(1982) findings of emotional expression imitation using slightly different rating categories. Anisfeld and colleagues (2001) and Heimann and colleagues (1989), among others, could not document imitation of MO or LP.

These nonreplications drew attention to important methodological variables and raised questions about possible limitations in the phenomenon. As Meltzoff and Moore (1983) pointed out, so many variations were used in lab environment, stimulus delivery, data scoring, and data analysis that comparisons across studies were difficult to make. The many challenges of assessing newborns includes their state and behavioral variability, their relatively limited visual acuity, their limited periods of alertness, their spontaneous movement patterns, and the fact that the imitative stimuli represent behaviors that are already in the infants' spontaneous behavioral repertoires.

Crucial methodological variables detailed by Meltzoff and Moore (1983) and Anisfeld and colleagues (2001) that must be considered when evaluating these papers involve stimulus delivery, behavior coding, and data analysis. In terms of stimulus delivery, the tightest designs required the experimenter to deliver the stimuli in a predetermined, randomized, and counterbalanced fashion at specific time intervals to rule out the possibility that the experimenter's delivery of the stimuli was being influenced by the infant's spontaneous movements. In terms of behavior coding, studies that code and analyze partial as well as complete demonstrations of the target behaviors have demonstrated more findings than those that require a complete replication of the target behavior. Other crucial coding variables include raters who are blind to the stimulus and who are coding the infant's actual behavior, rather than force classifying them into a set of predetermined variables (e.g., corners of mouth up as opposed to forced classification as happy or sad). Finally, in terms of analysis, the necessary comparisons involve comparing the frequency of the targeted behavior in the target experimental condition against the frequency of the same behavior in another experimental condition rather than a baseline condition (this guards against the response reflecting a general behavioral arousal (see Jones, 1996).

Replication efforts have highlighted several important points: How limited is the response, how automatic versus volitional is the response, and how specific is the response. A behavior that is limited to a single behavior or two, that appears quite automatic, and that occurs in response to many different types of stimuli in addition to human models, does not seem to meet the criteria for an imitation.

First is the issue of limitations in the infant's imitative repertoire. Several of the aforementioned authors (Anisfeld et al., 2001; Jones, 1996; Kaitz et al., 1988) have argued that response is limited primarily to only one behavior—tongue protrusion—and thus can be more parsimoniously explained as a fixed action pattern, or reflexive action, than an indication of the capacity for imitation in general. Thus, the number of movements that neonates will imitate is an issue. However, at least three rigorous studies have replicated Meltzoff and

Moore's findings of imitative responses for multiple behaviors in the first 6 months of life. All studies used standardized stimulus delivery, raters blind to hypotheses and conditions, infant behavioral codings rather than forced judgments, and group analyses comparing frequencies across experimental conditions. Vintner (1986) demonstrated both TP and hand open–close using a highly standardized delivery (though it is not stated that the two behaviors modeled were randomly varied). Fontaine (1984) demonstrated imitation of several different oral behaviors (but no imitation of manual behaviors) in 2-month-olds. Thus, both mouth and manual movement imitations have been demonstrated in several extremely rigorous studies.

The second issue concerns the volitional aspect of the imitation. Even though developmentalists recognize some behavior in neonates that is not reflexive (e.g., attentive gaze), it is difficult to attribute intentions to movement patterns of newborns. However, the pattern of the response in these early infant imitation studies does not fit the pattern of automatic or reflexive movements in several ways. First, an automatic behavior generally follows the stimulus immediately. However, the infants in these studies produce the behavior after the stimulus has ended, during the response periods, and can do so even if their ability to respond immediately to the stimulus is blocked, as with a pacifier in the Meltzoff and Moore (1977) study. Second, a reflex or automatic behavior should weaken or habituate over multiple elicitations. Yet these responses appear stronger over multiple stimuli and in one study have been shown to gradually strengthen or improve in accuracy. Experimenters (Kugiumutzakis, 1999; Meltzoff & Moore, 1992) describe "effortful" behavior from the infants as they carry out the imitations, which we have also seen in our lab. As Pennington (personal communication, December 27, 2005) has pointed out, all behavior is determined by a neural response to an antecedent stimulus. At a neural level, operational definitions of voluntary or involuntary behavior become very difficult. Characteristics like flexibility, effortfulness, and latency appear more useful constructs than intentionality.

A third issue concerns the specificity of the response. Evidence that TP occurs nondiscriminately comes from three experiments by Jones (1996). The first experiment demonstrated that 4-week-olds increased both TP and MO when engaged with interesting visual stimuli (in this case, blinking lights). However, only TP appeared to be influenced by the level of engagement of the infant with the stimulus. The second experiment demonstrated that 4-week-olds spent more time looking at an adult modeling TP than an adult displaying MO, and interpreted this finding to mean that TP is the more interesting stimulus to the baby. These two observations lead to the hypothesis that TP could occur more often in the TP than the MO condition due to increased infant attention and arousal in the TP condition. The third, longitudinal study of two infants examined weekly from 3 weeks to 30 weeks demonstrated that TP occurred at higher rates than mouth openings in the presence of interesting graspable objects dangling in front of the babies. Furthermore, as soon as the babies could reach for and grasp the objects, TP (but not MO) ceased almost entirely. She interpreted her data as suggesting that TP, including that which occurs under imitative conditions, reflects interest in the visual stimulus and is due to, and a kind of preparation for, later oral exploration (see also Nagy & Molnar, 2004). However, finding that TP occurs nonspecifically in conditions of infant arousal does not rule out the possibility that it can also occur as an imitative behavior. Newborns have limited motor control, and the mouth is likely to be an area of relatively great motor control for them. Finally, demonstration that another behavior occurs more often than TP in a contrasting experimental condition helps allay the concern that the matching responses of the infant are nonspecific responses. The demonstrations of multiple behaviors described previously address this concern.

To summarize the replication study findings, the variation in infant response from one lab to another likely reflects the instability of state and behavioral control of the human neonate as well as methodological differences across labs. Studies using methods that provide more support to the infant's attentional state tended to report more examples of imitation. However, even under the most rigorous methods of stimulus delivery, behavior measurement, and analysis, several independent labs have demonstrated that infants in the first month of life produce behaviors that appear to be imitative rather than fixed action patterns. The evidence supports the interpretation that very young infants are capable of providing an imitative response to several differing behaviors. However, it does not support the interpretation that infants are capable of a vast number of imitative responses, or that this is a robust part of their behavioral repertoire. As one reads the papers in this area, the inconsistent response patterns of the infants and the elaborate methods that have been developed to elicit this behavior give one the sense of a fragile response pattern, an incipient or rudimentary potential, a starting state and beginning point of self–other correspondence and an ability that will become wonderfully elaborated in the next 18 months.

We next consider the various interpretations of neonatal imitation and the underlying mechanisms. As Maratos (1998) stated, "the phenomenon of neonatal imitation of certain models is currently widely accepted and not challenged any more, and the still-animated theoretical discussions concern its meaning and importance for developmental psychological theories" (p. 147).

INTERPRETATIONS OF THE PHENOMENON

Developmental psychology has a very long experience with the challenge of interpreting behavior, and, as with many other developmental phenomena, infant responses to adult models have been subject to both rich and lean interpretations. The leanest interpretations of neonatal imitation, already touched on in this chapter, suggest that TP is the only behavior that replicates consistently across studies, and as such can be explained more parsimoniously as a somewhat automatic response, akin to a reflex or fixed action pattern, present at birth but disappearing over time, eventually replaced by higher-level, volitional, truly imitative behavior (Anisfeld et al., 2001; Heyes, 2002; Kaitz et al., 1988). Recent findings that nonhuman neonatal primates respond imitatively to models of TP (Bard & Russell, 1999; Myowa-Yamakoshi, 2000) could be considered to add weight to this argument. However, stating that a behavior is a fixed action pattern does not explain the behavior or the underlying mechanism involved.

Richer interpretations suggest that newborns are capable of making a variety of effortful, intentional, and goal-directed efforts to imitate the adult's specific behavior. The argument that neonatal responses are similar in kind to more mature imitative displays has been made most strongly by Meltzoff and Moore (1997) based on (1) the intentional nature of the infants' acts; (2) deferred imitation of the acts; (3) and the range and number of the acts. The evidence supporting this interpretation was discussed above.

How does a newborn produce an imitative response to a behavior the infant cannot see himself or herself make? Meltzoff and Moore suggest that the underlying mechanism involves an amodal representational system (active intermodal mapping [AIM]) present at birth that supports mapping of self and other's bodies. In their 1997 paper, Meltzoff and Moore lay out their model in a very detailed fashion. They suggest that the infant uses three main processes to produce the imitative response. First involves correspondence of body parts involving the infant's perceptual system ("organ identification" in their terminology). Second involves a comparative process across bodies using the AIM representational system. Matches are identified and mismatches are corrected through the third process, the infant's action system, which activates action patterns resulting from previous motor learning via circular reactions ("body babbling") occurring both prior to and after birth. They suggest that the infant's awareness of configural body matching provides a "like me" experience of self and other. According to Meltzoff and Moore, theirs is not an unduly nativist theory but, rather, a developmental theory built from some capacities present at birth that develop and gradually result in a restructuring of imitation over the first 18 months of life in accord with other developments in the infant's knowledge of self and other, gained through experience and cognitive development. Meltzoff and Decety (2003) make explicit reference to everyday experiences of the young infant, both imitative and self-experiences that provide opportunities to map bodily actions to psychological experiences.

The potential impact of early infant imitation abilities on psychosocial development was first realized in a landmark publication by Daniel Stern (1985). He integrated the early infant imitation findings with other research concerning early infant abilities to suggest a series of phases of interpersonal development, beginning with early imitation and pattern recognition as starting points, leading to milestones involving shared affect at a dyadic level, shared affect, attention and intentions at a triadic level, and eventual development of theory of mind.

Findings that both imitation and theory of mind were severely affected in autism led Rogers and Pennington (1991) to suggest that difficulty in imitation and formation of bodily self–other correspondences was a possible starting point for the cascade of social impairments seen in autism, including dyadic relations, triadic relations, and theory of mind, adding further weight to Stern's hypothesis concerning the potential importance of imitative behaviors in later human social relatedness. A similar line of thought was suggested by Meltzoff and Gopnik (1993), that the like-me experience of early imitation provides a basis of simulation for all other self–other experiences. This line of reasoning was further developed and tied to the exciting research on mirror neuron systems by Williams, Whiten, Suddendorf, and Perrett (2001), who suggested that the mirror neuron system, rather than the AIM mechanism, may be the mechanism for early imitation, and deficits in that system may be the cause of the difficulties with self–other mappings, and the resulting interpersonal deficits, in autism.

Empirical support for Meltzoff and Moore's theory requires both multiple examples of such cross-modal or intermodal processing and continuity of effects across development. Evidence includes cross-modal responses in very young infants involving in a visual–tactile cross-modal matching task demonstrated by Meltzoff and Borton (1979), though the amount of empirical support for both this task and the underlying hypothesis of amodal or cross-modal capacities in neonates has been questioned (Maurer, Stager, & Mondloch, 1999). A further problem for the theory, as discussed in the next section, is the sparse evidence to support continuities between neonatal imitation and later social–cognitive development.

The AIM approach has also been criticized as not fitting well with the current data on imitation from animal studies (definitions of imitation and TP in animals), mimicry studies (especially the importance of facial mimicry on social relations [Chartrand & Bargh, 1999]), and brain imaging studies (especially MN system findings in human imitation; Heyes, 2001). However, recent descriptions of the AIM theory demonstrate new integrations of the theory with research findings in all these areas (Meltzoff & Decety, 2003). Heyes (2001, 2002) has offered a leaner, alternative model, the Associative Sequence Learning model to explain imitative development in infancy. She rejects the interpretation of neonatal matching responses as true imitation. Rather, she suggests that imitation develops over time, as associations between sensory and motor representations of movements become linked through coactivation in experiences like mirrors, being imitated, observation of one's own movement, and so on (and that, at the neuronal level, some canonical neurons acquire a mirroring function through such experiences). The model suggests that once these associations are in place, via a general learning mechanism rather than a specialized imitation mechanism (Brass & Heyes, 2005), they would occur relatively automatically through coactivation, not only in imitative situations but in response to various observed actions (thus also allowing for interpretation of failed intentions or invisible goal states, for instance) and thus would need to be actively inhibited. The model suggests that co-ordination of first- and third-person information is quite important in building a theory of other minds, but that imitation is only one of various kinds of experience that provide this input, and thus does not have a privileged role in theory of mind development. Heyes fits this model to autism by suggesting that lack of attention to others in both dyadic and triadic interactions reduces the experiences needed to create the coactivated sensory–movement associations. The ASL model is compatible with studies of both mimicry and intentional imitation. Furthermore, the model is consistent with research on mirror neurons, brain activation patterns, and observational learning.

To conclude this section, we have discussed leaner and richer interpretations of the neonatal imitation studies. The leanest interpretations, those that consider neonatal matching responses to be fixed action patterns, do not seem to account well for the findings. However, the rich interpretations of early infant imitation rest strongly on developmental continuities between early infant imitation and later self–other capacities. What is the empirical support for these hypothesized continuities? We turn now to the evidence concerning continuities in imitation from the first month of life.

DEVELOPMENTAL CONTINUITIES AND DISCONTINUITIES

Demonstrating continuity over time between early infant responses and later intentional imitation and markers of social cognition would provide important support for the richer interpretations of early infant imitation. What is the evidence of continuity over time in imitative development? Unfortunately, most of the longitudinal studies of neonatal imitation have not been carried out over long enough periods of time to shed light on this question. Furthermore, most have analyzed the data cross-sectionally and have not examined individual patterns of performance over time.

The first longitudinal study (Maratos, 1982) examined imitation of a large number of behaviors over the first 6 months of life. Longitudinal examination of the group data revealed a decrease in imitative mouth and head responses between 2 and 4 months, and an increase in vocal responses from 2 to 5 months followed by decrease after 5 months. Maratos interpreted these data as demonstrating the presence in neonates of early reflexive or primary circular reaction imitative patterns (as described by Piaget, 1962) that demonstrate discrimination and intersensory coordination capacities and serve to elicit and maintain social–communicative interactions. She suggested that developmental discontinuity and reorganization occurs around 3 months of age in which early infant imitative responses are gradually replaced by more socially effective but later maturing smiles and vocal behaviors, followed by development of intentional imitation skills in the second half of the first year and beyond.

Several other longitudinal studies replicated Maratos's finding of declines in imitation of mouth and tongue movements between 2 and 4 months (e.g., Abranavel & Sigafoos, 1984; Kugiumutzakis, 1999). Kugiumutzakis (1999) carried out a rigorous longitudinal study examining imitation skills of infants every 2 weeks from birth to 6 months of age. Administration and scoring approaches were generally well standardized and used appropriate controlled methods. The longitudinal curves that mapped the frequencies of several different imitative oral, motor, and vocal behaviors demonstrated varying onset, offset, and peaks for various behaviors across this period. The author interpreted this to mean that, while imitations of individual behaviors wax and wane, the capacity to respond imitatively does not diminish.

Meltzoff and Moore (1992) responded to the inability of other researchers to document imitations in 3-month-olds with a study of imitation at 6 and 12 weeks using new methodology. The method involved two models: mother and stranger, who were attired differently, entered and existed the room via different routes and performed different gestures (MO or TP). Both a group of 32 6-week-olds and a different group of 16 9- to 12-week-olds displayed significantly more TP in the targeted experimental condition compared to the opposite condition. The older infants (but not the 6-week-olds) also displayed significantly more MO in the targeted than the contrast condition. Because no longitudinal data were provided, neither the question of individual consistency and stability of response nor the question of a decrease in frequency across the first 3 months was addressed. Furthermore, variations in method across these age periods makes comparisons of frequencies across the age periods uninformative. Meltzoff and Moore shared Maratos's hypothesis that apparent decreases or dropoffs in imitative behavior in these older infants was due to their replacement by newer and powerfully effective social behaviors like vocalizing and smiling.

Užgiris (1973) reported a longitudinal study of 12 infants beginning at 1 month of age and continuing across the first 2 years of life. The study used a Piagetian framework to examine both vocal and gestural imitation. Tasks were administered and coded by one experimenter. Behaviors consistently imitated in the first 2 months of life involved cooing vocalizations, while gestural imitations were not observed in at least half of the group until 6 months of age (although tongue movements were observed earlier and were reported informally). Užgiris observed that infants imitated behaviors already in their repertoire, and that older infants imitated novel acts more easily when acts are directed to an object rather than a gesture. She also addressed individual differences in overall imitative capacities, observing that "there was considerable consistency in the infants' behavior" (p. 601). Once an infant imitated an action, he or she tended to imitate that action in later testings. Furthermore, infants who were earlier to imitate actions at one level tended to be early to imitate actions at subsequent levels, and infants showed individual consistency across vocal and gestural imitations.

The only papers to report on consistency and stability of response at an individual level over time were published by Mikael Heimann. Heimann and colleagues (1989) examined 32 infants at 2–3 days, 3 weeks, and 3 months of age (23 infants completed the experiment) on imitation of TP, MO, and LP. Stimuli were administered according to a random schedule, but the number of presentations was not fixed. Coders blind to the stimulus and hypotheses coded all behaviors, as well as infant states. Almost no LP responses were seen so analysis of that behavior was not carried out. There was a significant increase of weak TP responses in the TP condition compared to the MO condition (more than half the sample showed this imitative response) at 2–3 days and 3 weeks, but not at 3 months, and the response frequency decreased significantly over time. (The frequency of MO was also higher in the TP than the MO condition, so the imitation effect was limited to TP.) When the data for individuals were examined across the three age periods, three of nine correlations were significant from 3 days to 3 weeks, but there were no significant correlations from 3 days to 3 months. The author interprets these as showing "no stability beyond the first three weeks of life" (Heimann et al., 1989, p. 98).

However, in a chapter that described additional analyses of these data, Heimann (1998) suggested that imitation in 3-month-olds showed a somewhat different pattern than in younger infants, involving a faster and more controlled response. Like Maratos (1982), he suggested a developmental change in imitation across this period, perhaps involving combined effects of cortical development, social experiences, and changes in motivational supports, among other possibilities. He also reported evidence of stability from 3 days to 3 months among a subgroup of infants categorized as high imitators as opposed to low imitators.

Heimann (1989) also examined relationships between early imitation and mother–child interaction patterns at 3 months of age using 6 minutes of a face-to-face mother–child interaction with the infant in a seat without toys. Of the 90 correlations run, 7 reached the $p < .05$ level of significance. Because this is only slightly more than would be expected by chance, interpretation needs to proceed cautiously. However, four of these significant correlations involved very similar relations: negative correlations between earlier imitative responses and amount of time that 3-month-olds spent averting gaze. Thus, less imitative infants showed more gaze aversion. The negative relation with gaze aversion may reflect lack of infant attention to the imitative stimulus. However, the method required the experimenter to continue to model until the infant attended to the stimulus. Thus, cessation of the model after infant attending appears to provide each infant with roughly the same exposure to the stimulus. This is an important finding, but understanding its full significance will require replication, examination of parental behavior, and longitudinal evidence of interactive differences over time.

Finally, Heimann (1998) described a 12-month assessment of these same subjects, using a variety of measures (i.e. temperament and language) including imitative tasks. There were no significant relations between neonatal imitation and any 12-month measures. Two significant positive correlations (total number not reported) were found between 3- month and 12-month imitative behaviors (but not other relations). Thus, Heimann has provided us with the first and only evidence to date of any longitudinal relations between early imitation and later imitation and other social responses. This is a slim empirical base for building rich and exciting hypotheses concerning the importance of early infant imitation to later interpersonal development. Additional longitudinal support is needed.

The foregoing studies have opened up several additional areas of inquiry for the next generation of infant imitation studies and theories. Particularly interesting questions concern the issue of mimicry, possible discontinuities in imitative development, and the effects of individual differences in imitative capacity, in both typical and atypical development. In the final section of this chapter, we turn to these current unanswered questions in early infancy imitation research.

CURRENT ARGUMENTS AND CRITICISMS THAT NEED ADDRESSING
Imitation versus Mimicry in Early Infant Imitation

Several of the critics of the neonatal imitation research suggest that the neonates' response is one of mimicry rather than imitation. In doing so, they appear to equate mimicry with a low-level response, akin to a reflex or fixed action pattern, and the assumption is that mimicry is unrelated to a volitional imitative response (see Nadel & Butterworth, 1999, for a rich discussion of the tendency in developmental psychology to devalue immediate imitation). This focus on classification of different types of matching behaviors has been a contribution of comparative psychology to the study of imitation in children, as demonstrated in a paper by Want and Harris (2002). They remind developmental psychologists that "what was once thought to have been the result of imitation, is now variously described as the result of local enhancement, stimulus enhancement, mimicry or emulation, rather than imitation. . . . While developmental psychology has been very good at mapping out children's proclivity to replicate the actions of others, it has often said little about how they do so" (p. 2). Want and Harris, among others (e.g., Tomasello, 1996), suggest that the term *imitation* be reserved for behaviors that involve understanding of both goals and means of the model. They further suggest that matching responses of infants below 13 months do not reflect intentional imitation but are the result of mimicry, defined as nonvolitional, automatic matching responses. However, this assumes, first, that mimicry is not related to means–end imitation, and second, it does not account for the proclivity or the power of gestural imitation in humans (Donald, 1991).

Mimicry is a powerful social phenomenon with a long history of research in social psychology. Mimicry may be a powerful contributor to interpersonal transmission of emotional states (emotional contagion; Hatfield, Cacioppo, & Rapson, 1994). Several developmental theorists have suggested that mimicry, or imitation of facial expressions, may be an important process underlying social relatedness and development of other mental state knowledge as well (Meltzoff & Gopnik, 1993; Rogers, 1999; Zajonc, Murphy, & Inglehart, 1989). Recent studies of mimicry have rekindled interest in this phenomenon (Chartrand & Bargh, 1999). Far from being a low-level response to be dismissed, mimicry appears to be an extremely important aspect of social relatedness to be studied and understood.

Is Mimicry Linked to Imitation?

We have no information regarding the relation of effortful imitation to mimicry in behavioral studies. (In fact, we have no information regarding the relations among the different kinds of matching behaviors specified by Want and Harris [2002] in human development. Examining the nature of these relations would provide evidence concerning the independence of these various behaviors.) However, functional brain studies are producing data that address this question. Current work in imitation neuroimaging research in humans demonstrates that some of the same neural areas are activated in conditions of action observation (which is likely the mimicry condition) and intentional imitation (Dapretto et al., 2006). Furthermore, electromyography (EMG) studies in social psychology indicate that observing other people activates unintentional motor mimicry in the observer (see Niedenthal, Barsalou, Winkielman, Krauth-Gruber, & Ric, 2005, for a recent review). This leads to the hypothesis that neural systems specifically activated during action–observation (and identical to those in intentional imitation conditions) also underlie mimicry responses—that mimicry and intentional imitation become the same response at the neural level, perhaps through a Hebbian learning process as suggested by Keysers and Perrett (2004).

A final concern that has been raised regarding the relations between mimicry and imitation deals with imitation of novel actions and movement patterns. Does the ability to imitate novel movements require a different underlying mechanism than mimicry? To what extent we are capable of imitating movements that are novel for us is an interesting question. When watching people, both infants and older humans, perform intentional imitative acts, one is impressed with the fact that, when a difficult novel movement is modeled, the subject tends to perform a simplified version of the action that is within his or her current repertoire. Indeed, for an amateur to learn a completely novel act via imitation—a dance move, an ice skater's spin, a trill played on the piano—requires breaking down the complex movement into its simple parts involving actions currently in one's repertoire, and then building up the complexity slowly, through trial and error, chaining and sequencing, and much practice—the same process that appears to underlie infant action learning. The challenge of novelty for our hypothesis concerning the relations of intentional imitation and mimicry may be more apparent than real. We imitate movements that are already in our repertoire, and when faced with novel movements, we either break them down into movements that are already in our repertoire and perform those or we laboriously go to work to master the novel movement, through trial and error, and repetition (and often, instruction, or pedagogy). Novel actions produced via imitation may be similar to novel language productions: "a new machine constructed of old parts" (Bates, 2004, p. 250).

How Does Mimicry Develop?

We have no studies, or developmental models, that consider how mimicry develops. In the area of motor learning, a behavior becomes automatic only after it is first acquired intentionally and volitionally. Learned motor skills such as driving or playing a sport or a musical instrument only slowly acquire automaticity as a result of mastery and developing expertise. Different neural activations, involving corticocerebellar circuits, occur during motor learning tasks involving new, effortful actions, than during skilled performance, which activates corticostriatal circuits (Lacourse, Orr, Cramer, & Cohen, 2005). It is possible that neural systems developed through imitative learning underlie mimicry, linking mimicry to intentional imitative development, particularly concerning facial, postural, and manual gestures. This might even be true of facial mimicry. Personal observations document that infant social smiles appear as an infant initiation well before they seem to occur automatically and responsively to others' directed smiles. Similarly, other infant expressions—disgust, mouth openings that anticipate a spoon—are initiated by infants before they became imitated or automatic. Neonatal facial imitation may be related to facial mimicry, but we do not yet have any evidence supporting this.

If mimicry follows mastery, this would support the idea that automaticity of perception–action responses is a result of advanced learning and practice rather than a starting-state capacity. The starting-state condition may involve effortful reproductions, like those described by some of the neonatal researchers. Is there any evidence linking mimicry to motor mastery? A recent neuroimaging study provides related evidence. Calvo-Merino, Glaser, Grezes, Passingham, and Haggard (2005) demonstrated mirror neuron (MN) activation to observation of actions (dance moves) mastered by the observers, but not to actions that were not part of their action repertoire.

If mimicry and imitation are so interdependent, then we can consider questions of development at the neural level as well as the behavioral level. In terms of the MN system, it is currently suggested by some that mirror neurons acquire and refine their perception–action-coupled firing properties and connections through experience (Keysers & Perrett, 2004; Meltzoff & Decety, 2003). The observation of several researchers that young infants can only imitate behaviors that are within their current repertoire, as well as the observation of neonates' gradual improvements in response accuracy during imitation experiments, may also speak to this notion of gradual acquisition or development of perception–action couplings.

Experiences that could develop and refine infant perception–action couplings are plentiful in typical infants' environments. Studies like Užgiris, Benson, Kruper, and Vasek (1989) and Pawlby's (1977), of maternal behavior, document the very strong tendency of parents to imitate their infant's behavior. Both sets of authors demonstrated that roughly 75% of the imitative rounds of behavior observed between mother and infants from early in life across the first year involved the mother's imitation of her baby's behavior. (Pawlby's comment that mothers seem unaware of this may indeed reflect the automatic nature of this imitative response of adults to young infants—mimicry in action.) Infants, moreover, are likely to discriminate adult imitations from early on, given their abilities to recognize novel stimuli and contingency (Field, Guy, & Umbel, 1985; Nadel, Carchon, Kervella, Marcelli, & Reserbat-Plantey, 2000) as well as their perception–action couplings Furthermore, variation in parental behavior in this domain may have important relations with infant imitative variability. The infant–parent dyad appears very well equipped to provide the infant with the inputs needed for the MN system to acquire, extend, and strengthen the infant's perception–action couplings.

In addition, infants' many opportunities to move their bodies and to experience multiple sensory inputs related to self-generated movement can provide experiences of simultaneous firing patterns needed to develop neural networks for the multisensory aspects of movements. Experiencing another's behavior, in any modality, can thus activate network responses of the infant in multiple modalities, providing sources for perception–action coupling of self and other across modalities (Neidenthal et al., 2005). Mirror exposure is a third source of multimodal feedback of self-movements for infants.

Thus, the newborn has (1) a number of movements involving TP, mouth activation, vocal, and hand movements, all of which have already provided the infant with multisensory input and perception–action couplings to start from; (2) sensitivity and preferences related to patterns, contingencies, and people; (3) some perception–action couplings that link self and other and are seen in initial capacity to imitate some responses; and (4) social partners who somewhat automatically respond to infant behaviors of many types by imitating (Pawlby, 1977; Užgiris et al., 1989). This is very fertile ground for acquisition and refinement of perception–action couplings involving MN systems that respond to other's familiar and novel actions with self-movements. The proposal here is that that mimicry develops as part and parcel of intentional imitation, over time, from repeated experiences and mastery of self–other mutual intentional imitation and self-experiences of multiple inputs related to movements and actions. Its presence may signal the completed coupling or achievement of fully attuned resonance of the observation–execution MN system for that particular meaningful act.

Is There a Loss of Early Imitation Around 3 Months?

Several pieces of evidence presented earlier suggest that there is indeed some kind of change occurring at 3 months. Heimann's (1989) findings concerning continuity in imitations before 3 months but lack of continuity from 1 month to 6 months is one such piece. This is accompanied by his additional finding of continuities between 3- and 12-month imitative data not seen between 1 and 12 months. Changes in infant social behavior from 1 to 3 months are a second set of observations along this line made by several researchers (Kugiumutzakis, 1999; Maratos, 1982). Third is the fact that, in demonstrating some facial imitation at 3 months, Meltzoff and Moore (1992) needed a very different procedure in order to elicit imitation. Thus, there seems to be a change in imitative response patterns at and after 3 months of age. Various causes for the change have been suggested by the authors reviewed previously, including a change from subcortical to cortical control of imitation (Heimann, 1991; Maratos, 1998), replacement behaviors based on reward patterns for infants (Maratos, 1982), increasingly sophisticated and differentiated social repertoires of infants regarding familiar and unfamiliar people (Meltzoff & Moore, 1992), and increasing capacity for inhibition (Decety, Chapter 11, this volume). A change in the nature of the response does not necessarily imply that the underlying imitative mechanism changes over time. However, it raises important questions that need to be answered in order for us to gain a more complete understanding of early imitation. Longitudinal studies that examine individual trajectories will be crucial for understanding the relations between early infant and later, toddler, imitation.

Individual Variation in Response

There is a wide range of individual variation in imitative responses produced in the various infant imitation experiments, as Meltzoff and Moore demonstrate in their reports of individual responses. Furthermore, many of the papers report that the data are not distributed normally. This variability of response may in fact be seen as supporting arguments that the behavior being examined is a volitional and discriminated response on the part of the infant. One would expect a reflexive behavior, like the Moro or the Gallant reflexes, to be much more consistently and rapidly expressed in newborns. One might expect that an evolutionarily important behavior would be more robust and generalized, and indeed imitation becomes pervasive in the infant repertoire in the toddler stage of development. However, a newborn has a very limited behavioral repertoire, and many evolutionarily important behaviors, such as tool use and language, are absent from the repertoire for many months after birth. Thus, the fragility of the imitative behavior early on does not indicate its lack of importance. On the contrary, its presence at all is an indicator of its potential importance. It would be helpful to have more information about the variability of responses, both within and across individual children, in the first months of life. What are the characteristics of more and less imitative infants? What are the typical responses of infants when alertness and attention are maximized? Is an imitative response produced by the majority of infants? For what behaviors, and at what ages? Fully understanding the phenomenon requires understanding of individual variation in its expression.

Does Early Imitation Influence Other Aspects of Child Development?

The final issue focuses on the contributions of early infant imitation, as opposed to imitative skills developing later in the first year, as a mechanism for early interpersonal development. There is a very solid body of evidence, reviewed by Masur (Chapter 2, this volume) and Charman (Chapter 5, this volume), of continuities between toddler imitation abilities and other developmental and social characteristics. Furthermore, Nadel and colleagues (1999) have provided a very clear hypothesis about the changing nature of imitation across the first year, developed from their rich history of studies in the social–communicative functions of young children's imitations. They suggest that early imitation underlies the shift from primary, or dyadic, to pragmatic, or triadic, communication, at the end of the first year. Further, they delineate two processes embedded in early imitation that facilitate this transition: mastery of interpersonal timing and topic sharing. This is the only theory put forward to account for changes in the nature of imitative behavior across the first year of life and deserves further study.

A challenge to the theories concerning the foundational role of neonatal imitation for later interpersonal development, both our own and others, is the lack of empirical evidence to support the models. Thus far only one author has published longitudinal studies that assess individual stability of imitative behavior from early infancy. The longitudinal evidence, reviewed previously, while supportive, is sparse and not strong. Heimann (1991) concludes that questions of stability are difficult to interpret from the existing data. He points out that changes in neural architecture may well account for lack of continuity in imitative response across the first year or two of life, but that long-term longitudinal studies are necessary to answer questions about the role of neonatal imitation in influencing interpersonal development across the first few years of life. However, even if neonatal imitation is not related to other infant behaviors, either concurrently or longitudinally, it may influence parental social engagement. Is it a prime mover of social development, or one of many infant characteristics that interact with others to affect social development? This remains a highly important area for further research.

CONCLUSION

There is solid evidence of the capacity of very young infants to imitate facial movements of models. Several different groups have demonstrated the phenomenon, for more than one behavior, with the most stringent experimental methodology and analytic approaches. It appears to be a volitional rather than reflexive response, though there is less evidence in this area. Furthermore, conceptualizing mimicry as a powerful social behavior and part of the continuum of imitative development via the MN system lessens the need to distinguish mimicry from imitation in newborns.

The issue of few or many different imitative behaviors in newborns, and the robustness versus the fragility of response, is important for answering questions concerning nativist versus developmental models of infant imitation, at the level of both neural systems and of overt behaviors. Fragile response patterns, and limited repertoire of imitative behaviors in newborns and very young infants, do not detract from arguments of the potential importance of early infant imitation for later social–emotional development. In fact, they support developmental models, by giving more opportunity for varying ontogenetic outcomes due to variance in starting states, variance in environmental affordances, and variances in individual learning styles and rates.

Neonatal imitation provides evidence of some perception–action couplings present at birth—a starting state for development of self–other mappings and coordinations. There is also evidence that adults are inclined to imitate infant behavior, providing the infant with many reciprocal experiences of perception–action relations across varying sensory modalities during a period of time when infants are rapidly gaining intentional control of their movements. In addition, infants see and feel themselves move, and thus provide themselves with multisensory information about the unity of self experiences, while building up neural networks for such perception–action couplings. If the MN networks acquire most of their functions through Hebbian learning experiences (Keysers & Perrett, 2004), starting-state potential and environmental affordances are available for the infant from birth.

In terms of mechanisms underlying early infant imitation, the multimodality perception–action couplings that the MN system affords is likely the neural mechanism underlying early imitation. If observation of a known movement directly activates the motor output system, then early imitation does not appear to require amodal or supramodal matching. Understanding how the MN system acquires its capacities will be a huge contribution to developmental psychology. Models that bridge MN research and imitative development have begun (Heyes, 2001; Keysers & Perrett, 2004). Thus far, discussions of MN function in general, and MN dysfunction in autism, have not taken a developmental perspective.

The extent to which early infant imitation directly contributes to later imitative development and development of other interpersonal skills—especially involving understanding of affective and mental states—is currently unknown and is an area ripe for longitudinal research efforts. There is evidence, as reviewed in this text, of the relations between imitative responses and other interpersonal relations, for toddlers and parents (Kuczynski, Zahn-Waxler, & Radke-Yarrow, 1987) and for adult interactive partners

(Chartrand & Bargh, 1999; Richardson, Marsh, & Schmidt, 2005; Sonnby-Borgstrom, Johsson, & Svensson, 2003). And, finally, there is the evidence of a trio of deficits involving imitation, mimicry (McIntosh, Reichmann-Decker, Winkielman, & Wilbarger, in press; Scambler, Hepburn, Rutherford, Wehner, & Rogers, in press), and theory of mind deficits in autism. It is these landmarks in imitation theory and research that have brought us to this current text. However, the links with early infant imitation have not yet been empirically demonstrated.

Several questions have been raised that are ripe for focused research. The longitudinal questions are paramount. We need longitudinal studies that test the relation of early imitation to later mental state development.

A second issue concerns the relations of the different types of matching responses in human development. Are gestural imitation, mimicry, emulation, and means–end imitation related in humans? One may pave the way for the other—in what order? They may all rely on MN system activation for their performance, and the differences so carefully articulated in the animal work may be more apparent than real when applied to human development.

In addition to understanding the relation of different types of imitative behaviors to each other, we need to understand the relations of these different types to differing strands of human social and cognitive development. Imitation is not all one thing, and its effects on development are probably also varied. Mimicry may be core to social communicative relations, while means–end intentional imitation may be core to apprenticeship functions involving tool use and instrumental learning. Both may be necessary to support pedagogical learning (Csibra & Gergely, in press). We need both cross-sectional and longitudinal studies that examine the development of different types of imitation as defined by comparative psychology and their relations to varying aspects of social–cognitive development.

Third, research needs to address the nature of the discontinuities in imitative performances across time. The differing patterns of performance shown by Kugiumutzakis (1999) are very interesting and probably contain important information for developmentalists concerning neural mechanisms, environmental affordances, and infant affect states and motivation. The early infant imitation studies suggest that imitative development is not a linear process.

Finally, studying imitative development in infants and young children with both typical and atypical development should be a very effective strategy in answering questions about developmental relations across abilities, and individual differences in both starting states and environmental supports. Children with autism and other developmental disorders will likely provide us with invaluable evidence to test theories concerning the role of early imitation to intersubjective development, including theory of mind. The current questions concerning neonatal imitation are not of its existence but of its impact.

ACKNOWLEDGMENTS

This effort was partially supported by funding from the National Institute of Child Health and Human Development (Grant Nos. U 19 HD35468-09 and HD36071) and the National Institute of Mental Health (Grant Nos. R01 MH068398 and MH 068232). The contributions of Debra Galik for manuscript preparation are gratefully acknowledged. The author is grateful to Justin Williams and Bruce Pennington for their critiques.

REFERENCES

Abravanel, E., & Sigafoos, A. D. (1984). Exploring the presence of imitation during early infancy. *Child Development, 55,* 381–392.

Alissandrakis, A., Nehaniv, C. L., & Dautenhahn, K. (2004). Towards robot cultures? Learning to imitate in a robotic arm test-bed with dissimilarly embodied agents. *Interaction Studies, 5,* 3–44.

Anisfeld, M., Turkewitz, G., Rose, S. A., Rosenberg, F. R., Sheiber, F. J., Couturier-Fagan, D. A., et al. (2001). No compelling evidence that newborns imitate oral gestures. *Infancy, 2,* 111–122.

Bard, K. A., & Russell, C. L. (1999). Evolutionary foundations of imitation: Social cognitive and developmental aspects of imitative processes in non-human primates. In J. Nadel & G. Butterworth (Eds.), *Imitation in infancy* (pp. 89–123). Cambridge, UK: Cambridge University Press.

Bates, E. (2004). Explaining and interpreting deficits in language development across clinical groups: Where do we go from here? *Brain and Language, 88,* 248–253.

Brass, M., & Heyes, C. (2005). Imitation: is cognitive neuroscience solving the correspondence problem? *Trends in Cognitive Sciences, 9,* 489–495.

Butterworth, G. (1999). Neonatal imitation: Existence, mechanisms, and motives. In J. Nadel & G. Butterworth (Eds.), *Imitation in infancy* (pp. 63–88). Cambridge, UK: Cambridge University Press.

Calvo-Merino, B., Glaser, D. E., Grezes, J., Passingham, R. E., & Haggard, P. (2005). Action observation and acquired motor skills: An fMRI study with expert dancers. *Cerebral Cortex, 15,* 1243–1249.

Chartrand, T. L., & Bargh, J. A. (1999). The chameleon effect: The perception–behavior link and social interaction. *Journal of Personality and Social Psychology, 76,* 893–910.

Chen, X., Striano, T., & Rakoczy, H. (2004). Auditory–oral matching behavior in newborns. *Developmental Science, 7,* 42–47.

Csibra, G., & Gergely, G. (in press). Social learning and social cognition: The case for pedagogy. In Y. Munakata & M. H. Johnson (Eds.), *Processes of change in brain and cognitive development XXI: Attention and performance.* Oxford, UK: Oxford University Press.

Dapretto, M., Davies, M. S., Pfeifer, J. H., Scott, A. A., Sigman, M., Bookheimer, S. Y., & Iacoboni, M. (2006). Understanding emotions in others: Mirror neuron dysfunction in children with autism spectrum disorders. *Nature Neuroscience, 9,* 28–30.

De Renzi, E., Motti, F., & Nichelli, P. (1980). Imitating gestures: A quantitative approach to ideomotor apraxia. *Archives of Neurology, 37,* 6–10.

Donald, M. (1991). *Origins of the mind.* Cambridge, UK: Harvard University Press.

Field, T. M., Guy, L., & Umbel, V. (1985). Infants' responses to mothers' imitative behaviors. *Infant Mental Health Journal, 6,* 40–44.

Field, T. M., Woodson, R., Greenberg, R., & Cohen, D .J. (1982). Discrimination and imitation of facial expression by neonates. *Science, 218,* 179–181.

Fontaine, R. (1984). Imitative skills between birth and six months. *Infant Behavior and Development, 7,* 323–33.

Hatfield, E., Cacioppo, J. T., & Rapson, R. L. (1994). *Emotional contagion.* New York: Cambridge University Press.

Heilman, K. M. (1979). Apraxia. In K. M. Heilman & E. Valenstein (Eds.), *Clinical neuropsychology* (pp. 159–185). New York: Oxford University Press.

Heilman, K. M., & Rothi, L. J. G. (1997). *Apraxia: The neuropsychology of action.* Hove, UK: Psychology Press.

Heimann, M. (1989). Neonatal imitation, gaze aversion, and mother–infant interaction. *Infant Behavior and Development, 12,* 495–505.

Heimann, M. (1991). Neonatal imitation: A social and biological phenomenon. In T. Archer & S. Hansen (Eds.), *Behavioral biology: Neuroendocrine axis* (pp. 173–186). Hillsdale, NJ: Erlbaum.

Heimann, M. (1998). Imitation in neonates, in older infants and in children with autism: feedback to theory. In S. Bråten (Ed.), *Intersubjective communication and emotion in early ontogeny* (pp. 89–104). Cambridge, UK: Cambridge University Press.

Heimann, M., Nelson, K. E., & Schaller, J. (1989). Neonatal imitation of tongue protrusion and mouth opening: Methodological aspects and evidence of early individual differences. *Scandinavian Journal of Psychology, 30,* 90–101.

Heyes, C. (2001). Causes and consequences of imitation. *Trends in Cognitive Sciences, 5,* 253–261.

Heyes, C. (2002). Transformational and associative theories of imitation. In K. Dautenhahn & C. L. Nehaniv (Eds.), *Imitation in animals and artifacts* (pp. 501–523). Cambridge, MA: MIT Press.

Jones, S. S. (1996). Imitation or exploration? Young infants' matching of adults' oral gestures. *Child Development, 67,* 1952–1969.

Kaitz, M., Meschulach-Sarfaty, O., Auerbach, J., & Eidelman, A. (1988). A reexamination of newborns' ability to imitate facial expressions. *Developmental Psychology, 24,* 3–7.

Keysers, C., & Perrett, D. I. (2004). Demystifying social cognition: A Hebbian perspective. *Trends in Cognitive Science, 8,* 501–507.

Kuczynski, L., Zahn-Waxler, C., & Radke-Yarrow, M. (1987). Development and content of imitation in the second and third years of life: A socialization perspective. *Developmental Psychology, 23,* 276–282.

Kugiumutzakis, G. (1999). Genesis and development of early infant mimesis to facial and vocal models. In J. Nadel & G. Butterworth (Eds.), *Imitation in infancy* (pp. 36–59). Cambridge, UK: Cambridge University Press.

Kuhl, P. K., & Meltzoff, A. (1996). Infant vocalizations in response to speech: Vocal imitation and developmental change. *Journal of the Acoustic Society of America, 100,* 2425–2438.

Lacourse, M. G., Orr, E. L. R., Cramer, S. C., & Cohen, M. J. (2005). Brain activation during execution and motor imagery of novel and skilled sequential hand movements. *NeuroImage, 27,* 505–519.

Lewis, M., & Sullivan, M. W. (1985). Imitation in the first six months of life. *Merrill-Palmer Quarterly, 31,* 315–333.

Liepmann, H., & Maas, O. (1907). Fall von linksseitiger Agraphie und Apraxio bei rechsseitiger lahmung. *Zeitschrift für Psychologie und Neurologie, 10,* 214–227.

Maher, L. M., & Ochipa, C. (1997). Management and treatment of limb apraxia. In L. J. G. Rothi & K. M. Heilman (Eds.), *Apraxia: The neuropsychology of action* (pp. 75–92). Hove, UK: Psychology Press.

Maratos, O. (1982). Trends in the development of imitation in early infancy. In T. G. Bever (Ed.), *Regressions in mental development: Basic phenomena and theories* (pp. 81–101). Hillsdale, NJ: Erlbaum.

Maratos, O. (1998). Neonatal, early and later imitation: Same order phenomena? In F. Simion & G. Butterworth (Eds.), *The development of sensory, motor, and cognitive capacities in early infancy* (pp. 145–160). Hove, UK: Psychology Press.

Maurer, D., Stager, C. L., & Mondloch, C. J. (1999). Cross-modal transfer of shape is difficult to demonstrate in one-month olds. *Child Development, 70*, 1045–1057.

McIntosh, D. N., Reichmann-Decker, A., Winkielman, P., & Wilbarger, J. L. (in press). When the social mirror breaks: Deficits in automatic, but not voluntary mimicry of emotional facial expressions in autism. *Developmental Science.*

Meltzoff, A., & Borton, R. W. (1979). Intermodal matching by human neonates. *Nature, 282*, 403–404.

Meltzoff, A., & Gopnik, A. (1993). The role of imitation in understanding persons and developing a theory of mind. In S. Baron-Cohen, H. Tager-Flusberg, & D. J. Cohen (Eds.), *Understanding other minds: Perspectives from autism* (pp. 335–366). Oxford, UK: Oxford University Press.

Meltzoff, A., & Moore, M. K. (1977). Imitation of facial and manual gestures by human neonates. *Science, 198*, 75–78.

Meltzoff, A., & Moore, M. K. (1983). Methodological issues in studies of imitation: Comments on McKenzie & Over and Koepke et al. *Infant Behavior and Development, 6*, 103–108.

Meltzoff, A. N., & Decety, J. (2003). What imitation tells us about social cognition: A rapproachment between developmental psychology and cognitive neuroscience. *Philosophical Transactions of the Royal Society of London B Biol Sciences, 29*, 491–500.

Meltzoff, A. N., & Moore, M. K. (1989). Imitation in newborn infants: Exploring the range of gestures imitated and the underlying mechanisms. *Developmental Psychology, 25*, 954–962.

Meltzoff, A. N., & Moore, M. K. (1992). Early imitation within a functional framework: The importance of person identity, movement, and development. *Infant Behavior and Development, 15*, 479–505.

Meltzoff, A. N., & Moore, M. K. (1997). Explaining facial imitation: A theoretical model. *Early Development and Parenting, 6*, 179–192.

Meltzoff, A. N., & Moore, M. K. (1999). Persons and representation: Why infant imitation is important for theories of human development. In J. Nadel & G. Butterworth (Eds.), *Imitation in infancy* (pp. 9–35). Cambridge, UK: Cambridge University Press.

Myowa-Yamakoshi, M. (2000). Evolutionary foundation and development of imitation. *Department of Behavioral and Brain Sciences, 17*, 349–367.

Nadel, J., & Butterworth, G. (1999). Immediate imitation rehabilitated at last. In J. Nadel & G. Butterworth (Eds.), *Imitation in infancy* (pp. 1–5). Cambridge, UK: Cambridge University Press.

Nadel, J., Carchon, I., Kervella, C., Marcelli, D., & Reserbat-Plantey, D. (2000). Expectancies for social contingency in 2-month-olds. *Developmental Science, 2*, 164–174.

Nadel, J., Guérini, C., Pezé, A., & Rivet, C. (1999). The evolving nature of imitation as a format for communication. In J. Nadel & G. Butterworth (Eds.), *Imitation in infancy* (pp. 209–234). Cambridge, UK: Cambridge University Press.

Nagy, E., & Molnar, P. (2004). Homo imitans or homo provocans? Human imprinting model of neonatal imitation. *Infant Behavior and Development, 27*, 54–63.

Niedenthal, P. M., Barsalou, L. W., Winkielman, P., Krauth-Gruber, S., & Ric, F. (2005). Embodiment in attitudes, social perception, and emotion. *Personality and Social Psychology Review, 9*, 184–211.

Pawlby, S. F. (1977). Imitative interaction. In H. R. Schaffer (Ed.), *Studies in mother–infant interaction* (pp. 203–223). Glasgow, Scotland: University of Strathclyde.

Piaget, J. (1962). *Play, dreams, and imitation in childhood.* New York: Norton.

Reissland, N. (1988). Neonatal imitation in the first hour if life: Observations in rural Nepal. *Developmental Psychology, 24,* 464–469.

Richardson, M. J., Marsh, K. L., & Schmidt, R. C. (2005). Effects of visual and verbal interaction on unintentional interpersonal coordination. *Journal of Experimental Psychology, 31,* 62–79.

Rizzolatti, G., & Craighero, L. (2004). The mirror-neuron system. *Annual Review of Neuroscience, 27,* 169–192.

Rogers, S. J. (1999). An examination of the imitation deficit in autism. In J. Nadel & G. Butterworth (Eds.), *Imitation in infancy* (pp. 254–283). Cambridge, UK: University of Cambridge Press.

Rogers, S. J., & Pennington, B. F. (1991). A theoretical approach to the deficits in infantile autism. *Development and Psychopathology, 3,* 137–162.

Scambler, D., Hepburn, S., Rutherford, M. D., Wehner, E., & Rogers, S. J. (in press). Emotional responsivity in children with autism, children with other developmental disabilities, and children with typical development. *Journal of Autism and Developmental Disorders.*

Smith, I. M., & Bryson, S. E. (1994). Imitation and action in autism: A critical review. *Psychological Bulletin, 116*(2), 259–273.

Sonnby-Borgstrom, M., Johsson, P., & Svensson, O. (2003). Emotional empathy as related to mimicry reactions at different levels of information processing. *Journal of Nonverbal Behavior, 27,* 3–23.

Stern, D. N. (1985). *The interpersonal world of the human infant.* New York: Basic Books.

Tomasello, M. (1996). Do apes ape? In C. M. Heyes & B. G. Galef Jr. (Eds.), *Social learning in animals: The roots of culture* (pp. 319–346). New York: Academic Press.

Užgiris, H., Benson, J. B., Kruper, J. C., & Vasek, M. E. (1989). Contextual influences on imitative interactions between mothers and infants. In J. J. Lockman & N. L. Hazen (Eds.), *Action in social context: Perspectives on early development.* New York: Plenum Press.

Užgiris, I. (1973). Patterns of vocal and gestural imitation in infants. In L. J. Stone, H. T. Smith, & L. B. Murphy (Eds.), *The competent infant: Research and commentary.* New York: Basic Books.

Užgiris, I. (1999). Imitation as activity: its developmental aspects. In J. Nadel & G. Butterworth (Eds.), *Imitation in infancy* (pp. 186–206). Cambridge, UK: Cambridge University Press.

Vinter, A. (1986). The role of movement in eliciting early imitations. *Child Development, 57,* 66–71.

Want, S. C., & Harris, P. L. (2002). How do children ape? Applying concepts from the study of non-human primates to the developmental study of "imitation" in children. *Developmental Science, 5,* 1–41.

Williams, J. H. G., Whiten, A., & Singh, T. (2004). A systematic review of action imitation in autistic spectrum disorder. *Journal of Autism and Developmental Disorders, 34,* 285–299.

Williams, J. H. G., Whiten, A., Suddendorf, T., & Perrett, D. I. (2001). Imitation, mirror neurons and autism. *Neuroscience and Biobehavioral Reviews, 25,* 287–295.

Zajonc, R. B., Murphy, S. T., & Inglehart, M. (1989). Feeling and facial efference: Implications of the vascular theory of emotion. *Psychological Review, 96,* 395–416.

Zentall, T. R. (2004). Action imitation in birds. *Learning and Behavior, 32,* 15–23.

CHAPTER 2

Vocal and Action Imitation by Infants and Toddlers during Dyadic Interactions

Development, Causes, and Consequences

ELISE FRANK MASUR

Experimental studies of imitation have uncovered evidence about diverse aspects of children's cognitive and imitative competence, including visual–motor coordination, memory, and acquisition of novel behaviors (e.g., Masur, 1993; McCall, Eichorn, & Hogarty, 1977; Meltzoff, 1988a, 1988b), to name just a few. Whereas experimental studies of imitation are designed to reveal what children of different ages *can* perform under controlled conditions, they cannot tell us what imitative behaviors children of different ages *do* employ during their everyday interactions. This question is important because imitation provides children a means for entering into social interchanges and for acquiring culturally relevant patterns of behavior, including language (Bloom, Hood, & Lightbown, 1974; Nelson, 1996; Tomasello, 1992; Užgiris, 1984). For answers to this question, observational studies of imitation during naturally occurring interactions are necessary. This chapter focuses on these studies, describing the course of imitation during dyadic interactions during the early years, especially our own studies of mother–child imitative interchanges from the end of the first to the end of the second year, a time of dramatic development in imitation and in language. Besides reviewing findings about changes in the amounts and kinds of behaviors—vocal as well as action—children imitate over time, we search for clues to understand the causes of individual differences in imitation and their consequences. We begin with a discussion of differences of perspective and process inherent in observational versus experimental studies of naturally occurring imitation.

CONTRASTS BETWEEN EXPERIMENTAL
AND OBSERVATIONAL APPROACHES

Differences in Purpose

Although the goals of investigations of experimental and naturally occurring imitation often overlap, their emphases are generally in divergent directions. Experimental studies are most often addressed to the question of children's competence: What are the limits of children's abilities at particular ages and under particular constraints, for example, after varying amounts of delay between presentation and permitted enactment (e.g., Meltzoff, 1988a, 1988b)? Such age comparisons are intended to reveal and index children's evolving capability along a presumed universal trajectory, emphasizing the first of McCall's (1981) "two realms of developmental psychology" (p. 1) by charting the developmental function. With a focus on marking developmental changes in highest levels of proficiency, experimental studies are frequently cross-sectional rather than longitudinal in design to avoid risking practice effects from repeated measurements. And although experimental researchers are mindful that children's elicited imitation involves both ability and willingness, their efforts are more likely to focus on motivating children's optimal performance to uncover their underlying facility through maximizing rapport (e.g., Masur, 1993) or presenting irresistibly attractive actions (e.g., Meltzoff, 1988a) than on exploring individual differences, which may be treated as error variance.

Although clearly interested in children's growing imitative proficiency as well, observational researchers generally concentrate on how children exercise and employ that ability: What are the amounts and kinds of imitative behaviors that infants and children of different ages produce during daily interactions with familiar social partners? Their focus is often also on delineating the range of individual variation in imitation among children and over time, sometimes in order to examine relations between individuals' imitativeness and their subsequent development in domains such as language (e.g., Masur & Eichorst, 2002; Snow, 1989a). Attention to the stability of individual children's or dyads' styles as well would place them within the second of McCall's (1981) two realms, for pursuing "the relative consistency of individual differences over age" (p. 3). Because of frequent interest in this question, observational studies are more likely than experimental ones to adopt a longitudinal approach (e.g., Eckerman, Davis, & Didow, 1989; Masur & Rodemaker, 1999; Užgiris, 1991). Furthermore, the emphasis on imitative use puts a premium on recording representative, rather than optimal, performance and on sampling typical, albeit less controlled, situations. This focus on representative performance also encompasses attention to the variety of behaviors performed. We have considered it important to investigate behaviors from both the vocal/verbal and the action domain in order to comprehend the range of children's imitative skill and choice. Similarly, even within the action domain, we have examined actions both with and without objects. Recognition of the issue of ecological range and validity necessarily prompts consideration not only of the physical environment but also of the interpersonal context—behaviors of interactive partners and their relations to children's acts. For these reasons, our own and others' studies have examined the development of, diversity in, and relations between children's and mothers' imitative behaviors during familiar dyadic situations over time (e.g., Folger & Chapman, 1978; Masur & Rodemaker, 1999; Snow, 1989a; Užgiris, 1991; Užgiris, Vasek, & Benson, 1984).

Differences in Method

In addition to differences in focus, studying infants' and toddlers' naturally occurring imitation presents methodological challenges not found in researching elicited imitation under controlled conditions. The most serious concerns the problem of defining imitation. Criteria adopted for identifying imitation can be analyzed in terms of researchers' judgments about the relation between modeled and responding behavior with respect to four interrelated dimensions—similarity versus dissimilarity, contingency versus independence, immediacy versus delay, and novelty versus familiarity (Masur, 1987; see also Whiten, Chapter 10, this volume, for other considerations, especially within the dimension of similarity/dissimilarity, in defining both human and nonhuman imitation). The requirements of similarity and contingency are common to both experimental and observational studies (Meltzoff & Moore, 1983; Užgiris, 1984). The first determination is whether the match between a model's behavior and a subsequent responder's act is exact or a close approximation, the standard our laboratory has always employed (Masur, 1987; Masur & Rodemaker, 1999). Other researchers, however, have sometimes chosen different standards for judging equivalence, even including children's performance of complete acts when only partial, unsuccessful ones are modeled (e.g., Meltzoff, 1995).

The second evaluation concerns whether the responder's action is contingent upon or evoked by the model's behavior, rather than occurring independently. This determination is easier to make in a laboratory where the likelihood of performing designated acts after modeling can be statistically compared with the probability in the absence of a model. In observational studies, researchers usually rely on calculating reliability between trained observers' judgments based on preestablished criteria. In our studies, when respondent behaviors qualified as exact copies or close approximations, coders then considered a number of factors, including attentional focus, behavioral change, and timing, in judging contingency (Masur & Rodemaker, 1999). Evidence that the imitator attended to—saw or heard—the partner's modeled behavior, from gaze patterns for example, was taken into account. A determination of contingency is clearer, for example, if the responder interrupts his or her ongoing behavior and shifts to matching the partner's act.

Another factor our coders considered, the timing between modeled and respondent acts, has a bearing on the general issue of immediacy versus delay. While delayed or deferred imitation is a significant accomplishment in its own right (Meltzoff, 1988a, 1988b), too great a delay during dyadic interaction raises questions about contingency. For this reason, and for practical considerations, immediate imitation has been overwhelmingly preferred in experimental as well as observational studies. The limits governing the boundaries of "immediate" have been inconsistent, however. The amount of elapsed time permitted between modeled and respondent acts has varied from as little as 2 to a much more typical 15 seconds in both experimental and observational studies of action imitation (e.g., Masur, 1993; Užgiris et al., 1984). For observational studies of verbal imitation, in contrast, the standard has sometimes involved the number of permitted intervening utterances, which has ranged from none to as many as five, rather than a time limit (Bloom et al., 1974; Ramer, 1976). To meet our goal of recording and comparing spontaneous vocal/verbal and action imitation, we have adopted a timing standard that could be applied equally across these domains. Thus, to be judged contingent, respondent matching behaviors also had to occur within 15 seconds of the modeled behavior.

The final issue, novelty versus familiarity, is relevant to the question of contingency as well. In addition to the privileged status that children's reproduction of novel behaviors holds theoretically (Meltzoff, 1988a; Piaget, 1962), replication of an act not previously present in a child's performance repertoire provides clear evidence of contingency, as it could only occur in response to the model's behavior. Furthermore, children's novel imitation is important to study because reproduction of novels acts affords children the opportunity to incorporate the culturally meaningful behaviors, including the linguistic ones, of the adults around them into their performance repertories (Nelson, 1996; Tomasello, 1992). Under controlled conditions, novel versus familiar actions can be determined in advance and presented systematically (Masur, 1993; Meltzoff, 1988a). During naturally occurring interchanges, however, the identification of novel behaviors is more difficult, sometimes requiring such additional procedures as maternal interviews, which we have needed to employ (Masur & Eichorst, 2002).

One other methodological issue deserves brief mention—the choice between counting instances and counting episodes. In experimental studies in which a predetermined number of discrete behaviors are modeled, researchers generally record each behavior as imitated or not by a given child (e.g., Killen & Užgiris, 1981). But during social interactions, children frequently engage in imitative bouts or games involving multiple rounds or turns, such as alternately banging a drum or throwing a ball (Eckerman et al., 1989; Masur, 1987; Užgiris et al., 1984). Because counting each imitative turn as a separate instance could artificially inflate a child's score, studies of naturally occurring imitation usually treat each multiround bout as a single imitative episode (e.g., Masur, 1987; Pawlby, 1977; Užgiris et al., 1984). Starting at the first modeled behavior and ending with the last matching turn, each episode is classified according to the modeled act and analyzed in terms of the first imitator. Imitative episodes are counted in all studies of dyadic imitation reviewed here.

THE DEVELOPMENTAL COURSE OF DYADIC IMITATION

In this section, we trace the development of dyadic imitation, especially mother–child imitative interactions, during the first 2 years of life. This overview is organized according to a set of questions about changes across each year. The first two concern amount and type of imitation: How does the frequency or rate of imitation change overall, and for mothers and children separately? What kinds of behaviors are imitated, and how does the type of imitation change over time? The last two questions shift from focusing on average developmental changes to investigating variation in imitative expression: What is the extent of individual differences in imitation? And, are there dyadic relations in imitative style with highly imitative mothers having highly imitative children?

Changes during the First Year of Life

Children's imitation during dyadic interactions with their mothers has been studied from the first months. Užgiris and her colleagues have conducted the most systematic and comprehensive set of investigations of the developmental course of mother–infant imitation during the first year of life (Užgiris, 1991; Užgiris, Benson, Kruper, & Vasek, 1989; Užgiris, Benson, & Vasek, 1983; Užgiris et al., 1984). In a series of studies, she and her colleagues examined matching episodes in both cross-sectional and longitudinal samples during mother–infant interactions lasting 9–12 minutes when the infants were ages 2–3 months, 5–6 months, 8–9 months, and 11–12 months. They analyzed imitation during face-to-face interchanges without toys in both cross-sectional and longitudinal samples and during interactions with toys in the cross-sectional sample, counting all vocal and motoric behaviors with the exception of smiles. Although the observations took place in a laboratory setting with mother and child positioned facing each other at eye level, the mothers were asked to "play with their infants the way they usually did" (Užgiris et al., 1989, p. 110) and left alone in the room with their infants.

Changes in Imitation Frequency and Type

Užgiris (1991; Užgiris et al., 1989) reported large gains in the average number of imitative episodes across the first year of life in both their cross-sectional and longitudinal analyses. For the 17 longitudinal dyads, the increase in imitative episodes more than tripled, from 6.4 episodes at 2½ months to 21.6 at 11½ months, a change from about one episode every 2 minutes to nearly two per minute for an average session of about 11 minutes (Užgiris et al., 1984). And the increase in frequency was paralleled by a growth in the lengths of imitative episodes. Episodes consisting of two or more rounds, where each partner performed the behavior at least twice, accounted for only 11% of episodes at 2½ months, but as much as 24% at 11½ months (Užgiris et al., 1984). When Užgiris and colleagues examined imitation by partner, they found that mothers' initial matching of their children's behaviors accounted for the overwhelming majority of all imitative episodes at each age, although the proportion of matching episodes initiated by infants more than doubled, from 12% at 2½ months to 28% at 11½ months.

Užgiris and her colleagues (1984) also addressed the question of the kinds of behaviors replicated by mothers and children at different ages. Separating episodes in the longitudinal study by vocal, motor, and combined behaviors, they reported considerably more imitation of motoric than vocal behavior at each age for infants and at all ages except 2½ months for mothers. The preponderance of action over vocal imitation by both partners was present in their cross-sectional laboratory study of face-to-face interactions without toys as well (Užgiris et al., 1989). The kinds of motoric behaviors copied also shifted with age, with mouth movements most common at the youngest age, gaze following and hand and finger movements increasing across the next two times of measurement, and conventionally meaningful acts and gestures like pointing, waving, and clapping more prevalent at the end of the first year (Užgiris et al., 1984).

Such a preference for action imitation by both partners was not replicated in two other studies examining mother–infant matching during the first year, which, in contrast to analyses by Užgiris and colleagues, included actions on objects but not gaze shifting. A small-scale longitudinal study by Pawlby (1977) found differential preferences in the kinds of behaviors replicated by mothers and infants. Pawlby videotaped eight mother–infant pairs in laboratory interactions weekly from 4 to 10 months of age, but her dyads were permitted two toys to play with as well. She also noted increased matching over time and greater imitation overall by mothers than infants. Like Užgiris and colleagues, she found infants more likely to imitate actions than sounds, and especially likely in the second half of the first year to repeat actions involving the objects more so than facial expressions. Unlike Užgiris, however, she reported that mothers were more likely to reproduce vocal behaviors than actions,.

A similar pattern of differential vocal versus action matching by partners was also found in a cross-sectional sample we observed during naturalistic free play and bath interactions in their homes (Masur, 1989). Among the 12 dyads with children ages 10–12 months, mothers matched almost twice as many behaviors overall as their infants, but the kinds of behaviors imitated differed. The infants produced more than twice as many total action imitations as vocal or verbal matches, while the mothers produced more than four times as many vocal/verbal as action repetitions. For both children and mothers, reproductions of actions involving objects greatly surpassed repetitions of gestures or actions without objects. For vocal imitations, mothers' reproductions of their children's discrete speech-relevant vowel sounds and consonant–vowel syllables exceeded repetitions of their children's words, conventionally communicative vocalizations (like engine or animal noises), or miscellaneous nonspeech sounds or laughter combined. Children's less prevalent vocal repetitions, however, were more than twice as likely to copy maternal words as other sounds.

Patterns of Individual Differences

The findings describing average developmental changes in matching or distinctions between mothers' and children's imitative preferences mask a great range of individual differences in imitation. For example, the frequencies of dyadic matching episodes ranged from 0 to 33 at 2½ months and from 9 to 34 at 11½ months in Užgiris and colleagues' (1984) longitudinal study. These variations were not stable throughout most of the first year, however; the correlation between frequencies of total dyadic imitative episodes was significant for the interval from 8½ to11½ months.

The question of dyadic correspondence—whether highly imitative mothers have highly imitative children—was addressed only in an analysis of vocal imitation involving 14 of the participants in Užgiris and colleagues' longitudinal sample. Broome and Užgiris (1985) reported a significant association between mothers' and children's vocal matching at 11½ months. Positive relations were also found in an analysis of 18 dyads from our cross-sectional sample, with children ranging from 10 to 14 months, between mothers' and children's reproduction of conventional vocalizations plus words and between mothers' replications of their children's discrete speech-relevant vocalizations, their most frequent type of imitation, and children's repetitions of mothers' actions on objects, their most prevalent imitation category (Masur, 1987). Thus, some correspondence between mothers' and children's imitativeness begins to appear at the end of the first or beginning of the second year.

Imitation in the First Year

In sum, these reports of imitation confirm that imitative episodes are an increasingly frequent part of unstructured dyadic interactions during the first year of life. Matching is more likely to be achieved by mothers' repeating their infants' acts than the reverse, but infants' replications also grow over time, illustrating their increasing participation in the interactions. Furthermore, the changing characteristics of behaviors infants replicated during these playful interchanges appear to parallel the progression in their independent capabilities toward more conventional sounds, gestures, and actions with and without objects. And, finally, by the end of the first year, the most imitative children are the ones with the most imitative mothers, indicating that stylistic differences among dyads are starting to emerge.

Developmental Changes from the End of the First Year to the End of the Second Year

The developmental pattern of children's spontaneous imitation evident during the first year is revolutionized during the second year as children begin to acquire language. The review of developmental trends in dyadic imitation during this pivotal period is based on analyses from our longitudinal sample of 20 mother–child dyads observed during natural interactions in their homes (Masur & Rodemaker, 1999). The participants, half girls and half boys and their mothers, came from lower-middle- to middle-class families living in suburban, small town, and rural areas near a state university campus about 65 miles west of Chicago. The families were recruited to participate in a more extensive longitudinal study of "infants' reactions to the people and objects in their environment" involving a number of developmental questions besides imitation (Masur & Rodemaker, 1999, p. 395). Except for three who joined the study at the second time of measurement, the dyads were visited in their homes at four ages that were chosen to coincide with the typical occurrence of several important imitative and language benchmarks: 10 months, when communicative gestures appear; 13 months, when first words and imitation of novel behaviors emerge; 17 months, when vocabulary acquisition accelerates; and 21 months, when production of two-word sentences and imitation of behavior sequences begin.

The children were visited twice at each age, in sessions about 1 week apart. During the first visit, mothers and children were videotaped during three naturalistic interactions, each with sets of toys provided: bathtime, a routine caretaking activity with an agenda; free play with a set of typical toys, a less structured social–interactive activity; and free play with a set of more novel toys, an activity designed to elicit teaching behaviors. Session order was counterbalanced across children, with bathtime occurring either first or third and free play with typical toys occurring either first or second. The first visit ended with a maternal interview focusing on children's language and behavioral development. The second visit involved an experimental imitation task, with the mothers serving as models. However, imitation was never mentioned during or in reference to the naturalistic interactions of the first visit.

We examined children's and mothers' imitation during the bathtime and free play with typical toys in sessions, each of which lasted about 14 minutes. Masur and Rodemaker (1999) provide a complete report of imitation during each interactive session; for our review here, data from the two contexts are combined. Observers reached reliability in identifying imitation according to the criteria of similarity, contingency, and immediacy described previously and marked imitative episodes, from the beginning of the modeled act through the last imitation of that act, on transcripts of the interactive sessions. The first imitator in each episode was recorded, and the episodes were classified in terms of the type of behavior modeled into one of four categories: verbal, including conventional words or phrases and conventionally meaningful vocalizations (e.g., *ball*, *thank you*, and *uh-oh*); vocal, including babbling and all other sounds and noises (e.g., *aah* and laughter); actions without objects, including gestures and head or hand motions (e.g., waving and clapping), but excluding subtle facial expressions and smiling as too difficult to discern on the videotapes and/or to evaluate for contingency; and actions with objects, including motor behaviors involving a toy or other object (e.g., throwing the ball and banging the drum).

Changes in Imitation Frequency and Type

Overall, spontaneous imitation grew dramatically from the end of the first to the end of the second year of life. For the two interactive contexts combined, dyads' rates of imitation rose from an average of about one episode every 3 minutes at 10 months to nearly two per minute at 21 months. The imitative rate during these interactions at 10 months was considerably less than the rate Užgiris (1991) reported during face-to-face laboratory interactions without toys at 11½ months, perhaps because of the competing agenda in the bath situation and the greater opportunity for nonimitative play afforded by the toys available during the free play session. But despite the modest rate of imitation at 10 months, spontaneous imitation increased greatly from the end of the first to the end of the second year, with average total matching episodes per dyad increasing more than fivefold from 10.73 at 10 months to 54.24 at 21 months. And this increment represented growth in the number of different behaviors copied, not just greater repetition of a limited repertoire of acts. Unique imitative episodes during the two sessions combined increased from an average of 8.80 at 10 months to 39.06 at 21 months and accounted for from 71% to 82% of the episodes at each age.

In these dyadic interactions, the rise in total imitation during the second year was evident in both partners' behavior (see Table 2.1). At the end of the first year, unlike Užgiris and colleagues (1984), we found slightly more matching episodes initiated by children than by mothers. And from the end of the first to the end of the second year, imitation by both partners climbed sharply, but mothers' gains outstripped children's. From 10 to 21 months, imitative episodes initiated by children more than tripled and those initiated by mothers multiplied more than sevenfold.

This expansion in both partners' imitation was due almost entirely to the extraordinary growth in verbal matching by the middle of the second year, a time when children's vocabularies are typically burgeoning (Goldfield & Reznick, 1990). While mothers' imitation of their children's actions with and without objects changed very little over time, their verbal imitation quadrupled from an extremely low average level at 10 months to 1.74 at 13 months, multiplied nearly eight times from 13 to 17 months, and then doubled again from 17 to 21 months. The developmental pattern for children was similar. While children's replication of actions on objects remained strong and relatively constant across the second year and their matching of actions without

TABLE 2.1. Mean Numbers (and Standard Deviations) of Children's and Mothers' Spontaneous Imitative Episodes in Four Categories during Natural Free Play and Bath Interactions Combined

			Imitation category		
	Vocal	Verbal	Actions without objects	Actions with objects	Total
At 10 months					
Children	0.34	0.48	0.10	4.91	5.83
	(0.74)	(1.05)	(0.22)	(2.10)	
Mothers	1.89	0.43	0.16	2.42	4.90
	(1.88)	(1.25)	(0.46)	(2.33)	
At 13 months					
Children	0.65	1.85	0.33	6.40	9.23
	(1.13)	(1.90)	(0.84)	(3.61)	
Mothers	3.88	1.74	0.13	2.81	8.56
	(4.34)	(1.96)	(0.41)	(1.53)	
At 17 months					
Children	0.40	8.41	0.58	5.46	14.85
	(0.53)	(9.99)	(1.21)	(3.23)	
Mothers	3.54	13.82	0.62	3.19	21.17
	(4.33)	(16.75)	(1.14)	(2.08)	
At 21 months					
Children	0.40	9.88	0.66	6.77	17.71
	(0.87)	(9.66)	(0.87)	(3.54)	
Mothers	3.44	27.66	1.64	3.79	36.53
	(4.02)	(21.47)	(2.52)	(2.95)	

objects remained very infrequent, their repetitions of mothers' conventional vocalizations plus words accelerated, with the greatest leap, more than four-fold, also from 13 to 17 months. Thus, while replication of object-related actions had been the first or second most frequent category for both partners at 10 and 13 months, by 17 months verbal imitation surpassed all other kinds for both mothers and children.

Patterns of Individual Differences

These general developmental trends, however, conceal striking differences among dyads and individuals. For example, although the total number of imitation episodes during the play and bath sessions combined averaged 36.02 per dyad at 17 months, one mother–child pair produced only 1, while another produced 112, or about 4 every minute. In the former dyad, the boy matched a single maternal act, while the boy in the highly imitative dyad child copied 46. Even among relatively imitative children, the kinds of behaviors they chose to reproduce varied. For the highly imitative boy, 83% of his matches were of conventional vocalizations and words and only 13% were of object-related actions. Another boy at the same age matched half as many behaviors overall, but only 35% of them were in the verbal category while 61% were actions on objects.

We can also ask whether these individual differences in imitative style were stable over time and within dyads. The correlations for children's and mothers' combined total, verbal, and object-related action imitation, presented in Table 2.2, point up the stability in children's and mothers' verbal imitation in particular. Children's tendencies to match their mothers' total and action behaviors remained stable from the end of the first through the middle of the second year, but only their imitation of conventional vocalizations and words was stable from both 13 to 17 and 17 to 21 months. Similarly, the high consistency in mothers' total imitativeness across each interval was clearly attributable to the strong stability in their verbal imitativeness.

The special nature of verbal imitation was evident in the analyses of dyadic relations as well. Correspondence between mothers' and children's imitation rates was not found for imitation of object-related actions, and relations between partners' total imitation frequencies at 17 and 21 months were due to their verbal matching: Mothers who copied more of their children's conventional sounds and words had children who produced more verbal imitation at the beginning, middle, and end of the second year. Thus, during the second year, verbal imitation becomes a familiar feature of the play and caretaking routines of some mother–child dyads. Marked individual differences in

TABLE 2.2. Pearson Product Correlations of Stability and Dyadic Correspondence in Children's and Mothers' Naturally Occurring Imitative Interactions

	Stability across time intervals		
	10–13 months	13–17 months	17–21 months
Total imitation			
Children	.68**	.50*	.27
Mothers	.52*	.63***	.73***
Verbal imitation			
Children	—	.66***	.39*
Mothers	—	.76***	.69***
Object-related action imitation			
Children	.72***	.66***	.32
Mothers	.14	.43*	.33

	Dyadic correspondence between children's and mother's imitation			
	At 10 months	At 13 months	At 17 months	At 21 months
Total imitation	.28	.27	.84***	.65***
Verbal imitation	—	.66***	.93***	.80***
Object-related action imitation	.18	.19	−.06	.18

Note.—indicates correlations not computed due to infrequent imitation.
*$p < .05$; **$p < .01$; ***$p < .0001$; all one-tailed.

children rates of vocal/verbal imitation and/or significant relations between mothers' and children's imitativeness have also been reported in a number of other studies (Bloom et al., 1974; Broome & Užgiris, 1985; Folger & Chapman, 1977; Snow, 1989a).

Imitation during the Second Year

Mother–child interactions during the second year provided the context for remarkable growth in matching behavior. Most notable was the extraordinary increase in both mothers' and children's imitation of their partners' conventional vocalizations and words. Yet, although the developmental function charts large average increments in verbal and total matching over this period, individuals and dyads often differed greatly. And these individual differences indexed relatively enduring imitative tendencies over time, especially in the verbal domain. More important, the frequency of children's verbal imitation from the beginning of the second year is related to that of their mothers'. These correlational findings do not prove a causal relation or indicate a direction of effect. Whether children are adopting an imitative style from observing their mothers' matching behavior is unknown. But some mother–child dyads are incorporating verbal imitation as a frequent component of their naturally occurring interactive interchanges. And high rates of verbal imitation, as we discuss below, are positive predictors for children's subsequent language competence (Masur & Eichorst, 2002; Snow, 1989a, 1989b), although we cannot yet determine whether such associations truly represent causal relations.

CHILDREN'S DYADIC IMITATION: CAUSES AND CONSEQUENCES

In this final section, we consider evidence and entertain hypotheses regarding the origins and outcomes of early imitation and, especially, of the individual differences in children's imitativeness during the first couple of years.

Influences on Children's Imitation

In our research, we have examined several factors that might have influenced the imitativeness of the children in our longitudinal sample. The first factor we considered was whether dyadic imitation might occur in response to requests for imitation by partners. Because Tamis-LeMonda and Bornstein (1991) had reported that mothers frequently requested play behaviors from their children, it seemed reasonable to investigate whether mothers might also solicit imitation and whether these solicitations might account for a substantial proportion of children's matching episodes. Accordingly, we searched the videotapes of the free-play sessions for all invitations to copy a modeled vocal, verbal, or object-related action behavior delivered by either partner verbally and/or nonverbally; we also noted whether or not the solicitation resulted in imitation.

Mothers did solicit imitation from their children (Masur & Rodemaker, 1999). But their solicitation of vocal/verbal behaviors was rare. Only five or fewer mothers requested vocal/verbal imitation at any age, and the average number of solicitations was considerably less than 1.0. Thus, we cannot attribute the children's growing verbal matching to this cause. Action imitation, however, presented a different picture. At each age, three-quarters or more of the mothers invited action repetition, and the number of invitations proffered averaged from 2.40 at 21 months to 3.76 at 10 months. Furthermore, about half of the maternal solicitation elicited an imitation. However, because many solicitations occurred in the midst of an ongoing imitative episode rather than at the beginning, only a small minority of all children's imitation episodes, from 17% to 27% at any age, could be attributable to maternal requests. Thus, solicitations failed to account for the majority of children's action matching as well. Incidentally, children's solicitations also failed to account for maternal matching. Children never solicited vocal/verbal imitation from their mothers, and their relatively rare action solicitations accounted for an even smaller proportion of mothers' matching episodes, 14% or less at each age (Masur & Rodemaker, 1999).

Because solicitation was not an adequate explanation for children's imitation, we have turned to other possible contenders. One clear possibility is maternal imitation. Such matching might provide a model for appropriate behavior during dyadic interactions that children can adopt themselves. As mentioned earlier, a positive relation between children's rates of vocal and/or verbal imitation and their mothers' rates has indeed been found in a number of studies, including our own (e.g., Broome & Užgiris, 1985; Folger & Chapman, 1978; Masur & Rodemaker, 1999; Snow, 1989a). But the absence of a similar correspondence between children's and mothers' action matching argues for exploring other influences as well, although maternal modeling of matching behavior, especially verbal matching, would need to be borne in mind when assessing such factors.

Accordingly, we have considered two additional influences, one interpersonal and the other intrapersonal (Flynn, Masur, & Eichorst, 2004). The interpersonal factor we explored was opportunity. Perhaps developmental changes in children's imitation may be a function of increasing opportunities for matching provided by their mothers over time. It is also possible that more or less matching by different children at a given age may be related to differences in the numbers of imitable behaviors their mothers perform. The intrapersonal factor we examined was disposition. Perhaps children's likelihood of engaging in action imitation is a reflection of the degree of their interest and involvement in object-related play in general, with those who perform more object-related play spontaneously more likely to match object-related actions by their mothers. Greater verbal imitation, in turn, might characterize the dyadic interactions of those children who are more spontaneously talkative or more linguistically adept.

To address these alternatives, we investigated the children's spontaneous object-related play and conversational production of conventional sounds and words as measures of their own dispositions to engage in these behaviors independently and their mothers' spontaneous motoric and verbal behaviors as an index of the opportunities provided by their partners in these domains (Flynn et al., 2004). For these analyses, we examined an 8-minute portion of the free-play sessions at each age in our longitudinal sample. From transcripts and the videos, observers coded the action and verbal productions of the participants, examining the dispositions displayed by the children and the imitative opportunities provided by their mothers.

The findings indicated that although both opportunity and disposition played a role in children's imitation, disposition was the stronger influence (Flynn et al., 2004). With respect to action imitation, despite overall declines in the object-related play behaviors mothers provided from 10 to 13 months and from 17 to 21 months the children as a group expanded the proportion of opportunities they copied during those intervals, generating increased action imitation. Influences on verbal matching were analyzed only at 17 and 21 months because children's verbal imitation was so infrequent at 10 and 13 months. Children's rates of matching at the middle and end of the second year were associated with both the verbal opportunities their mothers made available and their own dispositions to participate conversationally in the interactions. However, when opportunity and disposition were each evaluated with mothers' modeling of imitation and the alternative factor controlled, only disposition remained a significant correlate of children's verbal imitation. In other words, when exposure to an imitative partner and available imitable opportunities are adjusted for statistically, then children's own spontaneous conversational expressiveness predicts their overall verbal matching. Yet, in naturally occurring dyadic interactions such factors are obviously never truly controlled. Children's developmental competence and interpersonal motivation and mothers' provision of imitable behaviors and modeling of an imitative style must combine to yield differences in children's verbal imitation. And because, as we shall discuss in the next section, children's differential imitation may have important consequences, means for promoting children's matching behavior deserve further inquiry.

Functions of Children's Naturally Occurring Dyadic Imitation

Questions about children's purposes in imitating during natural interactions and the consequences of their doing so have been addressed by numerous researchers. The answers they have proposed generally emphasize either imitation's social aspect or its cognitive aspect, although Užgiris (1981) pointed out that imitation involves simultaneously both the social-interpersonal and the cognitive-intrapersonal domain.

Social Consequences

From a social perspective, we can note that when children participate in imitative interactions, their matching behavior can "communicat[e] mutuality and shared understanding with another person" (Užgiris, 1981, p. 1). Imitation can be a means for children to respond to another, take an interactive or conversational turn, and sustain a verbal or motoric interchange (Bloom, Rocissano, & Hood, 1976; Keenan, 1974; Užgiris, 1984). Thus, imitation may serve as an occasion for children to practice and develop their interactive skills. In fact, some have proposed that the process of matching may support children's development of social understanding more broadly. As long ago as 1895, Baldwin suggested that children's imitation may foster their knowledge of self and others: "My sense of myself grows by imitation of you, and my sense of yourself grows in terms of my sense of myself. Both ego and alter are thus essentially social; each is a socius and each is an imitative creation" (p. 338). Such a viewpoint is echoed in more recent statements by Meltzoff (1990) that "imitative interactions provide infants with a unique vehicle for elaborating the similarity between self and other and for understanding that others, like the self, are sentient beings with thoughts, intentions, and emotions" (p. 141).

Although direct evidence that children's imitation may express or promote their social relations is difficult to come by, a comparison of the matching behavior of the children in our longitudinal sample (Masur & Rodemaker, 1999) with the imitative performance of peer dyads of similar ages supports that inference. Eckerman and colleagues (1989) studied a longitudinal sample of 14 dyads of peers—5 female, 4 male, and 5 mixed—who were initially unfamiliar with each other. They were observed during 16-minute interactions in a laboratory playroom at five ages, the first two of which at 16 and 20 months approximate the 17- and 21-month measurement points in our sample. Several findings showed the mother–child dyads to be imitatively advanced. For example, the rate of imitation per minute in our mother–child dyads at 21 months was about twice that observed in the peer dyads at 20 months, although peer imitation more than reached the frequency of mother–child imitation by 28 months. Also, using a standard of five unique nonverbal imitative interactions, Eckerman and colleagues considered 7 of their 14 dyads to have adopted imitation as a "widely applied behavioral strategy" (p. 446) by 20 months, while 9 of 17 mother–child dyads already reached that criterion during the free play sessions at 10 months of age.

Furthermore, multiround interchanges also appeared sooner and more frequently in mother–infant than peer interactions. Eckerman and colleagues (1989) reported only eight interactions involving imitation, mostly nonverbal, lasting three or more turns after the modeled act in the peer dyads at 16 months and 12 at 20 months. However, 17 interactions of this length or longer by 12 mother–child dyads occurred as early as 10 months and 23 by 17 dyads occurred at 13 months. While such extended bouts involving verbal imitation were rare in the peer interactions, 12 mother–child dyads produced 27 at 17 months and 15 dyads produced 42 at 21 months (Masur & Rodemaker, 1999).

Studies examining mother–child and peer dyadic interactions in the same children are needed to determine whether the imitative practices children observe and practice during naturally occurring exchanges with their mothers are the very ones they then extend to initiate and maintain social encounters with peers. It is possible that action matching with mothers may be the primary prerequisite to the kinds of nonverbal imitative interchanges with peers that Eckerman and Didow (1996) consider the foundation for developing coordinated social activity with agemates.

Cognitive Consequences

Children's imitation may serve as a means to express or promote cognitive as well as social development. Experimental research demonstrates that qualitative changes in children's imitative performance signal developmental changes in their cognitive competence (Masur, 1993; McCall et al., 1977; Meltzoff, 1988a, 1988b). But imitation may play a role as instigator, not just indicator, of cognitive development. It is a strategy children can recruit for learning and incorporating new behaviors into their performance repertoires. Such behaviors may be linguistic or motoric, arbitrary or culturally meaningful, modeled by adults or by peers, observed in day-care centers or at home (e.g., Bloom et al., 1974; Hanna & Meltzoff, 1993; Snow, 1981).

Although the findings from naturalistic observational studies are correlational rather than causal, and thus necessarily circumstantial rather than direct, they strengthen the argument that children's imitation can function as a cognitive facilitator. Two analyses from our longitudinal study of mother–child dyads bolster that argument, the first focusing on children's imitation of actions on objects and the second on their matching of conventional sounds and words. In the action domain, one measure of children's cognitive advancement is the level of their play with objects. Belsky and Most (1981) have described 12 developmental levels in children's play, ranging from mouthing and simple manipulation of objects (e.g., touching and looking) through investigation of the properties of objects singly and in inappropriate or appropriate combination (levels 3–6), to simple and increasingly complex scenarios of pretend symbolic play (levels 7–12). Although it seems eminently reasonable that the qualitative nature of parents' play interactions with their children should be related to, even predictive of, the children's developmental play levels, researchers have so far failed to discover those associations (Bornstein & Tamis-LeMonda, 1995). Instead of looking at all mothers' and children's play during interactive sessions as others had done, however, we have conducted a preliminary study to examine the play levels of mothers' and children's imitations of actions on objects specifically (Masur, 1997). We believe this study to be the first to concentrate on qualitative, rather than quantitative, aspects of children's spontaneous action imitation.

As part of a more comprehensive project, we coded the developmental play level of each of the children's, and of their mothers', imitative episodes of actions on objects during the free-play interactions with their mothers (Masur, 1997). From these, we derived scores for average and for highest levels of play exhibited imitatively by each child at 10, 13, 17, and 21 months of age. Then we analyzed whether these two qualitative assessments of children's action matching were related to their imitative experience. Like others who had examined nonimitative play levels, we found the average levels of imitative play displayed by the children and their mothers to be unrelated. In contrast, the highest levels exhibited by children and mothers were positively related at 21 months. More important, the highest levels of play demonstrated imitatively by the children at 17 and 21 months were related to their overall frequencies of object-related action imitation at those ages. That is, children who engaged in more action imitation overall with their mothers also imitated more developmentally advanced behaviors. Children's highest levels of imitative action play at 13 and at 21 months were also positively related to the frequencies with which the mothers imitated their children's object-related actions at those times. Although these preliminary analyses are not definitive, they suggest that greater exposure to and practice of action imitation in general are associated with higher developmental levels of imitative play. Whether these higher levels of imitative play in turn predict, or even possibly facilitate, higher levels of nonimitative independent play merits further study.

The evidence of a predictive relation between children's imitation and their later competence is even stronger from the verbal domain. As a beginning, one might point to the many studies reporting correlations between children's verbal imitation at one age and their vocabulary levels at a later age (e.g., Bates, Bretherton, & Snyder, 1988; Snow, 1989a, 1989b). Unfortunately, these kinds of studies are inadequate in two respects as evidence to support the argument that children' verbal imitation might foster their language development. First, the same studies that show sequential associations between imitation and vocabulary also find concurrent links as well. Before accepting the sequential relations as evidence, one would need to control for the influence of the children's initial lexical levels.

Second, studies like these have calculated relations between children's total verbal imitation and their later vocabularies. However, children's verbal matching includes replication both of words well practiced and familiar and of those novel or previously unknown. We have already seen that verbal imitation may serve such social and conversational goals as acknowledging the partner or sustaining the interchange. Perhaps any relation between imitation and language growth is attributable merely to greater interactive engagement by highly imitative children. If so, then children's imitation of familiar words should be just as predictive of their later language levels as their imitation of novel words. However, if imitation is serving as a strategy for children to acquire new, linguistically meaningful behaviors, then only reproduction of words not previously present in their productive repertoires, not replication of established words, should predict their later vocabularies.

We had, in fact, shown such a relation between children's imitation of novel, but not familiar, words during an experimental task and their later vocabulary levels (Masur, 1995). But why should children's imitation of a few novel words in a controlled context be associated with their later vocabularies? That link is difficult to interpret unless children's performance in an experimental situation is a reflection of their usual imitative behavior. Thus, we set out to discover whether children's spontaneous verbal matching of novel, rather than familiar, words during play and bath session with their mothers would predict their subsequent lexicons (Masur & Eichorst, 2002). For these analyses, we took advantage of the language interview we had conducted with the mothers in our longitudinal sample to evaluate the familiarity or novelty of the conventional vocalizations and words the children copied during the free play and bath sessions at 13 and 17 months. Both children's observed and reported noun and non-noun vocabularies were assessed at 17 and 21 months.

Because children's frequencies of novel or familiar imitation were related to their concurrent vocabulary levels at both ages, all the sequential analyses we computed controlled statistically for the children's initial lexicons (Masur & Eichorst, 2002). First, in agreement with results from previous studies, we found relations between children's total verbal imitation at 13 months, including matching of novel and familiar words as well as those whose status could not be determined, and their subsequent reported and observed lexicons at 17 and 21 months. More important, when novel and familiar word imitation at 13 months were examined separately, it was only children's replication of words outside their productive repertoires, not their repetition of known words, that significantly predicted their subsequent noun and non-noun reported and observed lexicons, even when earlier lexical levels were taken into account. Similarly, with initial vocabularies controlled, the children's novel, but not familiar, verbal matching at 17 months forecast their reported and observed noun vocabularies at 21 months. Thus, the children who copied more of the novel words their mothers uttered during natural play and bath interactions were the ones whose language advanced most. Although the relations remain correlational, these findings support the argument that children may use imitation as a potent strategy for knowledge acquisition, in this case for incorporating novel words into their language repertoires (Masur & Eichorst, 2002).

CONCLUSION

We have traced the development of children's spontaneous vocal/verbal and action matching behavior during naturally occurring interactions with their mothers from the beginning of the first to the end of the second year of life. Although children's imitation grows substantially during the first year, it is during the second year that the nature of children's imitation changes dramatically, shifting in emphasis from action to verbal matching in parallel with their burgeoning linguistic skills. During this period, as children and mothers participate in myriad everyday encounters, these partners gradually create together a style of interacting. For many dyads, that style encompasses recurrent imitation. During these routine interchanges with their mothers, many children observe and practice matching of diverse vocal, verbal, and action behaviors. The imitative expertise children develop with their mothers may in turn be available for later application in their interactions with peers. Children's imitation during these dyadic interactions may also serve them as a means to acquire meaningful linguistic forms, initiating them into knowledge of the world. We agree with Nelson (1996) that imitation's "critical role in human cognition and communication development in the early years should be widely recognized, not only for learning language but also for learning the ways and meanings of the culture, and thus furnishing the mind" (p. 102). It is within the familiar contexts of naturally occurring interactions with nurturing caregivers that this learning can take place.

ACKNOWLEDGMENTS

Some of the research studies reviewed in this chapter were conducted with the support of National Institute of Child Health and Human Development Grant No. HD37587. I would like to thank Jennifer E. Rodemaker, Doreen L. Eichorst, Valerie Flynn, many undergraduate assistants over the years, and the mothers and children participating in our research studies.

REFERENCES

Baldwin, J. (1895). *Social and ethical interpretations in mental development.* New York: Macmillan.

Bates, E., Bretherton, I., & Snyder, L. (1988). *From first words to grammar: Individual differences and dissociable mechanisms.* Cambridge, UK: Cambridge University Press.

Belsky, J., & Most, R. K. (1981). From exploration to play: A cross-sectional study of infant free play behavior. *Developmental Psychology, 17,* 630–639.

Bloom, L., Hood, L., & Lightbown, P. (1974). Imitation in language development: If, when, and why. *Cognitive Psychology, 76,* 380–420.

Bloom, L., Rocissano, L., & Hood, L. (1976). Adult–child discourse: Developmental interaction between information processing and linguistic knowledge. *Cognitive Psychology, 8,* 521–552.

Bornstein, M. H., & Tamis-LeMonda, C. S. (1995). Parent–child symbolic play: Three theories in search of an effect. *Developmental Review, 15,* 382–400.

Broome, S., & Užgiris, I. C. (1985, March). *Imitation in mother–child conversations.* Paper presented at the biennial meeting of the Society for Research in Child Development, Toronto.

Eckerman, C. O., Davis, C. C., & Didow, S. M. (1989). Toddler's emerging ways of achieving social coordinations with a peer. *Child Development, 60,* 440–453.

Eckerman, C. O., & Didow, S. M. (1996). Nonverbal imitation and toddler's mastery of verbal means of achieving coordinated action. *Developmental Psychology, 32,* 141–152.

Flynn, V., Masur, E. F., & Eichorst, D. L. (2004). Opportunity versus disposition as predictors of infants' and mothers' verbal and action imitation. *Infant Behavior and Development, 27,* 303–314.

Folger, J. P., & Chapman, R. S. (1978). A pragmatic analysis of spontaneous imitation. *Journal of Child Language, 5,* 171–183.

Goldfield, B., & Reznick, J. S. (1990). Early lexical acquisition: Rate, content, and the vocabulary spurt. *Journal of Child Language, 17,* 171–183.

Hanna, E., & Meltzoff, A. N. (1993). Peer imitation by toddlers in laboratory, home, and day-care contexts: Implications for social learning and memory. *Developmental Psychology, 29,* 701–710.

Keenan, E. (1974). Conversational competence in children. *Journal of Child Language, 1,* 163–184.

Killen, M., & Užgiris, I. C. (1981). Imitation of actions with objects: The role of social meaning. *Journal of Genetic Psychology, 138,* 219–229.

Masur, E. F. (1987). Imitative interchanges in a social context: Mother–infant matching behavior at the beginning of the second year. *Merrill-Palmer Quarterly, 33,* 453–472.

Masur, E. F. (1989). Individual and dyadic patterns of imitation: Cognitive and social aspects. In G. E. Speidel & K. E. Nelson (Eds.), *The many faces of imitation in language learning* (pp. 53–71). New York: Springer-Verlag.

Masur, E. F. (1993). Transitions in representational ability: Infants' verbal, vocal, and action imitation during the second year. *Merrill-Palmer Quarterly, 39,* 437–456.

Masur, E. F. (1997, April). *Quality of play during mothers' and infants' object-related imitation.* Paper presented at the biennial meeting of the Society for Research in Child Development, Washington, DC.

Masur, E. F., & Eichorst, D. L. (2002). Infants' spontaneous imitation of novel versus familiar words: Relations to observational and maternal report measures of their lexicons. *Merrill-Palmer Quarterly, 48,* 405–426.

Masur, E. F., & Rodemaker, J. E. (1999). Mothers' and infants' spontaneous vocal, verbal, and action imitation during the second year. *Merrill-Palmer Quarterly, 45,* 392–412.

McCall, R. B. (1981). Nature–nurture and the two realms of development: A proposed integration with respect to mental development. *Child Development, 52,* 1–12.

McCall, R. B., Eichorn, D. H., & Hogarty, P. S. (1977). Transitions in early mental development. *Monographs of the Society for Research in Child Development, 42*(3, Serial No. 171).

Meltzoff, A. N. (1988a). Infant imitation after a 1-week delay: Long-term memory for novel acts and multiple stimuli. *Developmental Psychology, 24,* 470–476.

Meltzoff, A. N. (1988b). Infant imitation and memory: Nine-month-olds in immediate and deferred tests. *Child Development, 59,* 217–225.

Meltzoff, A. N. (1990). Foundations for developing a concept of self. In D. Cicchetti & M. Beeghly (Eds.), *The self in transition* (pp. 139–164). Chicago: University of Chicago Press.

Meltzoff, A. N. (1995). Understanding the intentions of others: Re-enactment of intended acts by 18-month-old children. *Developmental Psychology, 31,* 838–850.

Meltzoff, A. N., & Moore, M. K. (1983). The origins of imitation in infancy: Paradigm, phenomena, and theories. In L. P. Lipsitt & C. K. Rovee-Collier (Eds.), *Advances in infancy research* (Vol. 2, pp. 266–301). Norwood, NJ: Ablex.

Nelson, K. (1996). *Language in cognitive development: Emergence of the mediated mind.* Cambridge, UK: Cambridge University Press.

Pawlby, S. J. (1977). Imitative interaction. In H. R. Schaffer (Ed.), *Studies in mother–infant interaction* (pp. 203–224). New York: Academic.

Piaget, J. (1962). *Play, dreams, and imitation in childhood.* New York: Norton.

Ramer, A. (1976). The function of imitation in child language. *Journal of Speech and Hearing Research, 19,* 700–717.

Snow, C. E. (1981). The uses of imitation. *Journal of Child Language, 8,* 205–212.

Snow, C. E. (1989a, April). *Imitation as one path to language acquisition*. Paper presented at the biennial meeting of the Society for Research in Child Development, Kansas City.

Snow, C. E. (1989b). Imitativeness: A trait or a skill? In G. E. Speidel & K. E. Nelson (Eds.), *The many faces of imitation in language learning* (pp. 73–90). New York: Springer-Verlag.

Tamis-LeMonda, C. S., & Bornstein, M. H. (1991). Individual variation, correspondence, stability and change in mother-toddler play. *Infant Behavior and Development, 14*, 143–162.

Tomasello, M. (1992). The social bases of language acquisition. *Social Development, 1*, 67–87.

Užgiris, I. C. (1981). Two functions of imitation during infancy. *International Journal of Behavioral Development, 4*, 1–12.

Užgiris, I. C. (1984). Imitation in infancy: Its interpersonal aspects. In M. Perlmutter (Eds.), *Minnesota Symposium on Child Psychology* (Vol. 17, pp. 1–32). Hillsdale, NJ: Erlbaum.

Užgiris, I. C. (1991). The social context of infant imitation. In M. Lewis & S. Feinman (Eds.), *Social influences and socialization in infancy* (pp. 215–251). New York: Plenum Press.

Užgiris, I. C., Benson, J. B., Kruper, J. C., & Vasek, M. E. (1989). Contextual influences on imitative interactions between mothers and infants. In J. J. Lockman & N. L. Hazen (Eds.), *Action in social context: Perspectives on early development* (pp. 103–127). New York: Plenum Press.

Užgiris, I. C., Benson, J. B., & Vasek, M. (1983, April). *Matching behavior in mother–infant interactions*. Paper presented at the biennial meeting of the Society for Research in Child Development, Detroit, MI.

Užgiris, I. C., Vasek, M. E., & Benson, J. B. (1984, April). *A longitudinal study of matching activity in mother–infant interaction*. Paper presented at the annual meeting of the International Conference on Infant Studies, New York.

CHAPTER 3

Instrumental, Social, and Shared Goals and Intentions in Imitation

MALINDA CARPENTER

In an imitation context, when a demonstrator says, "Do this," the first thing a potential imitator has to figure out is, "What, exactly, does she mean by 'this'?" In even the simplest of demonstrations, there are always multiple possible answers to this question: Reproduce the same end, use the same means, the same body part, the same force, the same angle, the same muscle movements, and so on. Bushnell (1998) has likened this to the "problem of reference" in language acquisition (which is, after all, another imitation context). There, a language learner must figure out exactly what out of countless possibilities a speaker is referring to when the speaker uses a novel word (Quine, 1960). The language learner can solve the problem of reference by using an understanding of the speaker's goals and intentions in the situation and an understanding of the speaker's communicative intentions toward the learner him- or herself, and by searching for relevant possibilities in the speaker's and learner's joint attentional focus or shared knowledge (Sperber & Wilson, 1986; Tomasello, 1999, 2003). In nonlinguistic imitation, similarly, in order to figure out what "this" in "Do this" refers to—or what an actor is trying to do in less elicited imitation contexts—learners must determine which of all the actions they see performed and all the results they see achieved are necessary for a "correct" reproduction. Here I attempt to show that learners can use exactly the same sorts of solutions as in language—an understanding of goals, intentions, and communicative intentions and joint attentional focus or shared knowledge—in nonlinguistic imitation to answer the question of what to imitate (see also Bushnell, 1998; Tomasello, Kruger, & Ratner, 1993).

Typically developing infants are already very good at flexibly answering the question of what to imitate by 12–18 months of age. Children with autism, on the other hand, show a pattern of results on imitation tests that suggests that they might not answer this question in the same way as other children. For example, recent reviews by Rogers, Cook, and Meryl (2005) and Williams, Whiten, and Singh (2004) have concluded that whereas children with autism as a group often do not show very pronounced deficits in tests involving imitation of actions on objects, they show consistent deficits in tests involving imitation of body and facial movements. In general, they are better at reproducing "meaningful" than "nonmeaningful" actions. Furthermore, when they reproduce a demonstrator's actions, these children often do not copy the particular way the demonstrator performed the action, and they sometimes make perspective reversal errors.

In this chapter, I compare how typically developing infants and children with autism answer the question of what to imitate, and I attempt to explain the pattern of weaknesses—and also relative strengths—seen in the imitation of children with autism. I selectively review the relevant literature in three areas. First, I explore to what extent children in each group can use an understanding of others' goals and intentions toward objects to infer what others are trying to do. Second, I discuss ways in which children might use an understanding of others' communicative intentions and shared goals in some situations to arrive at a solution in a more collaborative way, *with* the demonstrator. Third, because in some imitation contexts it is not so much the goals and intentions of the demonstrator that are important but those of the learner, I discuss how the answer to the question of what to imitate can, in addition, depend on whether the learner's own goal at the moment is an instrumental or a social one (Užgiris, 1981, 1984). (Other factors such as task structure and difficulty are involved as well but will not be discussed here; see, e.g., Bauer & Hertsgaard, 1993; Harnick, 1978; Sibulkin & Užgiris, 1978; Travis, 1997.) I conclude that it is the shared, social aspects of imitation that are most affected in children with autism but that a combination of all three factors best explains the pattern of results these (and other) children show across different types of imitation tests.

UNDERSTANDING OF OTHERS' GOALS AND INTENTIONS TOWARD OBJECTS

A potential imitator can gather several different sources of information from a demonstration (see Call & Carpenter, 2002; Carpenter & Call, 2002). Some of these sources of information, actions and results, are directly observable, but one, the goal, is only inferrable. That is, one can observe the demonstrator's body movements (actions) and the changes in the environment that those body movements bring about (results). From these and other sources of information, it is often possible to infer the goal of the demonstrator, the mental representation of the result that he or she wants to achieve.

There are many advantages to being able to use an understanding of others' goals to interpret a demonstration instead of copying all the actions and/or results one sees. For example, demonstrators often perform accidental, irrelevant, or unsuccessful actions, so being able to filter these out and hone in on just those actions that are relevant to achieving the goal would result in more efficient and conventional performance on the part of the learner. In addition, if learners know the goal of an action, they can achieve the same end even when there are dissimilarities in body size, situation, or constraints between themselves and the demonstrator (Nehaniv & Dautenhahn, 2001). Finally, sometimes the same two demonstrations can have different goals underlying them (see, e.g., Meltzoff, Gopnik, & Repacholi, 1999), and conversely two different demonstrations can have the same goal underlying them (see, e.g., Meltzoff, 1995). This means that relying on surface aspects of the demonstration and copying all actions and results can be misleading and result in imitation of either superfluous or insufficient elements of the demonstration.

Not only is understanding others' goals useful, so too is understanding others' intentions. Simply put, a goal is the mental representation of the desired end result and an intention is the mental representation of the means or plan of action the actor has chosen and committed him- or herself to in order to achieve the desired end (Bratman, 1989). That is, to achieve a goal, the actor can consider various means, taking into account his or her own knowledge and skills and any constraints present in the situation, and evaluating each means rationally with respect to the goal, and then choose one of the means as his intention or plan of action (Tomasello, Carpenter, Call, Behne, & Moll, 2005). Sometimes the goal is more important, and it does not matter so much how one goes about achieving it, but sometimes the means is an integral part of the goal, as when it is important to the actor that something be done in a particular way. Imitators must understand this in order to determine whether the means the demonstrator used is important and necessary to copy. Only learners who ask *why* a demonstrator performed an action in a particular way can appropriately decide whether or not to perform the same action when it is their turn. The ability to infer and use others' goals and intentions—interpreting others' behavior instead of responding based on the surface level of observable actions and results—thus allows learners to respond flexibly, copying actions in some cases and results in others.

Some animals mostly copy actions only and some mostly copy results only (see, e.g., Carpenter & Call, in press, for a review). Some—most notably humans—take others' goals into account when deciding whether to copy actions or results or both. Here I briefly review evidence suggesting that, already beginning around their first birthdays, typically developing human infants can infer others' goals and intentions, and that they use this ability to respond flexibly and appropriately in imitative contexts.

Typically Developing Infants

Typically developing infants apparently begin to understand other people as goal-directed agents at some point between 6 and 9 months of age (e.g., Behne, Carpenter, Call, & Tomasello, 2005; Csibra, Gergely, Bíró, Koós, & Brockbank, 1999; see Tomasello et al., 2005, for a review). By 12 months of age, infants can use this understanding in imitation contexts to determine what a demonstrator is trying to do and then respond appropriately by copying some aspects of the demonstration over others. Sometimes infants copy the results others achieve, sometimes they copy the actions others perform, and sometimes they do both (or even neither), and these responses can all be "correct" from the point of view of the demonstrator, depending on the demonstrator's goals.

The best evidence of infants' understanding of others as goal-directed agents comes from tests involving failed attempts and accidents, because there is a mismatch between the demonstrator's goal and what actually happens, and infants can show what they understand the demonstrator to be doing by either copying what they see (the demonstrator's surface behavior) or producing the action or result that the demonstrator meant to perform (his or her underlying goal). With regard to failed attempts, when a demonstrator tries unsuccessfully to achieve some result, 15- and 18-month-olds do not copy exactly what the demonstrator does. Instead, they produce the result the demonstrator intended to produce, and they do this as often as in a condition in which the demonstrator completed the result successfully (Meltzoff, 1995; see also Johnson, Booth, & O'Hearn, 2001). Somewhat older children can also see the same action as either a failed attempt or a playful action, depending on the emotional expressions and vocalizations of the demonstrator during and after the demonstration (Meltzoff et al., 1999; Rakoczy, Tomasello, & Striano, 2004). With regard to accidents, when an adult performs two actions, one action accidentally ("Whoops!") and one action intentionally ("There!"), 14- to 18-month-old infants usually reproduce only the intentional one (Carpenter, Akhtar, & Tomasello, 1998).

Infants this age thus do not simply copy the actions or the results they see. Instead, they see demonstrators' actions as goal-directed and adopt and strive toward the same goal as the demonstrator, adapting their own actions along the way. They can come up with new actions (see also Meltzoff et al., 1999), filter out unintended actions, and produce results that they have never seen completed. They can see two identical actions as having different underlying goals and two different demonstrations as having the same underlying goal.

In another interesting type of study, in contrast, the demonstrator fully achieves his or her goal—there are no failed attempts or accidents—and the question is whether or not the infant copies the means the demonstrator used. In this type of study, children see a demonstrator use the same particular action in both of two different conditions, but they copy it in one condition but not the other.

One set of these studies involves goal inference and illustrates that when children do not see any other salient goal, they assume that what the demonstrator is doing—the particular action he or she is using—*is* the goal. For example, 2-year-old children who watched an adult pulling a pin out of a box with large twisting motions before opening a door on the box were more likely to copy the (unnecessary) twisting motions than were children in other conditions in which the adult had first done something to the box (or to other boxes) that allowed children to infer that her goal was to open the box (Carpenter, Call, & Tomasello, 2002). In the first case, when the twisting motions were the first thing children saw, children apparently assumed that what the adult was doing was simply twisting the pin (and were then surprised to see the box open at the end). In the second case, though, they saw pulling out the pin merely as a means to the end of opening the box and thus mostly set about opening the box themselves in the most direct way possible, by pulling the pin straight out. Similar results have been found with 12-month-old infants: If 12-month-olds watch an adult make a toy mouse hop to the center of a table, they will make the mouse hop on the table too. But if they see the adult make the mouse hop in exactly the same way, to the same location, but there is a little house in that location, then infants simply pick up the mouse and put it directly into the house without making it hop (Carpenter, Call, & Tomasello, 2005; see also Bekkering, Wohlschläger, & Gattis, 2000, for the same type of study with older children). Infants and young children are thus more likely to copy the exact way the demonstrator performed an action if they do not see any salient end result—that is, if that particular action appears to be an end in and of itself.

A second set of these studies involves infants' understanding that others choose means rationally, and infants' search for the reasons *why* others act as they do. For example, the preliminary results of a study by Behne, Carpenter, van Veen, and Tomasello (2006) suggest that if 18-month-olds see an adult performing an unusual action (e.g., illuminating a light with her forearm) while the adult is looking at what he or she is doing, infants often copy this unusual action. However, if infants see the adult perform the exact same action but while he or she is bending down and looking for another toy on the floor, they often do not copy the unusual action, instead illuminating the light themselves with their hand. This study shows that infants copy what a demonstrator does depending on whether or not he or she chose to do the action. Another study shows further that infants take into account the specific reasons why a demonstrator chose to use a particular action. Gergely, Bekkering, and Király (2002) showed 14-month-old infants an adult using a highly unusual action to turn on a light panel: The adult bent over and pressed the panel with her head. Infants copied this unusual action in this situation. However, in a condition in which the adult performed the exact same action (also in an intentional way) but with her hands occupied (she was holding onto a blanket around her shoulders), infants did not copy the head action, instead turning on the light with their hands. Apparently, in the latter condition, infants saw the unusual action, knew that it was not the normal way to do things, wondered why the adult chose this way to do it, and decided it was done because the adult's hands—the more normal thing to use—were unavailable. This constraint did not apply to them; thus, when it was their turn to operate the light panel, they used their hands. In the first condition, however, infants could not find a good answer to the question of why the adult chose the unusual action so they figured there must be a good reason for this choice and copied it themselves. Results from our laboratory show that 12-month-olds show the same understanding on a different but analogous task (Schwier, van Maanen, Carpenter, & Tomasello, in press). Tomasello and colleagues (2005) have taken the results of these studies as evidence that 1-year-old infants understand not just that others have goals but also that others form intentions rationally—that they choose action plans based on some reason that takes into account the current state of the environment and the actor.

In summary, by approximately 1 year of age, infants have some basic understanding of others' goals and intentions and can use this understanding to interpret others' behavior and decide which aspects of it they should copy. They can use a variety of social and contextual sources of observable information to infer others' goals and intentions (see Carpenter & Call, in press).

Children with Autism

Relatively few studies have directly investigated what children with autism understand about others' goals and intentions. In studies that did not use imitation as a response measure, findings are mixed. For example, Phillips, Baron-Cohen, and Rutter (1998) tested children on a target shooting game and found that children with autism were less able than children with other developmental delays to identify which target they had intended to hit in some conditions. However, Russell and Hill (2001) found no differences between children with autism and typically developing children matched on mental age on this and another task, when children were asked to report both their own and another person's intended target. Other studies have found that children with autism are less able than children without autism to use others' gaze direction to determine their goals (Baron-Cohen, Campbell, Karmiloff-Smith, Grant, & Walker, 1995), but on one of these tasks mixed results are found (i.e., Phillips, Baron-Cohen, & Rutter, 1992, and Roeyers, van Oost, & Bothuyne, 1998, vs. Carpenter, Pennington, & Rogers, 2002, and Charman et al., 1997).

Two studies have directly tested the understanding of others' failed attempts in children with autism using an imitation paradigm. Both used the general procedure of Meltzoff (1995) in which children are shown an adult trying unsuccessfully to achieve some result. In the first study, Aldridge, Stone, Sweeney, and Bower (2000) used one condition of Meltzoff's (1995) procedure with young children with autism and found no impairment for these children on this task. However, Aldridge and colleagues compared children with autism to typically developing infants matched on a nonverbal measure of object concept and all but three of these infants were younger than 12 months old and thus would not be expected to pass this test (Bellagamba & Tomasello, 1999). Aldridge and colleagues also only presented children with one of Meltzoff's conditions, the condition in which the failed attempt was shown, and thus could not directly address possible alternate explanations such as stimulus enhancement. In the other study, Carpenter, Pennington, and Rogers (2001) used Meltzoff's full procedure (although within subjects) and compared children with autism to children with other developmental delays matched on chronological and verbal and nonverbal mental age (all ≥ 16 months). They too found no clear autism deficit on this task: The pattern of results for children with autism did not differ from that of the children with other developmental delays, and both groups showed a pattern of results that was similar to that of the typically developing 18-month-olds from Meltzoff's study in the key conditions. However, for children with autism there were no differences between the condition in which the failed attempt was shown and a control condition in which the adult simply manipulated the object, limiting what could be concluded from this study.

Sally Rogers and colleagues (Colombi, Rogers, & Young, 2005; Rogers, 2005) have since replicated these results more convincingly, but still we must be cautious in claiming that children with autism understand others' failed attempts and thus goals because all these studies have used the same task, that of Meltzoff (1995), and there are potential problems with Meltzoff's task when it is used in isolation. That is, Huang, Heyes, and Charman (2002) claim and provide evidence that even typically developing children could have been using nonsocial information instead of an understanding of the adult's unfulfilled goal in Meltzoff's failed attempt condition. That is, children could have achieved the "correct" response in this test by using an understanding of the objects' affordances or spatial contiguity cues suggested by the adult's behavior. This is not a problem for typically developing infants because there is plenty of other evidence that they understand others' goals (and failed attempts in particular). This evidence comes both from (1) nonimitative tasks (e.g., Behne, Carpenter, Call, & Tomasello, 2005) and (2) a variety of other types of imitation tasks in which the *same* actions and results are shown in different conditions (with the only difference between conditions being social or contextual information about the adult's goal or intention), so nonsocial, action- or object-based alternate explanations are less plausible (e.g., Behne et al., 2006; Carpenter, Akhtar, & Tomasello, 1998; Carpenter, Call, & Tomasello, 2002, 2005; Gergely et al., 2002; see Carpenter, Pennington, & Rogers, 2003; Tomasello & Carpenter, 2005b, for more discussion of this). Without such clear supporting evidence for children with autism, we cannot yet make any firm conclusions about their understanding of others' goals.

We also do not know much about these children's understanding of others' intentions or rational choice of means. Young children with autism may understand others' actions as a means to an end (that is one possible interpretation of a study by Carpenter, Pennington, & Rogers, 2002, in which children copied an adult's head touch action and looked expectantly to the light that was about to come on), but this does not necessarily mean they know that others can choose means rationally according to the situation in which they find themselves. There are preliminary indications that these children do not show the same difference in responding that typically developing 12- and 14-month-old infants show in the studies that we have taken as evidence for understanding others' intentions (Gergely et al., 2002; Schwier et al., in press). Instead, children with autism copy the demonstrator's action equally frequently in both conditions (Somogyi et al., 2005).

In summary, more work needs to be done on understanding of others' goals and intentions in children with autism, in both imitation and non-imitation contexts. In imitation contexts, more different tasks are needed, especially tasks like those used with typically developing infants, which keep the actions and results constant across conditions while varying only information about the demonstrator's goal or intention. More investigation into whether children with autism understand others' intentions along with their goals would also be interesting because intentions are less easily inferrable from observable behavior than goals. An understanding of others' goals but not intentions would allow children to pass tests such as that of Meltzoff (1995) but would mean that they would not see the importance of the means the demonstrator chose to achieve his or her goal, and thus they would not necessarily copy this means (except when it suited them to do so—see below).

COLLABORATIVE IMITATION: SHARING GOALS AND UNDERSTANDING COMMUNICATIVE INTENTIONS

The preceding discussion has shown that typically developing infants, at least, can use various types of observable information to infer a demonstrator's goals and intentions toward the object the demonstrator is acting on, and then can use this inference to answer the question of what to imitate when it is their turn to act on the object themselves. In many cases, children are able to infer others' goals and intentions toward objects even when children are watching from the outside, as it were, and even when the demonstrator is not aware that the children are watching (much as children can learn novel language by overhearing speech that is not directed to them; Akhtar, Jipson, & Callanan, 2001). But in other cases, the children themselves are an integral part of the demonstration. This can happen in at least two ways. First, the demonstration can occur in the context of an already shared interaction between the child and the demonstrator. In this case, if children are already sharing goals with the demonstrator—if they are engaging in joint attentional and joint intentional interaction with him or her—then there are in effect no goals to infer because children know that the demonstrator's goals are the same as the children's own.

Second, the demonstrator can actively provide observable cues concerning his or her goals and intentions toward children themselves: his or her "communicative intentions." In human communication, Sperber and Wilson (1986) argued that speakers help listeners comprehend their message by providing ostensive-communicative cues that tell listeners that the speaker thinks what will follow is relevant for them. In turn, listeners recognize speakers' ostensive-communicative cues and make relevant assumptions and inferences about the speakers' intentions. This type of communication is thus a collaboration because both speaker and listener are working together, helping each other so that the listener comprehends the speaker's meaning (Clark, 1996; Tomasello et al., 2005). The same processes may be at work in a certain type of collaborative imitation situation in which the demonstrator is deliberately trying to show the learner how to do something and signals to the learner what he or she wishes him or her to do using ostensive-communicative cues such as meaningful eye contact, meaningful looks to parts of the object or his or her own body, gestures such as pointing or tapping, exaggerated actions and facial expressions, and of course verbal hints such as "Watch" or "Do it like *this*." These types of cues can help highlight and frame some aspects of the demonstration, marking the important parts as *for* the observer and so *relevant* for him or her (Bushnell, 1998; Gergely & Csibra, in press). When the demonstrator manifests his or her communicative intentions in this way, in effect the demonstrator is inviting the learner to adopt and share his or her goal (note that this does not necessarily mean that the demonstrator intends the learner to copy him or her exactly). If the learner makes the relevant assumptions and inferences and then adopts and shares the demonstrator's goal, checking with the demonstrator for feedback along the way, then the end result is a collaborative interaction very similar to the collaborative interaction that occurs in linguistic communication.

Typically Developing Infants

Infants begin sharing goals with others basically as soon as they are able to understand others' goals, by age 9 months (see Tomasello et al., 2005, for a review). Somewhat older infants imitatively learn novel language better when they are in joint attentional engagement when the novel word is presented, because when they are already sharing attention and goals, determining the adult's referent is easier because infants are already attending to the relevant parts of the situation (Tomasello, 2003; Tomasello & Farrar, 1986). Infants begin to engage in joint attention before they begin to imitate others' actions on objects (Carpenter, Nagell, & Tomasello, 1998), so it is likely that the benefits of joint attentional frames also apply to nonlinguistic imitation situations as well.

By age 14 months, infants show that they understand something about others' communicative intentions as well. Behne, Carpenter, and Tomasello (2005) first had an adult engage 14-, 18-, and 24-month-old children in a visible hiding game, in which children saw in which of two containers a toy was placed. Then, the adult hid the toy in such a way that the children did not know which of two containers it was in. The adult then either pointed to one of the two closed containers or alternated gaze between the child and one of the containers. When she did this in an ostensive, communicative way, children at all ages chose the container she indicated and found the toy. Although at first glance this task seems trivially easy, results from similar studies of chimpanzees show that it is not (see Call & Tomasello, 2005, for a review). Participants in this task must follow the adult's gaze and pointing gestures to one of the containers (that is something chimpanzees can do), but then, in addition, they must see the adult's gestures as "for them" and as relevant to their previous shared interaction, and on the basis of this further infer that the toy is hidden in the container the adult indicated (all things chimpanzees apparently do not do). It is important to note that children in Behne and colleagues' study did not do this when the adult did not provide ostensive-communicative cues. When she performed very similar surface behaviors in an absent-minded, distracted, noncommunicative way (e.g., she held out her index finger in the same place—at the midline across her body—but looked down as if inspecting her arm), children chose the correct container only at chance levels. Thus, by 14 months of age, infants know when adults are trying to tell them something, and are good at inferring adults' communicative intentions based on what is relevant in their current or previous joint attentional and joint intentional interactions.

In nonlinguistic imitation situations, the only studies that have directly tested the effect of ostensive-communicative cues are as yet unpublished ones. For example, Gergely and colleagues (reported in Gergely & Csibra, in press, and Király, Csibra, & Gergely, 2004) investigated whether infants would copy an unusual demonstration more when ostensive-communicative cues were present than when they were not. In both of two of their conditions, they showed 14-month-old infants an adult touching her head to a light panel to turn it on (while her hands were free). In one condition, the adult did this with full ostensive-communicative cues: She first established eye contact with the infant, and then looked at the object, saying, "Look, I'll show you something!" (as in Gergely et al., 2002), and 60% of infants copied the head touch action. In the other condition, the adult provided none of these cues, instead simply walking into the room and performing the demonstration without ever looking at or communicating with the infants (infants' attention was attracted by a sound coming from the light box to ensure that they watched the demonstration). In this condition, in contrast with the first one, infants only very rarely copied the head touch action. Thus, infants apparently took the adult's ostensive-communicative cues in the first condition as a sign that what was to follow was "for them" and worthy of imitation.

Finally, there is preliminary evidence from our laboratory that suggests that 12- and 18-month-old infants can see the collaborative structure of some imitative interactions, inferring the adult's intention toward them, reversing roles, and redirecting the action back toward the adult. For example, after showing the child how to place a toy on a plate, the adult held out the plate and waited for the child to place the toy on it twice. Then, in the role-reversal imitation test, the adult switched objects with the child, giving the plate to the child, and waited for the child to hold the plate out to her so that she could place the toy on it. Some 12- and 18-month-olds reversed roles in this way, also looking to the face of the adult in expectation of her fulfilling her role (Carpenter, Tomasello, & Striano, 2005).

Children with Autism

With regard to shared goals, children with autism have severe deficits in the ability or motivation to engage in joint attentional interaction with other people. Compared to other children, they initiate fewer episodes of joint engagement by looking to others or pointing declaratively (e.g., Charman et al., 1997; Lewy & Dawson, 1992; Mundy, Sigman, Ungerer, & Sherman, 1986) and they have more difficulty following others' gaze direction and pointing gestures (e.g., Baron-Cohen, 1989; Leekam, Baron-Cohen, Perrett, Milders, & Brown, 1997). Furthermore, whereas typically developing infants begin to engage in joint attention before they begin to imitate others' actions on objects (Carpenter, Nagell, & Tomasello, 1998), young children with autism may show a different pattern, some of them apparently copying others' actions on objects before they begin engaging in joint attention (Carpenter, Pennington, & Rogers, 2002). Without the benefit of a shared context with joint attention and joint intentions, inferring relevant aspects of a demonstration would be all the more difficult.

With regard to communicative intentions, as a group, people with autism have difficulty with many aspects of communicative intentions even as adults, both in their own communication and in understanding and drawing relevant inferences from the communication of others (e.g., Happé, 1993; Surian, Baron-Cohen, & Van der Lely, 1996; see Sabbagh, 1999, for a review). Children with autism also have difficulty with many of the basic abilities that underlie understanding of others' communicative intentions. For example, they are less responsive to speech and other social stimuli than are children without autism (Dawson, Meltzoff, Osterling, Rinaldi, & Brown, 1998; Klin, 1991). In particular, one of the clearest signalers of communicative intent is ostensive eye contact. Individuals with autism pay less attention to others' eyes and have more difficulty detecting when others make eye contact with them than do nonautistic individuals (Klin, Jones, Schultz, Volkmar, & Cohen, 2002; Senju, Yaguchi, Tojo, & Hasegawa, 2003). They also have trouble understanding the "language of the eyes," or how various intentions or other mental states can be inferred from information contained in the eye region of the face (Baron-Cohen et al., 1995; Baron-Cohen, Wheelwright, & Jolliffe, 1997). In language-learning situations, these children do not use adults' gaze direction to imitatively learn a novel word; instead they learn the novel word for the object they themselves were looking at when the word was uttered (Baron-Cohen, Baldwin, & Crowson, 1997). In nonlinguistic imitation contexts, if children with autism do not pick up on or realize the significance of demonstrators' ostensive eye contact, they miss out on an important channel of information that is available to nonautistic individuals as extra help in framing important aspects of the demonstration and thus in answering the question of what to imitate.

Finally, children with autism also do not collaborate in the same way as do typically developing infants in some imitation tasks. Carpenter, Tomasello, and Striano (2005) included a small group of children with autism in one of their collaborative role reversal imitation tests. In this case, the adult hid a toy under a cloth for the child to find it and then gave the toy and cloth to the child to see if the child would reciprocate and hide the toy for the adult. We found that the children with autism did hide the toy, but, unlike 18-month-old typically developing infants and matched children with other developmental delays, they did not look to the face of the adult in expectation of her fulfilling her role. They did not perform the action *for* the adult, as she had done for them. There are also many other examples of difficulties with reversals that do not involve looking to the other person. That is, when they copy others' gestures, children with autism often show an interesting pattern of errors. Ohta (1987), Whiten and Brown (1998), Smith and Bryson (1998), and Hobson and colleagues (Hobson & Lee, 1999; Meyer & Hobson, 2004) all have reported that children with autism sometimes reproduce actions exactly as they see them, without switching perspectives. For example, when the modeled action was "waving with the open palm facing the subject," some children with autism waved with their own palm facing themselves, as opposed to with their palm facing the experimenter.

More research is needed regarding these children's understanding of communicative intentions and their ability to collaborate with others (in and out of imitative contexts). In terms of intervention, it might help to focus more training efforts on noticing and interpreting common ostensive-communicative signals. And, a possible practical implication of the preceding discussion is that it may help if imitation researchers scaffold the test context more for children with autism, making it clear somehow (if not verbally then through the preceding activities) whether children should "do as the adult does" or just "have a turn" to play with the object as they choose. For example, Whiten and Brown (1998) reported more copying by children with autism when imitation was elicited—when children were specifically trained and then asked to "Do as I do"—than in a more spontaneous context (although there was a clear confound of type of task in this comparison). Still, as discussed at the beginning of this chapter, even in the "Do as I do" context, the correct response is ambiguous and will have to be inferred by the imitator.

CHILDREN'S OWN INSTRUMENTAL VERSUS SOCIAL GOALS

Along with children's ability to infer others' goals and intentions toward objects, and their ability to collaborate with others in imitation by sharing goals and reading others' communicative intentions toward them, another factor is important in determining which aspects of a demonstration children are likely to copy. This involves why the child is imitating in the first place, that is, the function of imitation for the child at the moment of the demonstration and response.

Užgiris (e.g., 1981, 1984) identified two functions of imitation in infancy (here modified slightly): an instrumental function in which the imitator learns something about the object or action in the demonstration, and a social function in which the focus is on the dyad and their interpersonal interaction. Užgiris saw the social function of imitation as a "means of communication with the partner," claiming that "the basic message that imitation conveys is mutuality or sharing of a feeling, understanding, or goal" and that "matching serves to affirm a shared state" (Užgiris, 1984, p. 25; see also, e.g., Nadel, Guérini, Pezé, & Rivet, 1999, for a similar view). Another social motive for imitation may be an affiliative one. That is, infants apparently identify with others early on, seeing themselves as *like* but *different* from others (Hobson, 1993; Meltzoff & Decety, 2003; Tomasello et al., 2005). One important social function of imitation may be to make oneself *more like* others.

Of course, the instrumental and social functions of imitation can co-occur, but which of them is most important to a learner at the moment of the demonstration and response may be the single most powerful determiner of which aspects of the demonstration the learner will copy. If the instrumental function of imitation is more important—if, for example, a child learns from a demonstration that one can open a container and retrieve a reward from inside—the child may not be so concerned about the exact way in which the demonstrator performed the action used to achieve the result, and thus may copy only those elements of the demonstration (if any) that are directly relevant to achieving this result. In contrast, if the social function of imitation is more important, the child may choose to perform the action the same way the demonstrator did, using the same means and even the same "style" (Hobson & Lee, 1999) that the demonstrator used.

Typically Developing Infants

A good indicator of whether the social function of imitation is important to infants is when they copy the particular way someone does something even though that particular way is clearly not necessary to achieve the same effect.

This would indicate that infants see the use of the same action as the adult as a goal in and of itself.

Young children often choose to adopt adults' means, even when they are not causally necessary. For example, Nagell, Olguin, and Tomasello (1993) showed that 2-year-old children copied an adult's flipping or no-flipping actions with a rake even when it resulted in less efficient performance on their part. Similarly, Whiten, Custance, Gomez, Teixidor, and Bard (1996) found that 2- to 4-year-old children copied the particular actions an adult used to open a box, even though these actions were not causally effective (see also Call, Carpenter, & Tomasello, 2005, for similar results with 2-year-olds on a different task). Sometimes, children may copy the adult's particular action even when they know for a fact that it is not necessary (i.e., after they have already achieved the same end themselves using a more efficient means; Gergely et al., 2002).

This kind of social motivation is particularly clear when it occurs spontaneously, with no real demonstration and expectation of a response. For example, I have recorded many observations of my own young son very deliberately copying such behaviors as unconscious body postures of people who were not interacting with him (e.g., hands on hips or chin resting in hands) and actions performed by oblivious peers (e.g., jumping on the couch in a particular way). And, of course, this type of imitation permeates the lives of older children and adults too, when we copy the way others dress, talk, and gesture, to name a few examples.

The importance of the social function of imitation is often dependent on the task and on one's social partner, and it may change with time, not only from moment to moment but also with development. These developmental changes may occur not just linearly but in one or more inverted U-shaped curves. One early peak in this social motivation may occur around age 18 months. For example, Gergely (2003) reports that whereas 14-month-olds copy the unusual head touch action an adult uses to turn on a light only when the adult apparently freely chose that action (in the "hands-free" condition), 18-month-olds often copy the unusual action regardless of the adult's reasons for performing it. But, of course, as discussed earlier, even 18-month-olds do not *always* copy exactly what adults do; sometimes they do what the adult intended to do instead (e.g., Carpenter, Akhtar, & Tomasello, 1998; Meltzoff, 1995).

Children with Autism

In their review of the autism imitation literature, Rogers and colleagues (2005) concluded that the social function of imitation may be more impaired in children with autism than the instrumental function of imitation, citing better performance on tasks involving objects—which may involve the instrumental function of imitation more than the social one—than on tasks involving more social aspects of imitation such as imitation of body and facial movements. But even within tasks involving actions on objects, there is evidence that the social function of imitation may not be so important to children with autism, when they choose not to copy the particular actions demonstrators use.

In some imitation studies of children with autism, means and end are not clearly dissociable, but in those in which they are, findings are mixed: In some tasks, children with autism copy the means the demonstrator used to achieve some end and in some tasks they do not. For example, Carpenter, Pennington, and Rogers (2002) found that young children with autism copied an adult touching her head to a box to turn on a light just as often as young children with other developmental delays but not autism (whereas they could just as easily—in fact much more easily—have used their hands). However, Williams and colleagues (2004) and Whiten and Brown (1998) reported a study by J. Brown showing that, unlike typically developing children, young children with autism were unlikely to copy the same method a demonstrator used to open a container (although older children and adults with autism did use the demonstrator's method).

The clearest differences between children with autism and other children are found in the imitation of action "style." That is, sometimes children go beyond choosing the same general means as an adult and adopt even the particular style the adult used. Hobson and Lee (1999) tested this directly by showing adolescents with autism demonstrations in which an adult used an unnecessary action style to achieve some effect (e.g., strumming a stick along a pipe rack gently vs. harshly). They found that although most participants reproduced the general effect of the demonstrations, participants with autism copied the style the adult used far less often than matched participants without autism.

In a recent study, Hobson and Meyer (Chapter 9, this volume) have teased apart means, ends, and style more systematically. They reported that when the style was the end or goal (and thus it was not really a "style" anymore), children with autism reproduced it as often as children in the control group. But when the style was the means to the end, or especially when the style was incidental to the means and end, then children with autism copied it less often than other children (who copied the style at similar levels across the different tasks and conditions).

The tendency of children with autism not to copy others' action styles could be related to impairments in identifying with others (in Hobson's sense of actively "connecting with" and assimilating others' attitudes; see Hobson & Meyer, Chapter 9, this volume) or, as we would argue, it could be a result of a general lack of a motivation to share experiences with others (Tomasello et al., 2005) or to be more like others. Again, the impairments in joint attentional engagement and declarative gestures in children with autism are relevant here: If one of the (social) functions of imitation is to "communicate mutuality and shared understanding" with each other (Užgiris, 1981, p. 1)—a kind of joint attentional and joint intentional engagement—then clearly children with autism would be expected to have difficulty with this type of imitation. Support for the idea that social imitation involves joint attention, or that both of these involve the same social motivation to share experiences with others, comes from findings that joint attention and imitation are correlated in children with autism. Various measures of joint attention are positively correlated with imitation of the same means to an end (Carpenter, Pennington, & Rogers, 2002), imitation of simple actions on objects and oral–facial movements (Rogers, Hepburn, Stackhouse, & Wehner, 2003), and imitation of self–other orientation (see Hobson & Meyer, Chapter 9, this volume). Joint attention is also correlated with copying others' means and style in children without autism (Carpenter, Tomasello, & Savage-Rumbaugh, 1995; Hobson & Meyer, Chapter 9, this volume).

Further support for a motivational problem in children with autism comes from Whiten and Brown's (1998) preliminary findings that these children *can* imitate, it is just that they do not spontaneously do so—although again note that there is a confound of the different tasks (which may tap into the different functions of imitation) used in this comparison. Still, these findings are reminiscent of similar findings in the area of gaze following: When asked, children with autism can report what the focus of others' gaze is, but they are unlikely spontaneously to follow it (Leekam et al., 1997).

More research is needed on the function of imitation for children with autism. Along with investigating performance on different types of actions across tasks (e.g., "meaningful" vs. not, actions on objects vs. gestures), more research attention to children's reproduction of different components *within* a task would be helpful. In particular, it would help to more systematically tease apart means, end, and style and to do this in various (instrumental and social; spontaneous and elicited) contexts, to investigate when and why children with autism copy others' actions. More work on developmental differences in the social function of imitation (see, e.g., Whiten & Brown, 1998) and the function of echolalia in these children also would be informative.

DISCUSSION

In summary, three main factors that determine which aspects of a demonstration a learner will copy include (1) the ability to infer others' goals and intentions toward objects, (2) the ability to collaborate with others in imitation by sharing goals and reading others' communicative intentions toward oneself, and (3) one's own social versus instrumental goals at the moment. There is evidence that typically developing 1-year-old infants already show both of the first two social-cognitive abilities and also a social motivation to share experiences and be more like others. These three factors in combination help explain the complex pattern of flexible and selective responses by typically developing infants and young children across imitation tests. For example, they help explain why children usually copy a demonstrator's actions but can override this when they know the demonstrator did not mean to or was forced to use those particular actions, or when the demonstration was not marked as "for them."

Children with autism, in contrast, may understand others' goals (but perhaps not intentions) toward objects, but it is unlikely that they have the same understanding of others' communicative intentions as typically developing children, or the same social goals and motivation to collaborate and share experiences with others. These three factors in combination thus also help explain both the relative strengths—in goal-directed, "meaningful," instrumental tasks involving actions on objects—and the weaknesses and errors found in these children's imitation, including problems with role reversal imitation and deficits in imitation of action style and body and facial movements, especially when these are "nonmeaningful." Incidentally, the three factors may also help explain some interesting similarities in the pattern of deficits that children with autism show in language and communication on the one hand and nonlinguistic imitation on the other. For example, these children make role-reversal errors both in language (e.g., pronouns and questions–answers) and in imitation; their speech is often described as "wooden" and lacking normal prosody and intonation, which is reminiscent of their lack of imitation of action style; and they both communicate and apparently also imitate more often for instrumental (imperative) than social (declarative) reasons (see, e.g., Sigman & Capps, 1997, for a review).

In the bigger picture of uniquely human cultural learning and transmission, it is interesting to note that the same three factors in combination also help explain differences compared with typically developing humans in which aspects of a demonstration chimpanzees, our nearest primate relatives, are likely to copy. That is, chimpanzees show some evidence of understanding others' goals but as yet no evidence of understanding others' intentions (Call, Hare, Carpenter, & Tomasello, 2004; Tomasello & Carpenter, 2005a). They also show little evidence of understanding of others' communicative intentions (see Call & Tomasello, 2005, for a review), and little evidence of a general motivation to share experiences with others in joint attentional engagement or by using declarative gestures (e.g., Tomasello & Carpenter, 2005a). And their pattern of responses on imitation tasks is in many ways similar to that of children with autism: they perform better on tasks involving instrumental use of objects, they usually copy the end result or goal of a demonstration and not the means or style the demonstrator used, and they do not engage in role reversal imitation in the same way that typically developing infants do (Tomasello & Carpenter, 2005a; see, e.g., Call & Carpenter, 2003, for a review).

Thus, to explain uniquely human aspects of cultural learning and transmission, all three factors together are necessary; any of them alone or in other combinations is not enough. First, an understanding of others' goals and intentions (Tomasello et al., 1993) (or that in combination with an understanding of others' communicative intentions) is not enough because it does not capture the full complexity of why we so often do things the way other members of our culture do. For example, we tend to dress similarly to others not, I think, because we know that they intentionally chose to wear those particular styles but instead because we want to be like them or show them that we are like them. Second, Gergely and Csibra (in press) have proposed that cultural learning is based on adults' teaching and children's understanding of adults' communicative intentions, and that this complementary system ensures cultural relevance and transmission. But that (or that in combination with a social motivation to copy what others do) is not enough because it does not tell learners exactly which aspects of the demonstration are relevant, or what they are relevant *for*. For example, in Carpenter, Call, and Tomasello's (2002) study, even though the experimenter provided children with full ostensive-communicative cues before the demonstration of how to open the test box, children were not able to open the box themselves unless prior to this demonstration they received information about what the experimenter was trying to do (i.e., that her goal was to open the box). Third, a social motivation to copy exactly what others do is obviously not enough because then learners would copy everything they saw in each demonstration, even accidental and irrelevant actions, and thus each learner would attach idiosyncratic and inefficient actions without learning conventional and functional uses. The combination of a social motivation to copy the way others do things and an understanding of others' goals and intentions is *almost* good enough—it would result in learners usually copying the way others do things but being able to override this in the case of accidental or goal-irrelevant actions—but it breaks down when the goal is "opaque" and not inferrable by the learner. Then an understanding of others' communicative intentions (and a helpful teacher) can provide learners with a solution to the question of what to imitate (Gergely & Csibra, in press).

In conclusion, imitation is multifaceted and imitators' social-cognitive understanding and social motivations affect what they will copy from a demonstration. A complex interplay of three main factors—an understanding of others' goals and intentions, the ability to collaborate with others by sharing goals and reading others' communicative intentions toward oneself, and one's own social versus instrumental goals at the moment—together help explain how typically developing infants, children with autism, and chimpanzees answer the question of what to imitate, and thus uniquely human skills of cultural learning and transmission.

ACKNOWLEDGMENTS

I thank Tanya Behne, Josep Call, Sally Rogers, Michael Tomasello, and Justin Williams for helpful comments on previous drafts.

REFERENCES

Akhtar, N., Jipson, J., & Callanan, M. A. (2001). Learning words through overhearing. *Child Development, 72,* 416–430.

Aldridge, M. A., Stone, K. R., Sweeney, M. H., & Bower, T. G. R. (2000). Preverbal children with autism understand the intentions of others. *Developmental Science, 3,* 294–301.

Baron-Cohen, S. (1989). Perceptual role taking and protodeclarative pointing in autism. *British Journal of Developmental Psychology, 7,* 113–127.

Baron-Cohen, S., Baldwin, D., & Crowson, M. (1997). Do children with autism use the speaker's direction of gaze strategy to crack the code of language? *Child Development, 68,* 48–57.

Baron-Cohen, S., Campbell, R., Karmiloff-Smith, A., Grant, J., & Walker, J. (1995). Are children with autism blind to the mentalistic significance of the eyes? *British Journal of Developmental Psychology, 13,* 379–398.

Baron-Cohen, S., Wheelwright, S., & Jolliffe, T. (1997). Is there a "language of the eyes"? Evidence from normal adults, and adults with autism or Asperger syndrome. *Visual Cognition, 4,* 311–331.

Bauer, P. J., & Hertsgaard, L. A. (1993). Increasing steps in recall of events: Factors facilitating immediate and long-term memory in 13.5- and 16.5-month-old children. *Child Development, 64,* 1204–1223.

Behne, T., Carpenter, M., Call, J., & Tomasello, M. (2005). Unwilling versus unable? Infants' understanding of intentional action. *Developmental Psychology, 41,* 328–337.

Behne, T., Carpenter, M., & Tomasello, M. (2005). One-year-olds comprehend the communicative intentions behind gestures in a hiding game. *Developmental Science, 8,* 492–499.

Behne, T., Carpenter, M., van Veen, A., & Tomasello, M. (2006, June). *From attention to intention: 18-month-olds use others' focus of attention for action interpretation.* Poster presented at the International Conference on Infant Studies, Kyoto, Japan.

Bekkering, H., Wohlschläger, A., & Gattis, M. (2000). Imitation of gestures in children is goal-directed. *Quarterly Journal of Experimental Psychology, 53A,* 153–164.

Bellagamba, F., & Tomasello, M. (1999). Re-enacting intended acts: Comparing 12- and 18-month-olds. *Infant Behavior and Development, 22,* 277–282.

Bratman, M. E. (1989). Intention and personal policies. *Philosophical Perspectives, 3,* 443–469.

Bushnell, E. W. (1998, July). *The imitative context for learning how to make objects work during infancy.* Paper presented at the ISSBD Meetings, Berne, Switzerland.

Call, J., & Carpenter, M. (2002). Three sources of information in social learning. In K. Dautenhahn & C. Nehaniv (Eds.), *Imitation in animals and artifacts* (pp. 211–228). Cambridge, MA: MIT Press.

Call, J., & Carpenter, M. (2003). On imitation in apes and children. *Infancia y Aprendizaje, 26,* 325–349.

Call, J., Carpenter, M., & Tomasello, M. (2005). Copying results and copying actions in the process of social learning: Chimpanzees (*Pan troglodytes*) and human children (*Homo sapiens*). *Animal Cognition, 8,* 151–163.

Call, J., Hare, B., Carpenter, M., & Tomasello, M. (2004). "Unwilling" versus "unable": Chimpanzees' understanding of human intentions. *Developmental Science, 7,* 488–498.

Call, J., & Tomasello, M. (2005). What do chimpanzees know about seeing revisited: An explanation of the third kind. In N. Eilan, C. Hoerl, T. McCormack, & J. Roessler (Eds.), *Issues in joint attention* (pp. 45–64). Oxford, UK: Oxford University Press.

Carpenter, M., Akhtar, N., & Tomasello, M. (1998). Fourteen- through 18-month-old infants differentially imitate intentional and accidental actions. *Infant Behavior and Development, 21,* 315–330.

Carpenter, M., & Call, J. (2002). The chemistry of social learning: Commentary on Want & Harris (2002). *Developmental Science, 5,* 22–24.

Carpenter, M., & Call, J. (in press). The question of "what to imitate": Inferring goals and intentions from demonstrations. In K. Dautenhahn & C. Nehaniv (Eds.), *Imitation and social learning in robots, humans and animals: Behavioural, social and communicative dimensions.* Cambridge, UK: Cambridge University Press.

Carpenter, M., Call, J., & Tomasello, M. (2002). Understanding "prior intentions" enables 2-year-olds to imitatively learn a complex task. *Child Development, 73,* 1431–1441.

Carpenter, M., Call, J., & Tomasello, M. (2005). Twelve- and 18-month-olds imitate actions in terms of goals. *Developmental Science, 8,* F13–F20.

Carpenter, M., Nagell, K., & Tomasello, M. (1998). Social cognition, joint attention, and communicative competence from 9 to 15 months of age. *Monographs of the Society for Research in Child Development, 63*(4, Serial No. 255).

Carpenter, M., Pennington, B. F., & Rogers, S. J. (2001). Understanding of others' intentions in children with autism and children with developmental delays. *Journal of Autism and Developmental Disorders, 31,* 589–599.

Carpenter, M., Pennington, B. F., & Rogers, S. J. (2002). Interrelations among social-cognitive skills in young children with autism and developmental delays. *Journal of Autism and Developmental Disorders, 32,* 91–106.

Carpenter, M., Pennington, B. F., & Rogers, S. J. (2003). Response to Silvio Loddo's commentary. *Journal of Autism and Developmental Disorders, 33,* 547–549.

Carpenter, M., Tomasello, M., & Savage-Rumbaugh, S. (1995). Joint attention and imitative learning in children, chimpanzees, and enculturated chimpanzees. *Social Development, 4,* 217–237.

Carpenter, M., Tomasello, M., & Striano, T. (2005). Role reversal imitation and language in typically-developing infants and children with autism. *Infancy, 8,* 253–278.

Charman, T., Swettenham, J., Baron-Cohen, S., Cox, A., Baird, G., & Drew, A. (1997). Infants with autism: An investigation of empathy, pretend play, joint attention, and imitation. *Developmental Psychology, 33*(5), 781–789.

Clark, H. (1996). *Uses of language.* Cambridge, UK: Cambridge University Press.

Colombi, C., Rogers, S., & Young, G. (2005, May). *Understanding intentions on objects, imitation, and social engagement in children with autism.* Paper presented at the International Meeting for Autism Research, Boston.

Csibra, G., Gergely, G., Bíró, S., Koós, O., & Brockbank, M. (1999). Goal attribution without agency cues: The perception of "pure reason" in infancy. *Cognition, 72,* 237–267.

Dawson, G., Meltzoff, A. N., Osterling, J., Rinaldi, J., & Brown, E. (1998). Children with autism fail to orient to naturally occurring social stimuli. *Journal of Autism and Developmental Disorders, 28,* 479–485.

Gergely, G. (2003). The development of teleological versus mentalizing observational learning strategies in infancy. *Bulletin of the Menninger Clinic, 67,* 113–131.

Gergely, G., Bekkering, H., & Király, I. (2002). Rational imitation in preverbal infants. *Nature, 415,* 755.

Gergely, G., & Csibra, G. (in press). Sylvia's recipe: Human culture, imitation, and pedagogy. In N. Enfield & S. Levinson (Eds.), *The roots of human sociality: Culture, cognition, and interaction.* Oxford, UK: Berg.

Happé, F.G.E. (1993). Communicative competence and theory of mind in autism: A test of relevance theory. *Cognition, 48,* 101–119.

Harnick, F. S. (1978). The relationship between ability level and task difficulty in producing imitation in infants. *Child Development, 49,* 209–212.

Hobson, R. P. (1993). *Autism and the development of mind*. Hillsdale, NJ: Erlbaum.

Hobson, R. P., & Lee, A. (1999). Imitation and identification in autism. *Journal of Child Psychology and Psychiatry, 40*, 649–659.

Huang, C., Heyes, C., & Charman, T. (2002). Infants' behavioral reenactment of "failed attempts": Exploring the roles of emulation learning, stimulus enhancement, and understanding of intentions. *Developmental Psychology, 38*, 840–855.

Johnson, S. C., Booth, A., & O'Hearn, K. (2001). Inferring the goals of a nonhuman agent. *Cognitive Development, 16*, 637—656.

Király, I., Csibra, G., & Gergely, G. (2004, May). *The role of communicative-referential cues in observational learning during the second year*. Poster presented at the 14th biennial International Conference on Infant Studies, Chicago.

Klin, A. (1991). Young autistic children's listening preferences in regard to speech: A possible characterization of the symptom of social withdrawal. *Journal of Autism and Developmental Disorders, 21*, 29–42.

Klin, A., Jones, W., Schultz, R., Volkmar, F., & Cohen, D. (2002). Visual fixation patterns during viewing of naturalistic social situations as predictors of social competence in individuals with autism. *Archives of General Psychiatry, 59*, 809–816.

Leekam, S., Baron-Cohen, S., Perrett, D., Milders, M., & Brown, S. (1997). Eye-direction-detection: A dissociation between geometric and joint attention skills in autism. *British Journal of Developmental Psychology, 15*, 77–95.

Lewy, A. L., & Dawson, G. (1992). Social stimulation and joint attention in young autistic children. *Journal of Abnormal Child Psychology, 20*, 555–566.

Meltzoff, A. (1995). Understanding the intentions of others: Re-enactment of intended acts by 18-month-old children. *Developmental Psychology, 31*, 1–16.

Meltzoff, A., N., & Decety, J. (2003). What imitation tells us about social cognition: A rapprochement between developmental psychology and cognitive neuroscience. *Philosophical Transactions of the Royal Society of London B, 358*, 491–500.

Meltzoff, A. N., Gopnik, A., & Repacholi, B. M. (1999). Toddlers' understanding of intentions, desires, and emotions: Explorations of the dark ages. In P. D. Zelazo, J. W. Astington, & D. R. Olson (Eds.), *Developing theories of intention: Social understanding and self-control* (pp. 17–41). Mahwah, NJ: Erlbaum.

Meyer, J. A., & Hobson, R. P. (2004). Orientation in relation to self and other. *Interaction Studies, 5*, 221–244.

Mundy, P., Sigman, M., Ungerer, J., & Sherman, T. (1986). Defining the social deficits of autism: The contribution of non-verbal communication measures. *Journal of Child Psychology and Psychiatry, 27*, 657–669.

Nadel, J., Guérini, C., Pezé, A., & Rivet, C. (1999). The evolving nature of imitation as a format for communication. In J. Nadel & G. Butterworth (Eds.), *Imitation in infancy* (pp. 209–234). Cambridge, UK: Cambridge University Press.

Nagell, K., Olguin, R., & Tomasello, M. (1993). Processes of social learning in the tool use of chimpanzees (*Pan troglodytes*) and human children (*Homo sapiens*). *Journal of Comparative Psychology, 107*, 174–186.

Nehaniv, C. L., & Dautenhan, K. (2001). Like me?—Measures of correspondence and imitation. *Cybernetics and Systems: An International Journal, 32*, 11–51.

Ohta, M. (1987). Cognitive disorders of infantile autism: A study employing the WISC, spatial relationship conceptualization, and gesture imitation. *Journal of Autism and Developmental Disorders, 17*, 45–62.

Phillips, W., Baron-Cohen, S., & Rutter, M. (1992). The role of eye contact in goal detection: Evidence from normal infants and children with autism or mental handicap. *Development and Psychopathology, 4*, 375–383.

Phillips, W., Baron-Cohen, S., & Rutter, M. (1998). Understanding intention in normal development and in autism. *British Journal of Developmental Psychology*, *16*, 337–348.

Quine, W. (1960). *Word and object*. Cambridge, MA: Harvard University Press.

Rakoczy, H., Tomasello, M., & Striano, T. (2004). Young children know that trying is not pretending: A test of the "behaving-as-if" construal of children's early concept of pretense. *Developmental Psychology*, *40*, 388–399.

Roeyers, H., van Oost, P., & Bothuyne, S. (1998). Immediate imitation and joint attention in young children with autism. *Development and Psychopathology*, *10*, 441–450.

Rogers, S. J. (2005, May). *Intentionality and imitation in early autism. From social resonance to agency: Multidisciplinary perspectives*. An international symposium organized by Jean Decety and Jacqueline Nadel, Paris, France.

Rogers, S. J., Cook, I., & Meryl, A. (2005). Imitation and play in autism. In F. R. Volkmar, R. Paul, A. Klin, & D. Cohen (Eds.), *Handbook of autism and pervasive developmental disorders* (3rd ed., pp. 382–405). Hoboken, NJ: Wiley.

Rogers, S. J., Hepburn, S. L., Stackhouse, T., & Wehner, E. (2003). Imitation performance in toddlers with autism and those with other developmental disorders. *Journal of Child Psychology and Psychiatry*, *44*, 763–781.

Russell, J., & Hill, E. L. (2001). Action-monitoring and intention reporting in children with autism. *Journal of Child Psychology and Psychiatry*, *42*, 317–328.

Sabbagh, M. A. (1999). Communicative intentions and language: Evidence from right-hemisphere damage and autism. *Brain and Language*, *70*, 29–69.

Schwier, C., van Maanen, C., Carpenter, M., & Tomasello, M. (in press). Rational imitation in 12-month-old infants. *Infancy*.

Senju, A., Yaguchi, K., Tojo, Y., & Hasegawa, T. (2003). Eye contact does not facilitate detection in children with autism. *Cognition*, *89*, B43–B51.

Sibulkin, A. E., & Užgiris, I. C. (1978). Imitation by preschoolers in a problem-solving situation. *The Journal of Genetic Psychology*, *132*, 267–275.

Sigman, M., & Capps, L. (1997). *Children with autism: A developmental perspective*. Cambridge, MA: Harvard University Press.

Smith, I. M., & Bryson, S. E. (1998). Gesture imitation in autism I: Nonsymbolic postures and sequences. *Cognitive Neuropsychology*, *15*, 747–770.

Somogyi, E., Aouka, N., Egyed, K., Krekò, K., Király, I., Gergely, G., & Nadel, J. (2005, August). *Developmental similarities and differences in the imitation of typical and autistic children*. Poster presented at the European Conference on Developmental Psychology, Tenerife, Spain.

Sperber, D., & Wilson, D. (1986). *Relevance: Communication and cognition*. Cambridge, MA: Harvard University Press.

Surian, L., Baron-Cohen, S., & Van der Lely, H. (1996). Are children with autism deaf to Griceian maxims? *Cognitive Neuropsychiatry*, *1*, 55–71.

Tomasello, M. (1999). *The cultural origins of human cognition*. Cambridge, MA: Harvard University Press.

Tomasello, M. (2001). Perceiving intentions and learning words in the second year of life. In M. Bowerman & S. C. Levinson (Eds.), *Language acquisition and conceptual development* (pp. 132–158). Cambridge, UK: Cambridge University Press.

Tomasello, M. (2003). *Constructing a language*. Cambridge, MA: Harvard University Press.

Tomasello, M., & Carpenter, M. (2005a). The emergence of social cognition in three young chimpanzees. *Monographs of the Society for Research in Child Development*, *70*(1, Serial No. 279).

Tomasello, M., & Carpenter, M. (2005b). Intention reading and imitative learning. In S. Hurley & N. Chater (Eds.), *Perspectives on imitation: From neuroscience to social sci-*

ence: Vol. 2. Imitation, human development, and culture (pp. 133–148). Cambridge, MA: MIT Press.

Tomasello, M., Carpenter, M., Call, J., Behne, T., & Moll, H. (2005). Understanding and sharing intentions: The ontogeny and phylogeny of cultural cognition. *Behavioral and Brain Sciences, 28,* 675–691.

Tomasello, M., & Farrar, M. J. (1986). Joint attention and early language. *Child Development, 57,* 1454–1463.

Tomasello, M., Kruger, A. C., & Ratner, H. H. (1993). Cultural learning. *Behavioral and Brain Sciences, 16,* 495–552.

Travis, L. L. (1997). Goal-based organization of event memory in toddlers. In P. W. van den Broek, P. J. Bauer, & T. Bourg (Eds.), *Developmental spans in event comprehension and representation: Bridging fictional and actual events* (pp. 111–138). Mahwah, NJ: Erlbaum.

Užgiris, I. C. (1981). Two functions of imitation during infancy. *International Journal of Behavioral Development, 4,* 1–12.

Užgiris, I. C. (1984). Imitation in infancy: Its interpersonal aspects. In M. Perlmutter (Ed.), *The Minnesota symposia on child psychology: Vol. 17. Parent–child interactions and parent–child relations in child development* (pp. 1–32). Hillsdale, NJ: Erlbaum.

Whiten, A., & Brown, J. D. (1998). Imitation and the reading of other minds: Perspectives from the study of autism, normal children and non-human primates. In S. Bråten (Ed.), *Intersubjective communication and emotion in ontogeny: A sourcebook* (pp. 260–280). Cambridge, UK: Cambridge University Press.

Whiten, A., Custance, D. M., Gómez, J. C., Teixidor, P., & Bard, K. A. (1996). Imitative learning of artificial fruit processing in children (*Homo sapiens*) and chimpanzees (*Pan troglodytes*). *Journal of Comparative Psychology, 110,* 3–14.

Williams, J. H. G., Whiten, A., & Singh, T. (2004). A systematic review of action imitation in autistic spectrum disorder. *Journal of Autism and Developmental Disorders, 34,* 285–299.

CHAPTER 4

Mimicry and Autism

Bases and Consequences of Rapid, Automatic Matching Behavior

ERIC J. MOODY
DANIEL N. McINTOSH

Early in the 20th century, psychologists noted that when someone sees another's facial expression, posture, or movement the observer tends to quickly produce a matching expression or movement (Lipps, 1907). This observation set the stage for investigations of rapid reactions to emotional or physical displays of others. Consistent with Lipps's idea that the observer's response is automatic, McDougall (1908) suggested that a model's pain display is an unconditioned stimulus for production of a matched response. The view that responses to others' emotional or physical displays are automatic and innate previewed a common theme in contemporary research on rapid matching reactions to others' expressions or movements (typically termed *mimicry*). Most current investigations of this phenomenon consider mimicry to occur very quickly, without conscious planning or control, and without explicit behavioral goals.

Starting around 1980, researchers using modern psychophysiological techniques documented that people automatically mimic very quickly and theorized that such mimicry may play a role in a number of important social–emotional processes. For example, some have proposed that mimicry is critical for social functioning, emotional contagion, and understanding of another person's state of mind (Decéty & Chaminade, 2003; Hatfield, Cacioppo, & Rapson, 1994; Iacoboni, 2005; Lakin & Chartrand, 2003; Sonnby-Borgstroem, 2002). Others report that mimicry increases prosocial behaviors such as helping and generosity (van Baaren, Holland, Kawakami, & van

Knippenberg, 2004). Mimicry may have been evolutionarily adaptive because it helped humans communicate and foster relationships (Lakin, Jefferis, Cheng, & Chartrand, 2003).

Parallel to this work investigating social–emotional concomitants of mimicry, autism researchers have documented an array of social and emotional deficits in people with autism spectrum disorders (ASD). Indeed, ASD is characterized in part by deficits in social perception, social cognition, and language delay (American Psychiatric Association, 1994). A striking feature of the disorder is that people with ASD do not engage in social life the way typically developing individuals do, showing serious difficulty with socioemotional functioning and imitative behaviors and often showing significant social impairment, repetitive routines, and social aloofness (Baron-Cohen et al., 1999, 2000; Fein, 2001; Hobson, 2004; Hobson & Lee, 1998; Liss et al., 2001; Wing & Gould, 1979).

That mimicry is emerging as a process important to some social–emotional processes impaired in ASD suggests that mimicry deficits may play a role in the autistic phenotype. Impairments in mimicry may mark underlying deficits, may influence more visible and complex social–emotional processes impaired in ASD, or both. This chapter considers ways in which understanding mimicry may lead to advances in understanding ASD. To that end, we first discuss what constitutes mimicry, including distinctions between mimicry and other forms of interpersonal matching such as *imitation*. Following this, we review what is known about mimicry and evidence for a mimicry deficit in autism. We then discuss what mimicry may tell us about autism and what the consequences of a mimicry deficit may be. We conclude by discussing future directions for research in mimicry and autism.

MIMICRY

Interpersonal Matching Phenomena

Mimicry is part of a larger family of interpersonal matching phenomena. There are numerous ways to classify matching behaviors (Williams, Whiten, & Singh, 2004). Scholars differ on whether there are boundaries between these phenomena and, if so, what these boundaries are. Whiten (Chapter 10, this volume) discusses work from evolutionary and comparative psychologists on imitation and its "cognitive kin," providing a useful framework for investigating phenomena ranging from behavior matching to theory of mind. Across distinctions, matching phenomena share the characteristic of an observer engaging in behaviors similar to that of a model. Despite this underlying similarity, we believe it is useful to keep in mind that matching behaviors may involve a variety of processes (e.g., cognitive, affective, and motor), and that causes and consequences of the most complex may differ significantly from those of the most simple. We agree with others (e.g., Nadel, Chapter 6, this volume; Whiten, Chapter 10, this volume) that the productive question is not whether individuals with autism match others' behaviors but, rather, what behaviors they match and why.

Forms of interpersonal matching include *emulation*, in which a person observes a model engage in a goal-directed behavior and then behaves to achieve the same goal, although not necessarily with the same actions as the model (Tomasello, 1990; Want & Harris, 2002; Williams et al., 2004). This sort of matching is overt, not automatic, and requires a good deal of cognitive development to complete. A simpler form of interpersonal matching is *imitation*, in which the observer attempts to copy the actions of the model rather than matching the outcome of the action by different means (see Whiten, Chapter 10, this volume). The literature contains many definitions of imitation (Noble & Todd, 2002), but phenomena labeled as imitation tend to be fairly overt, may occur after a delay of at least several seconds, and, most important, are often defined as requiring the observer not only to copy the movements of the model but also to understand the effects of these movements on the environments and the intentional relations among the movements and effects (Noble & Todd, 2002; Tomasello, 1996). Nadel (Chapter 6, this volume) also stresses that imitation is not automatic but instead selective. That is, Nadel proposes that even from infancy, humans choose *which* stimuli to imitate, suggesting that imitation is purposeful.

In contrast to imitation, this chapter focuses on one of the simplest of the interpersonal matching phenomena: When an observer automatically, unintentionally, and quickly matches the movements of a model. Following common usage in psychophysiological investigations of rapid facial reactions, we use the term *mimicry* to describe this automatic behavior (Bush, Barr, McHugo, & Lanzetta, 1989; Hess & Blairy, 2001; Hess, Philippot, & Blairy, 1999; McIntosh, in press; Neidenthal, Brauer, Halberstadt, & Innes-Ker, 2001; Sonnby-Borgstroem, 2002).

Although mimicry is similar to the most basic level of imitation identified by Whiten (Chapter 10, this volume), there are important differences. The similarity lies in mimicry and imitation both involving matching. As specified by Whiten, imitative copying includes, at minimum, repeating the spatiotemporal shape of the model's actions. This shape matching is basic to mimicry. As commonly discussed in their respective literatures, however, mimicry and imitation differ in important ways. For example, all the phenomena identified by Whiten are forms of social learning. Mimicry, in contrast is a low-level phenomenon that is not necessarily a form of social learning. Relatedly, there is no intentional, goal-directed, functional component to mimicry; it does not involve acting on the world, or toward a particular goal, or in relation to objects. Moreover, the literature on mimicry is inconclusive as to whether the phenomenon is even *copying* of another's facial expression or is instead an affective process (Hess, Philippot, & Blairy, 1998). If mimicry is *not* copying but rather the result of the affective responses of the observer, then the behaviors typically labeled mimicry (perhaps more appropriately referred to as *rapid facial reactions*) can occur to nonfacial stimuli such as spi-

ders, snakes, and flowers (Dimberg, 1986; Dimberg & Thell, 1988). Therefore, although mimicry is similar in some surface features to imitation, it may
be most appropriately located "off the chart" of Whiten's taxonomy of imitation and social learning phenomena. Determination of the processes that lead
to mimicry is a central question in mimicry research; because this has implications for what a mimicry deficit in autism means, this chapter concentrates on
the current thinking regarding potential underlying processes responsible for
the matching of facial expressions.

The importance of avoiding premature closure as to the underlying
nature of mimicry is emphasized by the history of research on animal imitation; identifying something as copying without contemplation of simpler alternative reasons for the existence of similar behaviors may preclude careful consideration of those alternatives and may lead to assuming more complexity
than exists (Noble & Todd, 2002). As Whiten (Chapter 10, this volume)
points out, not all observations of apparent behavior matching and social
learning are really copying of another individual; some reflect simpler processes. For example, comparative psychologists have contrasted with imitation a more stimulus-driven phenomenon termed *stimulus enhancement*
(Noble & Todd, 2002; Spence, 1937). This occurs when an observer attends
to a model's behavior, so that the model's action draws the observer's attention to a relevant object, task, or location, thus increasing the likelihood of the
observer behaving in a manner similar to the model's. We see mimicry as
another example of a simple process. As discussed in current investigations of
social–emotional processes, mimicry differs from both imitation (as mimicry is
automatic, rapid, and not goal oriented) and stimulus enhancement (as mimicry does not involve directing attention to an object, task, or location, or
behaviors that would be generated based on such a shift in attention).

Conflating the variety of matching behaviors can lead to confusion, as the
distinctions mapped by differing terms may be significant in understanding
processes in typically and atypically developing humans (Whiten, Chapter 10,
this volume). The problem of conflating these terms and concepts becomes
apparent when viewed in light of current understanding of autism. Recently,
investigators have begun to differentiate between a more affective process
related to social exchanges with a second process involving "a more exec-
utively constructed, cognitively mediated, intentional imitation system" (Rogers, Hepburn, Stackhouse, & Wehner, 2003, p. 777). Rogers and colleagues
(2003) theorize that those with autism may use the second but *not* the first
(less complex) system. We believe distinctions such as those made by Noble
and Todd (2002), Rogers and colleagues (2003), and Whiten (Chapter 10, this
volume) are critical and concur that there are likely multiple mechanisms
causing apparent matching behavior; we believe that what is likely to be the
more primitive system (the automatic, rapid one potentially involving basic
affective processes) corresponds to what many social and emotion psychologists term *mimicry*. Only by distinguishing among these processes can their
role in autism become clear and can investigations elucidate the processes

involved in social phenomena. In light of the need for a clear understanding of what mimicry is, we next detail the mimicry process.

Mimicry Defined

The basic phenomenon of mimicry starts when an observer witnesses a model make some rudimentary action, such as a smile, and then spontaneously and very rapidly matches the model's actions. There are several characteristics of mimicry that set it apart from other ways in which people behaviorally match models.

First, mimicry occurs rapidly. For example, Dimberg (1982) has found that when an observer witnesses a picture of someone making a happy expression, the muscles responsible for smiling (*zygomaticus major*) will have an increased level of activity within 1,000 milliseconds (ms). If, however, the same person witnesses an angry expression, the muscles that are responsible for knitting the brow (*corrugator supercilli*) will have greater activity levels within this time frame. The mimicry literature includes studies investigating mimicry within the first second after a face is viewed (Dimberg, 1982, 1988) to reactions occurring within a few seconds after stimulus onset (Sonnby-Borgstroem, 2002; Thunberg & Dimberg, 2000), and sometimes including a couple of minutes after stimulus onset (McIntosh, 2006). We focus on the earliest reactions because we believe that the reactions during the first 1,000 ms (1) may be particularly reflective of the primitive process identified by Rogers and colleagues (2003); (2) are more likely than later responses to be influenced by fewer and more basic phenomena; (3) may be especially important for subsequent emotional, cognitive, and behavioral phenomena; and (4) are the least likely to overlap with other matching phenomena.

Second, perhaps due to the modern focus on very quick responses, or the historical understanding of the phenomenon as innate or unconditioned (Lipps, 1907; McDougall, 1908), mimicry is typically conceptualized and operationalized as automatic. Its automaticity is underscored by the fact that people mimic stimuli that are shown suboptimally. For example, several groups have found rapid facial reactions when observers were shown pictures of facial expressions for only a few dozen milliseconds or less, well below the level at which people consciously recognize the expression (Dimberg, Thunberg, & Elmehed, 2000; Rotteveel, de Groot, Geutskens, & Phaf, 2001).

The third characteristic of mimetic reactions as currently studied is that they are specific. From the previous examples and others (Dimberg, 1982, 1988; Lundqvist & Dimberg, 1995; McIntosh, 2006; McIntosh, Reichmann-Decker, Winkielman, & Wilbarger, 2006), participants' reactions are usually seen in specific muscles that corresponded to the stimulus presented as opposed to generalized activity increases in all muscles. That is, smiling, which is caused by the zygomaticus major muscles, leads to activity over the zygomaticus muscle in the observer and not the corrugator muscle, which knits the brow.

Fourth, mimetic reactions may be extremely subtle and not always observable with the unaided eye. Indeed, the typical paradigm for studying mimicry records the observers' facial movements using electromyography (EMG). This procedure uses surface electrodes placed over specific facial muscle groups to record the slight electrical changes over the muscles when they activate. EMG has the virtues of being able to assess very small movements within milliseconds after an observer views a facial expression.

Finally, just as emulation and imitation may not involve emotional matching, it is important to note that observed mimicry is not *necessarily* reflective of an affective response. The mimicry literature itself is ambiguous about this point. Some investigations of facial mimicry treat the reactions as automatic, nonaffective motor responses (Bavelas, Black, Chovil, & Lemery, 1988; Chartrand & Bargh, 1999) that, via facial feedback processes (McIntosh, 1996), can *cause* an emotional reaction in the observer (Hatfield et al., 1994; Lipps, 1907; McIntosh, Druckman, & Zajonc, 1994). Others have viewed facial response as *consequences* or markers of affective reactions of the observers to the emotional stimuli (Cacioppo, Martzke, Petty, & Tassinary, 1988; Winkielman & Cacioppo, 2001). That is, some view these rapid facial reactions as the result of the affective state of the observer caused by the situation the observer is in. This is not emotional contagion because the observer has not simply caught the model's emotion. Instead, the observer is experiencing endogenous emotions caused by the situation, which includes (but is not determined by) the other's emotional display. In this framing, the observer's facial reactions simply accord with the observer's emotions. The potential relation between mimicry and emotions in the observer is discussed in more detail later. However, to avoid presupposing a particular relation between observers' emotions and their facial actions, similar to Hess and Blairy (2001), we believe it is most clear to define mimicry as the behavior, and reserve other terms (e.g., *contagion* and *empathy*) for the emotional state of the observer rather than the facial expressions.

Research on Mimicry

Given the characteristics listed previously, mimicry is generally studied in a controlled laboratory setting (but see Hinsz & Tomhave, 1991, as an example of field documentation of mimicry). A typical paradigm involves a participant sitting in a chair before a computer screen. Photographs of stimuli (typically facial expressions such as scowling and smiling) are displayed in sequence. While the participant watches the screen, EMG is used to measure the changes in muscle activity. As evident from this paradigm, almost all research has examined facial responses to seeing the facial expressions of others; thus, this chapter necessarily focuses on facial mimicry (but see Berger & Hadley, 1975, for an example of nonfacial mimicry).

Mimicry appears to be a fairly robust phenomenon, with a number of researchers reporting mimetic reactions in typical samples (Bush et al., 1989;

Dimberg, 1982; Dimberg et al., 2000; Hess & Blairy, 2001; McIntosh, 2006; Sonnby-Borgstroem, 2002). Research on mimicry was limited before the 1980s (Bavelas, Black, Lemery, & Mullett, 1986). Early work was conducted by Berger and Hadley (1975), who recorded EMG activity in the arms and lips of observers watching videotapes of arm wrestling and stuttering. They found greater EMG activity in observers' muscles corresponding to the muscles being used by the performers than in muscles not corresponding to muscles being used by the performers. Vaughan and Lanzetta (1980, 1981) reported that a model's facial display of pain instigated congruent facial activation in an observer. Mimicry of positive expressions was found by Bush and colleagues (1989), who reported that participants exposed to smiling faces displayed greater zygomaticus and *orbicularis oculi* (narrows eyes, as when smiling) compared to those who did not see such faces.

Interest in mimicry as a process foundational to social and emotional development was increased by reports of facial matching in neonates. Infants are equipped with a high degree of facial neuromuscular maturity and are able to produce a wide variety of facial expressions (Stern, 1983). Both human and nonhuman primate infants appear to possess innate and early responses to facial expression (Brothers, 1989). A number of studies have demonstrated that neonates match facial expressions (e.g., Field, Woodson, Greenberg, & Cohen, 1982; Meltzoff & Moore, 1977; Reissland, 1988), although this conclusion is controversial (Koepke, Hamm, Legerstee, & Russell, 1983; McKenzie & Over, 1983; see Meltzoff & Moore, 1983, for reply; see also Kaitz, Meschulach-Sarfaty, Auerbach, & Eidelman, 1988). If infants do mimic, it provides support for the position that such matching is a basic response and raises the question of what deficits in such a response might mean. Such questions may echo those raised in prior considerations of mimicry; as early as 1937, deficits in facial mimicry were noted in certain psychopathologies such as schizophrenia (e.g., Abashev-Konstantinovsky, 1937). Next we discuss evidence for a mimicry deficit in autism and then consider the implications of such a deficit.

MIMICRY AND AUTISM SPECTRUM DISORDERS

There has been notable work investigating imitation deficits in ASD. For this type of interpersonal matching, the evidence is good that there is some type of deficit in those with ASD (Rogers, 1999; Williams et al., 2004). For example, Smith and Bryson (1998) found that children with autism imitated single postures much worse than typically developing children. Also, Roeyers, van Oost, and Bothuyne (1998) found that 5-year-old children with autism imitated novel procedural tasks unreliably whereas typically developing children did not.

Although such findings suggest a general deficit in interpersonal matching in ASD and thus that mimicry may also be impaired, the features of mimicry discussed previously differentiate it from more general matching phenomena. Because imitation is a more complex behavior than mimicry, it may be that the imitation deficit is due to impairments in those processes that do not overlap with mimicry processes. For example, if the deficit is related to the intentionality component of imitation, then mimicry may remain unaffected. Thus, it is possible there could be an imitation deficit in ASD where there is no mimicry deficit. Nonetheless, in addition to the general imitative deficit in autism, the presence of social–emotional deficits that are theoretically connected to mimicry, and (as discussed later) theorized impairments in the affective, motor, and perception–action processes foundational to mimicry, suggest that there could be a deficit.

Using the standard mimicry paradigm discussed earlier, McIntosh and colleagues (2006) investigated whether individuals with ASD show a mimicry deficit. A group of high-functioning adolescents and adults with ASD and a group of typically developing individuals matched on gender, verbal ability, and chronological age were presented with a series of still photographs of neutral and emotional facial expressions. As the participants were viewing the series of faces, EMG was measured over their cheek and brow regions. Facial activity between 200 to 600 ms after stimulus onset was examined for the presence of mimicry. Mimicry was demonstrated by participants' facial muscle activity being more congruent (e.g., smiled when the stimulus was a smiling face) than incongruent (e.g., furrowing the brow when the stimulus was a smiling face). The group with ASD did not automatically mimic facial expressions whereas the typically developing group did. However, both groups were successful in intentionally matching facial expressions upon request.

Despite this evidence that individuals with autism show a mimicry deficit, the picture is likely more complex than simply a relative absence of mimicry in those with autism. Indeed, the question is likely more one of *what* individuals mimic, and why. In addition to the lack of typical mimicry of emotional facial expressions indicated in the aforementioned studies, some people with autism show echolalia, which involves repeatedly matching the verbal behavior of another. That is, people with autism sometimes evidence *too much* matching behavior. One likely explanation for this pattern is that both the absence of facial mimicry and the presence of echolalia stem from a dysfunction of matching systems (Williams, Whiten, Suddendorf, & Perrett, 2001). However, another possibility emerges when considering theorized foundations for mimicry. The facial mimicry deficit may not be related to other behavioral matching dysfunctions (such as, for example, the imitation deficit or echolalia) but, instead, may reflect a deficit in emotional processes. This would be consistent with the discussion of two possible systems made by Rogers and colleagues (2003). The observed deficit in mimicry of emotional expressions may not be related to dysfunctions of neural or psychological processes of matching but, rather, of underlying affective processes. Thus, understanding the meaning for autism of a deficit in mimicking emotional facial expressions will require additional research in understanding mimicry. In the following sections, we discuss in more detail theories of mimicry and how they may relate to issues in understanding autism.

Implications of a Mimicry Deficit

At one level, finding a mimicry deficit in ASD is consistent with the broader work exploring imitation in ASD. Both reveal deficits in interpersonal matching; however, we believe that the differences discussed earlier between mimicry and other matching phenomena make a mimicry deficit particularly interesting in understanding ASD.

The first reason that a mimicry deficit may be useful in understanding ASD is that other forms of matching may look unimpaired or differentially impaired because individuals with ASD are able to employ compensatory strategies that obscure the deficit. Because forms of matching that are not spontaneous, not as quick, or not as specific may be generated by a broader selection of mechanisms, there is more opportunity for someone to develop unique ways of solving problems (compensatory strategies), which may impair our ability to understand the underlying processes affected in the disorder. For example, Alderidge, Stone, Sweeny, and Bower (2000) found that preverbal children with autism were better than cognitive age-matched controls at inferring intention in imitation tasks. One possible explanation for this pattern of findings was that the children with autism were able to use object affordances when imitating with objects to counteract their imitative deficit. Although the authors reject this explanation because object affordances did not help the typically developing children and some children with autism were unable to correctly perceive the correct affordance, given that the children with autism were better at the tasks than typically developing children, it could be that some of the children with autism used compensatory strategies. This would be consistent with the view of Rogers and colleagues (2003) that people with autism may use only the more complex, cognitive process of imitation and the suggestion of Kasari, Chamberlain, and Bauminger (2001) that children with autism may develop compensatory strategies. A deficit in mimicry, however, is far less likely to be hidden by compensatory strategies as it is so quick and occurs outside one's awareness.

The second reason a mimicry deficit is particularly interesting is because mimicry is so rapid, it may be less influenced by learning, social motivation, and socialization than are other matching phenomena. With fewer potential influences on mimicry, deficits may be more likely to be closely tied to underlying processes involved in matching behavior. Matching that operates on longer time scales may be based on a wider array of cognitive/affective processes and neurological substrates. For example, when someone imitates a set of actions, phrases, or postures as she is engaged in a conversation, her desire to have a specific type of relationship with the other person may alter the interaction. In addition, there may be executive mechanisms involved that allow her to understand the meaning of the gestures or tone the other person is using and allows her to plan and execute appropriate replies to enable imitative gestures. Examinations of the role of executive function in imitation deficits seen in ASD (Rogers & Bennetto, 2000) and research that has found deficits in ASD samples on tests of frontal functioning (Ozonoff et al., 2004) are consistent with this view. Executive functions like planning and means–end reasoning may play less of a role in mimicry. Due to the fewer likely influences on mimicry as compared to other interpersonal matching phenomena, a mimicry deficit points to more specific underlying processes that may be impaired in ASD. Understanding what mechanisms are involved in mimicry may suggest processes that may be impaired in ASD. We consider these in the next section.

Mechanisms of Mimicry and Processes in Autism

In previous sections, we discussed what automatic mimicry looks like at a behavioral level—it is a quick, spontaneous, specific, and often subtle matching of a simple behavior. This definition begs the questions of what the fundamental nature of the phenomenon is and what mechanisms support it. There is disagreement in the literature regarding the mechanisms of mimicry. Specifically, literature on facial mimicry generally falls into two camps regarding assumptions about the underlying mechanism of this phenomenon: (1) it is a nonaffective motor response that may lead to emotional processes or (2) it is a display of the affective state of the observer. These two bodies of research have not been able to (and for the most part, have not attempted to) rule out the alternative perspective; moreover, these perspectives are not mutually exclusive. Mimicry could be the result of both motor-related and affective mechanisms. Because these differing understandings of the processes underpinning mimicry have differing implications for autism, research determining the nature of mimicry may help illuminate the nature of ASD. In this chapter, we focus primarily on questions related to mimicry and refer only briefly to potential connections with autism. Developing and empirically exploring each of these connections in more detail will both address key questions in mimicry research and point toward the meaning of a mimicry deficit in autism.

Motor and Perception–Action Processes

Several researchers view facial mimicry as an automatic, nonaffective reaction (Bavelas et al., 1986; Chartrand & Bargh, 1999; Hoffman, 1984). Hess and colleagues (1999) have described this perspective's take on mimicry as a primitive motor code. For scholars who take this perspective, mimetic reactions are automatically and unconsciously generated and have no direct affective underpinnings. Rather, they are simple motor actions, and several mechanisms may play a role in this phenomenon such as cognitive schemas (e.g., Carver, Ganellen, Froming, & Chambers, 1983), neurological processes (e.g., Goldenberg & Hagmann, 1997; Iacoboni et al., 1999), or both. In other words, the mimetic reaction is thought of as a response to simply witnessing a facial expression that involves no affective or higher cognitive processes. However, the current evidence cannot confirm that this is the case.

Whatever the underlying mechanism(s), much research dating back to the turn of the 20th century (Lipps, 1907) has been used to support the automatic, nonaffective perspective, especially within the context of research addressing broader social–emotional processes. In these approaches, mimetic reactions are thought of as automatic motor or perception–action processes that lead to emotional phenomena (Hatfield et al., 1994). More recent arguments based on perception–action processes also suggest that mimicry is automatically and nonaffectively generated (e.g., Chartrand & Bargh, 1999; Lakin & Chartrand, 2003). Carver and colleagues (1983) suggest that when people observe someone make an action, this activates interpretive schemas. Because these schemas have substantial overlap with behavioral schemas (responsible for motor production) it is likely that they will be activated at the same time when observing actions. Indeed, there appears to be such a coactivation (Calvo-Merino, Glaser, Grezes, Passingham, & Haggard, 2004). This again suggests that mimicry is an automatic, nonaffective output.

This view of mimicry as simple perception–action matching or motor output has been connected with potential basic deficits in autism. Rogers (1999) contends that because people with ASD have general motor problems, they may be unable to effectively mimic other people's emotional expression, which prevents them from benefiting from the afferent feedback that informs them of what other people are feeling. Two lines of neurological research support the idea that motor or motor-related processes are involved in mimicry and thereby provide a connection between mimicry deficits and neurological dysfunctions in autism. For some time the possibility of cerebellar dysfunction has been considered in autism research; more recently there has been excitement about the existence of mirror neurons and their role in behavioral matching phenomena and autism. We briefly discuss each below.

Rogers's (1999) suggestion that mimicry deficits seen in ASD come from motor problems fits well with the view that the cerebellum helps coordinate automatic movements (Martin, Goldowitz, & Mittleman, 2003; Nair, Purcott, Fuchs, Steinberg, & Kelso, 2003; Turner, Desmurget, Grethe, Crutcher, & Grafton, 2003). Given that one of the most consistent neural anatomical findings in people with autism is cerebellar abnormalities such as decreased numbers and density of Purkinje cells, which are the neural output from the cerebellum to the neocortex (Courchesne, 1995; Hashimoto, Tayama, Murakawa, & Yoshimoto, 1995; Palmen, van Engeland, Hof, & Schmitz, 2004; Williams, Hauser, Purpurda, DeLong, & Swisher, 1980), and decreased vermis size (Courchesne, Yeung-Courchesne, Press, & Hesselink, 1988; Kleiman, Neff, & Rosman, 1992), a theory of autism based on dyspraxia seems viable. However, as some studies have found that people with autism have typical motor activation in the cerebellum in functional magnetic resonance imaging (fMRI) studies (Allen & Courchesne, 2003) and can adapt to motor tasks at normal rates (Mostofsky, Bunoski, Morton,

Goldberg, & Bastian, 2004), there is no consensus that cerebellar abnormalities play a direct role in the motor deficits of ASD.

More recently, the discovery of *mirror neurons* (MN) has suggested that dysfunctions in this class of cells may relate to autism deficits by disrupting perception–action connections. MNs have been linked to several cognitive functions that are deficient in those with autism, such as empathy (Gallese, 2001), imitative behavior (Iacoboni et al., 1999), and language in typical populations (Rizzolatti & Arbib, 1998) and have been hypothesized to play a role in the atypical executive and affective symptoms seen in those with ASD (Williams et al., 2001; but see Avikainen, Kulomaeki, & Hari, 1999, for an example of typical MN activity in people with Asperger's syndrome). Despite the connection with imitative behavior (Iacoboni et al., 1999; Whiten, Chapter 10, this volume), it is unclear whether MNs are directly involved in mimicry. MNs seem particularly relevant to goal-oriented behaviors (Rizzolatti & Arbib, 1998; Rizzolatti, Craighero, & Fadiga, 2002); MN activation is typically seen when the action being observed has a specific goal. Because mimicry differs from imitation in part due to the former's absence of clear goal orientation, the association of MNs with imitation or ASD does not necessarily indicate that they are associated with mimicry.

Note that, consistent with a MN approach, there is activation of the same brain regions during both the subjective experience of and perception of affective states such as disgust (insula) and pain (anterior cingulate cortex and anterior insula) (Gallese, Keysers, & Rizzolatti, 2004). Gallese and colleagues (2004) point out that these regions are fundamentally motor structures, involved in emotional expression and action control. The processes or mechanisms leading to this neurological mirroring are not yet clear. One possibility is that it is *part of* or the *result* of a perceptual–motor process, as proposed in this section. This view is consistent with the idea that mimicry is an example of a perceptual–motor process that leads to shared emotion. Although this work shows activation during emotion perception in motor centers tied to the emotional experience, whether and how mimicry or actual facial action is involved is not known. Future work should examine the degree to which perceptual–action processes tied to MNs are linked specifically to mimicry (see Decety, Chapter 11, this volume, for more detail regarding MNs).

A second possibility for the matching activation discussed by Gallese et al. (2004) is that the emotional correspondence precedes the matching of facial expression. In this case, the question of what causes the emotional correspondence is unanswered. Regardless of mechanism, however, the activation of a matching emotional experience initiated by perceiving another's emotion may cause a quick matching facial expression. This perspective is consistent with the affective view of mimicry discussed later.

To summarize a simplified version of this view, it may be that cerebellar, MN, or other neural abnormalities in people with ASD cause motor or perception–action integration difficulties impairing processes underlying mimicry. The resultant mimicry deficit could then lead to some of the impairments in more complex social emotional processes seen in autism. In this view, a mimicry deficit both points to motor or perception–action impairments (e.g., in MNs) as a primary source of deficits in ASD, and also may underlie other impairments.

Affective Processes

In contrast to the idea that mimicry is nonaffective motor action, several researchers consider the observed rapid facial responses as a readout of a person's affective states (Cacioppo et al., 1988; Dimberg, 1986; Dimberg, Hansson, & Thunberg, 1998; Winkielman & Cacioppo, 2001). The mimetic actions are seen as reflections of emotions in the model eliciting similar feelings in the observer. If seeing another person smiling makes a person happy, then an increase in the activity over the zygomaticus major muscle (the muscle that causes smiling) results from this emotion. In this perspective, the microexpressions documented in mimicry research represent an underlying affective process.

The research pointing to an affective basis to mimicry has emerged more recently than the work supporting the other perspective and comes mainly in the form of studies demonstrating how rapid facial reactions can be manipulated by affective variables. For example, Moody, McIntosh, Mann, and Weisser (2006) found that in typically developing individuals the emotions of the observer influenced the rapid facial reactions to pictures of emotional expressions. In particular, when participants were put into a heightened state of fear, they responded with *fear* expressions to anger faces but not to neutral faces. That is, they had an emotion-appropriate reaction to a threat stimuli rather than automatically matching the presented facial expression. This suggests that the rapid facial response to the emotional expression of another is not completely or primarily a motor or response matching action but is, instead, part of an emotional reaction. As the display of an angry face did not always result in a matching reaction in the observer, these data argue that there is an affective component to mimicry.

With this view of mimicry as an affective phenomenon, a mimicry deficit in those with ASD is both consistent with extant autism research on emotional impairments in ASD and provides information that may help clarify the nature of these deficits. Regarding the consistency with previous work, individuals with autism show a number of deficits in emotional processes, including in the perception and understanding of emotions, the generation of emotional expressions and gestures, and the regulation and coordination of emotions, especially in social contexts (Celani, Battacchi, & Arcidiacono, 1999; Dawson, Webb, Carver, Panagiotides, & McPartland, 2004; Hobson, 1991, 1995; Kasari & Sigman, 1996; Rogers & Pennington, 1991). Regarding observed deficits in the perception of emotional facial expressions in particular, Gross (2004) notes that the pattern of difficulty seen in people with autism may be related to them having a dysfunction of the "primary emotional system" (p. 478), and thus using only learned strategies in categorizing such expressions. This view is consistent with seeing affective dysfunctions as underlying deficits in mimicry of emotional facial expressions.

Additional support for a mimicry deficit being affective in nature comes from evidence of dysfunction of neurological regions serving affect in ASD. An affect-based perspective on mimicry predicts that poor functioning of brain regions related to affect would impair the quick facial reactions to emotional faces. The amygdala, for example, appears to be an essential structure for processing information about faces, assignment of affective significance to stimuli, and organization of defensive or aversive responses (Adolphs, Tranel, Damasio, & Damasio, 1995; Young et al., 1995). Some studies of individuals with autism have shown a lack of typical activation of the amygdala for emotional expressions (Critchley et al., 2000; Hazenedar et al., 2000), faces (Pierce, Muller, Ambrose, Alleen, & Courchesne, 2001), and eye gaze (Baron-Cohen et al., 2000). (However, structural studies are not consistent, as there are reports of both enlarged and reduced amygdala in people with ASD [Aylward et al., 1999; Bauman & Kemper, 1985].) A deficit in mimicry of emotional facial expressions is consistent with both the behavioral research and the neurological findings of atypical amygdala. In this view, the mimicry deficit in ASD may be a marker for impairment in affective processes rather than difficulties with self–other matching of movements or gestures. Indeed, in this perspective, the term *mimicry* may be more misleading than descriptive; here, the facial reaction is emotional, not matching.

Consequences of Mimicry

Regardless of the underlying cause for a mimicry deficit in ASD, several social–emotional functions thought to be impaired in autism have also been linked to mimicry in typical populations. A mimicry deficit may thus underlie impairments in these functions. In this section, we review the social functions related to mimicry, and discuss how impairments in these processes may be evident in ASD. Although these similarities cannot themselves indicate that a mimicry deficit in autism is responsible (in whole or in part) for impairments in these more complex social–emotional processes, consideration of these parallels can focus research examining these links and supports further investigation of the connections between mimicry and ASD.

Emotional Contagion

One of the first social–emotional outcomes to be associated with mimicry was emotional contagion: when an observer experiences the emotions of the observed (Hatfield et al., 1994; Lipps, 1907; Lundqvist & Dimberg, 1995; McIntosh, 2006; McIntosh et al., 1994; Vaughan & Lanzetta, 1981). One commonly theorized route for contagion is mimicry. This putative process starts with the observer witnessing a facial action and then, through a simple perceptual–motor reaction, automatically copying the expression. The consequent emotional facial expression is then theorized to cause a corresponding change in emotion in the observer, perhaps via self-perception, conditioning, activation of affect programs, or role-playing processes (McIntosh, 1996). Thus, most descriptions of this phenomenon assume that some important portion of the initial facial reaction of the observer is *not* the result of affect and that the initial facial reaction creates a change in the emotion of the observer. This traditional statement of the connection rests on the assumption that mimicry itself is not (solely) an affective output, and follows James's (1950/1890) suggestion that facial action leads to the emotion rather than the emotion leading to the facial action.

There is substantial evidence that contagion occurs (Hatfield et al., 1994; McIntosh et al., 1994). It is implicated in social processes such as helping (e.g., Batson & Coke, 1983; Krebs, 1975), avoidance of people in distress (Berger, 1962; Stotland, 1969), and the quality of interpersonal relationships (Levenson & Gottman, 1983, 1985). To the degree that individuals with ASD have a mimicry deficit, this could generate impairments in these processes. Moreover, without mimicry, those with ASD may not be able to catch others' emotions, and this may have particularly negative effects if occurring early in development (Rogers, 1999). It could lead to difficulty understanding that other people's emotions are the same as one's own and thereby limit the ability to form distinctions between self and others. Clearly, such a deficit could contribute to the social and emotional problems seen in ASD.

It is important to note, however, that mimicry is not the only possible way in which people can be influenced by the emotions of those around them (McIntosh et al., 1994). For example, one possibility is that due to classical conditioning or cognitive appraisal, the observed person's emotional state may trigger a corresponding state in the observer (consider your emotional state generated by watching a smiling versus a scowling police officer, spouse, or stranger approach you). A second alternative is that the observer may respond emotionally to imagining him- or herself in the situation of the observed person. Thus, a mimicry deficit may impair only one route by which a model's emotions influence an observer's. As people with autism can respond with congruent emotions to the emotions of those around them (Merges, 2003), the degree of impairment in contagion may be less than any deficit in mimicry.

Due in part to its connection with emotional contagion, mimicry has also been theorized to be a mechanism involved in empathy (Chartrand & Bargh, 1999; Hoffman, 1984; Sonnby-Borgstrom, Jonsson, & Svensson, 2003). Empathy has been defined as "an emotional response that stems from another's emotional state or condition, and involves at least a minimal degree of differentiation between self and other" (Eisenberg & Fabes, 1990, p 132). An important difference between empathy and emotional contagion is that in empathy the emotional states between the observer and the model do not necessarily have to match (Baron-Cohen & Wheelwright, 2004; McIntosh et al., 1994). Current evidence cannot support a causal role of mimicry in empathy (Hess et al., 1999). Future examination may establish connections between empathy and mimicry via emotional contagion; however, the relative complexity of empathy may limit the functional role of mimicry.

Emotion Perception

Individuals with ASD have been shown to have deficits in emotion perception (Celani et al., 1999; Dawson et al., 2004; Gross, 2004; Hobson, 1991; Hobson, Ouston, & Lee, 1988; Kasari & Sigman, 1996; Ozonoff, Pennington, & Rogers, 1990). A mimicry deficit may be associated with such deficits, as mimetic processes appear to influence the perception of emotion in typically developing individuals (Neidenthal et al., 2001). These findings suggest that mimicry may sway how people see emotional stimuli and have interesting implications for people with ASD. For example, if mimicry was impaired from a very early age, this could lead to stable shifts in how individuals perceive emotional expressions.

Social-Cognitive Functioning

Mimicry may have consequences for cognitive functioning. For example, a prominent theory of how the brain forms representations is *embodiment theory* (Barsalou, 1999, 2003; Johnson, 1987; Thompson & Varela, 2001). This theory suggests that all cognition is represented by multimodal sensory/motor activation; thought processes are not simple abstract patterns of activation but are, rather, based on sensory and motor patterns of activation. Thus, bodily states, actions, and perceptions influence cognition. If true, then motor movements, including mimicry, could influence how people represent the world; the motor output generated by mimicry could be an important factor in altering thought processes, perhaps to support social interactions. A mimicry deficit in those with ASD could help explain some of the deficits seen in autism.

The idea that cognition is embodied is consistent with *simulation theory's* account of the social deficits seen in ASD, which has emerged as an alternative theory to *theory of mind* (TOM). Although a detailed discussion of "mind-reading" processes such as simulation theory and TOM is beyond the scope of this chapter (see Decety, Chapter 11, this volume, and Williams & Waiter, Chapter 15, this volume, for a more detailed discussion of the bases of the development of understanding of other's minds), it is worth noting that simulation theory suggests that we use our own cognitive and affective mechanisms to simulate situations other people are in (Gordon & Barker, 1994). This allows us understand what other people are thinking and feeling in the same way that we understand our own mental states (Gallese et al., 2004). One way that our brains may simulate is through embodiment processes. That is, we may embody the actions of other's in the same way we embody our own sensory/motor states. Thus, our mimetic actions may tell us something of other people's mental or affective states by directly influencing how we think. Without mimicry, people may have difficulty understanding the mental states of others as is seen in those with autism.

Summary

Across our discussion of mimicry and social processes, a recurring theme has been that the physical action of mimicry is tied to social and emotional processes. Given that mimicry seems to be related to so many social–emotional phenomena, it seems likely that mimicry could be a vital component of social development. We believe that systematic study of how mimicry is involved in social–emotional phenomena and social development is warranted and may lead to a better understanding of the bases for some social–emotional processes in ASD.

FUTURE DIRECTIONS

We have argued that mimicry is an important avenue of study in autism research, because mimicry may be important for typical social–emotional processes that appear impaired in autism, and because it may point to underlying deficits in motor, perception–action, or affective systems. Progress in determining the role of mimicry in autism will require both basic research focused on understanding mimicry and research exploring connections between mimicry and autism. Next, we describe four broad questions that we believe would be informative in understanding the role of mimicry in autism.

First, we need to gain a clearer understanding of what mimicry is in typical populations (i.e., how does mimicry typically function?). We need to know how mimicry varies within typical populations, and what psychological or neurological differences associate with these variations so that we can have a clear idea of what factors and processes contribute to mimicry. Determination of whether people with autism mimic postures or nonfacial actions might help determine the degree to which the phenomenon relies on affective changes in the observer (i.e., do people with autism mimic nonemotional bodily changes as typically developing people do? [Berger & Hadley, 1975]). Reflecting the current discussions within the mimicry literature, we have focused on motor, perception–action, and affective processes here. In addition to exploring these possibilities, researchers should not forget that a mimicry deficit in autism may also be the result of social attentional and motivational processes that are important for typical social functioning (Pessoa, McKenna, Gutierrez, & Ungerleider, 2002). Impairments or delays in these areas have been implicated in autism (Osterling & Dawson, 1994; Whiten & Brown, 1999); indeed, social motivational impairments are likely part of the autism phenotype (Dawson et al., 2002). In addition to exploration of the processes on which we focused, work examining the role of attention to faces and social motivation in the development and process of mimicry is thus also important.

Second, we need to have a clearer understanding of how strong a role mimicry plays in typical social functioning. Associations between mimicry and many social phenomena have been postulated, but research documenting such associations remains scattered (Hess et al., 1999). Third, we need to determine the sources of mimicry. Is it innate or does it develop? If it develops, how does that occur?

The three aforementioned points deal with the need to understand how mimicry functions and develops. The fourth issue is investigation of causal links that have been proposed between mimicry and ASD. The cascade of developmental deficits based on poor mimicry has so far only been studied indirectly (e.g., cross-sectional correlations and associations). The mimicry literature has for the most part used adult samples; additional work documenting the presence and correlates of mimicry in younger samples and examining what precedes evidence of a mimicry deficit and what is longitudinally predicted by such a deficit will be important steps in determining whether mimicry is significant in the development of the social emotional deficits seen in the autistic phenotype.

CONCLUSIONS

Mimicry has been studied independently of autism for decades, even though the work on understanding other interpersonal matching processes in autism has been ongoing for at least 15 years. However, there are some general conclusions that we can make. First, typically developing people mimic; this is a fairly robust phenomenon. Second, people with autism appear *not* to mimic emotional facial expressions. The reasons for the particular deficit and its relation to other emotional or matching impairments (such as the excessive vocal mimicry of echolalia or the social learning deficits in imitation) need further exploration. Third, mimicry is related to social–emotional phenomena in typical populations. Finally, given the previous three conclusions, research on mimicry may lead to a better understanding of ASD, either by pointing to more basic impairments or through providing additional understanding of a process that is connected to the social–emotional deficits seen in ASD. The task of unraveling the link(s) between mimicry and autism is clearly a difficult one. It needs to be informed by ongoing research on the nature of mimicry, on other matching phenomena in ASD, and on other social–emotional processes in ASD. However, it will likely provide new insight into a disorder that has baffled researchers for half a century, and on a process that increasingly appears to be fundamental to typical human social functioning.

ACKNOWLEDGMENTS

Preparation of this chapter was supported in part by a grant from the National Alliance for Autism Research to Daniel N. McIntosh. We appreciate the feedback of Sally Rogers and Justin Williams, John Agnew, Paula Beall, Catherine Reed, and Rob Roberts on earlier versions of this chapter.

REFERENCES

Abashev-Konstantinovsky, A. L. (1937). Motor disorders in schizophrenia. *Sovetskaya Psikhonevrologiya*, (3), 100–107.

Adolphs, R., Tranel, D., Damasio, H., & Damasio, A. R. (1995). Fear and the human amygdala. *Journal of Neuroscience, 15*(9), 5879–5891.

Alderidge, M. A., Stone, K. R., Sweeney, M. H., & Bower, T. G. R. (2000). Preverbal children with autism understand the intentions of others. *Developmental Science, 3*(3), 294–301.

Allen, G., & Courchesne, E. (2003). Differential effects of developmental cerebellar abnormality on cognitive and motor functions in the cerebellum: An fMRI study of autism. *American Journal of Psychiatry, 160* 262–273.

American Psychiatric Association. (1994). *Diagnostic and statistical manual of mental disorders* (4th ed.). Washington, DC: Author.

Avikainen, S., Kulomaeki, T., & Hari, R. (1999). Normal movement reading in Asperger subjects. *Neuroreport, 10*(17), 3467–3470.

Aylward, E. H., Minshew, N. J., Goldstein, G., Honeycutt, N. A., Augustine, A. M., Yates, K. O., et al. (1999). MRI volumes of amygdala and hippocampus in non-mentally retarded autistic adolescents and adults. *Neurology, 53*, 2145–2150.

Baron-Cohen, S., Ring, H., Wheelwright, S., Bullmore, E., Brammer, M., Simmons, A., et al. (1999). Social intelligence in the normal and autistic brain: An fMRI study. *European Journal of Neuroscience, 11*, 1891–1898.

Baron-Cohen, S., Ring, H. A., Bullmore, E. T., Wheelwright, S., Ashwin, C., & Williams, S. C. R. (2000). The amygdala theory of autism. *Neuroscience and Biobehavioral Reviews, 24*(3), 355–364.

Baron-Cohen, S., & Wheelwright, S. (2004). The empathy quotient: An investigation of adults with Asperger syndrome or high functioning autism, and normal sex differences. *Journal of Autism and Developmental Disorders, 34*(2), 163–175.

Barsalou, L. W. (1999). Perceptual symbol systems. *Behavioral and Brain Sciences, 22*(4), 577–660.

Barsalou, L. W. (2003). Situated simulation in the human conceptual system. *Language and Cognitive Processes, 18*(5), 513–562.

Batson, C. D., & Coke, J. S. (1983). Empathic motivation of helping behavior. In J. T. Cacioppo & R. E. Petty (Eds.), *Social psychophysiology: A sourcebook* (pp. 417–433). New York: Guilford Press.

Bauman, M., & Kemper, T. L. (1985). Histoanatomic observations of the brain in early infantile autism. *Neurology, 35*(6), 866–874.

Bavelas, J. B., Black, A., Chovil, N., & Lemery, C. R. (1988). Form and function in motor mimicry: Topographic evidence that the primary function is communicative. *Human Communication Research, 14*(3), 275–299.

Bavelas, J. B., Black, A., Lemery, C. R., & Mullett, J. (1986). "I show how you feel": Motor mimicry as a communicative act. *Journal of Personality and Social Psychology, 50*(2), 322–329.

Berger, S. M. (1962). Conditioning through vicarious instigation. *Psychological Review*, 69(5), 450–466.

Berger, S. M., & Hadley, S. W. (1975). Some effects of a model's performance on an observer's electromyographic activity. *American Journal of Psychology*, 88(2), 263–276.

Brothers, L. (1989). A biological perspective on empathy. *American Journal of Psychiatry*, 146(1), 10–19.

Bush, L. K., Barr, C. L., McHugo, G. J., & Lanzetta, J. T. (1989). The effects of facial control and facial mimicry on subjective reactions to comedy routines. *Motivation and Emotion*, 13(1), 31–52.

Cacioppo, J. T., Martzke, J. S., Petty, R. E., & Tassinary, L. G. (1988). Specific forms of facial EMG response index emotions during an interview: From darwin to the continuous flow hypothesis of affect-laden information processing. *Journal of Personality and Social Psychology*, 54, 592–604.

Calvo-Merino, B., Glaser, D. E., Grezes, J., Passingham, R. E., & Haggard, P. (2004). Action observation and acquired motor skills: An fMRI study with expert dancers. *Cerebral Cortex*, 15(8), 1243–1249.

Carver, C. S., Ganellen, R. J., Froming, W. J., & Chambers, W. (1983). Modeling: An analysis in terms of category accessibility. *Journal of Experimental Social Psychology*, 19(5), 403–421.

Celani, G., Battacchi, M. W., & Arcidiacono, L. (1999). The understanding of the emotional meaning of facial expressions in people with autism. *Journal of Autism and Developmental Disorders*, 29(1), 57–66.

Chartrand, T. L., & Bargh, J. A. (1999). The chameleon effect: The perception–behavior link and social interaction. *Journal of Personality and Social Psychology*, 76(6), 893–910.

Courchesne, E. (1995). New evidence of cerebellar and brainstem hypoplasia in autistic infants, children and adolescents: The MR imaging study by Hashimoto and colleagues. *Journal of Autism and Developmental Disorders*, 25(1), 19–22.

Courchesne, E., Yeung-Courchesne, R., Press, G. A., & Hesselink, J. R. (1988). Hypoplasia of cerebellar vermal lobules VI and VII in autism. *New England Journal of Medicine*, 318(21), 1349–1354.

Critchley, H. D., Daly, E. M., Bullmore, E. T., Williams, S. C. R., Van Amelsvoort, T., Robertson, D. M., et al. (2000). The functional neuroanatomy of social behaviour: Changes in cerebral blood flow when people with autistic disorder process facial expressions. *Brain*, 123(11), 2203–2212.

Dawson, G., Webb, S., Schellenberg, G. D., Dager, S., Friedman, S., Aylward, E., et al. (2002). Defining the broader phenotype of autism: Genetic, brain, and behavioral perspectives. *Development and Psychopathology*, 14(3), 581–611.

Dawson, G., Webb, S. J., Carver, L., Panagiotides, H., & McPartland, J. (2004). Young children with autism show atypical brain responses to fearful versus neutral facial expressions of emotion. *Developmental Science*, 7(3), 340–359.

Decéty, J., & Chaminade, T. (2003). Neural correlates of feeling sympathy. *Neuropsychologia, Special Issue on Social Cognition*, 41, 127–138.

Dimberg, U. (1982). Facial reactions to facial expressions. *Pscyhophysiology*, 19(6), 643–647.

Dimberg, U. (1986). Facial reactions to fear-relevant and fear-irrelevant stimuli. *Biological Psychology*, 23(2), 153–161.

Dimberg, U. (1988). Facial electromyography and the experience of emotion. *Journal of Psychophysiology*, 2(4), 277–282.

Dimberg, U., Hansson, G., & Thunberg, M. (1998). Fear of snakes and facial reactions: A case of rapid emotional responding. *Scandinavian Journal of Psychology*, *39*(2), 75–80.

Dimberg, U., & Thell, S. (1988). Facial electromyography, fear relevance and the experience of stimuli. *Journal of Psychophysiology*, *2*(3), 213–219.

Dimberg, U., Thunberg, M., & Elmehed, K. (2000). Unconscious facial reactions to emotional facial expressions. *Psychological Sciencee*, *11*(1), 86–89.

Eisenberg, N., & Fabes, R. A. (1990). Empathy: Conceptualization, measurement, and relation to prosocial behavior. *Motivation and Emotion*, *14*(2), 131–149.

Fein, D. (2001). The primacy of social and language deficits in autism. *Japanese Journal of Special Education*, *38*(6), 1–16.

Field, T. M., Woodson, R., Greenberg, R., & Cohen, D. (1982). Discrimination and imitation of facial expressions by neonates. *Science*, *218*, 179–181.

Gallese, V. (2001). The "shared manifold" hypothesis: From mirror neurons to empathy. In E. Thompson (Ed.), *Between ourselves: Second-person issues in the study of consciousness*. (pp. 33–50). Charlottesville, VA: Imprint Academic.

Gallese, V., Keysers, C., & Rizzolatti, G. (2004). A unifying view of the basis of social cognition. *Trends in Cognitive Sciences*, *8*, 396–403.

Goldenberg, G., & Hagmann, S. (1997). The meaning of meaningless gestures: A study of visuo-imitative apraxia. *Neuropsychologia*, *35*(3), 333–341.

Gordon, R. M., & Barker, J. A. (1994). Autism and the "theory of mind" debate. In G. Graham & G. L. Stephens (Eds.), *Philosophical psychopathology* (pp. 163–181). Cambridge, MA: MIT Press.

Gross, T. F. (2004). The perception of four basic emotions in human and nonhuman faces by children with autism and other developmental disabilities. *Journal of Abnormal Child Psychology*, *32*(5), 469–480.

Hashimoto, T., Tayama, M., Murakawa, K., & Yoshimoto, T. (1995). Development of the brainstem and cerebellum in autistic patients. *Journal of Autism and Developmental Disorders*, *25*(1), 1–18.

Hatfield, E., Cacioppo, J. T., & Rapson, R. L. (1994). *Emotional contagion*. New York: Cambridge University Press.

Hazenedar, M. M., Buchsbaum, M., Wei, T., Hof, P., Cartwright, C., Bienstock, C., et al. (2000). Limbic circuitry in patient with autistic spectrum disorders studied with positron emission tomography and magnetic resonance imaging. *American Journal of Psychiatry*, *157*, 1994–2001.

Hess, U., & Blairy, S. (2001). Facial mimicry and emotional contagion to dynamic emotional facial expressions and their influence on decoding accuracy. *International Journal of Psychophysiology*, *40*(2), 129–141.

Hess, U., Philippot, P., & Blairy, S. (1998). Facial reactions to emotional facial expressions: Affect or cognition? *Cognition and Emotion*, *12*(4), 509–531.

Hess, U., Philippot, P., & Blairy, S. (1999). Mimicry: Facts and fiction. In P. Philippot & R. S. Feldman (Eds.), *The social context of nonverbal behavior* (pp. 213–241). New York: Cambridge University Press.

Hinsz, V. B., & Tomhave, J. A. (1991). Smile and (half) the world smiles with you, frown and you frown alone. *Personality and Social Psychology Bulletin*, *17*(5), 586–592.

Hobson, P. (2004). *The cradle of thought: Exploring the origins of thinking*. New York: Oxford University Press.

Hobson, R. P. (1991). Methodological issues for experiments on autistic individuals' perception and understanding of emotion. *Journal of Child Psychology and Psychiatry and Allied Disciplines*, *32*(7), 1135–1158.

Hobson, R. P. (1995). The intersubjective domain: Approaches from developmental psychopathology. In T. Shapiro & R. N. Emde (Eds.), *Research in psychoanalysis: Process, development, outcome* (pp. 167–192). Madison, CT: International Universities Press.

Hobson, R. P., & Lee, A. (1998). Hello and goodbye: A study of social engagement in autism. *Journal of Autism and Developmental Disorders, 28,* 117–127.

Hobson, R. P., Ouston, J., & Lee, A. (1988). What's in a face? The case of autism. *British Journal of Psychology, 79*(4), 441–453.

Hoffmann, M. L. (1984). Interaction of affect and cognition on empathy. In C. E. Izard, J. Kagan, & R. B. Zajonc (Eds.), *Emotion, cognition and behavior* (pp. 103–131). New York: Cambridge University Press.

Iacoboni, M. (2005). Understanding others: Imitation, language, and empathy. In S. Hurley & N. Chater (Eds.), *Perspectives on imitation: From cognitive neuroscience to social science: Vol. 1. Mechanisms of imitation and imitation in animals* (pp. 77–99). Cambridge, MA: MIT Press.

Iacoboni, M., Woods, R. P., Brass, M., Bekkering, H., Mazziotta, J. C., & Rizzolatti, G. (1999). Cortical mechanisms of human imitation. *Science, 286,* 2526–2528.

James, W. (1950). The emotions. In *The principles of psychology* (Vol. 2, pp. 442–485). New York: Holt. (Original work published 1890)

Johnson, M. (1987). *The body in the mind: The bodily basis of meaning, imagination, and reason.* Chicago: University of Chicago Press.

Kaitz, M., Meschulach-Sarfaty, O. Auerbach, J., & Eidelman, A. (1988). A reexamination of newborns' ability to imitate facial expressions. *Developmental Psychology, 24*(1), 3–7.

Kasari, C., Chamberlain, B., & Bauminger, N. (2001). Social emotions and social relationships: Can children with autism compensate? In J. A. Burack & T. Charman (Eds.), *Development of autism: Perspectives from theory and research* (pp. 309–323). Mahwah, NJ: Erlbaum.

Kasari, C., & Sigman, M. (1996). Expression and understanding of emotion in atypical development: Autism and down syndrome. In M. Lewis & M. W. Sullivan (Eds.), *Emotional development in atypical children* (pp. 109–130). Hillsdale, NJ: Erlbaum.

Kleiman, M. D., Neff, S., & Rosman, N. P. (1992). The brain in infantile autism: Are posterior fossa structures abnormal? *Neurology, 42*(4), 753–760.

Koepke, J., Hamm, M., Legerstee, M., & Russell, M. (1983). Neonatal imitation: Two failures to replicate. *Infant Behavior and Development, 6*(1), 97–102.

Krebs, D. (1975). Empathy and altruism. *Journal of Personality and Social Psychology, 32*(6), 1134–1146.

Lakin, J. L., & Chartrand, T. L. (2003). Using nonconscious behavioral mimicry to create affiliation and rapport. *Psychological Science, 14*(4), 334–339.

Lakin, J. L., Jefferis, V. E., Cheng, C. M., & Chartrand, T. L. (2003). The chameleon effect as social glue: Evidence for the evolutionary significance of nonconscious mimicry. *Journal of Nonverbal Behavior, 27*(3), 145–162.

Levenson, R. W., & Gottman, J. M. (1983). Marital interaction: Physiological linkage and affective exchange. *Journal of Personality and Social Psychology, 45*(3), 587–597.

Levenson, R. W., & Gottman, J. M. (1985). Physiological and affective predictors of change in relationship satisfaction. *Journal of Personality and Social Psychology, 49*(1), 85–94.

Lipps, T. (1907). Das wissen con fremden ichen. In T. Lipps (Ed.), *Psychologische untersuchungen* (Vol. 1, pp. 694–722). Leipzig: Engelmann.

Liss, M., Harel, B., Fein, D., Allen, D., Dunn, M., Feinstein, C., et al. (2001). Predictors and correlates of adaptive functioning in children with developmental disorders. *Journal of Autism and Developmental Disorders, 31*(2), 219–230.

Lundqvist, L.-O., & Dimberg, U. (1995). Facial expressions are contagious. *Journal of Psychophysiology*, 9(3), 203–211.

Martin, L. A., Goldowitz, D., & Mittleman, G. (2003). The cerebellum and spatial ability: Dissection of motor and cognitive components with a mouse model system. *European Journal of Neuroscience*, 18(7), 2002–2010.

McDougall, W. (1908). *An introduction to social psychology.* Boston: Luce.

McIntosh, D. (2006). Spontaneous facial mimicry, liking and emotional contagion. *Polish Psychological Bulletin*, 37, 31–42.

McIntosh, D., Reichmann-Decker, A., Winkielman, P., & Wilbarger, J. L. (2006). When the social mirror breaks: Deficits in automatic, but not voluntary mimicry of emotional facial expressions in autism. *Developmental Science*, 9(3), 295–302.

McIntosh, D. N. (1996). Facial feedback hypotheses: Evidence, implications, and directions. *Motivation and Emotion*, 20(2), 121–147.

McIntosh, D. N., Druckman, D., & Zajonc, R. B. (1994). Socially induced affect. In D. Druckman & R. A. Bjork (Eds.), *Learning, remembering, believing; enhancing human performance* (pp. 251–276, 364–371). Washington, DC: National Academy Press.

McKenzie, B. E., & Over, R. (1983). Young infants fail to imitate facial and manual gestures. *Infant Behavior and Development*, 6(1), 85–95.

Meltzoff, A., & Moore, K. (1977). Imitation of facial and manual gestures by human neonates. *Science*, 198, 75–78.

Meltzoff, A. N., & Moore, M. K. (1983). Methodological issues in studies of imitation: Comments on McKenzie & Over and Koepke et al. *Infant Behavior and Development*, 6(1), 103–108.

Merges, E. M. (2003). Emotion contagion in children with autism: The effect on affect and behavior. *Dissertaion Abstracts International, Section B: The Sciences and Engineering*, 6(6-B), 2930.

Moody, E. J., McIntosh, D. N., Mann, L. J., & Weisser, K. R. (2006). *The influence of affect on rapid facial reactions to faces.* Manuscript under review.

Mostofsky, S. H., Bunoski, R., Morton, S. M., Goldberg, M. C., & Bastian, A. J. (2004). Children with autism adapt normally during a catching task requiring the cerebellum. *Neurocase*, 10(1), 60–64.

Nair, D. G., Purcott, K. L., Fuchs, A., Steinberg, F., & Kelso, J. A. S. (2003). Cortical and cerebellar activity of the human brain during imagined and executed unimanual and bimanual action sequences: A functional MRI study. *Cognitive Brain Research*, 15(3), 250–260.

Neidenthal, P. M., Brauer, M., Halberstadt, J. B., & Innes-Ker, A. H. (2001). When did her smile drop? Facial mimicry and the influences of emotional state on the detection of change in emotional expression. *Cognition and Emotion*, 15(6), 853–864.

Noble, J., & Todd, P. M. (2002). Imitation or something simpler? Modeling simple mechanisms for social information processing. In K. Dautenhahn & C. L. Nehaniv (Eds.), *Imitation in animals and artifacts* (pp. 423–439). Cambridge, MA: MIT Press.

Osterling, J., & Dawson, G. (1994). Early recognition of children with autism: A study of first birthday home videotapes. *Journal of Autism and Developmental Disorders*, 24(3), 247–257.

Ozonoff, S., Cook, I., Coon, H., Dawson, G., Joseph, R. M., Klin, A., et al. (2004). Performance on Cambridge Neuropsychological Test automated battery subtests sensitive to frontal lobe function in people with autistic disorder: Evidence from the collaborative programs of excellence in autism network. *Journal of Autism and Developmental Disorders*, 34(2), 139–150.

Ozonoff, S., Pennington, B. F., & Rogers, S. J. (1990). Are there emotion perception deficits in young autistic children? *Journal of Child Psychology and Psychiatry and Allied Disciplines, 31*(3), 343–361.

Palmen, S. J. M. C., van Engeland, H., Hof, P. R., & Schmitz, C. (2004). Neuropathological findings in autism. *Brain, 127,* 2572–2583.

Pessoa, L., McKenna, M., Gutierrez, E., & Ungerleider, L. G. (2002). Neural processing of emotional faces requires attention. *Proceedings of the National Academy of Sciences, 99*(17), 11458–11463.

Pierce, K., Muller, R., Ambrose, J., Alleen, G., & Courchesne, E. (2001). Face processing occurs outside of the fusiform "face area" in autism: Evidence from functional MRI. *Brain, 124,* 2059–2073.

Reissland, N. (1988). Neonatal imitation in the first hour of life: Observations in rural Nepal. *Developmental Psychology, 24*(4), 464–469.

Rizzolatti, G., & Arbib, M. A. (1998). Language within our grasp. *Trends in Neurosciences, 21*(5), 188–194.

Rizzolatti, G., Craighero, L., & Fadiga, L. (2002). The mirror system in humans. In M. I. Stamenov & V. Gallese (Eds.), *Mirror neurons and the evolution of brain and language.* (pp. 37–59). Amsterdam: Benjamins.

Roeyers, H., Van Oost, P., & Bothuyne, S. (1998). Immediate imitation and joint attention in young children with autism. *Development and Psychopathology, 10*(3), 441–450.

Rogers, S. J. (1999). An examination of the imitation deficit in autism. In J. Nadel & G. Butterworth (Ed.), *Imitation in infancy* (pp. 254–283). New York: Cambridge University Press.

Rogers, S. J., & Bennetto, L. (2000). Intersubjectivity in autism: The roles of imitation and executive function. In A. M. Wetherby & B. M. Prizant (Eds.), *Autism spectrum disorders: A transactional developmental perspective* (pp. 79–107). Baltimore: Brookes.

Rogers, S. J., Hepburn, S. L., Stackhouse, T., & Wehner, E. (2003). Imitation performance in toddlers with autism and those with other developmental disorders. *Journal of Child Psychology and Psychiatry, 44*(5), 763–781.

Rogers, S. J., & Pennington, B. F. (1991). A theoretical approach to the deficits in infantile autism. *Development and Psychopathology, 3*(2), 137–162.

Rotteveel, M., de Groot, P., Geutskens, A., & Phaf, R. H. (2001). Stronger suboptimal than optimal affective priming? *Emotion, 1*(4), 348–364.

Smith, I. M., & Bryson, S. E. (1998). Gesture imitation in autism. I: Nonsymbolic postures and sequences. *Cognitive Neuropsychology, 15*(6), 747–770.

Sonnby-Borgstroem, M. (2002). Automatic mimicry reactions as related to differences in emotional empathy. *Scandinavian Journal of Psychology, 45*(5), 433–443.

Sonnby-Borgstrom, M., Jonsson, P., & Svensson, O. (2003). Emotional empathy as related to mimicry reactions at different levels of information processing. *Journal of Nonverbal Behavior, 27*(1), 3–23.

Spence, K. W. (1937). Experimental studies of social learning and higher mental processes in infra-human primates. *Psychological Bulletin, 34,* 806–850.

Stern, D. (1983). The infant's repertoire. In W. Damon (Ed.), *Social and personality development: Essays on the growth of the child* (pp. 4–16). New York: Norton.

Stotland, E. (1969). Exploratory investigations of empathy. In L. Berkowitz (Ed.), *Advances in experimental social psychology* (Vol. 4, pp. 271–314). New York: Academic Press.

Thompson, E., & Varela, F. J. (2001). Radical embodiment: Neural dynamics and consciousness. *Trends in Cognitive Sciences, 5*(10), 418–425.

Thunberg, M., & Dimberg, U. (2000). Gender differences in facial reactions to fear-relevant stimuli. *Journal of Nonverbal Behavior, 24*(1), 45–51.

Tomasello, M. (1990). Cultural transmission in the tool use and communicatory signaling of chimpanzees? In S. T. Parker & K. R. Gibson (Eds.), *"Language" and intelligence in monkeys and apes: Comparative developmental perspectives* (pp. 274–311). New York: Cambridge University Press.

Tomasello, M. (1996). Do apes ape? In C. M. Heyes & B. G. Galef, Jr. (Eds.), *Social learning in animals: The roots of culture* (pp. 319–346). San Diego, CA: Academic Press.

Turner, R. S., Desmurget, M., Grethe, J., Crutcher, M. D., & Grafton, S. T. (2003). Motor subcircuits mediating the control of movement extent and speed. *Journal of Neurophysiology, 90*(6), 3958–3966.

van Baaren, R. B., Holland, R. W., Kawakami, K., & van Knippenberg, A. (2004). Mimicry and prosocial behavior. *Psychological Science, 15*(1), 71–74.

Vaughan, K. B., & Lanzetta, J. T. (1980). Vicarious instigation and conditioning of facial expressive and autonomic responses to a model's expressive display of pain. *Journal of Personality and Social Psychology, 38*(6), 909–923.

Vaughan, K. B., & Lanzetta, J. T. (1981). The effect of modification of expressive displays on vicarious emotional arousal. *Journal of Experimental Social Psychology, 17*(1), 16–30.

Want, S. C., & Harris, P. L. (2002). How do children ape? Applying concepts from the study of non-human primates to the developmental study of "imitation" in children. *Developmental Science, 5*, 1–13.

Whiten, A., & Brown, J. D. (1998). Imitation and the reading of other minds: Perspectives from the study of autism, normal children and non-human primates. In S. Bråten (Ed.), *Intersubjective communication and emotion in early ontogeny* (pp. 260–280). New York: Cambridge University Press.

Williams, J., Whiten, A., & Singh, T. (2004). A systematic review of action imitation in autistic spectrum disorder. *Journal of Autism and Developmental Disorders, 34*(3), 285–299.

Williams, J. H. G., Whiten, A., Suddendorf, T., & Perrett, D. I. (2001). Imitation, mirror neurons and autism. *Neuroscience and Biobehavioral Reviews, 25*(4), 287–295.

Williams, R., Hauser, S., Purpurda, D., DeLong, R., & Swisher, C. (1980). Autism and mental retardation. *Archives of Neurology, 37*, 749–753.

Wing, L., & Gould, J. (1979). Severe impairments of social interaction and associated abnormalities in children: Epidemiology and classification. *Journal of Autism and Developmental Disorders, 9*(1), 11–29.

Winkielman, P., & Cacioppo, J. T. (2001). Mind at ease puts a smile on the face: Psychophysiological evidence that processing facilitation elicits positive affect. *Journal of Personality and Social Psychology, 81*(6), 989–1000.

Young, A. W. A., Aggleton, J. P., Hellawell, D. J., Johnson, M., Broks, P., & Hanley, J. R. (1995). Face processing impairments after amygdalotomy. *Brain, 118*(1), 15–24.

CHAPTER 5

Imitation and
the Development of Language

TONY CHARMAN

Before using words, children acquire a repertoire of conventional sounds and gestures to express intentions and to communicate. Some of these sounds and gestures develop from the ritualization of functional actions such as reaching, while others involve the imitation of actions that have conventional or agreed-on meanings, such as waving bye-bye, nodding, or pointing. At least three aspects of imitation are relevant to appreciating its role in the development of spoken language (Nadel & Butterworth, 1999). First, imitation is a form of social learning that involves observing others, listening to others, and learning from others. Second, imitation involves the acquisition of novel responses on the basis of social experience and reinforcement. Third, imitation can provide evidence that a child is able to form internal representations of the actions they observe and reproduce these representations in their own actions. Each of these aspects develops within the to-and-fro flow of social communication and the development of shared meanings (Bates, Benigni, Bretherton, Camaioni, & Volterra, 1979). These observations also apply to the development of spoken language. That is, children learn the meaning of words by observing how other people use them (for the purposes of communication). They then reproduce, or imitate, words they have learned the meaning of for the same purpose—to communicate. Imitation and language appear to be connected at the core level of developing understanding. For children with autism, the development of both imitation and spoken language is typically delayed and also deviates from the pattern seen in typical development.

At first glance the role of imitation in the ontogeny of the social and communicative impairments that characterize individuals with autism presents something of a conundrum. On one hand the phenomenon of echolalia, whereby some children with autism repeat back to the speaker a word or phrase, seems to suggest an intact capacity in the child's ability to imitate, at least for language. On the other hand, many parents of preschoolers with autism report that their children do not copy everyday household activities such as vacuuming and using a hammer and nail that appear to come so naturally to typically developing toddlers. Indeed, deficits in imitation form part of the characteristic behavioral profile of preschoolers with autism (Charman & Baird, 2002; Rogers, 2001). To understand this apparent contradiction one needs to understand the role of imitation in social, communication, and language development and in particular the psychological mechanisms that underlie the capacity for imitation. Imitation has long been a topic of interest in developmental psychology. More recently, it has been a focus of empirical activity and theoretical interest in several fields of scientific endeavor, including developmental psychopathology, cognitive neuroscience, comparative psychology, and ethology. The purpose of this chapter is to explore this common ground between action–imitation and language development. I ask what developmental processes are common to action–imitation and the development of verbal skills. In what ways is imitation necessary for language development and on what processes are imitation and language both commonly dependent?

I review both historical and more recent work from a number of these fields with a focus on the role of imitation in the development of language and communication. I also highlight aspects of the atypical development of imitation in children with autism that reflect broader (i.e., non-language-specific) impairments in social communication that define the disorder.

THE PIAGETIAN VIEW: LET'S START AT THE BEGINNING

The first comprehensive and authoritative developmental theory giving imitation a central role in the development and onset of language was Piaget's (1945/1962; Piaget & Inhelder, 1966/1969). Piaget described how body, facial, and vocal imitation developed throughout the six stages of sensorimotor development. No true imitation was possible in stage I (0–1 months) and any pseudo-imitative responses were considered reflexes. Sporadic imitation of "circular reactions" occurred during stage II (1–5 months) when an adult modeled behaviors that had just been displayed by the baby. During stage III (6–9 months), simple sounds and manual gestures that were already within the repertoire of the infant could be imitated. Critically, Piaget argued that these could be accomplished on the basis of an *intra*modal (within-modality) matching process. During stages IV and V (9–18 months), two critical aspects of early imitation begin to emerge. First, infants begin to imitate facial gestures that require *inter*modal (cross-modality) matching that is beyond the cognitive abilities of younger infants. Second, although not fully established before stage VI (18–24 months), the infant becomes capable of deferred imitation. Both of these landmark achievements require increasing representational capacity on the part of the infant whereby he or she is able to form, manipulate, store, and retrieve cognitive representations or symbols. Piaget linked this to the concurrent development of symbolic play and spoken language, both of which he also argued require such representational skills.

While other theorists, notably Werner and Kaplan (1963) and Vygotsky (1934/1986), argued for a greater role for social interaction between children and adults in the development of such symbolic skills, Piaget's theory was the dominant one within developmental psychology at the time. For Piaget, representation begins when there is simultaneous differentiation and coordination between signifiers (the internal representation) and the signified (the content of the action). Imitation involves the first demonstration of such a differentiation between the observable action and the mental image or internalization of it. Under Piaget's account, such representational abilities underlie deferred imitation (the later reproduction of an earlier-observed action), the object concept, symbolic play, and spoken words.

Subsequent to Piaget's account, several strands of research emerged that all addressed the same question: What is the association between aspects of nonverbal communication and representational development in infancy and (later) language development? Each strand adopted a slightly different focus both in terms of the form of nonverbal communicative behavior that was studied and in terms of the extent to which the social and communicative context was emphasized. The Piagetian tradition outlined previously concentrated on symbolic (pretend) play and deemphasized the social and communicative context. Another tradition emphasized the role of joint attention, that is, how children learn to attend to objects and events that adults attend to, in language development (Bates et al., 1979; Bates, Thal, Whitesell, Fenson, & Oakes, 1989; Bruner, 1975a, 1975b; Tomasello, 1988; Tomasello & Farrar, 1996; Tomasello & Todd, 1983). A second psycholinguistic tradition (see below) also placed the social–communicative infant–caregiver dyad firmly in the center of things but focused on the link between immediate and deferred imitation of gestural communication and the emergence of language (Bates et al., 1979, 1989).

LANGUAGE DEVELOPMENT: PRAGMATICS VIEW

There is empirical evidence that reveals a remarkable coincidence in timing between the development of imitation skills and language onset in the first 2 years of life (for reviews, see Bates & Dick, 2002; Fenson et al., 1994). It appears that nonverbal gestures develop hand-in-hand with verbal communication skills and thus that the temporal coincidence is close. For example, babbling usually onsets between the age of 6–8 months and has been linked to the onset of rhythmic hand clapping and banging (Locke, 1993). Between 6 and 10 months of age typically developing children begin to understand spoken words and at the same time deictic (e.g., showing and pointing) and conventional gestures (e.g., waving bye-bye) begin to emerge (Bates et al., 1979).

The coincidence of emergence between gestural communication and language continues, at least for a period, after spoken language emerges. For example, the modal age for first spoken words is around the child's first birthday and about the same time children begin to produce functional or appropriate actions on objects (e.g., drinking from a toy cup) in their play, often initially in imitation of adult models of such acts and then increasingly spontaneously and generatively (Bates et al., 1989; Fenson et al., 1994). Typically, word combinations begin to appear between the middle of a child's second year of life and his or her second birthday, and around the same time gestures and words are also used in combination (Capirci, Iverson, Pizzuto, & Volterra, 1996). Naturally, the developmental tenet that temporal coincidence does not in any way imply a causal link between two phenomena applies. Nonetheless, what captured Piaget's interest was how to explain the apparent association between the two phenomena—gestures on the one hand, language on the other—that share common functions (communication and social interaction) but take very different forms. As we shall see later on, verbal imitation also plays a role in the development of language. However, in the nonverbal modality of social interaction and communication, imitation of gestures helps "bridge" the divide between receptive reference of symbols (word comprehension) and active reference of symbols (word production) (Volterra & Erting, 1990).

Whereas several aspects of Piaget's theory and timeline have been overtaken by subsequent work (see below), his writings and those of his contemporaries within the developmental psychology field laid the groundwork in terms of delineating the critical competencies that are required by most infants throughout the relatively short period of infancy. They also provided a nomenclature to describe the cognitive processes that underlie imitation. Two critical advances, now both considered landmarks, changed the majority view within the developmental field. The first was a series of empirical studies conducted by Meltzoff and his colleagues and the second was an establishment of *psycholinguistic* theory firmly within a social context, most notably in the writings of Bruner and Bates. The next two sections of the chapter will outline each of these advances, in turn.

MELTZOFF'S CHALLENGE TO PIAGET: LET'S START AT THE BEGINNING (AGAIN)

Meltzoff and Moore's (1977, 1983) seminal finding that neonatal infants could imitate certain facial gestures launched a series of studies whose outcomes both overturned the timetable and challenged the content of Piaget's account of infant cognitive development. According to Meltzoff and Moore (1977) this suggested that the effect was not simply an arousal reaction but evidence that neonates were making specific (*inter*modal) mappings between the modeled facial gestures of the experimenter and their own executed motor responses. They developed a theoretical model of infant facial imitation that

involves what they called active intermodal mapping (AIM). The critical process involves matching to target, whereby the infant's self-produced movements provide proprioceptive feedback that can be compared with the visually
specified target. Some innate propensity to social motivation—as evidenced by
the innate preference for faces or biological motion (de Haan & Nelson,
1999)—presumably underlies the recruitment of this cognitive system when
neonates are faced with an adult. Meltzoff further extended his model to
include oral, visual, and speech perception production mapping in infants in
the first few months of life (Kuhl & Meltzoff, 1996; Meltzoff & Borton,
1979; see Meltzoff, 1999, 2002, for reviews). This timetable of representational development was revolutionary compared to that set out by Piaget,
whereby the infant is not capable of such complex representational thought
until around 18–24 months of age.

Meltzoff then initiated a series of experiments with older infants that
investigated their imitation of modeled actions on objects in order to test
whether a similar adjustment to Piaget's timetable for deferred imitation was
required (see Meltzoff, 2002). Using an "observation only" design, Meltzoff
(1988a, 1988b) demonstrated that 9-month-old infants were able to reproduce actions on objects they have observed following a 24-hour delay, compared to 18 months of age under Piaget's sensorimotor timetable. Other studies have demonstrated some facility for deferred imitation in infants as young
as 6 months of age (Barr, Dowden, & Hayne, 1996). Perhaps the most
remarkable description is of 14-month-old children reproducing the modeled
action of leaning forward and touching a box with their forehead in order to
illuminate it (Meltzoff, 1988b). This action was not produced by any children
in the control group who had not seen the demonstration of the (deliberately)
unusual method of lighting the box. Notably this particular response was also
produced by very few children with autism in one of our own studies
(Charman et al., 1997).

What is striking when conducting this experiment with typically developing infants is how often reproduction of this unnecessary and certainly somewhat unusual action is accompanied by cries of laughter from the infants and
lots of eye contact with the adult. As we shall see later, in the real-world imitation is fun and sociable and reveals to us the thought processes and social
motivations of the infant. It is also noticeable in the "light box" paradigm that
sometimes children push the top of the box with their hand in order to illuminate the box and only then, as their second action, do they reproduce the
modeled forehead "bow." Other infants reproduce the bow first and then go
on to use their hand to illuminate the box on the second attempt. Imitation is
a context and an activity through which infants learn about both people and
things.

Further decoupling of memory and representation of actions occurs as
infants become able to transfer across contexts and generalize to objects of
different color and size (see Meltzoff, 2002, for a review). More direct evidence also emerged that these developing cognitive abilities were associated

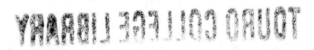

with infants' emerging language abilities. In a series of studies, Gopnik and Meltzoff (1986, 1987) demonstrated that during the second year of life differ-ent aspects of object representation can show considerable decalage and, fur-thermore, that specific aspects of object concept are related to specific lan-guage accomplishments. Thus, the onset of object permanence skills and the onset of infants' use of disappearance words are more closely yoked in time than object permanence and success/failure words (Gopnik & Meltzoff, 1986). Conversely, the onset of the ability to solve means–ends tasks is specifi-cally yoked to the infants' use of success/failure words. A second study pro-vided evidence that the naming explosion was linked to infants' ability to cate-gorize objects (Gopnik & Meltzoff, 1987). These studies indicated that different aspects of infants' emerging understanding of objects were more closely linked to specific aspects of language than to each other. Under Meltzoff's thesis, a *supra*modal ("higher-level," modality unconstrained) matching system underlies the imitation of gestures, sounds, and actions on objects, and imitation itself is necessary for language learning.

THE PSYCHOLINGUISTIC APPROACH TO INFANT LANGUAGE AND COGNITION

While Meltzoff's search started and then developed from his attempts to under-stand neonatal imitation and ended up as an account of how infants learn lan-guage (and indeed to read intentions and then to mentalize; see Meltzoff, 2002), at the same time a somewhat different theory was under development that attempted to explain the problem first articulated by Wittgenstein (1953): How can a child learn a word when no nonlinguistic procedures can unambiguously illustrate its reference? Bruner (1975a, 1975b) outlined a psycholinguistic approach that established continuities between prespeech communication and language. Similar to Meltzoff's conclusions, Bruner (1975a) said: "To master language a child must acquire a complex set of broadly transferable or genera-tive skills—perception, motor, conceptual, social, *and* linguistic—which when appropriately coordinated yield linguistic performances" (p. 256, emphasis in original). Such processes help the infant acquire language because they are used by the infant in communicative exchanges with her caregiver as the infant enters into social exchanges and intentionally laced communication about the objects and about the social world:

> For if the child, say, already knows (as we shall see) many of the conventions for give-and-take exchanges and how to conduct them by appropriate, nonlinguistic signalling, he is equipped better to interpret or "crack the code" of linguistic utterances used as regulators of such exchanges. (Bruner, 1975a, p. 261)

Critical to this process, "conversations" during the first year of life between the infant and his or her caregiver involve both partners using gesture, posture, and nonword vocalizations for the purposes of bringing the other partner's attention to an object or action or state. A second critical aspect is deixis—the *function* of pointing or *specifying from the perspective of a participant* in an act of speech or writing. This requires the infant use of spatial, temporal, and interpersonal contextual features of situations to guide joint attention or joint action. It is only through a history of multiple interpersonal exchanges that the infant is ready and able to understand that the words that accompany such nonlinguistic interchanges "stand for" events, actions, and objects. That is, conventional symbols can only be learned when the infant has already established a rich nonlinguistic "vocabulary" for communicative interchange.

Empirical evidence to support Bruner's thesis was soon available. Bates and colleagues demonstrated that linguistic and nonlinguistic social cognitive skills, including communicative gestures, words, and the imitation of actions, were highly related to each other at the end of the first year of life, and further that infants' imitation ability predicted the later nonlinguistic gestural competence and their spoken language ability (Bates et al., 1979, 1989). Bates and colleagues (1979) produced some of the first empirical evidence that demonstrated longitudinal associations between joint attention abilities, including protodeclarative pointing and following eye gaze, and later language ability (followed later by Carpenter, Nagell, & Tomasello, 1998; Mundy & Gomes, 1998; Tomasello & Farrar, 1986). Bates and colleagues (1989) found that in typically developing infants "imitating gestures with objects" (functional play acts) at 13 months of age was associated with expressive language ability 9 months later.

JOINT ATTENTION

Over the next two decades a significant body of evidence emerged that the child's exposure to activities involving joint attention and joint engagement, and the degree to which adult language is sensitive to the child's focus of attention in the language learning situation, are important for word learning and for promoting general linguistic competence (e.g., Tomasello & Farrar, 1986; Tomasello & Todd, 1983). This pattern of findings was confirmed in a recent longitudinal study that followed 24 infants at monthly intervals from 9 to 15 months of age (Carpenter, Nagell, & Tomasello, 1998). Carpenter, Nagell, and Tomasello (1998) measured a wide range of social cognitive skills, including imitation of arbitrary actions and imitation of instrumental actions. The former but not the latter were related to the age of emergence of referential language (see also Meltzoff, 1995). Similarly, imitative learning was associated with the infant following an adult's point toward an object. Carpenter, Nagell, and Tomasello concluded that in order to learn referential words, infants must be able to imitate sounds that are only arbitrarily connected to their reference and, furthermore, that both the imitation of arbitrary actions and point following involve the infants in following the adult's intention. Carpenter, Nagell, and Tomasello's longitudinal study provided evidence that in typically developing infants, imitation, joint attention, joint engagement, and understanding other's intentions are all associated with later language ability

MEANS–GOALS AND INTENTIONALITY

Another aspect of the psycholinguistic approach is the recognition that what is represented in an imitative context goes beyond the symbolic or cognitive level and involves some representation of the internal states of the child's imitative partner. Carpenter and Call (2002) elucidated a theoretical framework for understanding the different sources of information that may influence an observer's response to any modeled act (see Whiten, Horner, Litchfield, & Marshall-Pescini, 2004, for an alternative framework). A modeled action produces at least three products: *goals* (the demonstrator's aim or intention), *actions* (motor patterns), and *results* (the transformed environment). Depending on the context, the object, the infant's motivation and understanding, the familiarity of the adult partner, and social cues the adult gives out, infants' attention can be differentially drawn to different aspects of the social learning situation. Meltzoff developed the "behavioral reenactment paradigm" to test whether the infant follows a model's actions or goals (intentions). Meltzoff (1995) found that at 18 months, infants copied the intended but unconsummated action (though see Huang, Heyes, & Charman, 2002, for an alternative, more conservative interpretation). Using the same paradigm, Bellagamba and Tomasello (1998) found that 18-month-old, but not 12-month-old, infants did likewise. Several other ingenious paradigms have been developed to test which of these sources of information infants respond to. Carpenter, Akhtar, and Tomasello (1999) showed that 18-month-olds copy intended but not "accidental" actions on objects and Bekkering, Wohlschläger, and Gattis (2000) showed that school-age children imitate motor patterns of a model dependent on what they perceive to be the model's goal. Recently, Tomasello, Carpenter, Call, Behne, and Moll (2005) have also highlighted the role of social motivation in drawing infants toward intentional understanding rather than the actions or the outcome. In essence, fully understanding the impairments in the development of imitation and spoken language in autism may also require us to understand the social impairment that lies at the core of autism (see Charman, 2005; Hobson, 1993; Hobson & Meyer, Chapter 9, this volume; Williams, 2005).

Infants might copy an action or a result but be oblivious to the demonstrator's goal. Although two studies have shown that children with autism do produce the intended but unconsummated act in Meltzoff's behavioral reenactment paradigm (Aldridge, Stone, Sweeney, & Bower, 2000; Carpenter, Pennington, & Rogers, 2001), it is possible that they are producing these responses using "lower level" nonintentional means such as stimulus enhancement and object affordance (Charman & Huang, 2002; Heyes, 2001; Williams, Whiten, & Singh, 2004). It may be that for children with autism, mapping the relation between the action, the goal, and the model's intention is more difficult and that, depending on the circumstances, merely being able to reproduce the action, the goal (or even the intention) is insufficient to be a proficient imitator in everyday life.

While in typical development learning about objects via imitation and communicating with people are closely tied together, albeit at a much earlier stage than Piaget originally envisaged, one should not assume that the same is necessarily true for children with autism. A good demonstration of this principle is the finding by Hobson and Lee (1999; see Hobson & Meyer, Chapter 9, this volume) that teenage children with autism reproduced the target action of arbitrary actions on objects (the goal) but not the "style" of the action. Interestingly, few of the participants with autism adopted the orientation to self that had been modeled with the objects. While by this stage in later childhood children with autism can reproduce simple actions (see also Charman & Baron-Cohen, 1994), they do not step inside the model's mind and body as much as other children, what Hobson has referred to as a "lack of identification." In understanding the profile of intact and impaired imitative responses that have been shown in various imitation paradigms employed with children with autism (see Williams et al., 2004, for a review), it is important to recognize that imitation is not all-or-none but more or less. A variety of social and nonsocial learning processes affect how children respond to what they observe and what motivates and drives their response.

Imitation plays a role, as do other preverbal social cognitive skills (in particular joint attention and joint action), in the "meld" of nonverbal communicative interaction that infants experience during the first and second year of life. By the time infants begin to talk they are well versed as communicators and social partners. At a cognitive level, infants require the capacity to represent symbolic referents in memory and use these in interchanges, at first in combination with the nonverbal precursors and then increasingly in isolation. However, another strand of theoretical and empirical work exists that would consider that this position overemphasizes the role of representational or symbolic thought. It places the development of these precursor social communicative abilities more centrally in the social I–Thou interchange, and it is to this literature I turn next.

THE DYADIC INTERCHANGE

A rich line of empirical studies that have adopted detailed analysis of infant–adult (usually caregiver) interactions has demonstrated that as well as copying adults, infants are sensitive to and engage in back-and-forth "protoconversations" from as young as 2 months of age (Bateson, 1975; Trevarthen, 1974). Theorists have taken the demonstration of neonatal imitation as evidence that newborns are "hardwired" to perceive, respond to, and relate directly to other persons (labeled "primary intersubjectivity") (Trevarthen, 1979). Throughout the first year of life, as described previously, infants gain an understanding of meaning via engaging in cooperative activities with caregivers in joint activity with objects and events in the world. This has been described by Trevarthen (1979) as "secondary intersubjectivity," which involves the infant actively coordinating his or her interests in objects with the attention and apparent intentions of the partner. One important characteristic of this coordination is the timing element that leads to a back-and-forth reciprocity between carer and infant.

Trevarthen, Kokkinaki, and Fiamenghi (1999) summarize several experimental studies that are examples of protoconversations that involve rhythmic attunement of mother and infant vocalizations in the first few months of life (e.g., Papousek, 1989), with the mother protracting, amplifying, and enhancing versions of the infant's sounds. Such exchanges are accompanied by other sympathetic reactions that are nonimitative such as smiles, mutual gaze, hand gestures, and affective vocal expressions. Stern has called these supportive emotional colored attunements (Stern, 1985). By 6 months of age, more extended and complex vocal and emotional interchanges are possible with teasing games, baby songs (nursery rhymes), and action games where the affect, the vocalizations, and the movements of the mother and child take on a shared rhythmic pattern (see Trevarthen et al., 1999, Figure 5.4). The infant will either alternate with the mother or coincide on emotional climaxes of excitement (Stern, 1975). Out of such exchanges grow imitation of gestures and sounds and the use of these and other prelinguistic devices to refer to objects and emotions (social referencing) during the second half of the first year of life (e.g., Bates et al., 1979; Carpenter, Nagell, & Tomasello, 1998, summarized earlier).

In addition to imitating there is the other side of being imitated. There are other sources of evidence that infants are aware of being imitated. Field (1977) found that 7-month-old infants looked more toward their mother when she imitated than when she interacted in another way. Nadel (2000, cited in Nadel, Guérini, Pezé, & Rivet, 1999) found evidence that infants as young as 2 months of age were aware of being imitated. As well as increased looking, Nadel found that infants smiled and vocalized more when the mother's behavior was contingent or imitative of the child's. Interestingly, there was considerable variability in how consistently these actions and reactions were shown both by parents and by children. Nadel also reported that at least one 2-month-old produced a sequence of imitate–imitated–imitate or "imitation in return," similar to the vocalization exchanges summarized by Trevarthen and colleagues (1999). Three-month-olds are already able to detect contingency between their own bodily movements and those display on a television screen (Rochat & Morgan, 1995). However, while 3-month-olds preferred contingency, 5-month-olds preferred noncontingency, as if fascinated by the unexpected view of their own movements (see Gergely & Watson, 1999, for a pilot study of contingency in young children with autism, which deserves further investigation).

The role of social interaction in imitation continues into the preschool years and includes the effects of being imitated by peers as well as adults (Eckerman, Davis, & Didow, 1989). Being imitated provokes a social response in typically developing children. For example, Eckerman and Stein (1990) showed that when 2-year-olds' actions on objects were imitated by an adult they not only continued to play with the object for longer but engaged in social imitative games and looked more to the adult who imitated them. Shared engagement in objects (toys) in joint play between infants and their mothers ("symbol-fused engagement") is also associated to individual differences in language onset and language facility at age 2½ (Adamson, Bakeman, & Deckner, 2004). Similar evidence is available for the effects of verbal imitation in sustaining verbal interaction (Bloom, Rocissano, & Hood, 1976; Snow, 1983). (See Masur, Chapter 2, this volume, for a review of imitation during the toddler period.)

These studies focus on the social *exchange* and the development of turn taking, rather than the somewhat more "unidirectional" approaches where adults elicit responses from children in the more experimental studies and are important reminders that during infancy infants are deeply involved in communicative exchanges with caregivers. It is through such exchanges that infants develop an increasing repertoire of prelinguistic communicative forms, including gestures, imitation, nonword vocalizations, and affective expressions, which are the building blocks from which spoken language develops in typical development. As Nadel summarizes:

> Turn-taking, topic-sharing, understanding the other's intentions, negotiating shared goals through codes and routines, all these features of verbal language are prepared by the use of the imitative system. The imitative language can therefore be seen as a semantic foundation for verbal language, in the same way in which Donald (1991) describes the mimetic stage of humankind, compared to the stage of spoken language. (2002, p. 58)

INTEGRATION BETWEEN COMPONENTS

It appears that the development of the system that is involved in recognition of self–other correspondence is an integrated supramodal system so that at the behavioral level, similar developments are seen to occur in the vocal, motor, facial, and affective modalities. In real life these modalities are not as separate as they are described in psychology textbooks but together rather they are all used in social communication. One important question for understanding imitation and language development in autism is whether the fundamental impairments in social communication development lies at the level of these individual components (or modalities) or rather from deficits in the supramodal integration required for the components to function together. A recent brain-based model of deficits in interconnectivity between different systems that are recruited for complex problem solving (which would include social situations) might lead researchers interested in early social communication impairments in autism to design studies to answer this question (Just, Cherkassky, Keller, & Minshew, 2004).

There is some evidence that imitation of actions on objects and affective responsivity are also associated in autism. Charman and colleagues (1997) found impairments in both action imitation and an impoverished response to a display of feigned distress in toddlers with autism and Dawson, Meltzoff, Osterling, Rinaldi, and Brown (1998; statistical association cited in Gopnik, Capps, & Meltzoff, 2000) found that performance on tests of imitation and affective responsivity was associated in preschoolers with autism. To a large extent, investigations of imitation abilities and emotional responsivity have been conducted separately to date in the autism field. Emphasizing the value of studying imitation in a more naturalistic social context, Nadel and colleagues (1999) found that within a sample of school-age children with autism, the amount of imitative behavior was strongly associated with the amount of nonimitative social behavior. The development of experimental paradigms that include vocal, motor, facial, and affective modalities might lead to a clearer understanding of how "imitation" might fractionate (if at all) in autistic development.

In another study that examined relationships between these processes within a sample of children with autism, Rogers, Hepburn, Stackhouse, and Wehner (2004) found that object and oral imitation were associated with symptom severity and initiation of joint attention skills, unlike imitation of manual (nonconventional) gestures, which was associated with expressive language ability. This latter finding is consistent with an earlier study by Stone, Ousley, and Littleford (1997) who demonstrated some specificity of longitudinal associations from 2 to 4 years of age between imitation of body movements but not actions on objects with later expressive language skills. Perhaps as suggested previously, the social-communication system is more fractionated in autism, though whether this is due to impairments in separable components of the system or impairments in integrative processing remains to be determined.

LINGUISTIC PROCESSING: A WORD ABOUT SPEECH

Imitation of actions and gestures alone is not sufficient for (spoken) language acquisition and learning the acoustics of speech and an infant's exposure to socially modulating vocal partners and verbal imitation play an important role too (Kuhl, 2000). For example, contingent vocalizations by mothers promote speech production (Goldstein, King, & West, 2003), and speech discrimination at 6 months of age predicts language competence at 2 years of age

(Tsao, Liu, & Kuhl, 2004). The debate between Skinner's (1957) operant view of language learning encapsulated in his book *Verbal Behavior* and Chomsky's (1957) nativist, modularist position has been overtaken by empirical evidence that infants undertake a perceptual learning process during which they detect patterns in speech input, exploit statistical properties of speech input, and are perceptually altered by exposure to speech (see Kuhl, 2000, for a review). Vocal imitation links speech perception and production from early in the first year of life and auditory, visual, and motor information are all employed in speech comprehension and production. However, perception is not sufficient and a social interest in speech is also fundamental to language learning (Liu, Kuhl, & Tsao, 2003).

What do we know about linguistic and social processing of speech in children with autism? We know that social orienting to speech is impaired in young children with autism (Dawson et al., 1998, 2004). There is also some tentative evidence that children with autism show a selective impairment in the attention they pay to speech sounds (Ceponiene et al., 2003; Gervais et al., 2004) and consequent lessened activation of brain regions that process speech such as the superior temporal sulcus (STS). Notably, the STS is also involved in the detection of biological motion and mentalizing (Frith & Frith, 1999). In a recent study, Kuhl, Coffey-Corina, Padden, and Dawson (2005) demonstrated both a lack of preference to orient to speech (vs. nonspeech sounds) and a diminished ability in speech discrimination in preschool children with autism. Furthermore, these two abilities were directly associated with one another in the sample of children with autism. Whether the lack of social salience of voices causes or is a consequence of abnormal speech discrimination remains to be determined. Either way, lack of attention to voices in the early years may also have a negative impact on language learning in children with autism, and further work on speech and sound processing in individuals with autism is much needed.

COMMON NEURAL BASES FOR IMITATION AND LANGUAGE

Since the first report that a brain system, dubbed the "mirror neuron system," was activated in the area F5 of monkey premotor cortex both when a goal-oriented action is performed and when the same action is observed (Rizzolatti, Fadiga, Gallese, & Fogassi, 1996), there has been surge of empirical studies and theoretical accounts of this phenomena in apes and in humans (for reviews, see Decety, Chapter 11, this volume; Rizzolatti & Craighero, 2004; Williams & Waiter, Chapter 15, this volume). Further evidence has been forthcoming that the human analogue of F5, Broca's area (Brodmann area 44), along with other areas of the right anterior parietal cortex, serves a mirror neuron function in both human and nonhuman primates, in that there are neurons that are activated both when observing and performing the same specific actions (see Decety, Chapter 11, this volume). Building on theories that postulate that speech evolved from gestural communication (e.g., Armstrong, Stokoe, & Wilcox, 1994; Corballis, 2002), Rizzolatti and Arbib (1998) developed a theory that the mirror neuron system is the neural system from which language evolved. This has been more fully articulated by Arbib (2005).

Rizzolatti and Arbib (1998) and Arbib (2005) suggest that when actions-on-objects are observed, information is processed simultaneously through the dorsal stream (where the visuospatial qualities of the object and associated action are processed) and ventral stream processes where the familiarities ("knowledge" or semantics) of the object observed actions are understood. Arbib suggests that the two streams are integrated within F5/Broca's area. Further information about biological motion and intentional action is processed through the STS and inferior parietal area where intention can be attributed to the action. Arbib suggests that the mirror neuron system would first be used to imitate actions-on-objects involving the development of semantic knowledge associated with an action repertoire. This would lay the foundations for action imitation in the absence of the objects themselves leading to pantomime and gestural communication. This system then increasingly incorporated facial and oral action to evolve speech.

Therefore, according to this model, language evolved atop of a neural system that first served a reach-to-grasp function, then an imitation, a gestural communication, and pantomime function before, most recently, serving a spoken language function. If this model is correct, then language develops using the same imitative processes. New words are understood in terms of their associated "affordances" and intentions. They are assimilated into the repertoire through a self–other matching process that relates their use in the observed context to their use in the preexisting repertoire.

There is good evidence that language development is dependent on the "mirror neuron" system. Broca's area was well established as a brain region involved in various aspects of language processing from studies of patients with brain lesions, long before the neuroscience revolution of the 1990s, with lesions to Broca's area causing a characteristic aphasia of speech output with relatively conserved comprehension (Geschwind, 1970). However, there is also evidence that Broca's area is involved in the production and recognition of motor actions. Left-hemisphere brain damage causes apraxia, and an inability to copy novel actions can accompany aphasia (Goldenberg & Strauss, 2002). There is also convergent evidence that Broca's area is involved in the production of sign language and lexical retrieval for both signed and spoken language, although its role in sign language comprehension is less certain (Corina et al., 1999).

The suggestion that the mirror neuron system serves imitation, gestural communication, pantomime, and language leads perhaps obviously to the idea that it might lie at the heart of autism. The functioning of this system in individuals with autism is now under investigation and may yield evidence for a brain basis for some of the characteristic social impairments of autism (Williams, Whiten, Suddendorf, & Perrett, 2001, Williams & Waiter, Chapter 15, this volume).

Williams (2005) suggests that Arbib has misplaced his emphasis on the object-oriented as opposed to the social functions of language in developing his model:

> During early hominid evolution, the representations being pantomimed through gestural communication (including facial expression) would have been concerned with mental states, including feelings and desires. Facial and manual gestures were being used by individuals to express both their own feelings, and what they thought others were feeling. (p. 147)

IMITATION AND LANGUAGE IN DIFFERENT CLINICAL GROUPS

This raises one question that has been little studied. Is there something different about the imitation abilities, or the structure and functioning of neural circuits that are recruited in imitation and social cognition, in those individuals with autism who do not have delayed language development, in particular children with Asperger syndrome? Williams and colleagues (2001; Williams & Waiter, Chapter 15, this volume) suggests that there may be further brain areas that serve "mirror neuron" functions that do not involve language. Frontal areas such as that which Williams and colleagues identified as serving a self–other matching function in joint attention autism may be an example of such an area.

Experimental studies will have to be designed to test such questions and if possible using prospective designs with early diagnosed children with autism spectrum disorders, comparing early versus late talkers. This will be important to avoid the ceiling effects of simple imitation tasks due to the likely advanced IQ of the children with autism with better language skills. One possibility is that the brain basis for imitative impairment might be different according to the IQ and language abilities of the group with autism studied. This might explain the intriguingly discrepant findings from two recent structural brain studies that used very similar methodology. Boddaert and colleagues (2004) showed that STS affected the lower-ability group, whereas Waiter and colleagues (2005) found the higher-functioning group to show gray matter differences in frontal and ventral temporal cortex.

Another piece of evidence that links language and imitation is the recent discovery that children with specific language impairment (SLI) also have motor coordination, praxis and imitation impairments. In one study, even children with intact motor abilities as measured by the Movement Assessment Battery for Children (Movement ABC; Henderson & Sugden, 1992) were found to be as impaired as children with developmental coordination disorder (DCD) in the production of meaningful, representational gestures (Hill, 1998;

Powell & Bishop, 1992; see Hill, 2001, for a review). The types of errors made in such tasks by children with SLI included "spatial orientation" errors where the mapping between the gesture demonstrated and that produced is impaired, suggesting that intermodal matching of the motor action seen and the motor action planned and produced is impaired (Hill, Bishop, & Nimmo-Smith, 1998). Given the evidence (reviewed earlier) for a crucial role of mirror neuron systems in language, imitation, and motor control abilities, developmental neuroscientific approaches to research might be able to establish whether abnormalities in the structure or function of this brain region play a role in the genesis of SLI. Intriguingly, there is also evidence that the genetic risk for susceptibility to SLI might overlap with that for motor impairment, thus tying speech and motor development together even further back in the pathway from genes to brain development to behavior (Bishop, 2002).

CONCLUSIONS: NEURAL VERSUS SOCIAL APPROACHES TO THE IMITATION DEFICIT IN AUTISM

In autism we know at a behavioral level that imitation abilities are associated with language abilities, with several studies demonstrating that early imitation competence predicts later language competence (Charman, 2003; Charman et al., 2003; Stone et al., 1997; Stone & Yoder, 2001; see Williams et al., 2004, for a review). There is also good evidence that vocal and gestural imitation are both longitudinally associated with language development (Carpenter, Nagell, & Tomasello, 1998; Hepburn & Stone, Chapter 13, this volume; Masur & Rodemaker, 1999). We know that imitation and language abilities develop at a delayed pace in autism. What we do not know is whether these associations hold for the *same reasons* as in typical development or whether a *different cognitive mechanism* is at work. Further delineation of the brain systems that are recruited for different types of real and imagined imitated actions (on objects, of gestures, of emotional expressions) will be required in order for us to test out some of the provocative but potentially illuminating hypotheses that emerge from the active inquiry into the roots of imitation in a diverse range of scientific fields.

For example, in autism is imitation and language mediated at a neurophysiological level by the same mirror neuron brain systems as in typical development or might alternative neural systems be recruited over development for such purposes? Alternatively, are the same systems recruited but their operation is disrupted due to imprecise representation or slow or reduced capacity processing? Neuroimaging is making it possible to delineate differences between brain systems serving mimicry, goal emulation, and intention reading that will make it possible to see how these functions are differentially affected in autism.

There is also considerable remaining work to be done in terms of the experimental study of imitation in autism. Do children with autism with intact structural language development have a better facility for imitation of gestures and words? Can intervention programs that focus on the development of gestural, emotional, and vocal imitation improve language ability in children with autism? The fact that impairments in social motivation and social communication skills are central to autism means that the study of imitation abilities might yield evidence of where the fundamental impairment that underlies the disorder is seated. For example, does impoverished social motivation lead to impairments in processing speech sounds or does a basic impairment in processing speech sounds reduce social motivation (Kuhl et al., 2005)?

We need to pursue uncovering the underlying impairments behind the imitation deficit in autism using both the neural–cognitive and the social–ecological approaches. We can hope that the next 10 years of research yield some findings that will enable us to understand as well as to ameliorate the imitation and social communication deficits in autism.

ACKNOWLEDGMENTS

I am grateful to Suparna Choudhury and this volume's two editors for insightful comments on earlier drafts of this chapter and for discussions on this topic over the years.

REFERENCES

Adamson, L. B., Bakeman, R., & Deckner, D. F. (2004). The development of symbol infused joint engagement. *Child Development, 75*, 1171–1187.

Aldridge, M. A., Stone, K. R., Sweeney, M. H., & Bower, T. G. R. (2000). Preverbal children with autism understand the intentions of others. *Developmental Science, 3*, 294–301.

Arbib, M. A. (2005). From monkey-like action recognition to human language: An evolutionary framework for neurolinguistics. *Behavioral and Brain Sciences, 28*, 105–124.

Armstrong, D. F., Stokoe, W. C., & Wilcox, S. E. (1994). Signs of the origin of syntax. *Current Anthropology, 35*, 349–368.

Barr, R., Dowden. A., & Hayne, H. (1996). Developmental changes in deferred imitation by 6- to 24-month-old infants. *Infant Behavior and Development, 19*, 159–170.

Bates, E., Benigni, L., Bretherton, I., Camaioni, L., & Volterra, V. (1979). *The emergence of symbols: Cognition and communication in infancy.* New York: Academic Press.

Bates, E., & Dick, F. (2002). Language, gesture, and the developing brain. *Developmental Psychobiology, 40*, 293–310.

Bates, E., Thal, D., Whitesell, K., Fenson, L., & Oakes, L. (1989). Integrating language and gesture in infancy. *Developmental Psychology, 25*, 1004–1019.

Bateson, M. C. (1975). Mother–infant exchanges: The epigenesis of conversational interaction. In D. Aronson & R. V. Rieber (Eds.), *Developmental psycholinguistics and communication disorders* (pp. 101–113). New York: New York Academy of Sciences.

Bellagamba, F., & Tomasello, M. (1999). Re-enacting intended acts: Comparing 12- and 18-month-olds. *Infant Behavior and Development, 22*, 277–282.

Bekkering, H., Wohlschlager, A., & Gattis, M. (2000). Imitation of gestures in children is goal-directed. *Quarterly Journal of Experimental Psychology Section A—Human Experimental Psychology, 53*, 153–164.

Bishop, D. V. M. (2002). Motor immaturity and specific speech and language impairment: Evidence for a common genetic basis. *American Journal of Medical Genetics (Neuropsychiatric Genetics)*, *114*, 56–63.

Bloom, L., Rocissano, L., & Hood, L. (1976). Adult–child discourse: Developmental interaction between information processing and linguistic knowledge. *Cognitive Psychology*, *8*, 521–551.

Boddaert, N., Chabane, N., Gervais, H., Good, C. D., Bourgeois, M., Plumet, M. H., et al. (2004) Superior temporal sulcus anatomical abnormalities in childhood autism: A voxel-based morphometry MRI study. *NeuroImage*, *23*, 364–369.

Bruner, J. S. (1975a). From communication to language. *Cognition*, *3*, 255–287.

Bruner, J. S. (1975b). The ontogenesis of speech acts. *Journal of Child Language*, *2*, 1–19.

Capirci, O., Iverson, J., Pizzuto, E., & Volterra, V. (1996). Gestures and words during the transition to two-word speech. *Journal of Child Language*, *3*, 645–675.

Carpenter, M., Akhtar, N., & Tomasello, M. (1998). Fourteen-through-18-month-old infants differentially imitate intentional and accidental actions. *Infant Behaviour and Development*, *21*, 315–330.

Carpenter, M., & Call, J. (2002). The chemistry of social learning. *Developmental Science*, *5*, 22–24.

Carpenter, M., Nagell, K., & Tomasello, M. (1998). Social cognition, joint attention and communicative competence from 9 to 15 months of age. *Monographs of the Society for Research in Child Development*, *63*, 1–143.

Carpenter, M., Pennington, B. F., & Rogers, S. (2001). Understanding of others' intentions in children with autism. *Journal of Autism and Developmental Disorders*, *31*, 589–599.

Ceponiene, R., Lepisto, T., Shestakova, A., Vanhala, R., Alku, P., Naatanen, R., et al. (2003). Speech–sound–selective auditory impairment in children with autism: they can perceive but do not attend. *Proceedings of the National Academy of Sciences*, *100*, 5567–5572.

Charman, T. (2005). Why do individuals with autism lack the motivation or capacity to share intentions? *Behavioral and Brain Sciences*, *28*, 695–696.

Charman, T. (2003). Why is joint attention a pivotal skill in autism? *Philosophical Transactions of the Royal Society of London Series B—Biological Sciences*, *358*, 315–324.

Charman, T., & Baird, G. (2002). Practitioner review: Diagnosis of autism spectrum disorder in 2- and 3-year-old children. *Journal of Child Psychology and Psychiatry*, *43*, 289–305.

Charman, T., & Baron-Cohen, S. (1994). Another look at imitation in autism. *Development and Psychopathology*, *6*, 403–413.

Charman, T., Baron-Cohen, S., Swettenham, J., Baird, G., Drew, A., & Cox, A. (2003). Predicting language outcome in infants with autism and pervasive developmental disorder. *International Journal of Language and Communication Disorders*, *38*, 265–285.

Charman, T., & Huang, C. T. (2002). Delineating the role of stimulus enhancement and emulation learning in the behavioral re-enactment paradigm. *Developmental Science*, *5*, 25–27.

Charman, T., Swettenham, J., Baron-Cohen, S., Cox, A., Baird, G., & Drew, A. (1997). Infants with autism: An investigation of empathy, pretend play, joint attention and imitation. *Developmental Psychology*, *33*, 781–789.

Chomsky, N. (1957). *Syntactic structures*. The Hague, The Netherlands: Mouton.

Corballis, M. C. (2003). From mouth to hand: Gesture, speech, and the evolution of right-handedness. *Behavioral and Brain Sciences*, *26*, 199–208.

Corina, D. P., McBurney, S. L., Dodrill, C., Hinshaw, K., Brinkley, J., & Ojemann, G.

IMITATION IN TYPICAL DEVELOPMENT

(1999). Functional roles of Broca's area and SMG: Evidence from cortical stimulation mapping in a deaf signer. *NeuroImage, 10*, 570–581.

Dawson, G., Meltzoff, A. N., Osterling, J., Rinaldi, J., & Brown, E. (1998). Children with autism fail to orient to naturally occurring social stimuli. *Journal of Autism and Developmental Disorders, 28*, 479–485.

Dawson, G., Toth, K., Abbott, R., Osterling, J., Munson, J., Estes, A., & Liaw, J. (2004). Early social attention impairments in autism: Social orienting, joint attention and attention to distress. *Developmental Psychology, 40*, 271–283.

de Haan, M., & Nelson C. A. (1999). Brain activity differentiates face and object processing in 6-month-old infants. *Developmental Psychology, 35*, 1113–1121.

Donald, M. (1991). *Origins of the modern mind: Three stages in the evolution of culture and cognition.* Cambridge, MA: Harvard University Press.

Eckerman, C., Davis, C., & Didow, S. (1989). Toddlers' emerging ways of achieving social coordinations with a peer. *Child Development, 60*, 440–453.

Eckerman, C. O., & Stein, M. R. (1990). How imitation begets imitation and toddlers generation of games. *Developmental Psychology, 26*, 370–378.

Fenson, L., Dale, P. S., Reznick, J. S., Bates, E., Thal, D., & Pethick, S. (1994). Variability in early communicative development. *Monographs of the Society for Research in Child Development, 59*, 1–173.

Field, T. (1977). Effects of early separation, interactive deficits, and experimental manipulations on infant–mother face-to-face interaction. *Child Development, 47*, 172–177.

Frith, C. D., & Frith, U. (1999). Interacting minds: A biological basis. *Science, 286*, 1692–1695.

Gergely, G., & Watson, J. S. (1999). Infants' sensitivity to imperfect contingency in social interaction. In P. Rochat (Ed.), *Early social cognition* (pp. 101–136). Hillsdale, NJ: Erlbaum.

Gervais, H., Belin, P., Boddaert, N., Leboyer, M., Coez, A., Sfaello, I., et al. (2004). Abnormal cortical voice processing in autism. *Nature Neuroscience, 7*, 801–802.

Geschwind, N. (1970). The organisation of language and the brain. *Science, 170*, 940–944.

Goldenberg, G., & Strauss, S. (2002). Hemisphere asymmetries for imitation of novel gestures. *Neurology, 59*, 893–897.

Goldstein, M. H., King, A. P., & West, M. J. (2003). Social interaction shapes babbling: Testing parallels between birdsong and speech. *Proceedings of the National Academy of Sciences, 100*, 8030–8035.

Gopnik, A., Capps, L., & Meltzoff, A. N. (2000). Early theories of mind: What the theory can tell us about autism. In S. Baron-Cohen, H. Tager-Flusberg, & D. Cohen (Eds.), *Understanding other minds: Perspectives from developmental cognitive neuroscience* (2nd ed., pp. 50–72). Oxford, UK: Oxford University Press.

Gopnik, A., & Meltzoff, A. N. (1986). Relations between semantic and cognitive development in the one-word stage: The specificity hypothesis. *Child Development, 57*, 1040–1053.

Gopnik, A., & Meltzoff, A. N. (1987). The development of categorization in the 2nd year and its relation to other cognitive and linguistic developments. *Child Development, 58*, 1523–1531.

Henderson, S. E., & Sugden, D. A. (1992). *Movement Assessment Battery for Children.* San Antonio, TX: Psychological Corporation.

Heyes, C. M. (2001). Causes and consequences of imitation. *Trends in Cognitive Science, 5*, 253–261.

Hill, E. L. (1998). A dyspraxic deficit in specific language impairment and developmental coordination disorder? Evidence from hand and arm movements. *Developmental Medicine and Child Neurology, 40*, 388–395.

Hill, E. L. (2001).Non-specific nature of specific language impairment: A review of the literature with regard to concomitant motor impairments. *International Journal of Language and Communication Disorders, 36,* 149–171.

Hill, E. L., Bishop, D. V. M., & Nimmo-Smith, I. (1998). Representational gestures in developmental coordination disorder and specific language impairment: Error-types and the reliability of ratings. *Human Movement Science, 17,* 655–678.

Hobson, R. P. (1993). *Autism and the development of mind.* London: Erlbaum.

Hobson, R. P., & Lee, A. (1999). Imitation and identification in autism. *Journal of Child Psychology and Psychiatry, 40,* 649–659.

Huang, C. T., Heyes, C. M., & Charman, T. (2002). Infants' behavioural re-enactment of failed attempts: Exploring the roles of emulation learning, stimulus enhancement, and understanding of intentions. *Developmental Psychology, 38,* 840–855.

Just, M. A., Cherkassky, V. L., Keller, T. A., & Minshew, N. J. (2004). Cortical activation and synchronization during sentence comprehension in high-functioning autism: Evidence of underconnectivity. *Brain, 127,* 1811–1821.

Kuhl, P. K. (2000). A new view of language acquisition. *Proceedings of the National Academy of Sciences, 97,* 11850–11857.

Kuhl, P. K., Coffey-Corina, S., Padden, D., & Dawson, G. (2005). Links between social and linguistic processing of speech in preschool children with autism: Behavioral and electrophysiological measures. *Developmental Science, 8,* F1–F12.

Kuhl, P. K., & Meltzoff, A. N. (1996). Infant vocalizations in response to speech: Vocal imitation and developmental change. *Journal of the Acoustical Society of America, 100,* 2425–2438.

Liu, H. M., Kuhl, P. K., & Tsao, F. M. (2003). An association between mothers' speech clarity and infants' speech discrimination skills. *Developmental Science, 6,* F1–F10.

Locke, J. (1993). *The child's path to spoken language.* Cambridge, MA: Harvard University Press.

Masur, E. F., & Rodemaker, J. E. (1999). Mothers' and infants' spontaneous vocal, verbal, and action imitation during the second year. *Merrill-Palmer Quarterly, 45,* 392–412.

Meltzoff, A. N. (1988a). Infant imitation after a 1-week delay: Long-term memory for novel acts and multiple stimuli. *Developmental Psychology, 24,* 470–476.

Meltzoff, A. N. (1988b). Infant imitation and memory: Nine-month-olds in immediate and deferred tests. *Infant Development, 59,* 217–225.

Meltzoff, A. N. (1995). Understanding the intentions of others: Re-enactment of intended acts by 18-month-old children. *Developmental Psychology, 31,* 838–850.

Meltzoff, A. N. (1999). Origins of theory of mind, cognition and communication. *Journal of Communication Disorders, 32,* 251–269.

Meltzoff, A. N. (2002). Elements of a developmental theory of imitation. In A. N. Meltzoff & W. Prinz (Eds.), *The imitative mind* (pp. 19–42). Cambridge, UK: Cambridge University Press.

Meltzoff, A., & Borton, R. (1979). Intermodal matching by human neonates. *Nature, 282,* 403–404.

Meltzoff, A. N., & Moore, M. K. (1977). Imitation of facial and manual gestures by human neonates. *Science, 198,* 75–78.

Meltzoff, A. N., & Moore, M. K. (1983). Newborn infants imitate adult facial gestures. *Infant Development, 54,* 702–709.

Mundy, P., & Gomes, A. (1998). Individual differences in joint attention skill development in the second year. *Infant Behavior and Development, 21,* 469–482.

Nadel, J. (2002). Imitation and imitation recognition: Functional use in preverbal infants and nonverbal children with autism. In A. Meltzoff & W. Prinz (Eds.), *The imitative mind* (pp. 42–62). New York: Oxford University Press.

Nadel, J., & Butterworth, G. (1999). Immediate imitation rehabilitated at last. In J. Nadel & G. Butterworth (Eds.), *Imitation in infancy* (pp. 1–5). Cambridge, UK: Cambridge University Press.

Nadel, J., Guérini, C., Pezé, A., & Rivet, C. (1999). The evolving nature of imitation as a format for communication. In J. Nadel & G. Butterworth (Eds.), *Imitation in infancy* (pp. 209–234). Cambridge, UK: Cambridge University Press.

Papousek, M. (1989). Determinants of responsiveness to infant vocal expression of emotional state. *Infant Behavior and Development, 12,* 507–524.

Piaget, J. (1945). *La formation du symbole chez l'enfant.* Neuchâtel: Delachaux et Niestlé.

Piaget, J. (1962). *Play, dreams and imitation.* New York: Norton. (Original work published 1945)

Piaget, J., & Inhelder, B. (1969). *The psychology of the child.* New York: Basic Books. (Original work published 1966)

Powell, R. P., & Bishop, D. (1992). Clumsiness and perceptual problems in children with specific language impairment. *Developmental Medicine and Child Neurology, 34,* 755–765.

Rizzolatti, G., & Arbib, M. A. (1998). Language within our grasp. *Trends in Neuroscience, 21,* 188–194.

Rizzolatti, G., & Craighero, L. (2004). The mirror-neuron system. *Annual Review of Neuroscience, 27,* 169–192.

Rizzolatti, G., Fadiga, L., Gallese, V., & Fogassi, L. (1996). Premotor cortex and the recognition of motor actions. *Brain Research: Cognitive Brain Research, 3,* 131–141.

Rochat, P., & Morgan, R. (1995). Spatial determinants in the perception of self-produced leg movements by 3-month-old to 5-month-old infants. *Developmental Psychology, 31,* 626–636.

Rogers, S. J. (2001). Diagnosis of autism before the age of 3. *International Review of Mental Retardation, 23,* 1–31.

Rogers, S. J., Hepburn, S. L., Stackhouse, T., & Wehner, E. (2004). Imitation performance in toddlers with autism and those with other developmental disorders. *Journal of Child Psychology and Psychiatry, 44,* 763–781.

Skinner, B. F. (1957). *Verbal behavior.* New York: Appleton Century Crofts.

Snow, C. E. (1983). Saying it again: The role of expanded and deferred imitations in language acquisition. *Children's Language, 4,* 29–58.

Stern, D. N. (1985). *The interpersonal world of the infant.* New York: Basic Books.

Stone, W. L., Ousley, O. Y., & Littleford, C. D. (1997). Motor imitation in young children with autism: What's the object? *Journal of Abnormal Child Psychology, 25,* 475–485.

Stone, W. L., & Yoder, P. J. (2001). Predicting spoken language level in children with autism spectrum disorders. *Autism, 5,* 341–361.

Tomasello, M. (1988). The role of joint attentional processes in early language development. *Language Sciences, 10,* 69–88.

Tomasello, M., Carpenter, M., Call, J., Behne, T., & Moll, H. (2005). Understanding and sharing intentions: The origins of cultural cognition. *Behavioral and Brain Sciences, 28,* 675–691.

Tomasello, M., & Farrar, M. J. (1986). Joint attention and early language. *Child Development, 57,* 1454–1463.

Tomasello, M., & Todd, J. (1983). Joint attention and lexical acquisition style. *First Language, 4,* 197–212.

Trevarthen, C. (1974, May). Conversations with a two-month-old. *New Scientist,* pp. 230–235.

Trevarthen, C. (1979). Communication and cooperation in early infancy: A description of primary intersubjectivity. In M. Bullowa (Ed.), *Before speech: The beginnings of communication* (pp. 321–348). New York: Cambridge University Press.

Trevarthen, C., Kokkinaki, T., & Fiamenghi Jr., G. A. (1999). What infants' imitations communicate: With mothers, with fathers and with peers. In J. Nadel & G. Butterworth (Eds.), *Imitation in infancy* (pp. 129–185). Cambridge, UK: Cambridge University Press.

Tsao, F. M., Liu, H. M., & Kuhl, P. K. (2004). Speech perception in infancy predicts language development in the second year of life: A longitudinal study. *Child Development, 75*, 1067–1084.

Volterra, V., & Erting, C. J. (1990). *From gesture to language in hearing and deaf children.* Berlin: Springer.

Vygotsky, L. (1934/1986). *Thought and language.* Cambridge, MA: MIT Press.

Waiter, G. D., Williams, J. H. G., Murray, A. D., Gilchrist, A., Perrett, D. I., & Whiten, A. (2005). Structural white matter deficits in high-functioning individuals with autistic spectrum disorder: A voxel-based investigation. *NeuroImage, 24*, 455–461.

Werner, H., & Kaplan, B. (1963). *Symbol formation: An organismic developmental approach to language and the expression of thought.* New York: Wiley.

Whiten, A., Horner, I., Litchfield, C. A., & Marshall-Pescini, S. (2004). How do apes ape? *Learning and Behavior, 32*, 36–52.

Williams, J. H. G. (2005). Language is fundamentally a social affair. *Behavioral and Brain Sciences, 28*, 146–147.

Williams, J. H., & Whiten, A., & Singh, T. (2004). A systematic review of action imitation in autistic spectrum disorder. *Journal of Autism and Developmental Disorders, 34*, 285–299.

Williams, J. H., Whiten, A., Suddendorf, T., & Perrett, D. I. (2001). Imitation, mirror neurons and autism. *Neuroscience and Biobehavioral Reviews, 25*, 287–295.

Wittgenstein, L. (1953). *Philosophical investigations* (G.E.M. Anscombe, Trans.). Oxford, UK: Basil Blackwell.

CHAPTER 6

Does Imitation Matter to Children with Autism?

JACQUELINE NADEL

Little attention has been given to the motives that lead developing human infants to imitate. Although numerous recent and seminal works have been devoted to theorizing or demonstrating the developmental role of imitation in the building of social cognition (Meltzoff, 2002; Meltzoff & Gopnik, 1993; Tomasello, 1998), we do not know much about what exactly are the here-and-now benefits of imitating for a young human being. We do not know whether the adaptive benefits change throughout the preverbal period of the imitator's development and what is the nature of these changes, if there are any. As Roessler (2002) put it, "one may be forgiven the impression that imitation matters a great deal more to developmental psychologists than to infants" (p. 137). This is even more obvious concerning children with autism. Whether or not they are able to imitate is of concern; what their use of imitation might be is ignored.

One of the many reasons for the neglect of a functionalist perspective in the study of imitation is a mismatch between methodological and theoretical stances: Infants are claimed to be stimulus-expectant and goal-directed agents, but experimental designs are rarely embedded in rich and meaningful social settings where infants can develop their own purposes and choose between several ways to fulfill those purposes. There is nothing to expect in such settings, nothing essential to gain or to lose (except the experimenter's esteem). A direct adaptive advantage is not at stake. It follows that infants behave according to what they understand they are expected to do, not as they would have intended to do. They imitate because there is nothing else to do in the design presented, or because they are asked to do so ("do like me" procedure). Does it mean that imitation is of little importance in their real life? Certainly not. It just means that through instruction procedures it is not possible to capture the essence of what makes imitation adaptive: Imitation is highly selective. It is not an automatic reaction like closing the eyes in front of a collapsing object, it is not an ad hoc response driven by special circumstances. Those who are imitated often did not initiate their being imitated. Spontaneous imitation is at will. It is not an answer. It is a choice.

In this chapter, I focus on the selective production of spontaneous imitations during infancy. I show for instance that as early as 2 months of age, young infants select among self-propelled stimuli those that they will match. With older infants, richly embedded settings that are ecologically valid allow to document the function of imitation in everyday life throughout the preverbal period. Two- to 4-year-old children meeting same-age partners without an adult present, share common topics based on imitating each other's actions (Eckerman, 1993). Doing so, they may somehow disturb the definition of imitation given by Whiten and Ham (1992) and adopted by numerous authors: "Individual B imitates individual A when B learns from A some part of the form of a behavior" (p. 247). For, if the toddlers learn something while matching familiar actions, it is about anecdotal postures, about different procedural signatures via which a similar action may be achieved by different persons. This certainly does not constitute an urgent purpose for imitation.

Rather the benefit may rely on the fact that imitation here involves an audience. Toddlers take advantage of the fact that the two facets of imitation (imitate and be imitated) provide two roles. By alternating the roles of model and imitator, they use reciprocal imitation as a genuine communicative system where there is no need of an arbitrary set of symbols, where events resemble events in the real world, where, to follow Donald's (1991) definition of the mimetic culture of our ancestor *Homo erectus*, "perceptual events can be modeled in self-initiated motor acts" (p. 198). In a sense, prelinguistic children generate a mimetic culture of their own, restricted to their age peers, which will vanish forever as soon as language is mastered. The momentary functional use of imitation represents a remarkable example of a transitory adaptation that works as a precursor of more sophisticated adaptation to social environment via symbolic languages. It parallels at a developmental level the evolutionary stages of humankind suggested by Donald. It is worth keeping this in mind when considering the communicative resources of a nonverbal child with autism.

In the second part of the chapter, I describe our experiments using similar settings with children with autism. We see that among nonverbal children with autism, many have primary functional uses of imitation and strongly respond to being imitated. In particular, imitation is especially efficient as a way to establish close relationships with a child with autism. I explain the power of "be imitated" as linked to its effect on a sense of agency. Through being imitated, low-functioning children with autism start to understand that they can be at the origin of intentional actions of others, which may provide a social meaning to their behavior. Repeated imitative sessions improve imitation, recognition of being imitated, and nonverbal communication. Based on these findings, I suggest that appropriate stimulation of imitation can be used to enhance autonomous adaptive actions in children with autism. Robots can help in this attempt when human features are too difficult to face.

EARLY SELECTIVE USE OF IMITATION

One of the most fascinating questions regarding imitation concerns how early its selective use appears. Considering the neonatal preference for human movements over physical movement (Slater, 1998), the claim that imitation is selective of biological movements, and, more specifically, of humans' movements, appears to be perfectly plausible. Meltzoff and Gopnik (1993) exploit this idea when they hypothesize that newborns use a primitive ability of perception–action coupling to draw equivalences between what they see and what they do, thus forming the concept of like-me entities, a "primer" in folk psychology. To date, however, not much work has been devoted to test the hypothesis that early imitation is selective of human movements.

Our contribution to this question is to propose to young infants different categories of self-propelled movements to imitate and see what happens. In a study in progress, 48 infants ages 8 weeks were filmed in a counterbalanced order in front of a female stranger protruding her tongue and of a robotic mouth protruding at the same speed and for the same duration a tongue similar in size to a human tongue. Seventeen infants were also presented a human mouth with protruding tongue, with other parts of the face hidden.

The infants' behavior informed us about several aspects of an early selective use of imitation. It is worth noticing that there have been several previous attempts to investigate whether early imitation is selective of human features or rather elective of affordant stimuli. Jacobson's (1979) study is the most famous of these attempts. Jacobson presented a black pen moving back and forth, close to the infant's mouth. She found that infants ages 6–14 weeks protrude their tongue as frequently in front of the moving pen than in front of a moving tongue. However, several concerns can be raised regarding the experimental procedure. The movement of the pen was generated by a human hand, which possibly weakens the distinction between physical and biological movement. Moreover, the pen moving very close to the infant's mouth may have automatically elicited mouth opening and tongue protrusion. Legerstee (1991) presented to 8-week-olds a puppet protruding a tongue and showed that infants do not imitate in this condition. Ikegami's (1984) infants did not imitate tongue protruding from a mask simulating a human face, but the mask may have generated gaze aversion, as it equates a still face.

Our procedure differs from previous studies insofar as the robotic mouth is self-propelled and thus there is no human involvement in the movement of the tongue. In addition, parameters such as the size of the tongue, the speed, and duration of protrusion were controlled. All sessions started with a still period, and only infants who had no spontaneous tongue protrusion during this period were included in the experiment. The first group was presented a robotic tongue protrusion first; the second group was presented first a human tongue protrusion performed by a stranger, face visible. As illustrated in Figure 6.1, we found a significant difference between the two conditions for the same infants.

Remarkably, infants that did not imitate the robotic tongue protrusion first, did imitate the stranger's tongue protrusion afterwards, and only one infant did imitate the robotic tongue after having imitated the stranger. This documents the early selective aspect of imitation. Seven of 17 infants ages 2 months protruded their tongue in front of a human mouth, thus suggesting that face processing is a facilitator but not a condition of imitation of tongue protrusion. We now start working with a new televised design where only mouth and tongue are visible for robotic as well as for human models.

Another test of the selective use of imitation is given by 24 6-month-olds who were presented the three conditions of tongue protrusion: robotic, mouth, and face of a stranger. Only 2 of the 24 children imitated the human tongue protrusions. At the same period, however, 6-month-olds are capable to imitate simple actions with objects like tapping, pushing, grasping, and raising to mouth (Dunst, 1980; Nadel & Potier, 2002). For some authors it demonstrates that early imitation is an automatic response rapidly disappearing (Anisfeld, 1979; Hayes & Watson; 1981; Heyes, 2001; Masters, 1979). For us and other authors (see Butterworth, 1999, for a review), it shows, rather, that imitation is a selective phenomenon with evolving targets (which implies inhibition as well): If we propose the same stimulus to imitate throughout the first

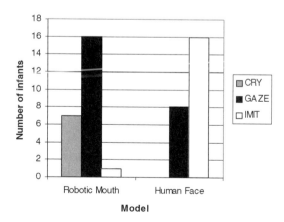

FIGURE 6.1. Two-month-olds imitate human tongue protrusion but do not imitate robotic tongue protrusion. The two exceptions found are due to previous imitation of human tongue protrusion. None of the infants imitated the robotic model when it was presented first.

6 months of life, we do not take into account the varying purpose underlying imitation and we certainly obtain a biased demonstration of imitation disappearance.

DIFFERENTIAL USE OF IMITATION ACCORDING TO CIRCUMSTANCES

Another way to highlight the selective aspect of imitation is to focus on its differential use according to circumstances.

At age 15 months, Gergely, Bekkering, and Király (2002) have given an elegant demonstration of a selective use of imitation. Adding a condition to Meltzoff's experiment with the magic box, they have shown that infants' imitation of a new procedure to fulfill a goal (i.e., light on a magic box with the head) is submitted to an examination of rationality. If there are other affordant means accessible to the infants (i.e., light on the magic box with the hands) but not to the experimenter (i.e., experimenter's hands occupied), infants use the simpler means and thus do not imitate. By contrast, if the simpler means are also accessible to the experimenter, the infants imitate the experimenter, as if they understood the experimenter's action as teaching a new procedure. This shows that imitation may be seen as an optional solution for a cognitive problem.

Another example of a differential use of imitation is the case of actions that fail to fulfill their goal. Meltzoff (1995) has shown that 18- months-olds understand intentions in others because they imitate the intended action rather than the failure of an experimenter. By contrast, Nadel has found that infants ages 18–24 months and even older infants imitate the failure acted by their same-age partner instead of the intended act (Nadel, 1986). This apparent contradiction can be explained by two different uses of imitation according to the circumstances. In Meltzoff experiment, there is a hierarchical relationship between an unacquainted adult and an infant. What the child understands is that there is a goal to achieve, whatever the issue of the adult's demonstration: The learning function of imitation is activated. In our experiments, there is no adult present, no instructions, and no hierarchical relationship between the infants. In this case, imitation is used as a mode of social interaction, a way to say, "I am interested in what you do, I am interested in you": The communicative function of imitation is activated.

To document the differential uses of imitation throughout early development, our group led a set of experiments (Baudonnière & Michel, 1988; Mertan, Nadel, & Leveau, 1991; Nadel, 1986; Nadel-Brulfert, & Baudonnière, 1982). Our interest for a functionalist perspective featured several specificities of our methodology. To study how, when, and at which end infants use imitation in their everyday life, we conceived an experimental setting designed in such a way that several purposes and several ways to fulfill those purposes were available. For instance, the infant could play alone with attractive toys, seek social company without the mediation of toys, and use toys to mediate their social encounters. The standardized experimental setting was embedded in a rich physical environment composed of 10 objects all in triplicate when three age-mates met or in duplicate in the case of dyadic meetings. Replacing the traditional asymmetric adult–infant dyad by a triad or dyad of same-age preverbal peers, we had in mind to evaluate the role of imitation when no instructions are given to infants meeting other infants without an adult present. How do infants adapt to a social environment via nonverbal communication? How important is imitation in such situations?

Because any definition of imitation is controversial, we defined imitation as performing similar actions while holding identical objects. Identical objects were supposed to label imitative actions insofar as they afford similar motor representations (Grèzes & Decety, 2002). We were able to show that the choice of an identical toy among all toys available is a good predictor of intentional imitation (Nadel, 1986). Using this setting and this definition of imitation, we compared the adaptive social behavior of infants facing infants ages 1–4 years. We obtained important information about differential uses of imitation. One set of information concerns the developmental changes in the use of imitation; another concerns how specific is the use of imitation as a communicative system.

IMITATION AS A COMMUNICATIVE SYSTEM: RISE, PEAK, AND DECLINE

After 12 months and up to 42 months, our group has shown that young children use more and more often imitation in a social context, especially in peer-age context. At 12 months, imitation of a peer-age partner was only 13% (mean % per child) of a 12-minute dyadic interaction session (Baudonnière & Michel, 1988); at 18 months, it increases to 25% (Baudonnière & Michel, 1988); at 21 months, it averaged 32% of session duration in triadic encounters (Mertan et al., 1991); at 30 months it came to a peak as a predominant means of exchange with 61% of the session time in triads (Nadel, 1986; Nadel-Brulfert & Baudonnière, 1982) and 70% in dyads (Nadel, 1986; Nadel & Fontaine, 1989). This selective use of imitation over all other nonverbal means of interaction declined abruptly a few months later with only 31% imitation in dyads of 42–46 months (Nadel & Fontaine, 1989), as Figure 6.2 shows. After 4 years, we noticed disappearance and even hostility toward imitation now considered as mockery.

The decline of imitation shown in 42- to 48-month-olds is of course indicative of a turning point in the use of imitation as a communicative tool. Eckerman (1993), observing groups in natural settings also acknowledged a peak of imitation at 30 months, and Abramovitch and Grusec (1978) in natural settings observed a progressive decrease of imitative behaviors from 2 to 5

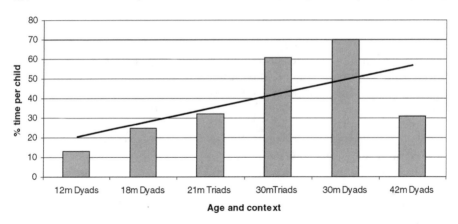

FIGURE 6.2. Evolving use of imitation as a communicative format.

years. More important, however, is that the decline of communicative imitation coincides with the mastery of language. How can we explain this coincidence?

Specific Use of Imitation as a Communicative System

We have claimed that, besides its use in cultural learning, imitation is also of use in preverbal communication. We have seen that the use of imitation for communicative purposes is a transitory one, increasing regularly from 12 to 36 months and then abruptly vanishing around 4 years. Such a developmental profile is in striking contrast with the lifelong use of imitation for learning purpose. Another main difference between the two functions of imitation concerns the goal to be achieved. We acquire our knowledge from more skillful agents: There is a hierarchical relationship between the imitative apprentices and the "teachers" (i.e., those who transmit knowledge, sometimes without any intention to do so). In the case of communication, any asymmetric relationship between partners immediately affects the ongoing interaction. What is at stake is sharing (Bruner, 1990). To learn, we have to anticipate and follow the intention of the model about a state of the world. What is at stake is an abstract relationship between means and end. The model is a vehicle of this relationship, nothing else, nothing more. By contrast, in case of communication, the benefit of imitation includes the two parties, the one who imitates and the one who is imitated. For imitation presents two facets that offer two roles: imitate and be imitated. The effect of "be imitated" has not a long history of developmental research, although Wallon (1942/1970) has given a thoughtful analysis of its role on self–other differentiation (see Nadel, 1994, for a review).

The interesting finding is that the infants take advantage of the two facets and alternate imitate and be imitated. This resembles turn taking, but it is more evolved than mere turn taking. Nine-month-olds take turns repeating their gestures after the mother has imitated them (Užgiris, 1984, 1989). Even 2-month-olds show reciprocal imitation when they face their mother live through our teleprompter design (Nadel, Revel, Andry, & Gaussier, 2004). The difference with role switching is that there needs to be an intentional engagement of the two parties to succeed in exchanging roles.

The intentional monitoring of role switching is highly representative of an understanding of others as subjects of a point of view. Imitation generates two points of view only. But these points of view are clearly opposite and exchangeable. They enable partners to get a similar phenomenological experience of relationships between action and perception. In other words, imitation affords the mechanism of shared motor representations. Last, but not least, alternating "imitate" and "be imitated" is a royal way to activate the difference between the by-product of self-agency (being aware that self-action is at the origin of what I see the other doing, when I am imitated) and the by-product of other-agency (being aware that what the other is doing is at the origin of self-action, when I imitate). Decety has elegantly and convincingly shed light on the mechanisms at the basis of this distinction. He has found a large overlap of neuronal activation in the two conditions, altogether with an important difference in parietal activation in case of imitation compared to recognition of "be imitated" (Decety, Chaminade, Grèzes, & Meltzoff, 2002; see also Decety, Chapter 11, this volume). When communicating via imitation, young children "play" at experiencing alternately the power of self-agency on other and the power of other-agency on self. Though far simpler than with a set of symbols, it resembles the pleasure of experiencing the power of mutually changing the other's mental state in the course of a discussion.

Let us add that children monitor synchrony, a major condition for shared experience, and build common topic via the use of identical items of an object (Nadel, 2002). We came then to the conclusion that imitation presents all the ingredients of a communicative system. It is generative and representational insofar as imitation creates gestural patterns that suggest sequences of events. It is intentional because imitation is self-initiated at will and is aimed at generating changes in mental states of others. But this communicative system is concrete, literal, and time-bound. It belongs to the episodic mentality theorized by Donald (1991) in our ancestor *homo erectus* and also in prelinguistic children. The arrival of symbolic language changes radically the means available to represent, recall, and suggest events. Why then keep such a heavy, rigid, and limited system to communicate? Communicating via imitation has no more reason to subsist, but it has had strong reasons to exist. Using imitation to communicate, children have gained the mastery of role switching, of self–other differentiation, of shared monitoring of dialogue, of sharing topics, of monitoring self-initiated actions in others, and thus of monitoring others' intention. If we can share topics via words is it not because we were previously able to share topics via similar actions upon similar objects?

Taking seriously the adaptive benefit of imitation for further communicative use of language, we now turn to investigate whether imitation may matter to nonverbal children with autism.

IMITATION AND AUTISM

Children with autism have long been said to be deeply and specifically impaired in imitation (DeMyer, Hintgen, & Jackson, 1981; Prior, 1979; Rogers, Benetto, McEvoy, & Pennington, 1996; Rogers & Pennington, 1991; Wing, 1976), but such a radical position is rarely held to date. There are two main reasons to be prudent in our statement on imitation in autism. A first reason of course is that there is no consensual definition of imitation. As thoroughly analyzed by Rogers (1999), "imitation is a molar construct" (p. 264) with such subcomponents as visual attention, cross-modal transfer, motor production, memory, representation, planning, representation of the body schema, and other capacities involving both cognitive and executive functions (see Gonzalez-Rothi, Ochipa, & Heilman, 1991, for a model). Rogers, Hepburn, Stackhouse, and Wehner (2003) call for "tasks that do not require children to imitate a model in order to perform the tasks, so that imitation and motor planning were not confounded" (p. 776). If we follow Smith and Bryson (1994), imitation may be rather diagnostic of basic problems in the development of action. Impaired imitation may also reflect problems of perception of movement (Gepner & Mestre, 2002).

As complex as it is, the construct of imitation is better understood if not considered as describing a unitary phenomenon but, rather, as resulting from a hierarchy of mechanisms involved in different types of reproductions that all react to the perception of goal-directed actions by the production of similar action. This leads many authors to now propose a continuum between low-level imitations that regroup all kinds of primitive matching behaviors and higher levels requiring motor representations, executive functions, and theory of mind. Our studies of infants of different ages show that while imitation of tongue protrusion declines and fairly disappears around 6 months, other and more sophisticated imitations continuously take place. High-level formats emerge from and are fed by low-level formats. This bottom-up perspective converges with current neuropsychological data that document the existence of a neuronal network accounting for shared motor representations indicative of a coupling between the action of an individual and the perception of another (Decety & Sommerville, 2003; Fadiga, Fogassi, Pavesi, & Rizzolatti, 1995; Jeannerod, 1997; Rizzolatti, Fadiga, Foggasi, & Gallese, 1996). It also opens avenues for the study and therapy of low-functioning children with autism.

Do Children with Autism Use Imitation?

Another reason to be prudent about the statement that children with autism are not able to imitate comes from the procedures used to assess imitation. Almost all procedures are instruction procedures and use a "do like me" instruction. There is no other purpose to fulfill in these conditions than to follow the experimenter's invitation to imitate or else to give up. Giving up does not mean being unable to imitate; it may also mean that the child does not understand the purpose of those imitations

Now, let us suppose that instead of eliciting imitation in a nonverbal child with autism via the classical request "do like me," you arrange a setting with two sets of identical objects, to generate similar affordant relationships between object and action, thus stimulating shared motor representations and favoring spontaneous imitation. Suppose now that one develops attractive actions without any request of the child. We will soon see even very low-functioning children picking up the similar object and attempting to imitate something. The elementary actions imitated are those of pushing, tracking, pulling, tapping objects, or turning a spoon in a cup. But lot of more complex ones are reproduced. Now we turn to imitate all the child does and we will observe mostly a change in the child's behavior, including intense gaze, smile, close proximity, or test of the imitator. We turn finally to demonstrate attractive actions, while asking the child to "do like me," and we will often find a change in the child's willingness to imitate.

We designed such a procedure as a three-step procedure. The first step, exploring spontaneous imitation, and the third step, exploring induced imitation, are composed of 10 comparable items with toys of similar attractiveness. The session lasts 12–15 minutes depending on how fast the child reacts to the experimenter's behavior. The exploration is still in progress. Three centers participated in the data collection. Sixty-five children with autism are now included in the study. We have computed the results for 36 of these children with autism, diagnosed according to DSM-IV (American Psychiatric Association, 1994) and the Childhood Autism Rating Scale (CARS; Schopler, Reichler, & Rochen-Renner, 1988). They are all ages 3–7 years and their developmental ages, as evaluated by Psychoeducational Profile—Revised (PEP-R; Schopler, Reichler, Basford, Lansing, & Marcus, 1988), the revised Binet–Simon scale (Zazzo, Gilly, & Verba-Rad, 1996), or the Kaufman Assessment Battery for Children (Kaufman, 1995), varied from 6 months to 65 months. All children with autism were able to spontaneously imitate at least simple familiar actions as 6- to 9-month-olds do. When the developmental age of the children was the criterion, instead of the chronological age, the developmental path of spontaneous imitation appeared to parallel the developmental path of typical young children during the first 2 years of life (Nadel et al., 2004). There was a significant correlation found between developmental age and scores of spontaneous imitations (Spearman rho = +857, $p < .001$).

Concerning imitation on request, however, the picture was heterogeneous: Some children who were good spontaneous imitators did not imitate when requested to do so and left the room, some had an equal score in the two conditions, and others who did not imitate spontaneously performed quite well when imitation was requested. Although not as informative as expected, these first results at least deliver the important message that elicited imitation only reveals part of the child's capacity to imitate. There was no significant relationship between scores for spontaneous imitation and scores for imitation on request.

Remarkably, children with autism displayed a selective use of spontaneous imitation: None of them spontaneously imitated meaningless gestures, which means that they did not display unintended and automatic imitation similar to echopraxia found in frontal patients (Lhermitte, Pillon, & Seradou, 1986). This suggests that scores of imitation on request give an incomplete appreciation of imitation capabilities, as they do not take into account the selective use of imitation.

Imitation recognition showed similar developmental steps in the 36 children with autism compared to typical infants. At a lower level of recognition, found after 6 months in typical infants, children with autism alternated visual control of their own movements to visual control of the experimenter's movements. More advanced indices of recognition included testing the intentionality of the imitator, like 14 months do (Meltzoff, 1990), or modeling playful behavior to meet the imitator's intentionality to communicate, as found after 18 months (Nadel, Guérini, Pezé, & Rivet, 1999). In all cases, the imitatee shows behavioral changes linked to being imitated. Those who did not test the experimenter but reciprocated imitation while smiling and approaching the experimenter showed an awareness of being imitated but probably did not understand the intentionality of the imitator. However, this basic response to being imitated is an encouraging first step toward an access to understanding intentionality. This was shown in a collaborative study with Field, Field, Sanders, and Nadel (2001). In this study, repeated sessions of being imitated during 1 week proved to significantly generate awareness/test of being imitated, increase imitation, enhance close proximity with the imitator, and decrease inactivity, as shown in Figure 6.3. These findings were recently replicated by Heimann, Laberg, and Nordoen (in press), who repeated imitative sessions three times in a day instead of a week.

How the awareness of being imitated can arise during repeated imitative sessions is to be linked to the discovery of self-agency. The early role of self-imitation ("ego imitation") in the development of agency has been recently grasped by Rochat (2002). Imitation of others combined with being imitated contributes to the distinction between perceptions caused by self and perceptions caused by the external world. Russel (1996) has highlighted the basic role of this distinction in understanding intentionality.

We tested the link between awareness of agency and the recognition of being imitated with 12 healthy young adults and 16 low-functioning children

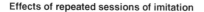

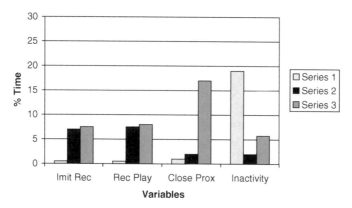

FIGURE 6.3. Effects of repeated sessions of imitation.

with autism who were presented two situations: (1) a situation in which they had to distinguish their own hand movements from prerecorded movements of another person and (2) a situation that they had to detect being imitated. Figure 6.4 illustrates the design we created to test awareness of agency (Libert, Revel, & Nadel, 2005). The subject is sitting in front of a table, hands hidden under the table, manipulating a wheel. Although reminiscent of Georgieff and Jeannerod's (1998) device, our design is simpler, because there is no assigned goal to the hand movements, and the prerecorded hand movements of another person are more easily recognizable as "not mine" because there is no concordance of goal and no synchrony of action.

The main strategy used by healthy controls to recognize self-generated hand movements consisted in systematically varying hand movements while gazing at the screen: 11 of the 16 children with autism showed this strategy, and stopped moving hands, like controls did, during the prerecorded session

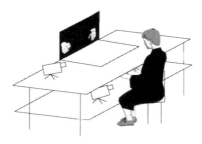

FIGURE 6.4. Device testing self-generated hand movements. From Libert, Revel, and Nadel (2005). Reprinted by permission of the authors.

of another's hand movements. Ten of these 11 children also recognized being imitated and tested their imitator. The five other children did not display any behavioral strategy and did not change behavior or express emotion during the prerecorded session, nor did they test their imitator or express any interest for her during their being imitated. The relationship between the two situations was highly significant and showed similar test strategies.

While acting, children with autism discover the external consequence of their action mirrored by another person. They perceive not only that they are the author of their actions but also that they are at the origin of the other's action, that they have a power over another person. But they have to perceive next that this power is restricted to the other's will, as the person is an agent.

A powerful test of the capacity of nonverbal children with autism to understand persons as intentional agents is our revisited version of the still face paradigm. (Nadel et al., 2000). The still face paradigm pioneered by Tronick (1982) is a three-episode situation in which mother first interacts with her infant, then poses a still face, and finally interacts again. The still face was designed to test whether young infants under 3 months of age are capable to detect noncontingent social behavior. A large number of studies using the still paradigm all converge to confirm the early sensitivity of the infant to mother's contingency. Interestingly, the still face design appears also to be a good tool to test other questions: When do children start forming a general concept of persons as interactive agents? Do low-functioning children with autism form such a general concept? To address these questions, we turned the "interaction–still face–interaction" procedure into a "still face–interaction–still face" procedure. Thus, instead of starting with an interactive partner, the session will start with a still partner, who will become animated during the interactive episode and will return to be inanimated during the second still face. Another difference with the classical design is that, instead of a close caregiver, the child will face a stranger. If children show negative reactions during the first episode of still face, in front of a still adult whom they have never met before, this means that they have identified the still person as an animated agent that should not be still and should behave contingently. If the child shows concern only during the second still face, after a contingent interaction with the adult, it means that he or she needs prior experience with persons before he or she will form expectancies about social behavior and willingness to share. Nonverbal children with autism involved in the pilot study and its replications (Escalona, Field, Nadel, & Lundy, 2002; Field et al., 2001; Nadel et al., 1999) displayed remarkably different behavior in the three episodes. They did not show any discomfort during the first still face of the stranger, reacted positively to her interaction during the second episode, and reacted negatively to the second still episode, initiating various attempts to make her interact again. A simple preference for animate stimulus will not lead the children to offer toys or to display positive social gestures toward the unacquainted adult during the second still face. An upset response to change will not explain why such children react positively to change from still to animate and negatively to change from animate to still. Taken together, these results rather show that low-functioning children with autism do not expect an unacquainted person to be a contingent agent prior to experiencing interaction with this person, but they can develop such expectancies after they have experienced the stranger as an interactive agent.

Other information provided by the revisited still face concerns the role of an imitative interaction: Imitative interaction was found to be a more powerful way of initiating emotional behaviors toward the stranger during the second still face than nonimitative contingent interaction (Escalona et al., 2002). Dawson and Adams (1984) and Tiegerman and Primavera (1981) had previously shown, in an experimental situation, the positive effect of being imitated on social gaze and motor activity. In our still experiments, being imitated led the children with autism to develop toward the unacquainted imitator affectionate initiations to interact, indicating that they understand her as an interactive agent.

Low-functioning children with autism produce spontaneous imitation assorted to their developmental level and linked to their own motives of action. They mostly recognize being imitated. Are they able to use the communicative function of imitation?

Eight dyads composed of a low-functioning child with autism and a low-functioning child without autism were observed in a setting with identical objects with no instructions about what to do. All children with autism imitated at least elementary familiar actions displayed by their partner. Some were able to imitate nonaffordant uses of objects with a communicative intent, as Figure 6.5 shows.

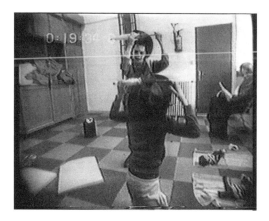

FIGURE 6.5. An example of the communicative use of spontaneous imitation in a dyad composed of two low-functioning and same-age children, one with a diagnosis of autism, the other not. This dyad was able to monitor synchrony and switch roles of imitator and imitatee.

Switching roles was observed in two dyads only. Those dyads were able to communicate fully via imitation. In the six other dyads, the child without autism never imitated the child with autism: The poor repertoire of actions displayed by the child with autism was certainly not attractive enough. Starting from these observations, we developed the notion of an ideal partner that will allow children with autism to exert the power of self-agency by displaying selective imitation, regardless of how attractive the child's behavior is. Robota, a doll-shaped robot designed by Billard and Mataric (2000) was considered as meeting this description. Robota mirrors the movements of the arm and head of the human partner but no other movements. Thus, the child with autism facing Robota can exert his or her capacity to recognize being imitated and select movements that are imitable by Robota (see Figure 6.6).

We suggest that the stimulation of spontaneous imitation and the recognition of being imitated can be used as a remediation to enhance autonomous actions. Imitation and recognition of being imitated develop when they are used. The enhancement of such experiences may be based on new technologies, such as robots or virtual experimenters. As first underlined by Dautenhahn (2003), robots are more predictable, more stable, and less complex than are human partners. Robots and virtual experimenters possibly meet more closely what children with autism can accept as a social environment. Another advantage is that they can be parameterized according to individual needs and can evolve in complexity in the course of a behavioral therapy

What is interesting in our experiment with Robota is that the children have to understand not only that they are at the origin of the movement of Robota (they thus have to develop a sense of self-agency), but also that a

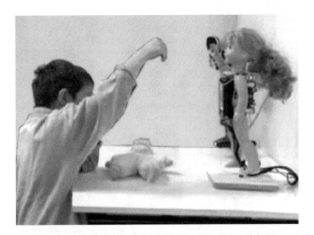

FIGURE 6.6. A child with autism moving his arm so as to be imitated by Robota.

unique category of movements can enhance Robota's movement (they have thus to develop intentional selection of own movements).

CONCLUDING COMMENTS

Does imitation matter to young children? Does imitation matter to children with autism? In an attempt to address these questions, we have designed ecologically valid settings allowing normal and clinical populations of children to behave as goal-directed agents that develop their own purposes, choose between several ways to fulfill those purposes, and build a context for their intended behavior. When possible, the examination of functional uses of imitation is facilitated by the presence of same-age partner(s) coupled with the absence of an adult in the setting. These settings, however, are not free settings. They are standardized kindergarten spaces arranged in a standardized way with standardized sets of identical objects, to propose a large but similar range of potentialities for social exchanges to all children of different ages and status. Although children do not receive any instructions about what to do in this space, the physical properties of the space itself afford dynamic interactions that can mediate social relationships in several ways, among which is an imitative way. For instance, the choice to handle identical toys and to develop similar actions with similar items is at will. The modes of exchanges developed, their frequency, and their duration are then representative of the main ends and privileged means at a given developmental period.

There is a golden age for the use of imitation. This golden age starts around 18 months and ends around 42 months. During this period, imitation serves two functions: learning (specially focused on motor strategies and language acquisition) and nonverbal communication. The extended use of imitation for communicative purpose was revealed in our settings. We were also able to acknowledge the disappearance of this transitory function of imitation when language is mastered.

Preverbal infants and nonverbal children with autism are able to share motor representations of simple actions afforded by familiar objects, via imitation and recognition of being imitated. They can also take turns, alternately initiating imitation of actions or imitating actions originated from the partner. Children with autism select meaningful actions rather than meaningless ones when spontaneous imitation is concerned. Many low-functioning children can learn turn taking when turns consist of simply matching what the other does or performing a simple action for the other to imitate. Imitation can fill the gap between solitary motor representations of action and shared arbitrary codes that allow us to inform about what we have in mind. With imitation, what we have in mind is observable actions. Maybe the episodic mentality described by Donald (1991), time-bound, literal, concrete, is at reach for low-functioning children with autism via imitation. Numerous examples of their expressions of pleasure when imitated and of their spontaneous use of imitation tend to support this hypothesis.

REFERENCES

Abramovitch, R., & Grusec, R. (1978). Peer imitation in a natural setting. *Child Development*, *49*, 60–65.

American Psychiatric Association. (1994). *Diagnostic and statistical manual of mental disorders* (4th ed.). Washington, DC: Author.

Anisfeld, M. (1979). Interpreting "imitative" responses in early infancy. *Science*, *205*, 214–215.

Baudonnière, P.-M., & Michel, J. (1988). L'imitation entre enfants au cours de la seconde anneé. *Psychologie Française*, *33*(1), 29–35.

Billard, A., & Mataric, M. (2000). Learning human arm movement by imitation: Evaluation of a biologically inspired connectionnist architecture. In *Proceedings of the First IEEE-RAS International Conference on Humanoid Robotics*. Cambridge, MA: MIT Press.

Bruner, J. (1990). *Acts of meaning*. Cambridge, MA: Harvard University Press.

Butterworth, G. (1999). Neonatal imitation: Existence, mechanisms and motives. In J. Nadel & G. Butterworth (Eds.), *Imitation in infancy* (pp. 63–88). Cambridge, UK: Cambridge University Press.

Dautenhahn, K. (2003). Roles and functions of robots in human society. Implications from research in autism therapy. *Robotica*, *21*, 443–452.

Dawson, G., & Adams, A. (1984). Imitation and social responsiveness in autistic children. *Journal of Abnormal Child Psychology*, *12*, 200–226.

Decety, J., Chaminade, T., Grèzes, J., & Meltzoff, A. (2002). A PET exploration of the neural mechanisms involved in reciprocal imitation. *NeuroImage*, *15*, 265–272.

Decety, J., & Sommerville, J. (2003). Shared representations between self and others: A social cognitive neuroscience view. *Trends in Cognitive Science*, *7*, 527–533.

DeMyer, M., Hintgen, J., & Jackson, R. (1981). Infantile autism reviewed: A decade of research. *Schizophrenia Bulletin*, *7*, 388–449.

Donald, M. (1991). *Origins of the modern mind*. Cambridge, MA: Harvard University Press.

Dunst, C. J. (1980). *A clinical and educational manual for use with the Užgiris and Hunt Scales of Infant Psychological Development*. Baltimore: University Park Press.

Eckerman, C. (1993). Imitation and toddlers' achievement of co-ordinated action with others. In J. Nadel & L. Camaioni (Eds.), *New perspectives in early communicative development* (pp. 116–138). London: Routledge.

Escalona, A., Field, T., Nadel, J., & Lundy, B. (2002). Imitation effects on children with autism. *Journal of Autism and Developmental Disorders*, *32*(2), 141–144.

Fadiga, L., Fogassi, L., Pavesi, G., & Rizzolatti, G. (1995). Motor facilitation during action observation: A magnetic simulation study. *Journal of Neurophysiology*, *73*, 2608–2611.

Field, T., Field, T., Sanders, C., & Nadel, J. (2001). Children with autism display more social behaviors after repeated imitation sessions. *Autism*, *5*(3), 317–323.

Georgieff, N., & Jeannerod, M. (1998). Beyond consciousness of external reality: A who system for consciousness of action and self-consciousness. *Consciousness and Cognition*, *7*, 465–477.

Gepner, B., & Mestre, D. (2002). Rapid visual–motion integration deficit in autism. *Trends in Cognitive Science*, *6*, 455.

Gergely, G., Bekkering, H., & Király, I. (2002). Rational imitation in preverbal infant. *Nature, 415,* 755.

Gonzalez-Rothi, L., Ochipa, C., & Heilman, K. (1991). A cognitive neuropsychological model of limb praxis. *Cognitive Neuropsychology, 8,* 443–458.

Grèzes, J., & Decety, J. (2002). Does visual perception of object afford action? Evidence from a neuroimaging study. *Neuropsychologia, 40,* 212–222.

Hayes, L., & Watson, J. (1981). Neonatal imitation: Fact or artefact? *Developmental Psychology, 17,* 655–660.

Heimann, M., Laberg, K., & Nordoen, B. (in press). Imitative interaction increases social interest and elicited imitation in nonverbal children with autism. *Infant and Child Development.*

Heyes, C. (2001). Causes and consequences of imitation. *Trends in Cognitive Sciences, 5,* 253–261.

Ikegami, K. (1984). Experimental analysis of stimulus factors in tongue protruding imitation in early infancy. *Japonese Journal of Educational Psychology, 32,* 117–127.

Jacobson, S. W. (1979). Matching behavior in the young infant. *Child Development, 50,* 425–430.

Jeannerod, M. (1997). *The cognitive neuroscience of action.* New York: Blackwell.

Kaufman, A. (Ed.). (1995). *L'examen psychologique de l'enfant K-ABC.* Paris: Editions La Pensée Sauvage.

Legerstee, M. (1991). The role of person and object in eliciting early imitation. *Journal of Experimental Child Psychology, 51,* 423–433.

Lhermitte, F., Pillon, B., & Seradou, M. (1986). Human autonomy and the frontal lobes. Part I: Imitation and utilization behavior: A neuropsychological study of 75 patients. *Annals of Neurology, 19,* 326–334.

Libert, G., Revel, A., & Nadel, J. (2005). *The development of a sense of agency: Its relationship with imitation recognition in low functioning children with autism.* Paper presented at the biennial meeting of the Society for Research in Child Development, Atlanta, GA.

Masters, J. (1979). Interpreting "imitative" responses in early infancy. *Science, 205,* 215.

Meltzoff, A. (1990). Foundations for developing a concept of self: The role of imitation in relating self to other and the value of social mirroring, social modeling and self-practice in infancy. In D. Cicchetti & M. Beeghly (Eds.), *The self in transition: Infancy to childhood* (pp. 139–164). Chicago: University of Chicago Press.

Meltzoff, A. (1995). Understanding the intention of others: Re-enactment of intended acts: by 18-month-old children. *Developmental Psychology, 31,* 838–850.

Meltzoff, A. N. (2002). Elements of a developmental theory of imitation. In A. N. Meltzoff & W. Prinz (Eds.), *The imitative mind: Development, evolution and brain bases* (pp. 19–41). Cambridge, UK: Cambridge University Press.

Meltzoff, A. N., & Gopnik, A. (1993). The role of imitation in understanding persons and developing a theory of mind. In S. Baron-Cohen, H. Flusberg, & D. J. Cohen (Eds.), *Understanding other minds: Perspectives from autism* (pp. 335–366). Oxford, UK: Oxford University Press.

Mertan, B., Nadel, J., & Leveau, H. (1991). The effect of an adult presence on communicable behavior among toddlers. In J. Nadel & L. Camaioni (Eds.), *New perspectives in early communicative development* (pp. 190–201). London: Routledge.

Nadel, J. (1986). *Imitation et communication entre jeunes enfants.* Paris: Presses Universitaires de France.

Nadel, J. (1994). The development of communication: Wallon's framework and influence. In A. Vyt, H. Bloch, & M. Bornstein (Eds.), *Early child development in the French tradition* (pp. 177–189). Hillsdale, NJ: Erlbaum.

Nadel, J. (2002). Imitation and imitation recognition: Functional use in preverbal infants and nonverbal children with autism. In A. N. Meltzoff & W. Prinz (Eds.), *The imitative mind: Development, evolution and brain bases* (pp. 42–62). Cambridge, UK: Cambridge University Press.

Nadel, J., Croué, S., Mattlinger, M.-J., Canet, P., Hudelot, C., Lecuyer, C., et al. (2000). Do autistic children have expectancies about the social behaviour of unfamiliar people?: A pilot study with the still face paradigm. *Autism, 2,* 133–145.

Nadel, J., & Fontaine, A.-M. (1989). Communicating by imitation: A developmental and comparative perspective. In B. H. Schneider, G. Attili, J. Nadel, & R. P. Weissberg (Eds.), *Social competence in developmental perspective* (pp. 131–166). Dordrecht: Kluwer.

Nadel, J., Guérini, C., Pezé, A., & Rivet, C. (1999).The evolving nature of imitation as a format for communication. In J. Nadel & G. Butterworth (Eds.), *Imitation in infancy* (pp. 209–234). Cambridge, UK: Cambridge University Press.

Nadel, J., & Potier, C. (2002). Imiter et être imité dans le développement de l'intentionnalité. In J. Nadel & J. Decety (Eds.), *Imiter pour découvrir l'humain* (pp. 83–104). Paris: Presses Universitaires de France.

Nadel, J., Revel, A., Andry, P., & Gaussier, P. (2004). Toward communication: First imitations in infants, low-functioning children with autism and robots. *Interaction Studies: Social Behaviour and Communication in Biological and Artificial Systems, 5*(1), 45–74.

Nadel-Brulfert, J., & Baudonnière, P. M. (1982). The social function of reciprocal imitation in 2-year-old peers. *International Journal of Behavioral Development, 5,* 95–109.

Prior, M. (1979). Cognitive abilities and disabilities in infantile autism: A review. *Journal of Abnormal Child Psychology, 7,* 357–380.

Rizzolatti, G., Fadiga, L., Fogassi, L., & Gallese, V. (1996). Premotor cortex and the recognition of motor actions. *Brain Research: Cognitive Brain Research, 3,* 131–141.

Rochat, P. (2002). Ego function of early imitation. In A. N. Meltzoff & W. Prinz (Eds.), *The imitative mind: Development, evolution and brain bases.* Cambridge, MA: Cambridge University Press.

Roessler, J. (2002). Some reasons to link imitation and imitation recognition to TOM: Reply to Jacqueline Nadel. In J. Dokic & J. Proust (Eds.), *Simulation and knowledge of action* (pp. 137–149). Amsterdam: John Benjamins.

Rogers, S. (1999). An examination of the imitation deficit in autism. In J. Nadel & G. Butterworth (Eds.), *Imitation in infancy* (pp. 254–283). Cambridge, UK: Cambridge University Press.

Rogers, S., Bennetto, L., McEvoy, R., & Pennington, B. (1996). Imitation and pantomime in high-functioning adolescents with autism spectrum disorders. *Child Development, 67,* 2060–2073.

Rogers, S., Hepburn, S., Stackhouse, T., & Wehner, E. (2003). Imitation performance in toddlers with autism and those with other developmental disorders. *Journal of Child Psychology and Psychiatry, 44*(5), 763–781.

Rogers, S., & Pennington, B. (1991). A theoretical approach to the deficits in infantile autism. *Development and Psychopathology, 3,* 137–162.

Russel, J. (1996). *Agency: Its role in mental development.* Hove, UK: Erlbaum.

Schopler, E., Reichler, R. J., Basford, A., Lansing, M. D., & Marcus, I. M. (1988). *Individual Psycho-Educational Profile.* Austin, TX: Pro-Ed.

Schopler E., Reichler R. J., & Rochen-Renner, B. (1988). *The Childhood Autism Rating Scale (CARS).* Chapel Hill, NC: Western Psychological Services.

Slater, A. (1998). *Perceptual development.* Hove, UK: Psychology Press.

Smith, I., & Bryson, S. (1994). Imitation and action in autism: A critical review. *Psychological Bulletin, 116*, 259–276.

Tiegerman, E., & Primavera, L. (1981). Object manipulation: An interactional strategy with autistic children. *Journal of Autism and Developmental Disorders, 11*, 427–438.

Tomasello, M. (1998).Emulation learning and cultural learning. *Behavioral and Brain Sciences, 21*, 703–704.

Tronick, E. (1982). *Social interchange in infancy*. Baltimore: University Park Press.

Užgiris, I. (1984). Imitation in infancy: its interpersonal aspect. In M. Perlmutter (Ed.), *Minnesota Symposium on Child Psychology* (Vol. 17, pp. 1–32). New York: Erlbaum.

Užgiris, I. (1999). Imitation as activity: Its developmental aspects. In J. Nadel & G. Butterworth (Eds.), *Imitation in infancy* (pp. 186–206). Cambridge, UK: Cambridge University Press.

Wallon, H. (1970). *De l'acte à la pensée*. Paris: Flammarion. (Original work published 1942)

Whiten, A., & Ham, R. (1992). On the nature and evolution of imitation in the animal kingdom: Reappraisal of a century of research. In P. Slater, J. Rosenblatt, C. Beer, & M. Milinski (Eds.), *Advances in the study of behavior* (pp. 239–283). San Diego, CA: Academic Press.

Wing, L. (1976). *Early childhood autism*. Oxford, UK: Pergamon.

Zazzo, R., Gilly, M., & Verba-Rad, M. (1966). *Nouvelle échelle métrique de l'intelligence*. Paris: Armand Colin.

CHAPTER 7

Imitation and Self-Recognition in Autism
In Search of an Explanation

MARK NIELSEN
THOMAS SUDDENDORF
CHERYL DISSANAYAKE

The observation that children with autism are deficient in their ability to imitate[1] dates back over 50 years (Ritvo & Provence, 1953). Recent reviews have outlined experimental evidence that these children do not imitate in the same way as do typically developing children (Rogers, 1999; Williams, Whiten, & Singh, 2004; Williams, Whiten, Suddendorf, & Perrett, 2001). Yet, as the chapters in this book attest, considerable debate remains over how best to define the imitation deficit in autism and the basis of this deficit. In this chapter we review two possible explanations for the imitative deficit shown by children with autism. The first is that it may reflect wider problems in their socioaffective and/or sociocommunicative abilities. The second is that there is a diminution or disruption in their ability to match seen and felt sensations. We review old and introduce new research with typically developing children and children with autism to evaluate these explanations.

Infants have been shown to copy simple but novel actions on objects from 6 to 9 months of age (Barr, Dowden, & Hayne, 1996; Meltzoff, 1988a, 1988b). Hence, quite early in life infants can use imitation as a means of acquiring new skills. However, children can also imitate others' actions on objects as a means of initiating and sustaining interaction, something they may not do until their second year (Užgiris, 1981). To illustrate this point we begin with a review of the development of an important, but largely neglected, aspect of imitation.

THE EMERGENCE OF SYNCHRONIC IMITATION IN THE SECOND YEAR

Toward the middle of the second year, typically developing children begin to coordinate their own actions with the thematic specifics of a social partner's play, which helps generate and sustain ongoing interaction (Eckerman, Davis, & Didow, 1989; Eckerman & Didow, 1989; Nadel & Baudonnière, 1980, 1982; Nadel, Baudonnière, & Fontaine, 1983; Nadel & Fontaine, 1989). Children show a preference for engaging with objects that are similar to ones chosen by their play partner and tend to use the common object in a similar way. When this copying behavior is performed in concert with the play partner and the partners do not solely adopt one role but alternate between model and imitator, it is referred to as synchronic imitation (e.g., Asendorpf & Baudonnière, 1993; Nadel, 2002).

In controlled studies of synchronic imitation, an adult experimenter continuously models simple actions on a series of objects (e.g., tapping a toy hammer on the ground) to children who have a duplicate of the object available to them (Asendorpf, Warkentin, & Baudonnière, 1996; Nielsen & Dissanayake, 2004). To be classified as synchronic imitation, children must not only reproduce the actions of the experimenter but do so continuously and simultaneously for a certain amount of time. Using this approach, a recent longitudinal study assessed 86 toddlers for synchronic imitation at intervals of 3 months from 12 to 24 months of age (Nielsen & Dissanayake, 2004). Toddlers sat on a play mat opposite an experimenter. The experimenter took an object and offered the toddler a duplicate of the object. The experimenter continuously modeled an action for 15 seconds and then performed a second action with the same object for a further 15 seconds. This procedure was repeated on an additional three objects. Toddlers were classified as imitating synchronically if they took the duplicate object and, while the experimenter was modeling the action, copied him continuously for at least 3 seconds (following Asendorpf et al., 1996). The duration of the sequence was coded for as long as the toddler maintained imitation of the modeled action and continued to look at the experimenter at least once every 10 seconds. Hence, for each session toddlers could engage in synchronic imitation from 0 to 120 seconds.

When ages 12 and 15 months, the infants exhibited little to no synchronic imitation (see Figure 7.1). It was not until 18 months of age that they began to exhibit sustained imitative sequences, and by the 24-month session toddlers were spending approximately one-third of the 120-second episode engaging in synchronic imitation with the experimenter. This finding is consistent with earlier research showing synchronic imitation of an experimenter by 18-month-olds (Asendorpf et al., 1996). Together, these studies suggest that typically developing children begin to exhibit synchronic imitation by 18 to 24 months of age. There are further ways in which imitation changes over the course of the second year. Consider the following studies.

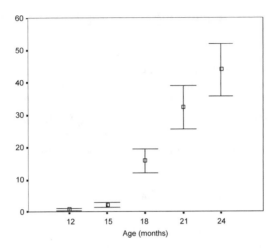

FIGURE 7.1. Mean duration (seconds) (and 95% confidence intervals) of synchronic imitation exhibited by the infants from 12 to 24 months of age. From Nielsen and Dissanayake (2004). Copyright 2004. Reprinted with permission from Elsevier.

COPYING OUTCOMES AND COPYING ACTIONS: DEVELOPMENTAL CHANGE IN TODDLER IMITATION

In a cross-sectional study of toddlers at ages 12, 18, and 24 months, an adult model demonstrated how a series of three novel boxes could be opened to obtain a desirable toy (Nielsen, in press). A different switch for each box had to be manipulated such that it disengaged a hidden latch and released the box's lid. In an experimental "object" condition, toddlers saw the model open each box by manipulating the switch using an arbitrary object (e.g., a plastic block). In this condition they could copy the model's behavioral means of activating the switches (i.e., use the object) or they could devise their own means (i.e., use their hands—something the model did not do). Two control conditions established that toddlers of all age groups could easily activate the switches by hand if shown how but that they would not spontaneously attempt to activate the switches, either by hand or by object, in the absence of modeling.

Surprisingly, when shown how to open the boxes using an object, 12-month-olds opened as many boxes as did 24-month-olds. However, examination of the results revealed that whereas the 24-month-olds typically attempted to open every box using an object, as was modeled to them, the 12-month-olds only attempted to open the boxes with their hands. Eighteen-month-olds showed reactions that were intermediate between the older and younger age groups. All age groups were equally successful at getting the boxes open, but because the 24-month-olds, and to a lesser extent the 18-month-olds, persisted in using the objects, their ability to activate the switches was diminished. With regard to achieving the modeled result (i.e., getting the boxes open), these children would have been better off employing their own behavioral means of activating the switches (i.e., their hands) and ignoring the actions used by the model.

In a subsequent study (Nielsen, in press), 12-month-olds did use an object in an attempt to activate the switches, but only when the model had success-fully used an object after first "attempting but failing" to activate the switches by hand. Thus, it appears that 12-month-olds did not fail to copy the model's object use because they could not use the object but, rather, because they did not interpret this action to be the most efficient alternative available (see also Csibra & Gergely, 2006; Gergely, 2003; Gergely, Bekkering, & Király, 2002; Gergely & Csibra, 2005).

When shown a model using an object to activate the switches, 24-month-olds persisted in using the object even if this action largely resulted in a failure to achieve the modeled outcome. The behavior of these toddlers is consistent with prior research showing that 2- to 4-year-old children will insist on copy-ing the behavioral means by which a model produced a particular goal, even if a more efficient method is available (Horner & Whiten, 2005; Nagell, Olguin, & Tomasello, 1993; Whiten, Custance, Gomez, Texidor, & Bard, 1996). In contrast, it was rare for 12-month-olds in the Object condition to attempt to touch a switch using an object; they used their hands instead. Thus, although these toddlers attempted to reproduce the result of the model's actions (i.e., opening the boxes), they did not copy the behavioral means used by the model (i.e., using an object). Surprisingly, it appears that 12-month-olds are more likely than 18- and 24-month-olds to devise their own ways of bringing about the outcome of another's actions.

To summarize, in these studies (Nielsen, in press; Nielsen & Dissanayake, 2004), unlike 18- to 24-month-olds, 12-month-olds do not synchronically imitate an adult model and they tend not to copy a model's specific actions (unless there is a logical reason to do so). A potential explanation for these changes in the way toddlers imitate is that through the second year the pri-mary motivation to imitate others' actions on objects changes from a need to fulfill a skill-acquisition function to a need to promote shared experience with others.

SKILL ACQUISITION AND SOCIAL INTERACTION: TWO FUNCTIONS OF IMITATION

As previously alluded to, Užgiris (1981) already argued that as children get older, their motivation to copy others changes according to two distinct func-tions of imitation: a cognitive function that promotes learning about events in the world and an interpersonal function that promotes children's sharing of experience with others (cf. Baldwin, 1894; Meltzoff, 1990; Meltzoff & Gopnik, 1993; Mitchell, 1987; Nadel, Guérini, Pezé, & Rivet, 1999;

Tomasello, 1999; Užgiris, 1981; Wallon, 1934). Užgiris suggested that young toddlers are primarily motivated to imitate in order to acquire new skills whereas older toddlers may imitate in the same context in order to satisfy social motivations. The emergence of synchronic imitation and "action imitation" (as opposed to "outcome imitation") in typically developing 2-year-olds may be due to these changes in toddlers' motivations to imitate rather than to changes in competence.

The actions we used in administration of the synchronic imitation task were simple (e.g., banging a hammer on the ground) (Nielsen & Dissanayake, 2004). Indeed, we noted that it was not uncommon for 12- and 15-month-old infants to reproduce the target actions of the experimenter during administration of the synchronic imitation task, but they did not copy the experimenter continuously and simultaneously. That is, they imitated but did not *synchronically* imitate. Therefore, the observed differences between the younger and older toddlers evident in Figure 7.1 cannot be attributed to changes in their ability to either produce or copy the modeled actions. Rather, if we accept Užgiris's (1981) argument, toddlers in the second half of their second year engage in synchronic imitation because they want to be social.

Užgiris (1981) also speculated that because young toddlers engage in imitation primarily to promote learning about events in the world, they will focus more on copying *what was done* rather than copying the *way it was done*. Older toddlers, by contrast, persist in copying the specifics of a model's actions in order to engage socially and to sustain interaction. This speculation is in line with the findings from Nielsen's (in press) study where 12-month-olds, unlike 18- to 24-month-olds, tended not to use the same behavioral means as another to bring about a modeled outcome.

Few studies have reported how manipulations in the level of social interaction provided by a model affect children's copying behavior. There is, however, some support for the notion that under certain circumstances children copy the specific actions of others to satisfy social motivations. Using an apparatus designed by Meltzoff (1988a), Gergely and Király (2004) had a model show 18-month-olds how to illuminate a plastic box by leaning forward and touching the top of it with her head. In one condition the model interacted with the toddlers and provided appropriate communicative–referential cues to accompany the demonstration (e.g., smiling, eye contact, and gaze shifting). In another condition the model was socially aloof and did not provide any communicative–referential cues. Toddlers who were shown the act by a socially engaging model predominantly copied her actions and attempted to illuminate the box using their head. Toddlers who saw a socially aloof model predominantly attempted to illuminate the box using their hands. Thus when the motivation for social interaction was reduced, 18-month-olds were more likely to reproduce the outcome of the model's actions but not the specific actions themselves (cf. Nielsen, in press, Experiment 3).

We are not suggesting that the instrumental function of imitation emerges prior to the social function. For example, neonates imitate a range of facial gestures, including emotional expressions (Field, Woodson, Greenberg, & Cohen, 1982; Legerstee, 1991; Meltzoff & Moore, 1977). As the actions that neonates copy are already within the newborn behavioral repertoire, it is not clear what sort of skill learning would be implicated in these acts. Indeed, Meltzoff and Moore (1992, 1995) argue that imitating is a powerful early means of social interaction. The social function of imitation is therefore likely to have been established well before the child's first birthday. What may happen is that around their first birthday children are making such rapid gains in motor skill development and in their ability to manipulate and understand the affordances of objects such that the skill acquisition function of copying takes temporary precedence (S. J. Rogers, personal communication, November 11, 2004). Copying in order to promote shared experience may then become more prominent as children develop other key social-cognitive skills during the second year, such as secondary representation (see pages 149–150) (Perner, 1991; Suddendorf & Whiten, 2001), joint attention (Carpenter, Nagell, & Tomasello, 1998; Corkum & Moore, 1995; Liszkowski, Carpenter, Henning, Striano, & Tomasello, 2004; Slaughter & McConnell, 2003),[2] and the capacity for reading intentionality into the behavior of others (Carpenter, Akhtar, & Tomasello, 1998; Meltzoff, 1995; Moore & Corkum, 1998; Repacholi & Gopnik, 1997).

What we wish to argue here is that children of different ages may imitate in order to satisfy different motivations. For some children, at certain ages and under certain circumstances, the prime motivation is to communicate and interact socially in order to promote shared experience with others. On the basis of this reasoning, one could expect that in children with autism, a disorder characterized by dysfunctions in social interaction, imitation should develop differently (e.g., Dissanayake & Sigman, 2000; Hobson & Lee, 1999; Moore, Hobson, & Lee, 1997; Sigman, Dissanayake, Arbelle, & Ruskin, 1997).

ACTION IMITATION IN CHILDREN WITH AUTISM

We have speculated that children with autism should show deficits in the exhibition of synchronic imitation (Nielsen & Dissanayake, 2003). However, no published research has used the previously outlined experimenter-elicited task to study synchronic imitation in children with autism (although see Nadel et al., 1999, for observational accounts). Given the "social motivation" argument outlined previously, children with autism could also be expected to focus more on reproducing the outcome of another's actions rather than the actions themselves. The two studies to have directly investigated this latter expectation have reported discrepant findings.

Whiten and Brown (1998) assessed imitation in adults with autism (mean chronological age [CA M] = 24 years, 8 months; mean mental age [MA M] = 6 years, 9 months), children with autism (CA M = 12 years, 1 month; MA M = 4 years, 9 months), children with mild learning difficulties (CA M = 11 years, 8 months; MA M = 6 years, 2 months), typically developing 5- to 6-year-olds (CA M = 5 years, 4 months; MA M = 5 years, 7 months) and typically developing 3- to 4-year-olds (CA M = 3 years, 4 months; MA M = 3 years, 6 months). They used a specially designed box (originally referred to as an artificial fruit; Whiten et al., 1996) that was kept shut by a series of pins, handles, and bolts, which could be disengaged using a range of manipulations that included poking and pulling. A desirable object could be retrieved once the box was opened. The participants were shown how the box could be opened using one of a number of possible methods. All participants attempted to open the box. Much like the 2-year-olds in the study by Nielsen (in press), although they could have devised their own strategies to open the box, both groups of typically developing children employed the method shown to them. In contrast, the children and adults with autism and those with learning difficulties were less inclined to copy the demonstrated method for opening the box. This finding indicates that the clinical participants did not focus on copying the specific actions used by others to bring about a particular outcome in the same way that the typically developing children did. However, more recent research suggests that children with autism do not always respond in this manner.

In a pilot study (Nielsen & Hudry, 2005) 17 children with autism and 9 children with Down syndrome were tested for imitation. As per the "object" condition of Nielsen (in press), an adult model demonstrated how a series of three novel boxes could be opened using an object to manipulate a switch. For each box we coded whether the children got the box open and whether they attempted to activate the box's switch using an object (as the model had done). The children were also assessed for communicative competency using the Communication subscale of the Vineland Adaptive Behavior Scale (Sparrow, Balla, & Cicchetti, 1984). Based on this score, the children with autism were divided into those with "high-functioning" communication skills and those with "low-functioning" communication skills. Our expectation was that the children with autism would respond in much the same way as typically developing 12-month-olds had done when tested on this task—they would ignore the model's object use and focus on opening the boxes using their hands. Contrary to this expectation, the "high-functioning" children imitated at ceiling (see Table 7.1). They opened significantly more boxes than both the low-functioning children and the children with Down syndrome. Furthermore, the high-functioning children successfully copied the technique used by the model—six of nine children opened all three boxes using an object. This finding may not be surprising given the chronological age and communicative ability of these children. However, although at lower levels than the high-functioning children, the low-functioning children not only opened some of the boxes but attempted to do so using an object. In fact, their copying behavior was similar to that of the typically developing 18-month-olds tested by Nielsen (in press). These data provide evidence that children with autism will copy not only the behavioral technique used by others to bring about a partic-

TABLE 7.1. Sample Characteristics and Copying Behavior of Children with Down Syndrome and Children with Autism

Condition	n	Chronological age	Communicative competency[a]	Mean number of boxes opened	Mean number of boxes where object placed to switch
Children with Down syndrome	9	72 months	31 months	1.77 (1.20)	2.44 (0.88)
"High-functioning" children with autism	9	69 months	46 months	2.78 (0.67)	2.67 (0.71)
"Low-functioning" children with autism	8	54 months	14 months	1.13 (0.99)	1.63 (1.51)

Note. From Nielsen and Hurdy (2005).
[a] As assessed through parent interview using the Communication subscale of the Vineland Adaptive Behavior Scale (Sparrow et al., 1984).

ular outcome but that they will do so at a level consistent with their communicative competency.

The reason for the discrepancy in the findings of Whiten and Brown (1998) and Nielsen and Hudry (2005) is not clear and more research into the tendency of children with autism to copy the specific actions of others is needed. Nevertheless, the results of Nielsen and Hudry provide preliminary evidence that children with autism can copy the specific technique used by a model in order to fulfill a social motivation like children without autism. This finding is in line with recent research demonstrating that although social responsivity is significantly correlated with imitation in children with autism, it does not contribute to the variance in imitation scores beyond overall developmental functioning (Rogers, Hepburn, Stackhouse, & Wehner, 2003). It is thus unlikely that any deficiency in imitation shown by children with autism can be solely explained by deficits in socioaffective and/or sociocommunicative functioning. Children with autism must display deficits in imitation for another reason—perhaps one more closely associated with dysfunction in cross-modal mapping.

THE IMITATION DEFICIT AND CROSS-MODAL MATCHING

It has been argued that the imitation deficit in children with autism may be due to a biological dysfunction that effects their ability to coordinate representations of self and other (Rogers & Pennington, 1991; Williams et al., 2001). A similar argument was put forward by Meltzoff and Gopnik (1993), who suggest that the deficits in imitation shown by children with autism may stem from an impairment in their ability to map externally perceived bodily movements to internal proprioceptive sensations. Meltzoff and Gopnik note that an impairment such as this could extend to the imitation of actions on objects as the acts of a model are seen from a different perspective than one's own acts.

In line with the aforementioned speculation, several studies have reported autism-related impairments in cross-modal mapping (Avikainen, Wohlschläger, Liuhanen, Hänninen, & Hari, 2003; Ohta, 1987; Whiten & Brown, 1998). For example, Ohta (1987) provided the first evidence of what has been termed "reversal errors." When shown a palm facing toward them, children with autism will copy this action according to their own perspective—they will hold their hand so that it also faces them. In contrast, age- and IQ-matched control children copy the action by holding their palm facing outwards. There appears to be a tendency for children with autism to copy the actions of a model according to their own perspective (and not the perspective of the model). This may be due to problems children with autism have in matching externally perceived movements to internal sensations, resulting in recourse to matching visual aspects of the model's actions to visual aspects of their own.

If the imitation deficit in children with autism is due to some form of cross-modal mapping, they should also show deficits in recognizing when they themselves are being imitated. That is, to recognize that they are being imitated, children need to appreciate that the actions of the imitator are in some way like their own actions. They need to match the seen actions of others to the felt actions of the self. To date, no deficits in this ability have been reported. Much like typically developing children in their second year (Eckerman & Stein, 1990; Meltzoff, 1990; Meltzoff & Decety, 2003), children with autism will repeat a particular gesture if it is being imitated[3] and they will look longer and smile more to an adult who imitates them than to an adult who does not (Dawson & Adams, 1984; Escalona, Field, Nadel, & Lundy, 2002; Field, Field, Sanders, & Nadel, 2001; Tiegerman & Primavera, 1984). These behaviors are not elicited to the same extent by an adult who acts contingently but does not imitate (Escalona et al., 2002; Field et al., 2001). However, no study has directly compared the responses of children with autism to being imitated with the responses of children without autism. Thus, although there is evidence that children with autism can detect being imitated, whether or not they do so in the same way as typically developing children remains to be established.

Many theorists have noted that there is a strong resemblance in the ability to imitate or to detect others' imitation of oneself and the ability to recognize oneself in a mirror (Gopnik & Meltzoff, 1994; Guillaume, 1926/1971; Meltzoff & Moore, 1999; Mitchell, 1993, 2002; Parker, 1991; Piaget, 1962; Suddendorf & Whiten, 2001). For example, Gopnik and Meltzoff (1994) suggest that in a similar manner to recognizing others' imitations of themselves, children use the correspondences between the proprioceptive sensations arising from their own bodies and the visual movements of their image in the mirror to recognize the association between their reflection and their own physical appearance. For Gopnik and Meltzoff, children can use "the perfect structural contingencies between their own proprioceptive image and the visual image in the mirror as a clue to the fact that even unfelt aspects of appearance . . . are part of the self" (p. 182).

The most widely used test of mirror self-recognition in young children is the "surprise-mark" test (Suddendorf, 1999) in which children are surreptitiously marked on a region of their face that cannot be seen directly. They are subsequently presented with a mirror and their reaction to the reflection is observed (Amsterdam, 1972; Gallup, 1970). While young infants tend to ignore the mark in the reflection, from around the middle of their second year children "pass" this task by investigating their own face in search of it (Amsterdam, 1972; Lewis & Brooks-Gunn, 1979; Nielsen, Dissanayake, & Kashima, 2003).

A number of correlational studies have reported positive associations between the exhibition of imitation and mirror self-recognition (Asendorpf & Baudonnière, 1993; Asendorpf et al., 1996; Hart & Fegley, 1994; Nielsen & Dissanayake, 2004). Hence, there is some support for the notion that imitation and mirror self-recognition draw on similar cognitive developments. However, as already noted, typically developing children can imitate others in their first year, well before they pass the mark test. Thus being capable of matching seen and felt movement cannot entirely account for the emergence of mirror self-recognition. Indeed, we have recently demonstrated that children also have to develop an expectation of what they currently look like (Nielsen, Suddendorf, & Slaughter, 2006)[4]. Nonetheless, when the opportunity to match across seen and felt movement is removed, such as in delayed video or photograph versions of the mark test, children have much greater difficulty passing (Povinelli, Landau, & Perilloux, 1996; Suddendorf, Simcock, & Nielsen, 2005; Suddendorf, 1999; Zelazo, Somerville, & Nichols, 1999). The ability to match their visual perceptions of the mirror image to their felt perception of their own actions may therefore be necessary but not sufficient for children's success on the surprise-mark test. By this reasoning, if children can pass the mirror version of the mark test they must be capable of recognizing the correspondence between felt and seen movements.

If the ability to match across seen and felt modalities is in some way disrupted in children with autism, one could therefore expect them to also show a diminished ability to self-recognize. In the following section we review such evidence, including new research on delayed video self-recognition.

SELF-RECOGNITION IN CHILDREN WITH AUTISM

A number of studies indicate that children with autism can recognize themselves in mirrors. As shown in Table 7.2, children with autism who are not severely cognitively impaired tend to pass the surprise-mark test (Dawson & McKissick, 1984; Ferrari & Matthews, 1983; Neuman & Hill, 1978; Spiker & Ricks, 1984). Their ability to self-recognize suggests that children with

TABLE 7.2. Details of Studies of Mirror Self-Recognition in Children with Autism

Study	n	Age range	% successful
Dawson & McKissick (1984)	15	4 years, 1 month, to 6 years, 8 months	87%
Ferrari & Matthews (1983)	15	3 years, 5 months, to 10 years, 4 months	53%[a]
Neuman & Hill (1978)	7	5 years, 5 months, to 11 years, 4 months	86%
Spiker & Ricks (1984)	52	3 years, 7 months, to 12 years, 8 months	69%

[a] The participants in Ferrari and Mathews (1983) who failed the mark test had mental ages below the developmental level at which many typically developing children recognize themselves and significantly lower than the children with autism who showed self-recognition.

autism can match across felt and seen modalities. However, the interaction provided by one's own mirror image is not identical to the interaction provided by another person. One's own felt movements and the movements in the mirror are perfectly matched (though inverted) both structurally and temporally. In imitation or imitation recognition the match between felt and seen behavior is by definition somewhat delayed. Thus, self-recognition of one's ongoing but delayed image would perhaps be a more appropriate analogue of imitation. We have recently investigated the ability of typically developing children to recognize themselves in an ongoing but 5-second-delayed video.

Thirty-six-month-old and 42-month-old typically developing children saw their video image on a large rear-projection screen (Experiment 3B, Suddendorf et al., 2005). By using dedicated computer software we were able to have the image of the children appear on the screen continuously but with a 5-second delay. That is, children could watch everything they did 5 seconds after it was done and test for contingency between their current movements and the movements of their image. By providing this opportunity for contingency testing, the setup contrasts with prior studies of delayed video self-recognition where children watch a previously recorded (e.g., 3 minutes old) video of themselves (Povinelli et al., 1996; Suddendorf, 1999; Zelazo et al., 1999). While viewing their ongoing but delayed video image, 62% of the 36-month-olds and 81% of the 42-month-olds passed an analogue of the surprise-mark test. Thus, this version of the test is clearly more difficult than the mirror version, which is passed by the majority of 24-month-olds, or live video versions, which are passed by about 30 months (Suddendorf et al., 2005). However, as just noted, the ongoing-but-delayed video test is easier for young children than tests using delayed, noncontingent video feedback (passed by about 48 months).

To establish whether children with autism can recognize themselves in delayed video feedback, we tested a group of 15 children with high-functioning autism (i.e., autism without associated intellectual disability) and a mental-age-matched group of 15 typically developing children (see Table

7.3), all between 5 and 9 years of age (Dissanayake & Suddendorf, 2005). All children in the control group passed this task. Eighty-three percent of autistic children also reached up for the surreptitiously placed sticker in their hair upon seeing the 3-minute-old video of themselves. The difference between the groups was not significant.

Children with autism can recognize images of themselves in mirrors and on delayed video. By implication we would expect them also to pass the slightly easier ongoing-delayed-video self-recognition task. However, this does not necessarily mean that self-recognition develops normally. In the aforecited studies of mirror self-recognition the youngest children were ages 3½ years (see Table 7.2)—and, as previously noted, the vast majority of typically developing children pass this task by 24 months of age. Similarly, in the study of delayed video self-recognition by Dissanayake and Suddendorf (2005) the children with autism and the typically developing children were between 5 and 9 years of age and performed close to ceiling. Pass rates may thus be due to the ages of the children tested, and it remains possible that children with autism are delayed in their development of both mirror and video self-recognition. Investigating self-recognition in younger children with autism is required to rule out this possibility.

This is important for another reason. Mirror self-recognition and synchronic imitation are part of a suite of cognitive developments that typically emerge in the second year of children's lives and are purported to depend on the development of a new level of representational capacity—the capacity to form secondary representations (Perner, 1991; Suddendorf & Whiten, 2001). Secondary representations permit children to hold in mind more than one model or representation of the world. For example, in pretend play, they have to represent the real world (e.g., mud) and the pretend world (e.g., a pie), and not confuse one for the other (i.e., not actually eating mud pies). Other expressions of secondary representation include passing tasks of hidden displacement, means–ends reasoning, understanding external representations (e.g., pictures), and understanding emotions and recognizing mental states (Suddendorf & Whiten, 2001). Children with autism show deficits in some realms of secondary representation (e.g., pretend play; Jarrold, 2003) but not in others (e.g., hidden displacement; Carpenter, Pennington, & Rogers, 2002). What we do not yet know is whether or not there is a developmental delay in

TABLE 7.3. Pass Rates on the Delayed-Video Self-Recognition Surprise-Mark Test

Design	n	Age (months)	% successful
3-minute delay	15 high-functioning autism	74–108 (M = 91)	83%
	15 typically developing	61–102 (M = 84)	100%

Note. From Dissanayake and Suddendorf (2005).

the emergence of secondary representation in children with autism. Testing across multiple realms of secondary representation in children younger than those previously tested would be required to answer this question.

Although there may still be some delays in the development of self-recognition, the finding that children with autism can pass both mirror and video versions of the surprise-mark test is problematic for any account of the imitation deficit that emphasizes a breakdown in matching felt to seen behavior. Moreover, recent research has shown that children with autism are able to integrate across visual and auditory modalities in speech perception (Williams, Massaro, Peel, Bosseler, & Suddendorf, 2004), providing further evidence that these children are unlikely to suffer from general deficiencies in cross-modal mapping. Although these data by no means rule out a developmental abnormality in matching in children with autism (e.g., a dysfunction in the mirror neuron system; Williams et al., 2001), they suggest that the apparent deficit in imitation in these children must be due to something more subtle than a disruption in their ability to match across seen and felt modalities.

CONCLUSIONS

Children with autism show signs of copying the outcome of a model's actions as well the specifics of those actions, of recognizing when they are being imitated, and self-recognition in both mirrors and delayed video. On the basis of these findings we have argued that the imitation deficit evident in children with autism cannot be entirely attributed to either social dysfunction or disruptions in their ability to identify a match between their own behavior and that of another (or that of their own image). It would seem that there must be some other reason for their imitation deficit. However, before any sound conclusions can be reached more research is needed.

Are children with autism capable of recognizing when they are being imitated in the same way as typically developing children? Experiments following the paradigm developed by Meltzoff (1990) are warranted. When assessed using the experimenter-elicited task outlined previously (Asendorpf et al., 1996; Nielsen & Dissanayake, 2004), will children with autism not only imitate an experimenter but synchronically imitate her as well? More research is also required into the tendency of children with autism to copy other's actions and outcomes. Do children with autism imitate a model differently depending on whether the model acts socially and interactively or is unsocial and aloof? Are deficiencies in imitation other than actions on objects (e.g., copying others' vocalizations or gestures) due to other causes entirely (e.g., a dysfunction in the mirror neuron system; Williams et al., 2001)? Are there delays in the emergence of abilities that children with autism have been shown not to be deficient in, such as self-recognition in mirrors and videos? Answers to these questions have the potential to better our understanding not only of imitation in children with autism but also of the normative development of imitation.

ACKNOWLEDGMENTS

Preparation of this chapter was supported by a University of Queensland Early Career Research Grant (No. 122524853) to Mark Nielsen and an Australian Research Council Discovery Grant (No. DP0208300) to Thomas Suddendorf.

NOTES

1. Although we acknowledge that debate remains over how best to use the term (Call & Carpenter, 2002; Want & Harris, 2002; Zentall, 2001), in this chapter we use "imitation" to refer very broadly to instances in which individuals reproduce actions or behaviors they have witnessed being produced by another (i.e., copying). Also, children can imitate many aspects of another's behavior, such as their vocalizations and gestures. We limit our discussion here primarily to the imitation of actions on objects.
2. It is nonetheless notable that the children assessed longitudinally for synchronic imitation in Nielsen and Dissanayake (2004) were also assessed for joint attention (Shafik-Eid, Dissanayake, & Nielsen, 2003) and we failed to find any reliable association between the emergence or exhibition of these two skills.
3. A captive chimpanzee has also shown these responses when being imitated (Nielsen, Collier-Baker, Davis, & Suddendorf, 2005)
4. We first established that 18- and 24-month-old toddlers were equally able to pass a novel leg version of the surprise mark test as they were at passing the standard face version (Nielsen et al., 2006; Study 1). We then demonstrated that when the reflection of their legs looked different from what they could have expected, children at these ages would typically fail the leg version of the mark test (Study 2)—unless they were given opportunity to update their expectations about what they look like (Study 3).

REFERENCES

Amsterdam, B. (1972). Mirror self-image reactions before age two. *Developmental Psychobiology, 5*, 297–305.

Asendorpf, J. B., & Baudonnière, P.-M. (1993). Self-awareness and other-awareness: Mirror self-recognition and synchronic imitation among unfamiliar peers. *Developmental Psychology, 29*, 88–95.

Asendorpf, J. B., Warkentin, V., & Baudonnière, P.-M. (1996). Self-awareness and other-awareness II: Mirror self-recognition, social contingency awareness, and synchronic imitation. *Developmental Psychology, 32*, 313–321.

Avikainen, S., Wohlschläger, A., Liuhanen, S., Hänninen, R., & Hari, R. (2003). Impaired mirror-image imitation in Asperger and high-functioning autistic subjects. *Current Biology, 13*, 339–341.

Baldwin, J. M. (1894). *Mental development in the child and the race.* New York: MacMillan.

Barr, R., Dowden, A., & Hayne, H. (1996). Developmental changes in deferred imitation by 6- to 24-month-old infants. *Infant Behaviour and Development, 19*, 159–171.

Call, J., & Carpenter, M. (2002). Three sources of information in social learning. In K.

IMITATION IN TYPICAL DEVELOPMENT

Dautenhahn & C. L. Nehaniv (Eds.), *Imitation in animals and artifacts* (pp. 211–228). Cambridge, MA: MIT Press.

Carpenter, M., Akhtar, N., & Tomasello, M. (1998). Fourteen- through eighteen-month-old infants differentially imitate intentional and accidental actions. *Infant Behaviour and Development, 21,* 315–330.

Carpenter, M., Nagell, K., & Tomasello, M. (1998). Social cognition, joint attention, and communicative competence from 9 to 15 months of age. *Monographs of the Society for Research in Child Development, 63*(4, Serial No. 255).

Carpenter, M., Pennington, B. F., & Rogers, S. J. (2002). Interrelations among social-cognitive skills in young children with autism. *Journal of Autism and Developmental Disorders, 32,* 91–106.

Corkum, V., & Moore, C. (1995). Development of joint visual attention in infants. In C. Moore & P. Dunham (Eds.), *Joint attention: Its origin and role in development* (pp. 61–84). Hillsdale, NJ: Erlbaum.

Csibra, G., & Gergely, G. (2006). Social learning and social cognition: The case of pedagogy. In Y. Munakata (Ed.), *Processes of change in brain and cognitive development. Attention and performance, XXI* (pp. 249–274). Oxford, UK: Oxford University Press.

Dawson, G., & Adams, A. (1984). Imitation and social responsiveness in autistic children. *Journal of Abnormal Child Psychology, 12,* 209–226.

Dawson, G., & McKissick, F. C. (1984). Self-recognition in autistic children. *Journal of Autism and Developmental Disorders, 14,* 383–394.

Dissanayake, C., & Sigman, M. (2000). Attachment and emotional responsiveness in children with autism. *International Review of Research in Mental Retardation, 23,* 239–266.

Dissanayake, C., & Suddendorf, T. (2005). *Delayed self-recognition in children with high-functioning autism and Asperger's disorder.* Manuscript in preparation.

Eckerman, C. O., Davis, C. C., & Didow, S. M. (1989). Toddlers' emerging ways of achieving social coordinations with a peer. *Child Development, 60,* 440–453.

Eckerman, C. O., & Didow, S. M. (1989). Toddlers' social coordinations: Changing responses to another's invitation to play. *Developmental Psychology, 25,* 794–804.

Eckerman, C. O., & Stein, M. R. (1990). How imitation begets imitation and toddlers' generation of games. *Developmental Psychology, 26,* 370–378.

Escalona, A., Field, T. M., Nadel, J., & Lundy, B. (2002). Brief report: Imitation effects on children with autism. *Journal of Autism and Developmental Disorders, 32,* 141–144.

Ferrari, M., & Matthews, W. S. (1983). Self-recognition deficits in autism: Syndrome-specific or general developmental delay? *Journal of Autism and Developmental Disorders, 13,* 317–324.

Field, T. M., Field, T., Sanders, C., & Nadel, J. (2001). Children with autism display more social behaviors after repeated imitation sessions. *Autism, 5,* 317–323.

Field, T. M., Woodson, R., Greenberg, R., & Cohen, D. (1982). Discrimination and imitation of facial expressions in neonates. *Science, 218,* 179–181.

Gallup, G. G., Jr. (1970). Chimpanzees: Self-recognition. *Science, 167,* 417–421.

Gergely, G. (2003). What should a robot learn from an infant? Mechanisms of action interpretation and observational learning in infancy. *Connection Science, 15,* 191–209.

Gergely, G., Bekkering, H., & Király, I. (2002). Rational imitation in preverbal infants. *Nature, 415,* 755.

Gergely, G., & Csibra, G. (2005). The social construction of the cultural mind: Imitative learning as a mechanism of human pedagogy. *Interaction Studies, 6,* 463–481.

Gergely, G., & Király, I. (2004, May). *The role of communicative–referential cues and teleological reasoning in observational learning of novel means during the second year.*

Paper presented at the XIV biennial meeting of the International Society of Infant Studies, Chicago.

Gopnik, A., & Meltzoff, A. (1994). Minds, bodies, and persons: Young children's understanding of the self and others as reflected in imitation and theory of mind research. In S. T. Parker, R. W. Mitchell, & M. L. Boccia (Eds.), *Self-awareness in animals and humans: Developmental perspectives* (pp. 166–186). New York: Cambridge University Press.

Guillaume, P. (1971). *Imitation in children* (2nd ed.). Menlo Park, CA: Benjamin/Cummings. (Original work published 1926)

Hart, D., & Fegley, S. (1994). Social imitation and the emergence of a mental model self. In S. T. Parker, R. W. Mitchell, & M. L. Boccia (Eds.), *Self-awareness in animals and humans: Developmental perspectives* (pp. 149–165). New York: Cambridge University Press.

Hobson, R. P., & Lee, A. (1999). Imitation and identification in autism. *Journal of Child Psychology and Psychiatry, 40,* 649–659.

Horner, V., & Whiten, A. (2005). Causal knowledge and imitation/emulation switching in chimpanzees (*Pan troglodytes*) and children (*Homo sapiens*). *Animal Cognition, 8,* 164–181.

Jarrold, C. (2003). A review of research into pretend play in autism. *Autism, 7,* 379–390.

Legerstee, M. (1991). The role of person and object in eliciting early imitation. *Journal of Experimental Child Psychology, 51,* 423–433.

Lewis, M., & Brooks-Gunn, J. (1979). *Social cognition and the acquisition of self.* New York: Plenum Press.

Liszkowski, U., Carpenter, M., Henning, A., Striano, T., & Tomasello, M. (2004). Twelve-month-olds point to share attention and interest. *Developmental Science, 7,* 297–307.

Meltzoff, A. N. (1988a). Infant imitation after a 1-week delay: Long-term memory for novel acts and multiple stimuli. *Developmental Psychology, 24,* 470–476.

Meltzoff, A. N. (1988b). Infant imitation and memory: Nine-month-olds in immediate and deferred tests. *Child Development, 59,* 217–225.

Meltzoff, A. N. (1990). Foundations for developing a concept of self: The role of imitation in relating self to other and the value of social mirroring, social modelling, and self practice in infancy. In D. Cicchetti & M. Beeghly (Eds.), *The self in transition: Infancy to childhood* (pp. 139–164). Chicago: University of Chicago Press.

Meltzoff, A. N. (1995). Understanding the intentions of others: Re-enactment of intended acts by 18-month-old children. *Developmental Psychology, 31,* 838–850.

Meltzoff, A. N., & Decety, J. (2003). What imitation tells us about social cognition: A rapprochement between developmental psychology and cognitive neuroscience. *Philosophical Transactions of the Royal Society of London B, 358,* 491–500.

Meltzoff, A. N., & Gopnik, A. (1993). The role of imitation in understanding persons and developing a theory of mind. In S. Baron-Cohen, H. Tager-Flusberg, & D. J. Cohen (Eds.), *Understanding other minds: Perspectives from autism* (pp. 335–366). New York: Oxford University Press.

Meltzoff, A. N., & Moore, M. K. (1977). Imitation of facial and manual gestures by human neonates. *Science, 198,* 75–78.

Meltzoff, A. N., & Moore, M. K. (1992). Early imitation within a functional framework: The importance of person identity, movement, and development. *Infant Behaviour and Development, 15,* 83–89.

Meltzoff, A. N., & Moore, M. K. (1995). Infants' understanding of people and things: From body imitation to folk psychology. In J. Bermúdez, A. J. Marcel, & N. Eilan (Eds.), *The body and the self* (pp. 43–69). Cambridge, MA: MIT Press.

Meltzoff, A. N., & Moore, M. K. (1999). Persons and representation: why infant imitation is important for theories of human development. In J. Nadel & G. Butterworth (Eds.), *Imitation in infancy* (pp. 9–35). Cambridge, UK: Cambridge University Press.

Mitchell, R. W. (1987). A comparative developmental approach to understanding imitation. In P. P. G. Bateson & P. H. Klopfer (Eds.), *Perspectives in ethology* (Vol. 7, pp. 183–215). New York: Plenum Press.

Mitchell, R. W. (1993). Mental models of mirror self-recognition: Two theories. *New Ideas in Psychology, 11,* 295–325.

Mitchell, R. W. (2002). Kinesthetic-visual matching, imitation, and self-recognition. In M. Bekoff, C. Allen, & G. Burghardt (Eds.), *The cognitive animal* (pp. 345–351). Cambridge: MIT Press.

Moore, C., & Corkum, V. (1998). Infant gaze following based on eye direction. *British Journal of Developmental Psychology, 16,* 495–503.

Moore, D. G., Hobson, R. P., & Lee, A. (1997). Components of person perception: An investigation with autistic, non-autistic retarded and typically developing children and adolescents. *British Journal of Developmental Psychology, 15,* 401–423.

Nadel, J. (2002). Imitation and imitation recognition: Functional use in preverbal infants and nonverbal children with autism. In A. Meltzoff & W. Prinz (Eds.), *The imitative mind: Development, evolution, and brain bases* (pp. 63–73). Cambridge, UK: Cambridge University Press.

Nadel, J., & Baudonnière, P.-M. (1980). L'imitation comme mode prépondérant d'échange entre pairs au cours de la troisième année [Imitation as a predominant mode for exchange among three-year-old peers]. *Enfance, 1–2,* 77–90.

Nadel, J., & Baudonnière, P.-M. (1982). The social function of reciprocal imitation in 2-year-old peers. *International Journal of Behavioural Development, 5,* 95–109.

Nadel, J., Baudonnière, P.-M., & Fontaine, A. M. (1983). Les comportements sociaux imitatifs [Imitative social behaviors]. *Recherches de Psychologie Sociale, 5,* 15–29.

Nadel, J., & Fontaine, A. M. (1989). Communicating by imitation: A developmental and comparative approach to transitory social competence. In B. H. Schneider, G. Attili, J. Nadel, & R. P. Weissberg (Eds.), *Social competence in developmental perspective* (pp. 131–144). Dordrecht, The Netherlands: Kluwer.

Nadel, J., Guérini, C., Pezé, A., & Rivet, C. (1999). The evolving nature of imitation as a format for communication. In J. Nadel & G. Butterworth (Eds.), *Imitation in infancy* (pp. 209–234). Cambridge, UK: Cambridge University Press.

Nagell, K., Olguin, R. S., & Tomasello, M. (1993). Processes of social learning in the tool use of chimpanzees (*Pan troglodytes*) and human children (*Homo sapiens*). *Journal of Comparative Psychology, 107,* 174–186.

Neuman, C. J., & Hill, S. D. (1978). Self-recognition and stimulus preference in autistic children. *Developmental Psychobiology, 11,* 571–578.

Nielsen, M. (in press). Copying actions and copying outcomes: Social learning through the second year. *Developmental Psychology.*

Nielsen, M., Collier-Baker, E., Davis, J. M., & Suddendorf, T. (2005). Imitation recognition in a captive chimpanzee (*Pan troglodytes*). *Animal Cognition, 8,* 31–36.

Nielsen, M., & Dissanayake, C. (2003). A longitudinal study of immediate, deferred, and synchronic imitation through the second year. *Interdisciplinary Journal of Artificial Intelligence and the Simulation of Behaviour, 1,* 305–318.

Nielsen, M., & Dissanayake, C. (2004). Pretend play, mirror self-recognition and imitation: A longitudinal investigation through the second year. *Infant Behavior and Development, 27,* 342–365.

Nielsen, M., Dissanayake, C., & Kashima, Y. (2003). A longitudinal investigation of self-other discrimination and the emergence of mirror self-recognition. *Infant Behavior and Development*, 26, 213–226.

Nielsen, M., & Hudry, K. (2005). *Do the means justify the ends? A new look at imitation in autism.* Manuscript in preparation.

Nielsen, M., Suddendorf, T., & Slaughter, V. (2006). Mirror self-recognition beyond the face. *Child Development*, 77, 176–185.

Ohta, M. (1987). Cognitive disorders of infantile autism: A study employing the WISC, spatial relationship conceptualization, and gesture imitations. *Journal of Autism and Developmental Disorders*, 17, 45–62.

Parker, S. T. (1991). A developmental approach to the origins of self-recognition in great apes. *Human Evolution*, 6, 435–449.

Perner, J. (1991). *Understanding the representational mind.* Cambridge, MA: MIT Press.

Piaget, J. (1962). *Play, dreams, and imitation in childhood.* New York: Norton.

Povinelli, D. J., Landau, K. R., & Perilloux, H. K. (1996). Self-recognition in young children using delayed versus live feedback: Evidence of a developmental asynchrony. *Child Development*, 67, 1540–1554.

Repacholi, B. M., & Gopnik, A. (1997). Early reasoning about desires: Evidence from 14- and 18-month-olds. *Developmental Psychology*, 33, 12–21.

Ritvo, S., & Provence, S. (1953). Form perception and imitation in some autistic children: Diagnostic findings and their contextual interpretation. *The Psychoanalytical Study of the Child*, 8, 155–161.

Rogers, S. J. (1999). An examination of the imitation deficit in autism. In J. Nadel & G. Butterworth (Eds.), *Imitation in infancy* (pp. 253–283). Cambridge, UK: Cambridge University Press.

Rogers, S. J., Hepburn, S. L., Stackhouse, T., & Wehner, E. (2003). Imitation performance in toddlers with autism and those with other developmental disorders. *Journal of Child Psychology and Psychiatry*, 44, 763–781.

Rogers, S. J., & Pennington, B. F. (1991). A theoretical approach to the deficits in infantile autism. *Development and Psychopathology*, 107, 147–161.

Shafik-Eid, R., Dissanayake, C., & Nielsen, M. (2003). *An investigation of early joint attention abilities in the development of social competence in preschool children.* Unpublished raw data.

Sigman, M., Dissanayake, C., Arbelle, S., & Ruskin, E. (1997). Cognition and emotion in children and adolescents with autism. In D. J. Cohen & F. R. Volkmar (Eds.), *Handbook of autism and pervasive developmental disorders* (2nd ed., pp. 248–265). New York: Wiley.

Slaughter, V., & McConnell, D. (2003). Emergence of joint attention: Relationships between gaze following, social referencing, imitation, and naming in infancy. *Journal of Genetic Psychology*, 164, 54–71.

Sparrow, S., Balla, D., & Cicchetti, D. (1984). *Vineland Adaptive Behaviour Scales—Interview Edition, Expanded Form.* Circle Pines, MN: American Guidance Service.

Spiker, D., & Ricks, M. (1984). Visual self-recognition in autistic children: Developmental relationships. *Child Development*, 55, 214–225.

Suddendorf, T. (1999). Children's understanding of the relation between delayed video representation and current reality: A test for self-awareness? *Journal of Experimental Child Psychology*, 72, 157–176.

Suddendorf, T., Simcock, G., & Nielsen, M. (2005). *Reflecting on the nature of visual self-recognition: A new developmental perspective.* Manuscript submitted for publication.

Suddendorf, T., & Whiten, A. (2001). Mental evolution and development: Evidence for secondary representation in children, great apes and other animals. *Psychological Bulletin, 127*, 629–650.

Tiegerman, E., & Primavera, L. H. (1984). Imitating the autistic child: Facilitating communicative gaze behavior. *Journal of Autism and Developmental Disorders, 14*, 27–38.

Tomasello, M. (1999). *The cultural origins of human cognition.* Cambridge, MA: Harvard University Press.

Užgiris, I. (1981). Two functions of imitation during infancy. *International Journal of Behavioral Development, 4*, 1–12.

Wallon, H. (1934). *Les origines du charactére chez l'enfant.* Paris: Boivin.

Want, S. C., & Harris, P. L. (2002). How do children ape? Applying concepts from the study of non-human primates to the developmental study of 'imitation' in human children. *Developmental Science, 5*, 1–13.

Whiten, A., & Brown, J. (1998). Imitation and the reading of other minds: Perspectives from the study of autism, normal children and non-human primates. In S. Bråten (Ed.), *Intersubjective communication and emotion in early ontogeny* (pp. 260–280). Cambridge, UK: Cambridge University Press.

Whiten, A., Custance, D. M., Gomez, J.-C., Texidor, P., & Bard, K. A. (1996). Imitative learning of artificial fruit processing in children (*Homo sapiens*) and chimpanzees (*Pan troglodytes*). *Journal of Comparative Psychology, 110*, 3–14.

Williams, J. H. G., Massaro, D. W., Peel, N. J., Bosseler, A., & Suddendorf, T. (2004). Visual-auditory integration during speech imitation in autism. *Research in Developmental Disabilities, 25*, 559–575.

Williams, J. H. G., Whiten, A., & Singh, T. (2004). A systematic review of action imitation in autistic spectrum disorder. *Journal of Autism and Developmental Disorders, 34*, 285–299.

Williams, J. H. G., Whiten, A., Suddendorf, T., & Perrett, D. I. (2001). Imitation, mirror neurons and autism. *Neuroscience and Biobehavioral Reviews, 25*, 287–295.

Zelazo, P. D., Somerville, J. A., & Nichols, S. (1999). Age-related changes in children's use of external representations. *Developmental Psychology, 35*, 1059–1071.

Zentall, T. R. (2001). Imitation in animals: Evidence, function and mechanisms. *Cybernetics and Systems, 32*, 53–96.

CHAPTER 8

Imitation, Theory of Mind, and Cultural Knowledge

Perspectives from Typical Development and Autism

EVA LOTH
JUAN CARLOS GÓMEZ

At the beginning of the film *2001: A Space Odyssey*, Stanley Kubrick ingeniously used one cut to represent human cultural evolution—from early tool use of sticks as clubs to modern 20th-century space shuttles. But human culture is not only "out there" in the form of material artifacts, institutions, or customs. In fact, a fairly recent and as yet marginal discipline—cultural psychology—emphasizes the role of culture in bringing about socially shared meanings (e.g., Bruner, 1990; Cole, 1996; Shore, 1996; Shweder, 1984; Wertsch, 1993): Cultural knowledge is seen as a prism through which all experiences are filtered. It influences how we perceive and interpret the world, it endows us with knowledge and expectations of what kinds of things happen in different events, which social behavior is "good" or "bad," permitted, allowed, or obligated. In this way, cultural knowledge is at the same time deeply social and cognitive. It is on the one hand shared by many people in one community and as such modulates many of our social interactions, yet on the other hand it is represented by individual minds.

No less intriguing than the phylogenetic evolution of culture is the ontogenetic acquisition of cultural knowledge; how children, over the course of their first years of life, come to, as Shweder (1991) put it, "think through culture."

The main aim of this chapter is to explore the role of different sociocognitive and socioperceptual skills in the acquisition of cultural knowledge by combining perspectives from typical development and autism. We focus mainly on imitation and theory of mind. Although imitation may be understood by some almost as synonymous to cultural or social learning (Rogers & Williams, Chapter 12, this volume), in this chapter, following current trends in comparative and developmental psychology, we use the term in a more specific sense to refer to one particular mechanism ("learning to do an act by seeing it done") whereby social learning may be achieved (Caldwell & Whiten, 2002; Tomasello, 1999; Whiten & Ham, 1992). Social learning (i.e., learning affected by the presence, behavior, or products of the behavior of another individual [Caldwell & Whiten, 2002]) may also be achieved through other mechanisms, such as emulation or stimulus enhancement. Imitation, however, is distinctive in requiring an ability to copy the observed action (Tomasello, 1999). Imitation in this sense has been frequently singled out as the key cognitive mechanism mediating culture and the transmission of social knowledge. This is especially so in views of culture as a collection of material skills. However, in the broader view of culture as a system of shared knowledge, imitation needs to coexist and collaborate with other cognitive abilities, among them—we argue—theory of mind (ToM), the ability to represent mental states, such as beliefs, intentions, or attention (Gómez, 2004; Premack & Woodruff, 1978).[1]

In the first part of this chapter, we look at different views on the relationship between the development of imitation and ToM in both normal development and autism. In the second part, we revisit imitation, ToM, and other socioperceptual and cognitive skills specifically with a view to their possible role in acquiring two key facets of cultural knowledge—social norms and event scripts. Again, a dual perspective is adopted, as we discuss findings from typical development and the as yet small body of research that has investigated cultural knowledge abnormalities in autism. We propose that cultural knowledge is both shaped by experience and shaping experience (i.e., influences how experiences are perceived and interpreted). Imitation, in collaboration with other early emerging socioperceptual skills, ToM, and language, enables children to directly and actively participate in cultural learning, as well as to acquire cultural knowledge vicariously, by building on others' experiences and knowledge. Profound deficits in these areas in autism create barriers for participation in the culture they grow up in and the acquisition of cultural knowledge.

IMITATION AND THEORY OF MIND: TYPICAL DEVELOPMENT

Two decades ago, Meltzoff and Moore (1983, 1977) stunned the developmental psychology community with the finding that literally newborn infants— some less than 1 hour old—could imitate a range of facial expressions, such as tongue protrusion, lip protrusion, and mouth opening. In combination with other reports about surprisingly sophisticated skills for social interaction in very young infants, such as "protoconversations" (e.g., Bates, 1979; Bateson, 1979; Stern, 1985; Trevarthen, 1979; Trevarthen & Aitken, 2001), these findings challenged both traditional Freudian and Piagetian views that saw infants as psychologically cut off from others, as not able to engage in meaningful social interactions until much later in their development. Instead, these findings suggested that at least the beginnings of imitation and social interaction are innate or "hard-wired." It seems that from the very beginning of life, infants have an innate ability to apprehend equivalences between self and other, between observed and executed acts.

In Meltzoff's view, neonatal imitation reveals something more—some kind of innate "starting state" mentalism that allows infants to recognize that other people are "like me." While infants are not born with an adult-like ToM, they are, from the start, equipped with a tool—imitation—to crack the problem of other minds as it allows them to put themselves in other people's mental shoes (Meltzoff, 2002). Different authors' theoretical positions of how children develop a ToM, what its earlier precursors or building blocks might be, and to what extent imitation is instrumental to this development are summarized in Figure 8.1.

In contrast to Meltzoff, others are more skeptical that newborn imitation reflects a level of mentalism with rudimentary introspective abilities or sophisticated cognitive skills or that it plays an instrumental role in developing it. Instead, they argue that innate attentiveness and reactivity to human face and voice (Johnson & Morton, 1991; Spelke, Phillips, & Woodward, 1995), paired with an innate sensitivity to temporal contingencies, may suffice to explain these early imitative interactions (e.g., Gergeley & Watson, 1999; Tomasello, 1999). Their skepticism rests, in part, on the gap between neonatal imitation and other ToM-related social behaviors (e.g., joint attention), which do not emerge until much later in the second half of infants' first year of life. The controversy about the true significance of neonatal imitation, therefore, remains.

However, there is consensus that in their second year of life, young children show more sophisticated forms of imitation. Whereas over the first months, they imitate *behaviors*, a series of studies has shown that from around 12 months, they now begin to imitate the *goals* behind behaviors. For example, in a now classic study, Meltzoff (1995) let 18-months-olds witness an actor unsuccessfully attempting to perform an act. In one instance he tried to pull two parts of an object apart but never quite succeeded. Infants subsequently imitated what the actor meant to do (i.e., his goal) just as well as a second group of children who had watched the actor successfully performing the act. In contrast, children did not tend to imitate the unsuccessful action after seeing it performed by a robot. This suggested that children selectively imitate other *people*. In another study, Carpenter, Akthar, and Tomasello (1998) demonstrated that infants from 14 months selectively imitated a model's *intentional* action (e.g., illuminating an object, which the model verbally marked by saying "there"), but not, when the same result was achieved *accidentially* (after she exclaimed "oops").

Author	Precursors and early social or cognitive abilities or predispositions necessary for theory of mind development	Imitation as *instrumental* in ToM development? − not instrumental; + instrumental; (+) instrumental among other processes
I. MODULARIST		
ToM as domain-specific, hard-wired (i.e., innate, matures more rather than being actively acquired by the child). Other modularists: Fodor, Chomsky, Spelke.		

Leslie (1994, 1987)	• **ToBy**, ~3–4 months: theory of body mechanism—infants' theory of physical bodies allows understanding of agents in a mechanical sense.
	• **ToMM**: theory of mind mechanism—two subsystems:
	  • **ToMM system 1** (~6–8 months): concerned with agents and goal-directed actions, enables, for example, gaze following.
	  • **ToMM system 2** (18–24 months): site of the ability to form M-representations (or metarepresentations), first evidenced in pretense.
	• A selection processor (performing a control function of selecting the appropriate counterfactual situation) is necessary to collaborate with ToMM to understand beliefs, does not mature before ~4 years.
		−

Baron-Cohen (1995)	• **ID**: Intentionality detector (~2 months)—reads goal direction into self-propelled motion. • **EDD**: eye-direction detector (~3 months)—detects presence of eyes, computes whether eyes are directed at self or other, infers that agent sees things. • **SAM**: shared attention mechanism (~9–12 months)—builds triadic relations between self, other and object, such as in joint attention. • **ToMM** (18–24 months, see Leslie's ToMM system 2).	−
Premack (1990)	From birth distinction between animate, self-propelled "objects" and inanimate objects. 1. Infant perceives motion changes in non-self-propelled objects in terms of causality and motion changes in self-propelled objects in terms of goal-directedness/intention. 2. Infants prefer other self-propelled objects over non-self-propelled objects. 3. When two self-propelled objects are perceived together, infants perceive one self-propelled object as intending to *affect* the other.	(−)*

(continued)

FIGURE 8.1. Different authors' views about the development of a theory of mind (ToM) and the role of imitation in it.

	4. In this case, infant expects the other self-propelled object to *reciprocate* with an act that preserves the same valence (positive/negative) as the original one. Transition from infant perception–interpretation to 4-year-olds conceptual–interpretation perhaps mediated by language.	
	*Neonate imitation would be the consequence of this rudimentary "end state" mentalism, rather than being instrumental for its development.	

II. THEORY–THEORY

This view draws parallels between theory change in science and cognitive development. Although the different theories are constructed for specific domains (e.g., folk physics and folk biology), the mechanisms underlying theory construction are thought to be the same. The child has a more active part in ToM development than in the modularist view.
Other theory–theorists: Carey, Keil.

Gopnik & Wellman (1994); Meltzoff & Gopnik (1993)	Children draw on their experience, including imitation, for theory building. • Infancy: Imitation provides "private tutorials" in common sense psychology, social interaction and communication • 2-year-old theory: psychological knowledge consists mainly of desires and perceptions, but not yet beliefs • 3-year-old theory (intermediate phase): Emergence of epistemic mental states (belief, think, know, remember) in language, but children's understanding of beliefs is largely nonrepresentational, belief contents as directly reflecting the world, modelled on the understanding of perception (see also Perner's "situation theory") • 4-year-old theory: unified representational model of the mind: interprets all psychological functioning as mediated by mental states, which are representations of reality and not reality itself	+

III DOMAIN–GENERAL

ToM as the result of domain–general reasoning abilities not specifically dedicated to reasoning about the social domain. Other domain–general theorists: Zelazo, de Loache, Piaget, Chandler, Flavell.

(Perner, 1988, 1993)	1 ."**Presentation**" (aka "primary representation"): young infants have a mental "model" of the world, albeit entirely determined by the perceptual input, and infants do not know *how* their "model" is related to reality. 2. "**Situation theorists**" (~2 years): children can form hypothetical and counterfactual representations, and can compare these models to the world and their previous knowledge base (enabling pretend play, understanding that dreams are not real). Children cannot yet represent this process of modeling, they cannot differentiate between the representational medium (i.e., the mind) and its representational content. "**Representation theorists**" (~4 years): child now understands representations as representations, hence can model the relationship between a model and what it models. Perner's metarepresentational stance is not specific to theory of mind, but incorporates a broader theory of knowledge (e.g., meta-memory)	–

(continued)

FIGURE 8.1. *(continued)*

IV: INFLUENCED BY PSYCHOANALYTIC THOUGHT		
Child–caregiver relationship as crucial for development. Other developmental psychologists inspired by psychoanalysis: Stern.		
Hobson (1993)	(Cognitive) ToM develops out of child's concept of "persons," which develops from the experience of affectively patterned personal relatedness. Imitation as part of the process (together with predisposition to facial and vocal expression, innate propensity to perceive appropriate emotional "meanings," "affective attunment," Stern, 1985) through which the infant's identification with the other is achieved. The emotional dimension of imitation helps to build interpersonal relationships between infant and caregiver.	+
V. SIMULATIONIST		
ToM as the result of mental simulation. Other simulation theorists: Gordon, Harris.		
Meltzoff (2002)	Newborn imitation reflects "starting state mentalism": Imitation as *the* main tool through which infants "crack the problem of other minds."	++
Trevarthen (1979); Trevarthen & Aitken (2001)	Significant role of imitation as part of infant–adult "protoconversations" (e.g., cooing, eye gaze, and understanding of temporal contingencies) that provide the innate foundation for social cognition. Emphasis on the intersubjective (i.e., socioemotional) and not only cognitive component of early imitative communication.	+
Tomasello (1999)	• ~0–9 months: Early imitative and affective interactions reflect infant's propensity for "identification" with others, which plays a crucial role in ToM development. Infant cannot yet introspect on intentional self states. • 9–14 months: Joint attention and imitation *reflect* infants' understanding of attention and intentions. • Imitation as the first form of *cultural learning*, which enables young children to learn *through* others. As such, imitation becomes more instrumental for children's sociocognitive development from 12–14 months.	(+)
Gallese & Goldman (1998); Gallese (2005)	Mindreading abilities rely on mental simulation; i.e., other people's mental states are represented by tracking and matching their states of mind with own resonant states. Propose that mindreading, as well as imitation abilities, might have evolved from more simpler mechanisms, specifically an action execution/ observation matching system that has its neural basis in the mirror neuron system of the premotor cortex.	+
VI. NEUROCONSTRUCTIVIST		
Johnson (1997, 2001)	Neuroconnectionionist: Infants as born with biases or a predisposition to attend, process and respond to social (over physical) stimuli, especially faces, but also speech, human movement, etc. These preferences shape subsequent learning. On the biological level, activity-dependent experiences influence aspects of postnatal functional brain development and plasticity, leading to specialization. Imitation probably as one manifestation of preferential interest in social stimuli.	(+)

(continued)

FIGURE 8.1. *(continued)*

Karmiloff-Smith (1998, 1992)	Gradual modularization of ToM built up from more basic attention biases that influence the storing of ToM relevant representations. Innate biological constraints are recognized, but less detailed and domain-specific than in the modularist view. A mechanism may be more relevant for one kind of input (e.g., social) than others (e.g., physical), but can also be used for other kinds of processing. Emphasis on the role of development itself, i.e., infants' progressive selection and processing of information in establishing domain-specificity. Imitation probably as one manifestation of preferential interest in social stimuli.	(+)
Gergeley (2002); Gergeley & Watson (1999); Csibra & Gergeley (1998)	• Self as "**physical agents**" (0–3 months): Differentiated representation of the body as a separate, integrated and dynamic entity that can cause physical changes in the environment. • Self as **"social agent"** (~0–6 months): Early imitative and affective interactions serve important evolutionary functions (e.g., affect regulation) but do *not* involve rudimentary starting state or end state mentalism. Contingency detection paired with social biofeedback, which serves as an emotional–intentional scaffolding environment, has a sensitization and representation-building function. Hence, imitation may be seen as indirectly instrumental. • **Teleological reasoning** (~9–12 months) based on (1) principle of rationality and (2) ability to represent goals. Teleological stance is a biological adaptation that may have developed independently from ToM to interpret goal-directed action. Understanding of intentional states emerges out of *teleological reasoning*. ~18–24 months: Understanding self and others as intentional mental agents	(+)

VII. EMBODIED COGNITION/COGNITIVE NEUROSCIENCE	
Assumes that it is not a pregiven mind that represents a pregiven world. Instead, the embodied cognition approach emphasizes that the development of cognitive processes is deeply rooted in the body's interactions with the world (Lakoff & Johnson, 1999; Varela, Thompson, & Rosch, 1991).	

Klin et al. (2003)	From the beginning, children show social motivations and visually focus on social aspects of the environment. Children's experiences and interactions with salient aspects of the world shape their learning and sociocognitive processes. Imitation is one important form through which children enact the social world and interact with others.	(+)

VIII. CULTURAL PSYCHOLOGY	

Bruner (2001)	Infant as proactively agentive, interested in the social world, of which imitation is one *manifestation*. This interest and active participation in the social world more generally, rather than imitation *per se*, drives young children's understanding of "simple" psychological states, such as shown in joint attention. At the same time, children's experiences and actions are shaped by intentional states. From 2–3 years, canonical narrative structures or event representations, structure children's "meaning-making processes" in their everyday activities and thereby foster ToM development.	(+)

FIGURE 8.1. *(continued)*

While during their first months infants "only" imitate behaviors already in their repertoire, they are now able to learn new things through imitation. In another well-known study (Meltzoff, 1988), infants watched an adult turning on a light, using the unusual strategy of leaning forward and touching a panel with her forehead. In this session, they were not allowed to manipulate the object. After 1 week, they were presented with the same scenario. Nearly two-thirds of the infants imitated the new head-touch behavior, although, of course, they could have used their hands if all they had represented was the goal of the behavior (what Tomasello, 1999, calls "emulation"). Infants, therefore, can achieve an adaptive balance between the coding of intentions beyond behavior and the coding of behavioral detail beyond intentions in an example of interaction between imitation and early ToM, namely, to read others' intentions.

This new progress in imitation occurs roughly over a period in which toddlers show other sociocognitive achievements: For example, they follow others' gaze to specific targets (e.g., Butterworth, 1991; Scaife & Bruner, 1975), they use pointing gestures to direct others' attention to some interesting object or event (Bates, 1976), they look to adults for checking their emotional reaction to novel objects or people (Campos & Sternberg, 1981). And, of course, infants begin to speak their first words. These accomplishments suggest that now they do indeed understand that others have "simple" psychological states (at the very least, those of attention and intention) that are directed at something and that can be shared.

Work by Baldwin (1995), Bloom (2000), and Tomasello (1992) suggests that children's understanding of speakers' attention and intention is behind their success in word learning—for Tomasello, a special form of "role-reversal imitation" (Tomasello & Carpenter, 2005). For example, Baldwin (1993) found that 18-month-olds correctly learned a novel word (e.g., "modi") by following the speaker's eye gaze to track what she was referring to (instead of associating the new word with a different novel object that the child had inspected when the word was uttered). In a series of elegant studies, Tomasello and colleagues engaged children of the same age in various games during which new words were introduced. Various social-pragmatic cues were provided to see whether children were sensitive to them in order to distinguish between multiple potential referents. Children learned words for intentional but not accidental actions or, in the context of a finding game, understood that of a series of novel objects, termination of the search and the speaker's smile indicated that he had found the "toma" (Tomasello & Barton, 1994).

In imitation, infants learn *through* adults; they use adults as a source of information to learn how to use objects. In addition, cultural learning is facilitated by the adult's willingness to *show* the infant the novel act (i.e., by a communicative context). Indeed, infants are less likely to imitate behaviors performed by an adult while ignoring them (Killen & Užgiris, 1981; cf. Tomasello, 1999). Humans may be the only species that spontaneously complement the imitative abilities of their offspring with "teaching" behaviors (Csibra & Gergeley, 2006; Strauss, Ziv, & Stein, 2002).

A number of authors have focused on joint attention (from around 12 months or earlier; Baron-Cohen, 1989, 1995) or pretend play (emerging around 18 months; see Leslie, 1987) as developmental precursors to the later developing ability to infer more complex mental states, such as beliefs. For some, these precursors are early manifestations of the basic theory of mind mechanisms of metarepresentation (e.g., Baron-Cohen, 1995; Leslie & Roth, 1993); for others building blocks toward metarepresentation (Gómez, Sarriá, & Tamarit, 1993; Hobson, 1993).

In this view, the relation between imitation and ToM is one of distinct abilities working together. However, it is possible to posit a more intimate relationship between both skills.

Theory of Mind as Imitation:
Simulation Theory and Embodied Simulation

According to the simulation theory, the basic mechanism behind the ability to understand other persons' mental states consists of simulating offline the mental states someone must be experiencing when engaging in a particular behavior or experiencing a particular situation. One mentally places oneself in the shoes of others and in this way "discovers" what the other must be thinking (Goldman, 1989; Gordon, 1996; Harris, 1992). This amounts to a sort of imitation of others' mental states that might emerge directly from the early ability to overtly imitate others' behaviors, postures, and expressions (Meltzoff, 2002).

Simulation theorists vary in their specification of the precise mechanisms responsible for mentalizing. Some authors suggest some automatic, largely unconscious processes of simulation (e.g., Gallese, 2005), whereas others refer to more conscious and explicit attempts at placing oneself in another's situation (Gordon & Cruz, 2003). Although originally a relatively marginal view, this approach received an important boost with the exciting discovery, first in macaque monkeys and later indirectly in humans, of "mirror neurons"— neurons that fire both to the execution and perception of one and the same action, such as grasping, tearing, holding, or manipulating an object (Rizzolatti, Fadiga, Gallese, & Fogassi, 1996; Rizzolatti, Fogassi, & Gallese, 2001; see also Gallese & Goldman, 1998). Although mirror neurons might appear to be ideally suited to provide the neural support for imitation, their discovery in macaque monkeys (a species with very poor imitation skills) prompted these authors to suggest that their primary role might be the understanding of others' actions in intentional goal-directed terms by coding the perceived actions in terms of the actions (and their underlying intentions) that one can perform oneself. This looks pretty much like the sort of mechanism that a simulation ToM would expect to be in place to implement mentalizing functions. Imitation itself and ToM would be a phylogenetically later emerging function.

What is more, a number of functional magnetic resonance imaging (fMRI) studies in humans now begin to show that parts of the same localized neural structures are activated respectively, when observing versus performing motor actions, when experiencing versus witnessing disgust (Wicker et al., 2003) when being touched versus observing someone else being touched (Keysers et al., 2004), or when experiencing versus witnessing pain (Singer et al., 2004).

In another recent fMRI study (Iacoboni et al., 2005), participants were shown a movie clip of a hand grasping a teacup (a stimulus that typically evokes activity in the human homologue of the mirror neuron system). However, in one condition this action was embedded in a context—a scene containing teapot, cup, etc.—which implies the intention to drink. The finding that the actions embedded in context elicited increased activity in mirror neuron areas compared to observing the same actions without context suggests that this system may indeed be implicated in coding the *social* intentions of others and not only in the understanding of localized motor intentions (see Jacob & Jeannerod, 2005).

Gallese (2005) proposed that the mirror neuron system might constitute the neural underpinning of "embodied simulation." Essentially, observing an action, emotion, or sensation in others constitutes a form of embodied simulation of that action, emotion, or sensation. Embodied simulation is automatic, unconscious, and prereflexive and gives us (i.e., the observer) an experiential first-person insight into other minds. This way, embodied simulation provides an elegant account for the link between first- and third-person experience without needing to evoke computational models, and it suggests that action and perception are related and grounded in the sensorimotor system.

Embodied simulation enabled by the mirror neuron system may then be the necessary but not sufficient prerequisite for imitation and more cognitively complex theory of mind abilities.

IMITATION AND THEORY OF MIND: THE CASE OF AUTISM

Autism is a pervasive developmental disorder, characterized on the basis of abnormalities in social and communication development, alongside repetitive interests and activities. The term *autism spectrum disorder* (ASD) emphasizes the vast differences between individuals with this condition both in terms of the way abnormalities in these three areas are manifested and in terms of level of intellectual abilities. While most individuals with ASD also have moderate to severe learning difficulties, the high end of the spectrum includes individuals with high-functioning autism and Asperger syndrome.

Over the past two decades, the ToM deficit (or "mindblindness") hypothesis has been the most influential neurocognitive account of *social* deficits in autism (Baron-Cohen, Leslie, & Frith, 1985). It seems that the *majority* of people with autism fail to understand that other people have different mental perspectives—for example, that their behavior can be motivated by "false beliefs." Most authors have viewed ToM deficits as essentially a *cognitive* deficit (e.g., Baron-Cohen, 1990; Leslie & Frith, 1990) while notably Hobson (1993) suggested that ToM deficits in autism are the result of primary emotional deficits in forming interpersonal relatedness. If (most) people with autism do not understand that others' actions are governed by their beliefs, intentions, and desires, the social world must be inherently unpredictable and confusing. This could explain why some people with autism are socially aloof and withdrawn but also why others make active attempts to engage with others, but often in profoundly odd ways. The work by Happé (1993, 1994) has shown that ToM deficits, especially difficulties inferring speakers' intentions, affect many aspects of nonliteral language (e.g., jokes, lies, and metaphors), where what is said differs from what is really meant.

However, one of the earliest criticisms had to do with timing. How can cognitive deficits in the ability to represent others' mental states at the level of false belief, which children typically develop around their fourth birthday, account for social deficits observed earlier in autism? This concern could be partially addressed by thinking of earlier occurring abnormalities in pre-linguistic communication skills—notably the joint attention behaviors and pretend play—as developmental *precursors* of the ability to represent mental states (e.g., Baron-Cohen, 1987, 1989; Charman et al., 1997; Leslie, 1987; Mundy, Sigman, Ungerer, & Sherman, 1986).

An alternative view to the issue of primary deficits in autism is imitation. Imitation deficits in autism were first reported by De Myer and colleagues (1972) but never gained much popularity until Rogers and Pennington (1991) proposed their hypothesis that imitation deficits might represent the *primary* deficit in autism, leading to a disruption in the ability to establish interpersonal relations with others (see also Meltzoff & Gopnik, 1993). Although results have not always been entirely consistent, three extensive reviews (Rogers, 1999; Rogers & Pennington, 1991; Smith & Bryson, 1994) conclude that the majority of studies between the 1970s and the late 1990s show that children with autism have important imitation deficits. Recently, Williams, Whiten, and Singh (2004) have also concluded that evidence points to a delayed development of action imitation in people with autism. And, interestingly, there are now two studies of which we are aware that provide evidence for dysfunctions in the mirror neuron system in high-functioning people with autism (Oberman, Hubbard, McCleery, Altschuler, Ramachandran, & Pineda, 2005; Théoret et al., 2005). For example, Oberman and colleagues (2005) found that people with autism showed mu-wave suppression (which is thought to be linked to mirror-cell activity) only when they performed an action, but unlike controls, not when the actions were imagined or observed.

Even the handful of studies that showed relatively *intact* imitation in autism (Carpenter, Pennington, & Rogers, 2001; Charman & Baron-Cohen, 1994; Morgan, Cutter, Coplin, & Rodriguez, 1989) leave to be explored whether people with autism truly imitate in the same way as people without autism and whether they would do so spontaneously and for the same reasons. All the aforementioned studies tested "instructed imitation," where a model demonstrated an action and the participant was instructed "now you." We know of the discrepancy between *ability* and day-to-day adaptive *performance* in autism in other areas. For example, success on experimental ToM tasks does not guarantee that people with ASD use mindreading abilities spontaneously to impose social meaning (Castelli, Frith, Happé, & Frith, 2002; Klin, 2000), pretend play can be fairly good in instructed and at the same time poor in spontaneous situations (Lewis & Boucher, 1988), and while people with ASD can easily geometrically trace what someone is looking at on demand they have difficulties with spontaneous gaze following (Leekam, Baron-Cohen, Perrett, Milders, & Brown, 1993).

In this regard, it remains to be established whether, for example, in social interactions, people with autism would display the "chameleon effect"—a tendency to match postures, mannerisms, facial expressions, and so on to that of one's interaction partner. Chartrand and Bargh (1999) have found such unintentional, "contagious" matching of motor behaviors especially in high-empathy individuals, and they also reported that it promoted positive feelings for one another in the interaction partners. Hobson and colleagues (Hobson & Lee, 1999; Hobson & Meyer, Chapter 9, this volume) emphasized that in situations in which people with autism could imitate upon request, this appeared to be restricted to the imitation of the model's *behavior*, without attempting to also imitate her *style* (i.e., the particular manner in which the action was performed). For Hobson, this reveals a lack of identification with the other person and their subjective experiences.

It is this spontaneous, interpersonal quality that seems characteristic of the imitation behavior even in young typically developing children and that may be lacking in autism, and that we argue might also be most fundamental to cultural learning.

Importantly, several studies suggest that the imitation deficits reported in autism seem to occur in concert with impairments in other sociocognitive abilities. Carpenter, Pennington, and Rogers (2002) found a strong intercorrelation between imitation deficits and impairments in joint attention, communicative gestures, gaze and point following, and referential language. Charman and colleagues (2003) examined longitudinal associations between diagnosis, joint attention, play, imitation abilities, and language outcome in infants with autism and pervasive developmental disorder. Language level at the age of 4 years was positively associated with joint attention and imitation abilities at 20 months, but not with play. Rogers, Hepburn, Stackhouse, and Wehner (2003) also found that in young children with autism of around 34 months, imitation skills were strongly correlated with autistic symptom severity and joint attention behaviors, even when developmental level and level of social cooperation were controlled for. Surprisingly, in contrast to Charman and colleagues' study, here imitation was not related to play or language development. These correlations with other skills (especially joint attention) leave open the question of which deficit is primary but from a cultural learning perspective offer a clear and consistent message that the earliest tools for cultural learning may be dramatically disrupted in children with autism.

WHAT IS CULTURAL KNOWLEDGE, AND HOW IS IT ACQUIRED?

According to the *Blackwell Dictionary of Sociology* (Johnson, 2000):

> [Culture is] the accumulated store of symbols, ideas, and material products associated with a social system, whether it be an entire society or a family . . . . Culture has both material and non-material aspects. Nonmaterial culture includes symbols as well as ideas that shape and inform people's lives in relation to one another and the social system in which they participate—attitudes, beliefs, values, and norms. (p. 73)

It is the nonmaterial aspect of culture that cultural psychologists and cognitive anthropologists have emphasized and that we here call cultural knowledge. Quinn and Holland (1987) defined cultural knowledge as "predisposed, taken-for granted models of the world that are widely shared (although not necessarily to the exclusion of other, alternative models) by the members of a society and that play an enormous role in their understanding of that world and their behaviour in it" (p. 4). More concretely, putting together concepts from different traditions, cultural knowledge includes (at least) the following:

- Shared cultural beliefs and belief systems purport to describe some aspect of collective reality, such as "the earth is round" (see Sperber, 1996, 1997). It is on the basis of these beliefs or belief systems that we construct the reality of everyday life (often without being aware that these "objective" realities are being socially constructed, Berger & Luckman, 1967).
- Social norms or rules associate people's behavior with rewards or sanctions. From the perspective of the social system (a particular culture or society) this serves the purpose of regulating behavior and appearance. In sociology, the concept of norms is closely related to that of social roles. Norms differ in terms of the severity of sanctions; some norms "must" be obeyed, such as laws; whereas customs or conventions "should" or "can" be followed.
- Event scripts or schemas are socially shared expectations of what normally happens in common and routine situations (including things that could, i.e., may or may not, happen). Event scripts provide an interpretive context and as such are a powerful tool in making sense of events, and of people, their mental states, and actions in different situations (Bruner, 1990; Schank & Abelson, 1977).

How would someone without cultural knowledge make sense of others' actions? This might be an easier thought experiment than to try and imagine what it would be like to lack ToM. In fact, it might not be unlike our experiences when traveling to a foreign country, where people have different, unfamiliar cultural customs and their behavior, their perceptions, and interpretations are governed by different meaning systems. Consider this fictitious example:

> "Imagine, you travelled through Tibet or India and observed someone carefully sliding a valuable object, like a precious stone or even a piece of jewellery into a river stream. This unlikely act itself begs for an explanation. It is likely that many of the explanations you generate involve theory of mind. Perhaps the person wants to hide something or play a trick, has lost his mind, is simply mad etc. . . ? Now, the same act was also observed by another Tibetan. In traditional Tibetan and Indian mythology, *Nagas* are mystical beings, half man, half snake, who dwell in water regions and are believed to control all natural phenomena, including the weather. A range of customs and practices serve the purpose of keeping the Nagas in a friendly mood. With this background knowledge in mind, the Tibetan might infer that by throwing this piece of jewellery in the stream, the actor performs a little ritual or offering by which he hopes to put himself and his family in favor, perhaps before embarking on a particularly difficult journey. Although both the Western and Tibetan observers can reasonably be credited with a theory of mind *capacity*, their interpretations of the activity are very different, and heavily depend on the degree of knowledge of the cultural frame in which the action took place. Moreover, once the Western observer was introduced to this belief or belief system, s/he might now also consider the actor's behaviour as meaningful (although s/he may not endorse the beliefs in the Nagas). Hence, the example highlights the relevance of cultural knowledge for the interpretation of experiences."

Cross-cultural differences in norms, beliefs, value systems, and scripts underscore that the *content* of cultural knowledge cannot be innate and must be acquired on the basis of specific *experiences* (Shore, 1996). However, so far, we know relatively little about the exact cognitive or social mechanisms through which children acquire cultural knowledge. A number of authors have emphasized that cultural knowledge cannot be fully grasped by means of logic and deduction, or solely through individual experiences of the world. Shweder (1984) argued that many cultural beliefs or customs are neither rational nor irrational (e.g., men don't wear skirts) but are best seen as "nonrational." Bruner (1986), too, challenged the preeminence of rational thought. He related mind and culture through narratives, which he proposed as the primary mode of thought in the service of the construction of meaning. And Lakoff and Johnson (1999) argued that metaphorical concepts, which are part of our everyday speech, affect the ways in which we think, perceive, and act. Taken together, children must rely on forms of social transmission of knowledge to acquire their cultures.

In the following sections, two important questions are considered: *When* and *how* (i.e., through what kind of social or cognitive mechanisms) do children acquire different facets of cultural knowledge?

When Do Young Children Show an Understanding of Cultural Knowledge?

Social Norms: Morals and Conventions and Deontic Reasoning

One prominent theory of moral development has been put forward by Kohlberg (1984). Building on previous work by Piaget (1932/1965) on children's stage-like cognitive development, Kohlberg (1984) suggested that children's understanding of moral obligations develops from their earlier understanding of social conventions.

A different influential approach was put forward by Turiel and colleagues (Turiel, 1983; see Nucci, 2002, for review). Instead of positing different levels, these authors suggested that the moral and the conventional represent two different domains of rule-based thinking. They argued that while morals may be universal across cultures (e.g., "you must not kill"), conventions can be accepted as being different between different cultures (for instance, it is okay in England to eat beef but not in most parts of India). Challenging Kohlberg's argument, children as young as 3–5 years old were found to already have an understanding of what an objective obligation is (e.g., Smetana & Braeges, 1990). They recognized that moral obligations cannot be altered by majority vote or different groups' preferences because they pertain to universal matters of human welfare and fairness, whereas conventional obligations can be changed, as they are context dependent (but see, for a critique, Shweder, Mahaptra, & Miller, 1987). Turiel and colleagues, however, left relatively unspecified what kind of cognitive abilities the child needs to bring along in order to understand and distinguish between morals or conventions.

A separate line of research has studied the development of deontic reasoning; the cognitive basis of the understanding of what one may, may not, can, or ought to do (e.g., Cummins, 1996; Jackendoff, 1999). From early on, children are confronted with social rules, of the type "all children must stay in the playground" or permission rules, which grant a particular action, provided a specified condition has been met, "if you clean up your room, you can watch TV."

It is now fairly well established that people reason about permission rules quite differently from the way they reason about the truth value of a conditional statement. The most widely used paradigm is the Wason Selection task (e.g., Cheng & Holyoak, 1985; Cosmides, 1989; Johnson-Laird, Legrenzi, & Sonino-Legrenzi, 1972). In the original version, participants are presented with four cards, all of which have a number on one side, and a letter on the other side (e.g., A, D, 4, 7). Their task is to turn around as many cards as necessary to prove whether or not the statement "If a card has a vowel on one side, then it has an even number on the other side" is correct. Most frequently, people choose A and 4 (p and q), while the actual correct solution, A and 7 (p and *not* q), is chosen rather rarely. Now consider how people reason when they are given the following variant: "If John stays overnight at his cabin, then he always comes home with a sack of garbage." Participants are asked to adopt the perspective of a wildlife protector and to make sure that John had obeyed the rule about garbage disposition. Participants typically choose "stayed overnight at his cabin" and "returned without a sack of garbage" (i.e., p and *not* q) (Cummins, 2000). It seems that the participants' performance is determined by the problem content, and not the logical structure of the task. When people reason about social rules, they spontaneously look for possible violations—which is what Cummins calls the deontic effect. It is, however, highly controversial how this deontic effect occurs. One account is that humans have a "cheater detection module," which has evolved in response to pressure to reason about social exchange (Cosmides, 1989; Cosmides & Tooby, 1992; Gigerenzer & Hug, 1992). Others argued that improved performance is due to higher familiarity with the problem content (Johnson-Laird et al., 1972) or evocation of pragmatic class-specific reasoning schemas (e.g., Cheng & Holyoak, 1985).

There is a small body of research that has investigated deontic reasoning in young children, often using simplified versions of the Wason Selection task (Cummins, 1996; Harris & Núñez, 1996, 1998; Keller, Gummerum, Wang, & Lindsey, 2004). Cummins (1996) showed the dissociation between truth testing and testing for norm violations in 3- to 4-year-old preschoolers. Harris and Núñez (1996, 1998) confronted 3- and 4-year-olds with permission rules of a type likely to be experienced in real life, such as "If Sally rides her bike, she must put her helmet on." The children were then shown four pictures of Sally walking wearing her helmet (not p, q), Sally riding her bike wearing her helmet (p and q), Sally riding her bike with no helmet (p, not q), and Sally walking with no helmet (not p, not q). The children were asked in which picture was Sally naughty? Most of the 3- and 4-year-olds pointed to the correct picture. The same finding was obtained when children were given totally new, unfamiliar rules. This condition rules out that children simply responded on the basis of experience with the familiar rule, without making a logical deduction. It seems therefore that from early on, children adopt the same distinctive way of reasoning about what is socially allowed and what not as adults.

Event Scripts

The notion of "scripts" was first developed by Schank and Abelson (1977). In the attempt to model complex processes such as text or language comprehension in artificial intelligence, Schank and Abelson faced the problem that people infer much more about a situation than what is literally said. Real-world based scripts were their proposed solution, defined as high-level schematically organized knowledge structures. As schemas in general, scripts or event schemas are thought to stand midway between immediate perceptual experiences and paradigmatic abstractions, where in a set of expectations, the whole (e.g., living room) implies certain components, but the components (e.g., tables and chairs) do not imply the whole. Event scripts comprise a sequence of actions that are organized within a particular spatial–temporal context and around goals and subgoals. In addition, events are represented in generalized terms and are hierarchically structured. The hierarchical structure refers to the description of actions and so-called props (objects, artifacts) at different levels of abstraction. At the highest level of abstraction are *scenes* (in the restaurant example, entering, ordering, eating, paying, leaving). At the next lower level, actions can be described as *slots*, such as "eating a main course." Slots can be expressed in terms of still more concrete examples, called *slotfillers*. For instance, a main course (slot) can mean different things at different occasions, such as spaghetti Bolognese or chicken curry (slotfillers). In addition, actions and props differ in terms of their importance for the event and the probability with which they occur; they can be either central (such as paying the bill or ordering in a restaurant) or optional (having pudding) to the event. Due to the interplay between central and optional acts and the relatively high-level representation, event scripts serve two main functions: they provide structure for new experiences and at the same time allow for a great deal of flexibility between different encounters with one event.

From the beginning of the 1980s, a systematic research program by Nelson and her colleagues has shown that already by the age of $2\frac{1}{2}$ to 3 years, typically developing preschoolers possess basic schematized knowledge of familiar and recurrent events in a script format (e.g., Nelson, 1986).

One common way to test script knowledge is to ask children to provide narratives (e.g., "What happens at the nursery?"). Preschoolers typically state that "they/you play" instead of using the "I" or "we" forms, and they describe events in the present instead of the past tense, which, together, indicate generality. In addition, they describe actions in their appropriate temporal/causal order, and at a relatively high level of abstraction. For example, children would state that during the break they "play" instead of spontaneously giving specific examples. Hudson (1988) found that already by around 4 years children distinguished between acts that are central (judged as occurring always) and those that are optional (judged as occurring sometimes). According to Nelson, scripts are derived from concrete experiences of events but are nonetheless abstractions from this experienced reality; people perceive the world in terms of regular "canonical" features and they notice and learn from anomalies and exceptions to expectations.

In sum, from preschool age children understand social experiences and act upon the social world on the basis of cultural knowledge, which specifies what people *should*, *must*, or *must not* do, and they have general expectations of what *will*, *might*, or *could* happen in different situations.

The Role of Early Socioperceptual and Sociocognitive Skills in the Acquisition of Cultural Knowledge

Children acquire culture both directly, through their personal experience, and vicariously, through communication and testimony, as they build their own knowledge upon that of others, their parents, peers, teachers, and past generations. In the following section, we consider the role of different socioperceptual and sociocognitive skills in enabling children to participate in their culture.

Direct Experiences

Perhaps nobody has elaborated more lucidly than Mead (1934) the view that mind and self develop out of social processes, out of intersubjective activity. Certainly the foremost form of "symbolic interaction" he emphasized is language, where a vocal gesture becomes symbolic in that it can predictably evoke the same meaning in others as in the one who is producing it. Mead, however, also stressed the roles of play and games in the emergence of self and the socialization process. The sort of play he referred to contains both aspects of symbolic and imitative play. Children play "mother–father–child," "teacher," "policeman," and so on and in this way literally take the roles of these others. By taking their roles, children elicit the same reactions in themselves as in others. He suggested that it is through this act of taking the role or attitudes of others that a reflective social self emerges as the child comes to view him- or herself from the standpoint of others. While during play, children act as though they were a specific other, taking a particular role at a time (a mother, doctor, nurse, etc.), games involve more complex forms of role playing. Here the child needs to take the attitude of all others involved in the game that must be in some definite relationship to one another and the overarching rule of the game. This organization of roles within rules creates a new unity of the "generalized other," through which, when internalized, the child perceives and judges her own behavior. Perhaps most important for the present argument is the notion that through these activities and interactions, children not only develop a reflective sense of their own self but, by enacting and reenacting cultural scenes, also acquire and consolidate their understanding of what different events entail, and to a certain extent what kinds of behavior, from the point of view of different roles, are normative or not. More recently, Tomasello and coworkers (Tomasello, 1999; Tomasello, Carpenter, Call, Behne, & Moll, 2005; Tomasello, Kruger, & Ratner, 1993) emphasized the role of intention reading, shared intentionality, and imitation as foundational skills for cultural transmission and cultural learning. They argue that these early emerging sociomotivational and sociocognitive skills enable diverse forms of cultural cognition, from the acquisition of language and use of linguistic symbols over the construction of social norms to the establishment of social institutions.

Observational studies by Nadel and colleagues have demonstrated that children spontaneously combine elements of pretend play, joint attention and imitation in their interactions. In one early study, Nadel-Brulfert and Baudonniere (1982) observed pairs of 30- to 42-month-old children left to their own devices in a room full of identical toys. The younger children used pointing gestures as an invitation to imitate actions involving identical objects. Or both partners simultaneously pretended to pour water into a cup to give their respective dolls a drink. By 42 months, children developed shared topics or stories that were mainly imitative, for instance, " 'My baby is thirsty'— 'yes, my baby is thirsty also' . . . 'It is vacation. I will put the picnic bag in the boat'—'yes, and I will wake the babies and dress them' . . . " (Nadel, Guérini, Pezé, & Rivet, 1999, p. 211).

Lakoff and Johnson (1999) stressed the role of *sensorimotor* experiences, in forming (and constraining) the (cultural) concepts and categories in which we think. They showed that a lot of our cultural knowledge is nonliteral, webs of beliefs or belief systems that take the form of "complex metaphors" such as "a purposeful life is a journey." They argued that these complex metaphors, which affect how we think and relate to others, are "anatomically" made up of diverse "primary metaphors," that is, culturally shared associations, such as "affection is warmth," "intimacy is closeness," "difficulties are burdens," and so forth.

In his narrative psychology, Bruner (1986, 1990) argued that culturally shared meanings (including script knowledge) are negotiated through shared modes of discourse, especially narrative activities. Telling little stories (for instance, about what happened throughout the day) serves two import functions: first, they are "exercises in canonical encoding, and, specifically, in the making of non-idiosyncratic and culture-embodying meanings" (Bruner & Feldman, 1993, p. 275). In other words, children strengthen their understanding of what different common and routine events entail. Second, by telling stories about what happened, children need to solve the puzzle why people behaved in certain ways. In this way, Bruner argued that narratives scaffold metacognitive thinking—theory of mind. Thus, Bruner predicts that driven by the narrative mode of thought, event knowledge and ToM develop in tandem.

Vicarious Experiences

Moreover, there are important facets of cultural knowledge that cannot be easily acquired on the basis of personal experiences—scientific knowledge, knowledge of historical events, or religious beliefs. Instead, this cultural knowledge is related to children formally (as in teaching) and informally through verbal communication. Different authors have highlighted the role of ToM in these processes.

Sperber (1996, 1997) distinguished between two types of cultural beliefs—intuitive and reflective beliefs—both of which can either be descriptive or normative. However, he argued that they fundamentally differ in the way they are acquired or represented. Intuitive beliefs (e.g., "charcoal is black") are acquired either through perceptual experiences or through inferences based on them; they are common and widely shared within and between cultures because as humans, we share a similar perceptual apparatus. Reflective beliefs (e.g., "God sees everything" and "there are male and female plants"), on the other hand, are acquired vicariously, communicated to us by others. These beliefs are often only half-understood ideas, beyond the realm of full understanding of the child or sometimes even the adult. Sperber argued that we hold these beliefs on the basis of trust in those who communicate them to us. They are reflectively represented in the sense that they are believed in virtue of second-order beliefs about them, and in this sense they require metarepresentation (the cognitive substrate underlying ToM—Leslie, 1987; Perner, 1991). Most of us believe that $e = mc^2$, not because we understand the formula but because Einstein and other scientists have told us, and we believe that what they say (or *think*, *know*) is right. We may believe that "God sees everything" because our parents and other "significant others" told us, and we believe that their beliefs are true.

Clément, Koenig, and Harris (2004) tested belief formation processes from others' testimony in preschoolers. Most 4-year-olds but only a few 3-year-olds showed "skeptical trust." They tended to check what other informants said against their own prior knowledge (where possible) and they did not indiscriminately trust any informant but, selectively, the one who had proved to be reliable in the past. The explanation discussed by the authors is that the 4-year-olds use their now emerging ToM capacity when acquiring new (cultural) knowledge, and recognize when an informant entertains or indeed seeks to create a false belief.

It is currently a matter of debate whether or not ToM and deontic reasoning are separate or interlinked cognitive domains. Some (Cummins, 2000; Jackendoff, 1999) view ToM and deontic systems as separate domains. While violations from rights or obligations can be directly detected in behavior, mental states need to be inferred. And although evidence that nonhuman primates understand mental states is thin (especially, at the level of false-belief understanding), there is evidence that primates, which live in societies that are structured in terms of dominance hierarchies, readily recognize when someone violates a social norm in situations, such as grooming, food sharing, or mating (see, e.g., de Waal, 1982). Others (Núñez & Harris, 1998; Wellman & Miller, 2005) suggested an intimate connection between the understanding of other minds and deontic concepts. Núñez and Harris pointed out that deontic rules apply to human agents who can deliberately break rules or obligations. Wellman and Miller (2005) argued for a (still relatively domain-specific) core human social reasoning system that encompasses and integrates deontic and ToM constructs as behavior is situated in a normative, rule-governed context.

Bloom (2004) pointed out that our abilities to put ourselves in others' shoes and to feel empathy are essential to both moral reasoning and to bring about moral changes in the course of history. To understand the Golden Rule, which is based on the principle of impartiality (e.g., "What you would that men should do to you, do ye also to them likewise"), it is necessary to see one's own actions from the perspective of the other. And while, for example, the principle of impartiality was once compatible with keeping slaves (because slaves were considered subhuman, hence outside the boundaries), empathy with those who do not fall into the moral circle may have motivated the search for rational arguments leading to changes in cultural beliefs, including laws.

It seems that ToM together with other related sociocognitive skills and verbal language is highly relevant for children to acquire cultural knowledge vicariously, in order to build up their knowledge on the experience and expertise of others, who communicate this knowledge to them.

Taken together, these different approaches converge insofar as they suggest that the processes underlying the acquisition of cultural knowledge cannot consist only of cold intellectual endeavors on the part of the child. Instead, they seem to be inseparable from children's day-to-day experiences with the social world. This naturally leads to the question of how advanced cultural knowledge may be affected in people with autism, who typically show impairments in their socioperceptual and sociocognitive skills.

DO PEOPLE WITH AUTISM HAVE DEFICITS IN CULTURAL KNOWLEDGE?

One of the major challenges for the ToM deficit hypothesis as a sufficient account of the social abnormalities of autism is the now fairly consistent findings documenting that high-functioning individuals with this disorder, especially those with Asperger syndrome, in fact quite often succeed on even complex ToM tasks in experimental situations. Still, these ASD ToM passers show clear social difficulties in real life (and, as most people who work with autistic persons agree, the more people involved and the less structured the situation, generally the more difficulties present). Partially in response to this challenge, recent research has shifted to the focus on socioperceptual skills and motivations, showing deficits in face perception (both in terms of recognition of person identity and emotion expression) on the behavioral level and at the neurofunctional level using fMRI techniques (e.g., Critchley et al., 2000; Hobson, 1986; Hobson, Ousten, & Lee, 1988; Schultz et al., 2000; see, for a recent review, Schultz, 2005). Dawson, Meltzoff, Osterling, Rinaldi, and Brown (1998) reported that young children with autism showed deficits in orienting to social stimuli, such as when being called by their name or in response to hand clapping, and that these deficits were related to joint attention impairments. Klin, Jones, Schultz, and Volkmar (2002, 2003) used eye-tracking technology to study visual fixation patterns when viewing naturalistic scenes on video. Both young toddlers with autism and adults with this condition were found to focus less often on actors' eyes (which convey the most diagnostic information about what the person is thinking or feeling) and instead more on the mouth region or context-irrelevant nonsocial objects in the background. These studies suggest that diminished social predisposition may be apparent from early on and a pervasive feature in autism.

One important implication of this approach is that people with autism may have a fundamentally different "topology of salience," a predisposition toward favoring objects relative to people (Klin et al., 2003). This would put children with autism on an entirely different developmental trajectory, including a diminished motivation to attend to or seek information from and through other people. As a consequence, virtually all the processes of cultural transmission and acquisition discussed in the previous section could be predicted to be derailed in autism.

Direct and Vicarious Experiences

Despite growing up in a rich cultural environment, the important deficits in imitation and symbolic play, language delays, and impaired narrative skills (e.g., Bruner & Feldman, 1993; Loveland, McEvoy, Kelley, & Tunali, 1990; but see Losh & Capps, 2003), obstruct children with autism in their opportunities for cultural learning. Parent reports and interviews, such as the Autism Diagnostic Interview, document well that in their everyday life, children with autism do not tend to role play or to reenact cultural scenes. They are often less interested in storybooks, drama, or comedy than factual information (and if they are interested in, say, storybooks or a particular TV show, then sometimes for idiosyncratic reasons), they do not tend to discuss with their parents what happened during the day, and so forth. Perhaps they are not tuned into Bruner's "narrative mode of thought." Interpreting discourse on the basis of rationality principles, assuming, for example, that people say things solely to state the truth, would make it inherently difficult to understand why one can sometimes make very different claims about the same issue when talking to different people in different situations (speaking to, say, a biologist or a feminist), namely, in order to make a particular point, justify something, convince someone, or distribute blame.

By definition, children with autism have language delays. Following the view advocated by Bloom, Baldwin, or Tomasello, abnormalities in language acquisition can—to some extent—be related to deficits in the joint attention skills and imitation. Indeed, using Baldwin's word-learning paradigm, Baron-Cohen, Baldwin, and Crowson (1997) reported that children with autism did not tend to use speaker's eye gaze as an index of the speaker's intention to refer.

Difficulties with the understanding of metaphors and other forms of nonliteral language, even in high-functioning people with autism, are well documented. Drawing on relevance theory, Happé (1993) has linked these difficulties to ToM deficits, in particular to problems tracking speakers' communicative intentions. For Lakoff and Johnson (1999), metaphors are not only a communicative or linguistic device but represent a fundamental category in which we think. Although more speculatively, this approach would generate important predictions for autism. They suggested that "primary metaphors," such as "affection is warmth" are formed by associating basic-level concepts with sensorimotor experiences. It is possible that because of different social or, in some cases, sensory experiences, children with autism may have difficulties understanding such primary metaphors as derived from their own experience, or also that impairments in imagination affect their ability to understand and form these semantic associations. There are interesting recent attempts to develop an embodied theory of concepts that links the representation of action and more abstract concepts, such as metaphors—via the role of imagination or action simulation in it—to the mirror neuron system; an area, which, as previously discussed, may well be affected in autism (Gallese & Lakoff, in press).

Moreover, ToM impairments could be predicted to have an impact, for example, on the understanding that justification of many social norms (at least in Western societies) refers to social consequences (e.g., doing such-and-such won't be good for you/the other person), to understand how different social events are linked, to distinguish between information that can and cannot be reasonably trusted, to monitor other people's social expectations of one's own behavior in different contexts, to internalize these expectations, and so on.

Finally, although our emphasis here has been on the role of *socio*-perceptual and *socio*cognitive skills in cultural learning, it should be borne in mind that this does not exclude the implication of other cognitive processes. For example, adaptive social understanding requires the ability to generalize information across different situations (of which one relevant cognitive process is categorization) and event scripts rely on the ability to form cognitive schemas. Therefore, neuropsychological abnormalities in executive functions (e.g., Rogers & Pennington, 1991), or perceptual or cognitive biases, such as weak central coherence (Frith, 1989; Happé, 1999), perceptual enhancement (Plaisted, 2001), or impairments in prototype formation (Klinger & Dawson, 2001) are also likely to affect the way cultural knowledge is acquired, represented, or used in different social situation.

Understanding Social Rules, Norms, and Morals

Do individuals with autism understand social rules and norms? There is ample clinical and anecdotal evidence, including Kanner's (1943) original observations, suggesting that people with autism *behave* as if oblivious to social norms. There is also some anecdotal evidence that people with autism have difficulties *understanding* social rules or generalizing them across different contexts (Williams, 1992).

In a more systematic study, Dewey (1991) has shown that people with ASD judge social situations quite differently from most of us. She presented seven young men with autism with a set of stories in which the protagonists displayed behaviors likely to be seen in people with autism. For example, in one story, a young man was feeding pigeons in a park and observed how a baby in a carriage began to cry, unnoticed by its mother who was swinging an older child nearby. As he had learned from his baby nephew that when he screamed, it sometimes meant that the diaper pin had opened, instead of bothering the mother, he quickly checked the baby's clothing for an open pin. Dewey asked her participants to rate the story characters' behavior on a scale ranging from "fairly normal behavior in that situation" to "shocking behavior." Her respondents with autism often revealed a disregard for the social context or social convention. For example, unlike the control participants, they did not rate the behavior of a stranger touching a baby as shocking. At the same time, the men with autism tended to judge conventional behaviors as eccentric or even shocking (e.g., wasting good food by throwing it on the ground for birds).

There are a number of more recent tasks that tap understanding of socially appropriate versus inappropriate behavior, such as Baron-Cohen, O'Riordan, Stone, Jones, and Plaisted's (1999) "Faux Pas" test, revealing deficits in people with high-functioning autism or Asperger syndrome. However, these tests are typically designed as more ecologically valid *theory of mind* tests, which means that from task failure it is hard to tell whether those with ASD perform poorly because of difficulties with the ToM component or because of difficulties in the understanding of social norms.

Blair (1996) used Smetana and Braeges's (1990) classic paradigm to investigate whether people with autism distinguish between moral and conventional transgressions. He subdivided his ASD group into those who failed versus those who passed false-belief tasks. Both ASD groups agreed that it was okay to break a convention (e.g., a child walking out of the classroom without permission) if, prior to that behavior, it had been established that "at this school anybody can do [so] if they want to." At the same time they felt it was not okay to hit another child (moral transgression), even if beforehand it had been established that this was allowed at that school. Blair concluded that appreciation of the moral/conventional distinction indicates that people with autism are sensitive to the distress of others, and that ToM is not a prerequisite for understanding morality. However, for the appreciation of moral/conventional transgressions it is perhaps more important to understand the actor's intentions, which typically develops earlier than understanding of beliefs, and which his ToM failers (with a mean age of 11.6 years) as well as Smetana and Braeges's 3-year-olds were able to appreciate.

Loveland, Pearson, Tunali-Kotoski, Ortegon, and Gibbs (2001) showed children with and without autism staged interactions between adults on video. The interactions were either appropriate or inappropriate, and half of them either contained verbalizations or were purely nonverbal. The participants were asked whether the interaction was okay or somehow wrong, and if wrong, what exactly was wrong and why. Both groups correctly identified the actors' appropriate behavior. However, both in the verbal and nonverbal situations, the controls detected the inappropriate behavior more often than those with autism. And while the control participants explained the inappropriate behavior more often on the basis of social norms or principles, the explanations offered by the autism group were more often inappropriate and did not reflect social awareness.

We recently devised a "social inference test" (Loth & Gómez, 2002) to explore whether ToM deficits had a developmental effect on the ability to predict and explain social norm-based behavior. To test social norm understanding as separate from online ToM abilities, the task was designed in a way that it was not necessary to impute a mental state to an agent in order to perform well. Participants were read short stories, for instance, about John getting ready for a wedding in the countryside. The question was, "What is John going to wear"? Participants were shown four pictures, in this example, of a wedding dress, a suit, a uniform, and a mountain jacket. For each picture they had to make a forced choice indicating whether the type of clothing was "yes, likely" or "no, unlikely." Participants were then asked to justify their choices, for example, why was a wedding dress un/likely? Responses were only coded if participants passed a memory control question, for example, "Where did John go?"

Twenty-one participants with ASD (between 8 and 28 years of age) took part in this study. As an index of their sociocognitive competencies, they were subdivided into ToM failers, first-order ToM passers, and advanced ToM passers. ToM abilities were tested using a standard "unexpected content" false-belief task (a version of the Sally-Ann paradigm; Baron-Cohen, Leslie, & Frith, 1985) and six of Happés Strange Stories, which tap understanding of irony, lie, white lie, jokes, persuasion, and double bluff. For example, in one vignette, a girl received a boring, old set of encyclopedias as a Christmas present, but she had really hoped for a rabbit. When her parents asked her how she liked her present, she replied, "It's lovely, thank you. It's just what I wanted." The participants were asked whether it was true what the character said, and to explain why she said it. A correct answer required appreciation that she did not say the truth because she wanted to spare her parents' feelings. The ASD group was compared separately to typically developing children and individuals with learning difficulties with similar verbal abilities. All participants in the control groups had passed the false-belief task.

Alternative hypotheses were considered: If social norm reasoning were developmentally independent from ToM or related sociocognitive abilities, ASD ToM-failers would be expected to perform comparable to controls with similar intellectual abilities. On the other hand, if ToM or associated abilities had a developmental effect on social norm acquisition, we would expect selectively ToM failers to show abnormalities. The results were clear-cut: The ASD ToM failers succeeded significantly less often than the typically developing children and children with learning difficulties in predicting the likely behavior of the protagonists.

On the prediction measure, there were no group differences between the ASD first-order ToM subgroup and their controls or between the ASD advanced ToM subgroup and their advanced ToM controls. However, all control groups mostly referred to a social norm or drew on real-world knowledge to justify their choices (e.g., "Men don't wear dresses") instead of attributing a particular mental state to the character. By contrast, the individuals with ASD gave significantly fewer social norm explanations than their respective controls. Instead, their responses often revealed that they had associated a particular place or object with a particular function, often disregarding the context, or they gave otherwise inappropriate explanations.

Correlation analyses yielded a significant relationship between social norm explanations and continuous ToM scores in the ASD group, both before and after the effect of verbal IQ was partialed out. This lends further support to our suggestion that sociocognitive abilities are implicated in the understanding of social norms and real-world knowledge, although our data do not allow us to specify whether this relationship is between metarepresentional theory of mind or is linked to other areas of sociocognitive/perceptual deficits in autism.

Event Scripts

Only a handful of studies have investigated script abnormalities in autism, and they have produced mixed results. This relative neglect is surprising, in view of the argument detailed in previous sections that scripts are essential in modulating social interaction and communication.

Loveland and Tunali (1991) invited individuals with autism and learning difficulties to participate in an acted-out "tea party" situation during which one of the experimenters talked about an unhappy experience (his stolen wallet). Like the controls, the children with autism behaved appropriately during the tea party. However, they were less likely to (spontaneously or even after prompting) comfort the experimenter for his stolen wallet, which Loveland and Tunali considered as a parallel "script." Volden and Johnston (1999) compared the event narratives (e.g., about going to the movies or the grocery store) of higher- and lower-functioning subgroups with ASD with those of verbal mental age-matched peers. Both ASD groups had difficulties generating references to central acts. Instead, they reported more acts that were irrelevant to the event. However, when they were shown short video clips and asked to predict the next core element, they performed comparable to the control group. On this basis the authors concluded that their participants with autism had appropriate "content" knowledge but lacked the "microlinguistic" skills to produce a coherent narrative.

Script impairments, on the other hand, were found in two other studies. Loveland and Tunali (1993) reported that a 10-year-old with pervasive developmental disorder did not succeed in explaining what generally happens when going on holidays. He started off describing what he planned to do in that year but soon switched to his own favorite topic—hotels. The authors suggest that he seemed unable to generalize different experiences and also showed lack of awareness of the kind of narrative structure he was asked to produce. Trillingsgaard (1999) hypothesized that the inability to form scripts might be related to ToM deficits because "the meaning of people's behaviour obviously requires common knowledge of the situations in which the behaviour takes place" (p. 45). She found that compared to controls, the scripts produced by a group of people with autism were significantly impoverished (all individuals with ASD passed first-order ToM tasks but fewer second-order ToM tasks than the controls). She also noted that although with increasing age the autistic children were able to appropriately sequence their scripts, these were more rigid and narrow, including less variety of options relating to actors, actions, and objects.

One of the limitations of most of the previous studies was that coding schemes tended to be fairly coarse. In addition, with the exception of Trillingsgaard's study, they were also exploratory in nature in that they did not depart from clear theoretical predictions whether and why scripts should be impaired in autism, in general or only certain facets of them. In a recent study (Loth, Gómez, & Happé, 2005) we reasoned that both sociocognitive/perceptual and other cognitive abnormalities putatively specific to autism affect particular aspects of event representation. We asked participants with ASD, those with learning difficulties, and typically developing children to produce narratives of familiar events—for example, going to a restaurant or celebrating Christmas. The prediction generated from Bruner's and other accounts stressing the role of active participation, enactment, and reenactment of events in forming implicit event representations was difficult to test here directly. However, more concrete predictions from a ToM perspective were that difficulties with the understanding of mental states would impair the ability to grasp the meaning of different events, in other words, why people participate in these events (e.g., people go to a restaurant because they *want* to have a good time, don't *feel* like cooking, etc.). It would also impair comprehension of how different "scenes" are linked or "enabled" through different subgoals. This account predicts differences in terms of event understanding between people with ASD, depending on their level of ToM competencies.

Moreover, we reasoned that in autism, specifically the hierarchical organization would be affected. From a comparative perspective, Mesoudi and Whiten (2004) recently argued for the adaptive value of hierarchical imitation, in other words, action imitation at a fairly high program level. Work by Bauer and Mandler (1989) and Whiten (2002) investigating imitation of hierarchical structures using reenactment paradigms showed that already children around 20 months selectively imitate actions with causal relations, leaving out unimportant and optional ones. In other words, hierarchical structuring seems to be a representational organization principle from very early on. We reasoned that in ASD, the hierarchical organization of scripts might be specifically impaired as a consequence of characteristic perceptual and cognitive biases. In particular, it has been suggested that autism may be characterized by weak central coherence—a cross-domain cognitive style affecting both perception and cognition by favoring local over global processing and reducing the normal tendency to integrate information in context (Frith, 1989; Happé, 1999). A local, detail-focused processing style might lead to a tendency to represent event actions and props at the level of low-level concrete examples—slotfillers—as opposed to higher-level slots. Second, difficulties to process information in context and for meaning might affect the distinction between aspects that are central versus optional to the event.

Initially, Frith and Happé (1994) argued that weak coherence might be a processing style pervasive in autism (i.e., to also characterize individuals with ASD who show ToM competencies). On this basis, abnormalities with the hierarchical organization, which would reduce the understanding of event variability, were predicted for all people with ASD.

For a first analysis, participants with ASD were again subdivided into ToM passers and ToM failers. The most striking finding was that seven of eight (87%) of the children with ASD who had failed ToM tasks seemed altogether to lack event scripts as a cognitive frame for their experiences. Their event narratives lacked generality, as they often talked about their own personal experiences, and most of them did not sequence different actions in the temporal or causal order in which they normally occur. This drastically contrasted with the performance of the typically developing children and the ones with learning difficulties, who gave evidence of generality, temporal–causal, and hierarchical organization. For instance, when asked "what happens normally when people go to a restaurant?" typically developing children would state "they go in and eat" (i.e., would describe actions at a fairly abstract level); in contrast, the ASD ToM failers tended to describe actions at a much lower level (e.g., stating " 'fish'n chips', they had beans, sausage and pie for dinner"). With the exception of one boy, none of the ASD ToM failers could explain why people go to restaurants or celebrate Christmas.

The narratives of the ASD ToM passers (comprising those who passed first- and those who passed second-order ToM tasks) showed relatively intact generality and causal–temporal organization. However, they, too, demonstrated significant abnormalities in the hierarchical organization. Compared to a control group, they still mentioned significantly more slotfillers. For example, when asked what a restaurant looks like, one participant with ASD insisted on Chinese lanterns, which he did not seem to consider as a variable detail, substitutable by other forms of lightning. ASD ToM passers also showed significant difficulties in appreciating the optional character of actions, stating, for example, that people *always* have starters in a restaurant.

The value of event scripts consists of both providing structure and accommodating variability across different experiences with an event. These results suggest that whereas lower-functioning individuals with ASD who fail ToM tasks have difficulties with both facets, high-functioning ASD ToM passers have more specific difficulties appreciating event variability. In a second analysis, the role of weak central coherence was examined. For each individual, a composite central coherence score was computed, based on the combined performance on two visuospatial and one verbal–semantic task tapping this construct. In contrast to Frith's original proposal, a weak coherence cognitive style was found to be not universal to the participants with ASD but characteristic for only 44% (see Loth et al., 2005b). Correlation and multiple regression analyses lent support to our predictions that weak coherence was related to (maladaptive) low-level slotfiller descriptions.

However, it cannot be ruled out that abnormalities in script narratives were influenced by verbal or narrative impairments. Therefore, in the next study we aimed to reduce the verbal production demands and to investigate more specifically whether abnormalities in the hierarchical organization of events affects appreciation of event variability (Loth, 2003; Loth & Gómez, 2004). The "Frequency Rating Task" consists of stories of the life of two characters: Dr. Smith and the teacher, Mrs. Jones. Dr. Smith is portrayed, for example, on the train to work and at work in the surgery. The sentences were composed of acts that are central, optional, or inappropriate to the events. Participants were asked to rate how doctors *normally* behave when they are in that situation, using a rating scale that ranged from always, most of the time, sometimes, rarely, to never. On the basis of a pilot study with university students it was established that correct ratings of a central act (e.g., "In the surgery, Dr. Smith examines a patient") were "always" or "most of the time." We considered the responses "most of the time," "sometimes," and "rarely" as acceptable for optional acts. Optional acts included acts that may or may not occur because they are peripheral to the event (e.g., "On the train, Dr. Smith is eating a sandwich") or very specific examples—"slotfillers" (e.g., "In the supermarket, Dr. Smith is putting orange juice in his cart"). Correct ratings of inappropriate acts ("In the surgery, Dr. Smith and his patient are eating sandwiches") were "rarely" and "never."

It was predicted that people with ASD would understand basic components of scripts, hence to give appropriate ratings for the central acts. However, we expected that the ratings of optional acts would be disturbed. If scripts were represented at the level of slotfillers and not of slots, changes in slotfiller occurrences might be perceived as a deviance from the script (as would for a typically developing child or adult changes in a whole slot). And if people with ASD have difficulties understanding the global meaning of the event and how actions are causally related, this, too, would disturb the ratings of optional acts. Finally, we also expected the group with ASD to have difficulties rating inappropriate acts, because their inappropriateness was due to being performed in the wrong context (it is possible that a doctor eats a sandwich on a train but to eat a sandwich with patients in the consulting room is not considered to be appropriate). Only participants who passed a pretest and thus showed that they understood the rating scale received the main task.

Unexpectedly, both participants with ASD and the controls made more mistakes rating optional items (i.e., they were rated as occurring always or never) than rating central or inappropriate items. However, the important finding was that the ASD group rated optional acts significantly more often incorrectly than the control groups. This was found when the ASD sample as a whole was compared to the control group and also when the ASD sample was split into low-IQ and norm-IQ subgroups and compared separately to controls of similar verbal abilities. There were no group differences on ratings of central or inappropriate acts. In addition, correlation analyses showed that in the ASD group only ToM, but unexpectedly neither central coherence nor VIQ scores, yielded a significant relationship to the number of inappropriately rated optional acts. Hence, it seems that ToM ability has a developmental effect on the understanding of event variability.

To examine the significance of abnormalities in event variability for the understanding of autistic symptoms in real life, we recently gave a modified version of this task to a group of norm-IQ boys with Asperger Syndrome (ages 8–16 years). Parents were asked to complete the Childhood Asperger Syndrome Test (CAST; Scott, Baron-Cohen, Bolton, & Brayne, 1999), which taps presence and absence of characteristic social and nonsocial autistic features. Preliminary correlation analyses between number of errors on the ratings of optional items and parents' ratings on the CAST revealed a strong and significant positive relationship.

The results of these script studies have important implications. As French (1985) speculated, both someone without an understanding of central script components and someone with a very rigid representation of events would behave inappropriately across different common and routine situations. Our findings highlight that attempts to "teach" individuals with autism event scripts can only be partially successful if the understanding of event variability is not specifically addressed. Script abnormalities and, in particular, abnormalities in the hierarchical representation may provide a possible link between social and nonsocial facets of this disorder. Script abnormalities would not only impair social understanding but might also shed light on the origins of the insistence on strict and inflexible routines—an important facet of repetitive behaviors. Our results suggest that such dysfunctional insistence on routines might be related to abnormalities in representing event variability. Things that *could* occur may be represented as if they *should* occur.

Taken together, the studies on social norms and event scripts suggest that in addition to difficulties understanding that others' behavior is motivated by their internal mental states, some people with ASD also show abnormalities in predicting and explaining behavior using cultural knowledge. Our work also emphasizes that there are clear differences between different individuals across the autism spectrum—higher- and lower-functioning individuals who pass versus fail ToM tasks. These abnormalities in the acquisition and representation of cultural knowledge may be developmentally related to abnormalities in the development of sociocognitive and/or perceptual skills. In our studies we found relationships with ToM competencies (at the level of false-belief understanding), yet further work is needed in order to specify whether abnormalities in other, earlier (but possibly related) socioperceptual/cognitive skills, such as imitation, are implicated in the difficulties found here.

GENERAL DISCUSSION: SPECULATIONS AND AN OUTLOOK TO THE FUTURE

In this chapter we attempted to bring together rather disparate literatures: perspectives from typical and atypical development of imitation as well as perspectives from embodied cognitive neuroscience and cultural psychology. When putting together these diverse literatures, speculatively the following picture seems to emerge: From the moment infants are born, they are typically endowed with some innate rudimentary skills that allow them to recognize people as distinct from inanimate objects, including some ability to imitate others. Over the first 2 years of their lives, young children use in coordination a number of sociocognitive skills (including joint attention, intention attribution, and imitation) that enable them to learn *through* others. Eventually, they develop a more full understanding of complex cognitive mental states, such as beliefs.

Currently, a number of different proposals regarding the significance of imitation behavior and its role in ToM development are being debated. One possible way in which imitation and ToM are related is that both abilities are rooted in "embodied simulation," which links action with perception and thus allows observers to attain some unconscious, prereflexive first-person insight into the actions, emotions, and sensations of others.

In our argument we put a great deal of emphasis on the notion that cultural knowledge is based on experience, and that the child recruits different emerging socioperceptual and sociocognitive skills in order to actively participate in cultural learning. Developmental studies suggest that typically developing children from preschool age understand different facets of cultural knowledge. They demonstrate basic script knowledge and are able to reason about social norms and rules. This provides children with a cognitive frame to anticipate, interpret, and evaluate new experiences, a mental guidebook to navigate the complex, ever-changing social world.

A large body of research documents that people with an autistic disorder show by and large imitation deficits and also characteristic delays in ToM development (with some individuals never gaining true insight that behavior is motivated by internal mental states). Based on the arguments about the role of these sociocognitive skills in cultural knowledge acquisition, cultural knowledge abnormalities were predicted for individuals with this condition. The majority of available studies that examined cultural knowledge in autism (until now exclusively in participants from middle childhood, and mainly adolescents and adults) suggest that their cultural knowledge in two key areas, social norms and scripts, is indeed impaired relative to their age and intellectual ability levels.

By combining perspectives from cultural psychology and cognitive development, it is suggested that cultural knowledge is both acquired on the basis of experiences and shapes in turn experiences in that it modulates "top-down" perception and interpretation of concrete social situations. There are two main implications for future work that flow from these arguments: First, it raises the questions of how different perceptual and cognitive processes (such as attention or memory) are influenced by context or conceptual information (here in particular cultural concepts) and whether there may be abnormalities in autism (Frith, 2003; Frith & Dolan, 1997). This approach would be compatible with recent developments in sociocognitive neuroscience that place stronger emphasis on experience as a fundamental factor in functional brain development (e.g., Gauthier, Skudlarski, Gore, & Anderson, 2000; Johnson, 2001). Second, the relationship between early social and cognitive competencies and the acquisition of higher-level cultural knowledge should be on the agenda for future research. This would have, not least, direct implications for teaching and intervention in young children with ASD. Moreover, by comparing and contrasting developmental patterns in typical and atypical development, we may attain a deeper understanding of the role of imitation and other sociocognitive and perceptual skills, not only for the understanding of other minds but also for the development of the understanding of the culture we live in, and through which we perceive and interpret the world, others', and our own actions.

One fundamental message is that, from the perspective of cultural knowledge, abilities such as imitation, joint attention, pretend play, ToM, or language, cannot be contemplated in isolation. They all play a role in bringing about the acquisition of the patterns of behaviors and representations that we call culture and that inform our ability to behave adaptively in our social and physical world. Because autism implies major deficits or abnormalities in several of these skills, adopting a cultural knowledge perspective could provide a unifying framework for understanding the diverse, yet at the same time converging, pattern of autistic disturbance. In the end what is affected, to a greater or lesser extent, in one way or another, is the ability to acquire culture, which modulates virtually every aspect of human cognition and behavior.

ACKNOWLEDGMENTS

We would like to thank Francesca Happé and Quinton Deeley for their helpful comments on an earlier version of this chapter. The empirical work summarized here would not have been possible without the help, commitment, and trust of individuals with an autistic condition, and those with learning difficulties and their teachers and parents, as well as a range of volunteers who acted as "controls." Eva Loth was supported by an ESRC postdoctoral fellowship while writing this chapter.

NOTE

1. In the following, the terms *theory of mind*, *mentalizing*, and *mindreading* are used interchangeably.

REFERENCES

Baldwin, D. A. (1993). Infants' ability to consult the speaker for clues to word reference. *Journal of Child Language, 20*, 395–418.

Baldwin, D. A. (1995). Understanding the link between joint attention and language acquisition. In M. K. Moore & P. J. Dunham (Eds.), *Joint attention: Its origins and role in development* (pp. 131–158). Hillsdale, NJ: Erlbaum.

Baron-Cohen, S. (1987). Autism and symbolic play. *British Journal of Developmental Psychology, 5*, 139–148.

Baron-Cohen, S. (1989). Perceptual role-taking and protodeclarative pointing in autism. *British Journal of Developmental Psychology, 7*, 113–127.

Baron-Cohen, S. (1990). Autism: A specific cognitive disorder of "mind-blindness." *International Review of Psychiatry, 2*, 79–88.

Baron-Cohen, S. (1995). *Mindblindness. An essay on theory of mind and autism.* Cambridge, MA: Bradford Book, MIT Press.

Baron-Cohen, S., Baldwin, D., & Crowson, M. (1997). Do children with autism use the Speaker's Direction of Gaze (SDG) strategy to crack the code of language? *Child Development, 68*, 48–57.

Baron-Cohen, S., Leslie, A., & Frith, U. (1985). Does the autistic child have a "theory of mind"? *Cognition, 21*, 37–46.

Baron-Cohen, S., O'Riordan, M., Stone, V., Jones, R., & Plaisted, K. (1999). Recognition of faux pas by normally developing children and children with Asperger syndrome or high-functioning autism. *Journal of Autism and Developmental Disorders, 29*(5), 407–418.

Bates, E. (1979). On the evolution and development of symbols. In E. Bates (Ed.), *The emergence of symbols: Cognition and communication in infancy* (pp. 1–32). New York: Academic Press.

Bateson, B. (1979). 'The epigenesis of conversational interaction': A personal account of research development. In M. Bullowa (Ed.), *Before speech: The beginning of human communication* (pp. 63–77). Cambridge, UK: Cambridge University Press.

Bauer, P. J., & Mandler, J. M. (1989). One thing follows another: Effects of temporal structure on 1- to 2-year-olds' recall of events. *Developmental Psychology, 25*(2), 197–206.

Berger, P. L., & Luckman, T. (1967). *The social construction of reality: A treatise in the sociology of knowledge.* New York: Anchor.

Blair, R. J. R. (1996). Brief report: Morality in the autistic child. *Journal of Autism and Developmental Disorders, 26*(5), 571–579.

Bloom, P. (2000). *How children learn the meaning of words.* Cambridge, MA: MIT Press.

Bloom, P. (2004). *Descartes' baby.* Cambridge, MA: Perseus/Basic Books.

Bruner, J. (1986). *Actual minds, possible worlds.* Cambridge, MA: Harvard University Press.

Bruner, J. (1990). *Acts of meaning.* Cambridge, MA: Harvard University Press.

Bruner, J. (2001). Human infancy and the beginnings of human competence. In J. A. Bargh & D. K. Apsley (Eds.), *Unraveling the complexities of social life: A festschrift in honor of Robert B. Zajonc* (pp. 133–140). Washington, DC: American Psychological Association.

Bruner, J., & Feldman, C. F. (1993). Theory of mind and the problem of autism. In S.

Baron-Cohen, H. Tager-Flusberg & D. J. Cohen (Eds.), *Understanding other minds: Perspectives from autism* (pp. 267–291). Oxford, UK: Oxford University Press.

Butterworth, G. (1991). The ontogeny and phylogeny of joint visual attention. In A. Whiten (Ed.), *Natural theories of mind: Evolution, development, and simulation of everyday mindreading* (pp. 223–232). Oxford, UK: Basil Blackwell.

Caldwell, C. A., & Whiten, A. (2002). Evolutionary perspectives on imitation: Is a comparative psychology of social learning possible? *Animal Cognition, 5,* 193–208.

Campos, J. J., & Sternberg, C. (1981). Perception, appraisal, emotion: The onset of social referencing. In M. Lamb & L. Sherrod (Eds.), *Infant social cognition: Empirical and theoretical considerations* (pp. 273–314). Hillsdale, NJ: Erlbaum.

Carpenter, M., Akhtar, N., & Tomasello, M. (1998). Fourteen- to 18-month-old infants differentially imitate intentional and accidental actions. *Infant Behavior and Development, 21,* 315–330.

Carpenter, M., Pennington, B. F., & Rogers, S. J. (2001). Understanding of others' intentions in children with autism. *Journal of Autism and Developmental Disorders, 31*(6), 589–599.

Carpenter, M., Pennington, B. F., & Rogers, S. (2002). Interrelations among social-cognitive skills in young children with autism. *Journal of Autism and Developmental Disorders, 32*(2), 91–106.

Castelli, F., Frith, C., Happé, F., & Frith, U. (2002). Autism, Asperger syndrome and brain mechanisms for the attribution of mental states to animated shapes. *Brain, 125*(8), 1839–1849.

Charman, T., & Baron-Cohen, S. (1994). Another look at imitation in autism. *Development and Psychopathology, 6,* 403–413.

Charman, T., Baron-Cohen, S., Swettenham, J., Baird, G., Drew, A., & Cox, A. (2003). Predicting language outcome in infants with autism and pervasive developmental disorder. *International Journal of Language and Communication Disorders, 38*(3), 265–285.

Charman, T., Baron-Cohen, S., Swettenham, J., Cox, A., Baird, G., & Drew, A. (1997). Infants with autism: An investigation of empathy, pretend play, joint attention, and imitation. *Developmental Psychology, 33*(5), 781–789.

Chartrand, T. L., & Bargh, J. A. (1999). The chameleon effect: The perception–behaviour link and social interaction. *Journal of Personality and Social Psychology, 76*(6), 893–910.

Cheng, P. W., & Holyoak, K. J. (1985). Pragmatic reasoning schemas. *Cognitive Psychology, 17,* 391–416.

Clément, F., Koenig, M., & Harris, P. L. (2004). The ontogenesis of trust. *Mind and Language, 19*(4), 360–379.

Cole, M. (1996). *Cultural psychology: A once and future discipline.* Cambridge, MA: Harvard University Press.

Cosmides, L. (1989). The logic of social exchange: Has natural selection shaped how humans reason? Studies with the Wason Selection Task. *Cognition, 31,* 187–276.

Cosmides, L., & Tooby, J. (1992). Cognitive adaptations for social exchange. In J. Barkow, L. Cosmides, & J. Tooby (Eds.), *The adapted mind: Evolutionary psychology and the generation of culture* (pp. 166–228). New York: Oxford University Press.

Critchley, H., Daly, E. M., Bullmore, E. T., Williams, S. C., Van Amelsvoort, T., Robertson, D. M., et al. (2000). The functional neuroanatomy of social behaviour: Changes in cerebral blood flow when people with autistic disorder process facial expressions. *Brain, 123*(11), 2203–2212.

Csibra, G., & Gergely, G. (1998). The teleological origins of mentalistic action explanations: A developmental hypothesis. *Developmental Science, 1*(2), 255–259.

Csibra, G., & Gergely, G. (2006). Social learning and social cognition: The case for pedagogy. In Y. Munakata & M. H. Johnson (Eds.), *Process of change in brain and cognitive development: Attention and performance* (Vol. 21, pp. 294–274). Oxford, UK: Oxford University Press.

Cummins, D. (1996). Evidence of deontic reasoning in 3-and 4-year-old children. *Memory and Cognition*, 24(6), 823–829.

Cummins, D. (2000). How the social environment shaped the evolution of mind. *Synthese*, 122, 3–128.

Dawson, G., Meltzoff, A. N., Osterling, J., Rinaldi, J., & Brown, E. (1998). Children with autism fail to orient to naturally occurring social stimuli. *Journal of Autism and Developmental Disorders*, 28(6), 479–485.

De Myer, M. K., Alpern, G. D., Barton, S., De Myer, W., Churchill, D. W., Hingtgen, J. N., et al. (1972). Imitation in autistic, early schizophrenic, and nonpsychotic subnormal children. *Journal of Autism and Childhood Schizophrenia*, 2, 264–287.

de Waal, F. (1982). *Chimpanzee politics: Power and sex among apes*. Baltimore: Johns Hopkins University Press.

Dewey, M. (1991). Living with Asperger's syndrome. In U. Frith (Ed.), *Autism and Asperger syndrome* (pp. 184–206). Cambridge, UK: Cambridge University Press.

French, L. A. (1985). Real-world knowledge as the basis of social and cognitive development. In J. B. Pryor & J. D. Day (Eds.), *The development of social cognition* (pp. 179–209). New York: Springer-Verlag.

Frith, C. (2003). What do imaging studies tell us about the neural basis of autism? *Novartis Foundation Symposium*, 251, 149–166.

Frith, C., & Dolan, R. J. (1997). Brain mechanisms associated with top-down processes in perception. *Philosophical Transactions of the Royal Society of London, B, Biological Sciences*, 352, 1221–1230.

Frith, U. (1989). *Autism. Explaining the enigma*. Oxford, UK: Blackwell.

Frith, U., & Happé, F. G. E. (1994). Autism: Beyond "theory of mind." *Cognition*, 50, 115–132.

Gallese, V. (2005). Embodied simulation: From neurons to phenomenal experience. *Phenomenology and the Cognitive Sciences*, 4, 23–48.

Gallese, V., & Goldman, A. (1998). Mirror neurons and the simulation theory of mindreading. *Trends in Cognitive Sciences*, 2, 493–501.

Gallese, V., & Lakoff, G. (in press). The brain's concepts: The role of the sensory-motor system in conceptual knowledge. *Cognitive Neuropsychology*.

Gauthier, I., Skudlarski, P., Gore, J. C., & Anderson, A. W. (2000). Expertise for cars and birds recruits brain areas involved in face recognition. *Nature Neuroscience*, 3(2), 191–197.

Gergely, G. (2002). The development of understanding self and agency. In U. Goswami (Ed.), *Blackwell handbook of childhood cognitive development* (pp. 26–46). Malden, MA: Blackwell.

Gergely, G., & Watson, J. (1999). Early socio-emotional development: Contingency perception and the social-biofeedback model. In P. Rochat (Ed.), *Early social cognition: Understanding others in the first months of life* (pp. 101–136). Mahwah, NJ: Erlbaum.

Gigerenzer, G., & Hug, K. (1992). Domain-specific reasoning: Social contracts, cheating, and perspective change. *Cognition*, 43, 127–321.

Goldman, A. (1989). Interpretation psychologised. *Mind and Language*, 4, 161–185.

Gómez, J. C. (2004). *Apes, monkeys, children, and the growth of mind*. Cambridge, MA: Harvard University Press.

Gómez, J. C., Sarriá, E., & Tamarit, J. (1993). The communicative study of early communication and theories of mind: Ontogeny, phylogeny, and pathology. In S. Baron-Cohen, H. Tager-Flusberg, & D. J. Cohen (Eds.), *Understanding other minds: Perspectives from autism* (pp. 397–426). Oxford, UK: Oxford University Press.

Gopnik, A., & Wellman, H. M. (1994). The theory theory. In L. A. Hirschfeld & S. A. Gelman (Eds.), *Mapping the mind: Domain specificity in cognition and culture* (pp. 275–293). Cambridge, UK: Cambridge University Press.

Gordon, R. M. (1996). "Radical" simulationism. In P. Carruthers & P. K. Smith (Eds.), *Theories of theories of mind* (pp. 11–21). Cambridge, UK: Cambridge University Press.

Gordon, R. M., & Cruz, J. (2003). *Encyclopaedia of cognitive science* (L. Nadel, Ed.). London: MacMillan.

Happé, F. G. E. (1993). Communicative competence and theory of mind in autism: A test of relevance theory. *Cognition, 48,* 101–119.

Happé, F. G. E. (1994). An advanced test of theory of mind: Understanding of story characters' thoughts and feelings by able autistic, mentally handicapped, and normal children and adults. *Journal of Autism and Developmental Disorders, 24*(2), 129–154.

Happé, F. G. E. (1999). Autism: Cognitive deficit or cognitive style? *Trends in Cognitive Sciences, 3*(6), 216–222.

Harris, P. L. (1992). From simulation to folk psychology: The case of development. *Mind and Language, 7*(1 & 2), 120–144.

Harris, P. L., & Núñez, M. (1996). Understanding of permission rules by pre-school children. *Child Development, 67,* 1572–1591.

Harris, P. L., & Núñez, M. (1998). Psychological and deontic concepts: Separate domains or intimate connection? *Mind and Language, 13*(2), 153–170.

Hobson, R. P. (1986). The autistic child's appraisal of expressions of emotion. *Journal of Child Psychology and Psychiatry, 27*(3), 321–342.

Hobson, R. P. (1993). Understanding persons: The role of effect. In S. Baron-Cohen, H. Tager-Flusberg, & D. J. Cohen (Eds.), *Understanding other minds: Perspectives from autism* (pp. 204–228). Oxford, UK: Oxford University Press.

Hobson, R. P., & Lee, A. (1999). Imitation and identification in autism. *Journal of Child Psychology and Psychiatry, 40*(4), 649–659.

Hobson, R. P., Ousten, J., & Lee, A. (1988). What's in the face? The case of autism. *British Journal of Psychology, 79,* 441–453.

Hudson, J. A. (1988). Children's memory for atypical actions in script-based stories: Evidence for a disruption effect. *Journal of Experimental Child Psychology, 46,* 159–173.

Iacoboni, M., Molnar-Szakacs, I., Vallese, V., & Buccino, G., Mazziotta, J. C., & Rizzolatti, G. (2005). Grasping the intentions of others with one's own mirror neuron system. *Public Library of Science Biology, 3*(3), 0529–0535.

Jackendoff, R. (1999). The natural logic of rights and obligations. In R. Jackendoff, P. Bloom, & K. Wynn (Eds.), *Language, logic and concepts: Essays in memory of John MacNamara* (pp. 67–95). Cambridge, MA: MIT Press.

Jacob, P., & Jeannerod, M. (2005). The motor theory of social cognition: A critique. *Trends in Cognitive Sciences, 9*(1), 21–25.

Johnson, A. G. (Ed.). (2000). *The Blackwell dictionary of sociology: A user's guide to sociological language, second edition* (2nd ed.). Oxford, UK: Blackwell.

Johnson, M. H. (1997). *Developmental cognitive neuroscience.* Oxford, UK: Blackwell.

Johnson, M. H. (2001). Functional brain development in humans. *Nature Reviews Neuroscience, 2,* 475–483.

Johnson, M. H., & Morton, J. (1991). *Biology and cognitive development: The case of face recognition.* Oxford, UK: Basil Blackwell.

Johnson-Laird, P. N., Legrenzi, P., & Sonino-Legrenzi, M. (1972). Reasoning and a sense of reality. *British Journal of Psychology, 63,* 395–400.

Kanner, L. (1943). Autistic disturbances of affective contact. *Nervous Child, 2*, 217–250.

Karmiloff-Smith, A. (1992). *Beyond modularity. A developmental perspective on cognitive science*. Cambridge, MA: MIT Press/Bradford Books.

Karmiloff-Smith, A. (1998). Development itself is the key to understanding developmental disorders. *Trends in Cognitive Sciences, 2*(10), 389–398.

Keller, M., Gummerum, M., Wang, X. T., & Lindsey, S. (2004). Understanding perspectives and emotions in contract violation: Development of deontic and moral reasoning. *Child Development, 75*(2), 614–635.

Keysers, C., Wickers, B., Gazzola, V., Anton, J.-L., Fogassi, L., & Gallese, V. (2004). A touching sight: SII/PV activation during the observation and experience of touch. *Neuron, 42*, 1–20.

Killen, M., & Užgiris, I. C. (1981). Imitation of action with objects: The role of social meaning. *Journal of Genetic Psychology, 138*, 219–229.

Klin, A. (2000). Attributing social meaning to ambiguous visual stimuli in higher-functioning autism and Asperger syndrome: The social attribution task. *Journal of Child Psychology and Psychiatry, 41*(7), 831–846.

Klin, A., Jones, W., Schultz, R., & Volkmar, F. (2003). The enactive mind, or from actions to cognition: Lessons from autism. *Philosophical Transactions of the Royal Society of London—B Series, 358*, 345–360.

Klin, A., Jones, W., Schultz, R., Volkmar, F., & Cohen, D. (2002). Visual fixation patterns during viewing of naturalistic social situations as predictors of social competence in individuals with autism. *Archives of Genetic Psychiatry, 59*, 809–816.

Klinger, L. G., & Dawson, G. (2001). Prototype formation in autism. *Developmental Psychopathology, 13*(1), 111–124.

Kohlberg, L. (1984). *Essays on moral development: Vol. 2. The psychology of moral development*. San Francisco: Harper & Row.

Lakoff, G., & Johnson, M. H. (1999). *Philosophy in the flesh: The embodied mind and its challenge to Western thought*. New York: Basic Books.

Leekam, S., Baron-Cohen, S., Perrett, D., Milders, M., & Brown, S. (1993). Eye-direction detection: A dissociation between geometric and joint attention skills in autism. *British Journal of Developmental Psychology, 15*, 77–95.

Leslie, A. M. (1987). Pretense and representation: The origins of "theory of mind." *Psychological Review, 94*, 412–426.

Leslie, A. M. (1994). ToMM, ToBy, and agency: Core architecture and domain specificity. In L. A. Hirschfeld & S. A. Gelman (Eds.), *Mapping the mind: Domain specificity in cognition and culture* (pp. 119–148). New York: Cambridge University Press.

Leslie, A. M., & Frith, U. (1990). Prospects for a cognitive neuropsychology of autism: Hobson's choice. *Psychological Review, 97*, 122–131.

Leslie, A. M., & Roth, D. (1993). What autism teaches us about metarepresentation. In S. Baron-Cohen, H. Tager-Flusberg, & D. J. Cohen (Eds.), *Understanding other minds: Perspectives from autism* (pp. 83–111). Oxford, UK: Oxford University Press.

Lewis, C., & Boucher, J. (1988). Spontaneous, instructed and elicited play in relatively able autistic children. *British Journal of Developmental Psychology, 6*, 325–339.

Loth, E. (2003). *On social, cultural and cognitive aspects of theory of mind in practice*. Unpublished doctoral thesis, University of St. Andrews, Scotland.

Loth, E., & Gómez, J. C. (2002, September). *The role of theory of mind in the acquisition of "cultural knowledge" in autism*. Paper presented at the annual conference of BPS Developmental Section, Brighton, UK.

Loth, E., & Gómez, J. C. (2004). *Autism and the role of cultural knowledge in theory of mind in practice*. Paper presented at the International Meeting for Autism Research, Sacramento, CA.

Loth, E., Gómez, J. C., & Happé, F (2005a). *Event representation in autism: The role of theory of mind and weak coherence.* Manuscript submitted for publication.

Loth, E., Gómez, J. C., & Happé, F. (2005b). *Weak coherence in autism spectrum disorders: Specificity, individual differences, and the relation between cognitive biases in the visual–spatial and verbal–semantic domains.* Manuscript submitted for publication.

Loveland, K. A., McEvoy, R. E., Kelley, M. L., & Tunali, B. (1990). Narrative story telling in autism and Down's syndrome. *British Journal of Developmental Psychology, 8,* 9–23.

Loveland, K. A., Pearson, D. A., Tunali-Kotoski, B., Ortegon, J., & Gibbs, M. C. (2001). Judgments of social appropriateness by children and adolescents with autism. *Journal of Autism and Developmental Disorders, 31*(4), 367–376.

Loveland, K. A., & Tunali, B. (1991). Social scripts for conversational interactions in autism and Down's syndrome. *Journal of Autism and Developmental Disorders, 21,* 177–186.

Loveland, K. A., & Tunali, B. (1993). Narrative language in autism and the theory of mind hypothesis: A wider perspective. In S. Baron-Cohen, H. Tager-Flusberg, & D. J. Cohen (Eds.), *Understanding other minds: Perspectives from autism* (pp. 247–266). Oxford, UK: Oxford University Press.

Losh, M., & Capps, L. (2003). Narrative ability in high-functioning children with autism or Asperger's Syndrome. *Journal of Autism and Developmental Disorders, 33*(3), 239–251.

Mead, G. H. (1934). *Mind, self and society.* Chicago: University of Chicago Press.

Meltzoff, A. N. (1988). Infant imitation after a one-week delay: Long-term memory for novel acts and multiple stimuli. *Developmental Psychology, 24,* 470–476.

Meltzoff, A. N. (1995). Understanding the intentions of others: Re-enactment of intended acts by 18-month-old children. *Developmental Psychology, 31,* 838–850.

Meltzoff, A. N. (2002). Imitation as a mechanism of social cognition: Origins of empathy, theory of mind, and the representation of action. In U. Goswami (Ed.), *Blackwell handbook of childhood cognitive development* (pp. 6–25). Malden, MA: Blackwell.

Meltzoff, A. N., & Gopnik, A. (1993). The role of imitation in understanding persons and developing a theory of mind. In S. Baron-Cohen, H. Tager-Flusberg, & D. J. Cohen (Eds.), *Understanding other minds: Perspectives from autism* (pp. 335–366). Oxford, UK: Oxford University Press.

Meltzoff, A. N., & Moore, C. (1977). Imitation of facial and manual gestures by human neonates. *Science, 198,* 75–78.

Meltzoff, A. N., & Moore, M. K. (1983). Newborn infants imitate adult facial gestures. *Child Development, 54,* 702–709.

Mesoudi, A., & Whiten, A. (2004). The hierarchical transformation of event knowledge in human cultural transmission. *Journal of Cognition and Culture, 4,* 1–24.

Morgan, S. B., Cutrer, P. S., Coplin, J. W., & Rodriguez, J. R. (1989). Do autistic children differ from retarded and normal children in Piagetian sensorimotor functioning? *Journal of Child Psychology and Psychiatry, 30,* 857–864.

Mundy, P., Sigman, M. D., Ungerer, J. A., & Sherman, T. (1986). Defining the social deficits in autism: The contribution of non-verbal communication measures. *Journal of Child Psychology and Psychiatry, 27,* 657–669.

Nadel, J., Guérini, C., Pezé, A., & Rivet, C. (1999). The evolving nature of imitation as a format of communication. In J. Nadel & G. Butterworth (Eds.), *Imitation in infancy* (pp. 209–234). Cambridge, UK: Cambridge University Press.

Nadel-Brulfert, J., & Baudonnière, P. M. (1982). The social function of reciprocal imitation in 2-year-old peers. *International Journal of Behavioural Development, 5,* 95–109.

Nelson, K. (1986). *Event knowledge: Structure and function in development.* Hillsdale, NJ: Erlbaum.

Nucci, L. P. (2002). The development of moral reasoning. In U. Goswami (Ed.), *Blackwell handbook of childhood cognitive development* (pp. 303–326). Malden, MA: Blackwell.

Núñez, M., & Harris, P. L. (1998). Psychological and deontic concepts: Separate domains or intimate connection? *Mind and Language, 13*(2), 153–170.

Oberman, L. M., Hubbard, E. M., McCleery, J. P., Altschuler, E. L., Ramachandran, V. S., & Pineda, J. A. (2005). EEG evidence for mirror neuron dysfunction in autism spectrum disorders. *Brain Research: Cognitive Brain Research, 24*(2), 190–198.

Perner, J. (1988). Developing semantics for theory of mind: From propositional attitudes to mental representation. In D. R. Olson, J. W. Astington, & P. L. Harris (Eds.), *Developing theories of mind* (pp. 141–171). Cambridge, UK: Cambridge University Press.

Perner, J. (1991). *Understanding the representational mind.* Cambridge, MA: MIT Press.

Perner, J. (1993). The theory of mind deficit in autism: Rethinking the metarepresentation theory. In S. Baron-Cohen, H. Tager-Flusberg, & D. J. Cohen (Eds.), *Understanding other minds: Perspectives from autism* (pp. 112–137). Oxford, UK: Oxford University Press.

Piaget, J. (1965). *The moral judgment of the child.* New York: Free Press. (Original work published 1932)

Plaisted, K. (2001). Reduced generalisation in autism: An alternative to weak central coherence. In J. A. Burack, T. Charman, N. Yirmiya, & P. R. Zelazo (Eds.), *The development of autism: Perspectives from theory and research.* Mahwah, NJ: Erlbaum.

Premack, D. (1990). The infant's theory of self-propelled objects. *Cognition, 36*, 1–16.

Premack, D., & Woodruff, G. (1978). Does the chimpanzee have a theory of mind? *Behavioral and Brain Sciences, 4*, 515–526.

Quinn, N., & Holland, D. (1987). Culture and cognition. In D. Holland & N. Quinn (Eds.), *Cultural models in language and thought* (pp. 3–40). Cambridge, UK: Cambridge University Press.

Rizzolatti, G., Fadiga, L., Gallese, V., & Fogassi, L. (1996). Premotor cortex and the recognition of motor actions. *Brain Research: Cognitive Brain Research, 3*, 131–141.

Rizzolatti, G., Fogassi, L., & Gallese, V. (2001). Neurophysiological mechanisms underlying the understanding and imitation of actions. *Nature Neuroscience Reviews, 2*, 661–670.

Rogers, S. (1999). An examination of the imitation deficit in autism. In J. Nadel & G. Butterworth (Eds.), *Imitation in infancy* (pp. 254–283). Cambridge, UK: Cambridge University Press.

Rogers, S. J., Hepburn, S. L., Stackhouse, T., & Wehner, E. (2003). Imitation performance in toddlers with autism and those with other developmental disorders. *Journal of Child Psychology and Psychiatry, 44*(5), 763–781.

Rogers, S. J., & Pennington, B. F. (1991). A theoretical approach to the deficits in infantile autism. *Development and Psychopathology, 3*, 137–162.

Scaife, M., & Bruner, J. (1975). The capacity of joint visual attention in the infant. *Nature, 253*, 265–266.

Schank, R., & Abelson, R. (1977). *Scripts, plans, goals and understanding.* Hillsdale, NJ: Erlbaum.

Schultz, R. (2005). Developmental deficits in social perception in autism: The role of the amygdala and fuisform face area. *International Journal of Developmental Neuroscience, 23*, 125–141.

Schultz, R., Gauthier, I., Klin, A., Fulbright, R., Anderson, A., Volkmar, F. R., et al. (2000). Abnormal ventral temporal cortical activity among individuals with autism and Asperger Syndrome during face discrimination. *Archives of General Psychiatry, 57*, 331–340.

Scott, F. J., Baron-Cohen, S., Bolton, P., & Brayne, C. (2002). The CAST (Childhood Asperger Syndrome Test): Preliminary development of a UK screen for mainstream primary-school-age children. *Autism*, 6(1), 9–31.

Shweder, R. A. (1984). Anthropology's romantic rebellion against the enlightment, or there's more to thinking than reason and evidence. In R. A. Shweder & R. A. LeVine (Eds.), *Culture theory: Essays on mind, self and emotion* (pp. 27–66). Cambridge, UK: Cambridge University Press.

Shweder, R. A. (1991). *Thinking through cultures*. Cambridge, MA: Harvard University Press.

Shweder, R. A., Mahapatra, M., & Miller, J. G. (1987). Culture and moral development. In J. Kagan & S. Lamb (Eds.), *The emergence of morality in young children* (pp. 1–83). Chicago: University of Chicago Press.

Shore, B. (1996). *Culture in mind: Cognition, culture, and the problem of meaning*. Oxford, UK: Oxford University Press.

Singer, T., Seymour, B., O'Doherty, J., Kaube, H., Dolan, R., & Frith, C. D. (2004). Empathy for pain involves the affective but not sensory components of pain. *Science, 303*, 1157–1162.

Smetana, J. G., & Braeges, J. L. (1990). The development of toddlers' moral and conventional judgments. *Merrill-Palmer Quarterly, 36*, 329–346.

Smith, I. M., & Bryson, S. E. (1994). Imitation and action in autism: A critical review. *Psycholocial Bulletin, 116*(2), 259–273.

Spelke, E. S., Phillips, A., & Woodward, A. L. (1995). Infants' knowledge of object motion and human action. In D. Sperber, D. Premack, & A. J. Premack (Eds.), *Causal cognition: Multidisciplinary debate* (pp. 44–78). Oxford, UK: Oxford University Press.

Sperber, D. (1996). *Explaining culture: A naturalistic approach*. Oxford, UK: Blackwell.

Sperber, D. (1997). Intuitive and reflective beliefs. *Mind and language, 12*(1), 67–83.

Stern, D. N. (1985). *The interpersonal world of the infant*. New York: Basic Books.

Strauss, S., Ziv, M., & Stein, A. (2002). Teaching as a natural cognition and its relations to preschoolers' developing theory of mind. *Cognitive Development, 17*, 1473–1487.

Theoret, H., Halligan, E., Kobayashi, M., Fregni, F., Tager-Flusberg, H., & Pascual-Leone, A. (2005). Impaired motor facilitation during action observation in individuals with autism spectrum disorder. *Current Biology, 8*(15), R84–85.

Tomasello, M. (1992). The social bases of language acquisition. *Social Development, 1*, 68–87.

Tomasello, M. (1999). *The cultural origins of human cognition*. Cambridge, MA: Harvard University Press.

Tomasello, M., & Barton, M. (1994). Learning words in non-ostensive contexts. *Developmental Psychology, 30*, 639–650.

Tomasello, M., & Carpenter, M. (2005). Intention reading and imitative learning. In S. Hurley & N. Chater (Eds.), *Perspectives on imitation: From cognitive neuroscience to social science: Vol. 2. Imitation, human development, and culture* (pp. 133–148). Cambridge, MA: MIT Press.

Tomasello, M., Carpenter, M., Call, J., Behne, T., & Moll, H. (2005). Understanding and sharing intentions: The origins of cultural cognition. *Behavioral and Brain Sciences, 28*, 675–735.

Tomasello, M., Kruger, A. C., & Ratner, H. H. (1993). Cultural learning. *Behavioural and Brain Sciences, 16*(3), 495–511.

Trevarthen, C. (1979). Communication and cooperation in early infancy: A description of primary intersubjectivity. In M. Bullowa (Ed.), *Before speech: The beginnings of human communication* (pp. 321–347). London: Cambridge University Press.

Trevarthen, C., & Aitken, K. J. (2001). Infant intersubjectivity: Research, theory, and clinical applications. *Journal of Child Psychology and Psychiatry, 42*(1), 3–48.

Trillingsgaard, A. (1999). The script model in relation to autism. *European Journal of Adolescent Psychiatry, 8*(1), 45–49.

Turiel, E. (1983). *The development of social knowledge: Morality and convention.* Cambridge, UK: Cambridge University Press.

Varela, F. J., Thompson, E., & Rosch, E. (1991). *The embodied mind: Cognitive science and human experience.* Cambridge, MA: MIT Press.

Volden, J., & Johnston, J. (1999). Cognitive scripts in autistic children and adolescents. *Journal of Autism and Developmental Disorders, 29*(3), 203–211.

Wertsch, J. V. (1993). A sociocultural approach to socially shared cognition. In L. B. Resnick, J. M. Levine, & S. D. Teasley (Eds.), *Perspectives on socially shared cognition* (pp. 85–100). Washington: American Psychological Association.

Wellman, H. M., & Miller, J. G. (2005). *Including deontic reasoning as fundamental to theory of mind.* Manuscript submitted for publication.

Whiten, A. (2002). Imitation of sequential and hierarchical structure in action: Experimental studies with children and chimpanzees. In K. Dautenhahn & C. L. Nehaniv (Eds.), *Imitation in animals and artifacts: Complex adaptive systems* (pp. 191–209). Cambridge, MA: MIT Press.

Whiten, A., & Ham, R. (1992). On the nature and evolution of imitation in the animal kingdom: Reappraisal of a century of research. In P. J. B. Slater, J. S. Rosenblatt, C. Beer, & M. Milinski (Eds.), *Advances in the study of behavior* (Vol. 21, pp. 239–283). San Diego, CA: Academic Press.

Wicker, B., Keysers, C., Plailly, J., Royet, J.-P., Gallese, V., & Rizzolatti, G. (2003). Both of us disgusted in my insula: The common neural basis of seeing and feeling disgust. *Neuron, 40,* 655–664.

Williams, D. (1992). *Nobody nowhere.* London: Doubleday.

Williams, J. H., Whiten, A., & Singh, T. (2004). A systematic review of action imitation in autism spectrum disorder. *Journal of Autism and Developmental Disorders, 34*(3), 285–299.

CHAPTER 9

Imitation, Identification, and the Shaping of Mind

Insights from Autism

PETER HOBSON
JESSICA MEYER

One of the most intriguing questions for developmental psychology, child psychiatry, and philosophy of mind is this: How does a young child become mentally connected to other people in such a way that over the course of early development, he or she develops an understanding of what it means to be a self in relation to other selves, and to have a mind that is both connected with and differentiated from the minds of others? It is one of the unique strengths of developmental psychopathology, with its insistence on integrating perspectives from typical and atypical development, that it allows us to address questions as fundamental but seemingly inaccessible as this, on the basis of new evidence as well as fresh theoretical insights. Through the unusual case of autism in particular, we may discern the nature and significance of otherwise elusive primary social-development determinants of interpersonal relations, psychological understanding ('theory of mind'), and, arguably at least, flexible, creative, symbolic thinking itself.

In this last sentence, we have jumped the gun—and in more than one respect. First, although we may indeed discern the nature and significance of primary deficits in interpersonal relations in the syndrome of autism and discover that this illuminates elusive aspects of typical development, it is by no means clear that so far we have achieved this goal. Indeed, a principal thrust of this chapter is to suggest a new way of looking at what is basic to autism and, correspondingly, what is pivotal for typical development. Second, there is a long way to go before we can be confident which aspects of developmental disability in autism give rise to other areas of impairment, and which exist alongside, interact with, or merely reflect different components of the syndrome. In this respect, our approach is forthright but qualified: We suggest how a child's behavior and thinking is indeed *shaped by* interpersonal processes—and suggest how in the relative absence of such processes in autism, thinking is constrained—but acknowledge that the evidence is inconclusive. Yet whatever caveats we may wish to introduce, the study of autism is already furthering our understanding of what it means to have full and truly interpersonal engagement with others, and revealing just how important such engagement is for cognitive/linguistic as well as social and cultural development.

Thus far, we have highlighted person-to-person connectedness, the development of self, the acquisition of interpersonal understanding, and social-developmental sources of flexibility in action and thinking. We argue here that a special quality of interpersonal engagement, allied with but not reducible to imitation, is critical for the development of human beings in each of these respects, and critically impaired in children with autism. Before we attempt to characterize more precisely what we mean by special quality, it is fitting to illustrate the kinds of phenomena any theory of the developmental psychopathology of autism needs to encompass, from clinical and experimental perspectives. Are there features of autism that lead one to wonder whether some specific aspect of self–other connectedness and imitation might underlie the range of social and cognitive abnormalities characteristic of the syndrome? If so, how far-reaching might the developmental implications of such an impairment prove to be?

CLINICAL PERSPECTIVES

We restrict our excerpts from clinical accounts of autism to just two seminal contributions to the literature: the classic account in which Kanner (1943) first delineated the syndrome, and then one of the least cited but most enlightening descriptions and theoretical explorations of the children's social impairments, the book that its author, Gerhard Bosch (1970; or perhaps his translator) dauntingly titled *Infantile Autism: A Phenomenological–Anthropological Investigation Taking Language as the Guide.*

From the plethora of clinical features of autism he documented, Kanner (1943) chose to highlight the children's "inborn autistic disturbances of affective contact" (p. 250) as pathognomonic. This is still a radical stance. Even though the narrowly cognitive and linguistic theories of autism that dominated academic psychology and psychiatry in the latter part of the 20th century have given way to perspectives that accord a place for primarily social impairments, it remains the case that for many researchers in the field, issues of "affective contact"—and note how the phase captures *what it is like* for a person to be in relation to another—are still of peripheral concern in theorizing about autism. Yet Kanner went further than this. He not only claimed that the children's impairment in affective contact was central to autism but also suggested that "further study of our children may help to furnish concrete criteria regarding the still diffuse notions about the constitutional components of emotional reactivity" (p. 250). Clearly, Kanner was alert to the need to explain what *does* give us the feeling of being in affective contact with other people, and to account for its relative absence in our own experience when relating to children with autism.

Then there were the additional "fascinating peculiarities" of autism, as Kanner called them, which might help us to think more deeply about the interconnectedness of psychological development. In discussing his 11 cases, for example, Kanner noted (among other things) how the children failed to assume an anticipatory posture to being picked up. They had difficulty in using language to convey meaning to others, although many could repeat nursery rhymes or even foreign-language (French) lullabies; they would often use sentences that were "parrot-like repetitions of heard word combinations" (p. 243), sometimes taking the form of delayed echolalia; their words were often used with inflexible meanings, and personal pronouns might be repeated just as heard, complete with echoed intonation and without adjustment to who was speaking. Some of the children were so unresponsive that they were considered deaf or hard of hearing; they had a wish to maintain sameness and displayed little variety in their spontaneous activity; and above all, they showed a "profound aloneness" in relation to others, such that "people, so long as they left the child alone, figured in about the same manner as did the desk, the bookshelf, or the filing cabinet" (p. 246).

What is striking about these clinical features, beyond the issue of affective contact? Well, what each seems to entail is not merely a lack of attentiveness or even affective responsiveness to other people but also a lack of *movement* into the stance, the attitude, or the communicative intention of the other. Take the example of children extending their arms to be picked up. On those occasions when parents lift their babies or toddlers from the floor, it is not merely the young child who (typically) offers his or her arms. The adult does so, too. In stretching forth his or her arms, the child is responding in kind to the actions shown *toward the self* by someone else. It is at least plausible that the child assimilates those actions into the child's own repertoire and proceeds to show similar actions *toward the other*. Or, again, what do we observe in the children's language and thought? They are good at remembering by rote, or repeating things exactly as heard: It is when they need to adjust their language (including the personal pronouns "I" and "you") according to the stance of the person-in-speaking (with a new "I" or "you") that they become stuck. It is in using language for communicating meaning to someone who needs enlightening or who will be available for contact—and whom the child appreciates to have exactly these qualities, both different from and similar to him- or herself—that the children have most difficulty. In thinking and relating to the world, as well as in communicating, it is when they need to move through alternative perspectives, the kinds of perspective that different people might have, that the children encounter severe problems. No wonder that children with autism are inflexible and rigid in their take on the world, if they are unmoved by others. Finally, in their relations with other people, it is not just that the children are inattentive; it is also that they are not involved with the attitudes of others in the same way or to the same extent as children without autism. This is the case, whether those attitudes are simply sentiments or outward-directed attitudes to things and events in the world, including attitudes toward the self.

Gerhard Bosch (1970) pinpoints more precisely just how the children's lack of interpersonal engagement is intimately bound up with their limited worldview. Bosch stresses how children with autism have a "delay in the constituting of the other person as someone in whose place I can put myself . . . and in the constituting of a common sphere of existence, in which things do not simply refer to me but also to others" (p. 89). He does not discount the fact that many children with autism *do* develop relationships that "without doubt may be termed personal" (p. 93), but when it comes to the kind of reciprocal relationship in which others' expressiveness is responded to as such, or where the child needs to establish a world as shared and at the same time experienced differently by others, profound difficulties arise. Bosch focuses on the children's struggles to comprehend and use personal pronouns and ties these in with their failure to grasp the distinction between themselves and others as agents responsible for actions, and as beings who can stand in a possessive relationship to things.

How does this picture differ from that of typically developing children or adults? When I see that it is you who acts, or you who possesses something, I comprehend this as you having the kind of ownership of the action or possession that I might have. When you seize something and insist: "Mine!", I can feel your possessive attitude, but feel it as yours. Therefore, it makes sense for me to use the very same word for *my* self-centered attitude toward things I consider as "Mine!". This simple example illustrates how each of us is naturally *identified with* other people through our engagement with their bodily expressed attitudes. As one facet of this, we have the propensity to be *moved toward adopting* others' attitudes, as those attitudes are directed toward the social and nonsocial world. If you screw up your face in disgust when you taste a peach, I am hardly likely to ask for a bite. Often we discover new meanings in things, through other people. In typical development, very young children do so too.

The point we take from Bosch (although he did not express it in these terms) is how fundamental such processes of identification are for aspects of self–other experience and understanding. Not only do they yield a grasp of the nature of human psychological perspectives—both one's own and those of others—but they result in constantly shifting orientations as one moves between one's own viewpoint and viewpoints adopted from and through others. Such processes are critical not only for taking part in reciprocal communication but also for acquiring flexibility in attitude, action, and thinking. The reason is that movements in attitude and takes on the world that occur *through* others become fluid and flexible movements that occur within the individual's own mind. In accordance with the ideas of Vygotsky (1978), interpersonal transactions become intraindividual mechanisms of thinking and moving in thought. Processes of identification mesh with, but are to be distinguished from, what customarily falls under the title of imitation. Some but only some forms of copying draw on identification; and from a complementary standpoint, imitation as usually defined represents only one among many domains in which identification is manifest. Therefore, if indeed it is the case that autism entails a characteristic deficit in identifying with others, we shall need to reconsider how far it would be accurate to pinpoint imitation (rather than identification) as basic to the disorder.

IMITATION, IDENTIFICATION, AND SELF–OTHER RELATIONS

In an early investigation that appeared just a decade after Kanner (1943) identified the syndrome of autism, Ritvo and Provence (1953) evaluated six children between the ages of 22 and 39 months. As well as focusing on the children's disturbance in human contact, they highlighted their "intense interest in certain toys . . . (with) . . . a constriction in the range of playthings the child uses and a difficulty in shifting from one plaything to another" (p. 156), and their unusual postures, rhythms, and motor patterns. The authors were impressed by the difficulty these young children showed in learning to play simple games dependent on "orientation to the human face and imitation of human movement" (p. 156). The mother of one of the children described how her young son could not learn how to play pat-a-cake in the usual way through watching her playing with him, and how she had to teach him to play the game by manipulating his hands physically. Upon discovering that all six of these children performed poorly on formal tests of imitation, Ritvo and Provence offered the following reflections:

> The process of imitation presupposes both a certain distance from and a certain closeness to the object (i.e. the person). In imitation the transformation of the self is carried out according to an image of the object or the nonself . . . the lack of differentiation of the representation of the self from the nonself suggests disturbances in processes of identification. . . . (pp. 159–160)

Despite the sporadic appearance of more systematic investigations of the profile of imitative strengths and limitations among children with autism, and in particular, the demonstration by DeMyer and colleagues (1972, 1974) that they are especially poor in imitating bodily movements, it was not until the late 1980s and early 1990s that a renewed focus on impaired socioemotional processes in autism (e.g., Dawson & Lewy, 1989; Fein, Pennington,

Markowitz, Braverman, & Waterhouse, 1986; Hobson, 1989a; Mundy & Sigman, 1989) prompted academic researchers to accord self–other connectedness and differentiation a pivotal role in theoretical accounts of the disorder.

Two integrative contributions with this focus appeared in close succession in the journal *Development and Psychopathology* (and see Meltzoff & Gopnik, 1994, for another closely related account). In a paper titled "On the Origins of Self and the Case of Autism," Hobson (1990) elaborated his view that impairments in intersubjectivity are of primary importance not only in explaining the children's difficulties in sharing experiences and in deriving concepts of the mind but also in acquiring a sense and understanding of self and others as individuated centers of consciousness and attitude. He referred to the children's "failure to identify with the personal meanings of those activities and attitudes of mind which normal children imitate" (p. 175). In parallel, Rogers and Pennington (1991) gave special prominence to ways in which deficits in imitation might make a distinctive contribution to the intersubjective impairment that characterizes autism and posited a fundamental disturbance in self–other representation. According to these authors' formulation, the foundation for the children's difficulties occurred in "forming and coordinating social representations of self and other at increasingly complex levels via amodal or cross-modal representational processes that extract patterns of similarity between self and other" (Rogers & Pennington, 1991, p. 157). Although the focus here is on what are generally (albeit controversially) considered the representational aspects of self–other coordination, it is also important that in subsequent reviews of this account, Rogers (1999; Rogers & Bennetto, 2000) has continued to stress how the thesis concerned "a core deficit in the capacity to imitate motor movements" (Rogers & Bennetto, 2000, p. 81). This emphasis on motor imitation is now complemented by consideration of emotional contagion. Meanwhile, Rogers and Bennetto (2000) are appropriately cautious in discussing whether other components of the model, and especially dyspraxia and/or impairment in executive functioning, are primary and whether they can explain the children's impaired intersubjective engagement.

In each case, phenomena of autism that had previously been considered in more or less separate compartments (partly in accord with traditional categories of cognitive, affective, and conative aspects of psychological functioning) were reconceptualized as manifestations of dysfunction in closely related *social* processes that have an intimate connection with imitation. Each was concerned to rethink the very nature of intersubjectivity, role taking, self-awareness, and cognitive flexibility, and to do so with reference to the abnormalities characteristic of autism.

Given the convergence between these two approaches with very substantial areas of overlap, it may be timely to explore some of the differences. These are largely matters of degree, but they bring into focus some subtle contrasts in philosophical as well as theoretical orientation that have far-reaching implications. Take one point of agreement and contrast: In an early chapter, Hobson (1989a) set the framework for his approach as follows: "The affective responsiveness between caretaker and infant, along with other kinds of attunement which are less recognizably affective in quality (such as certain imitative motor patterns), are especially important for the reason that the infant finds in and through his caretaker patterns of action and feeling in which he himself can participate" (p. 30). The emphasis here is on the kind of infant *experience* in which there is both connectedness and separateness from another person prior to conceptual representation of self and other. Rogers deals with these issues, too, and her more recent thinking reflects her shared concern with the affective dimension of interpersonal synchrony. Yet whereas Hobson's (e.g., 1993) emphasis has been on the significance of identification (and its relative lack in autism) as the affect-imbued psychological process that entails both subjective connectedness and differentiation—and critically, that serves to *move* a child to assume another person's psychological orientation and at the same time bring this in relation to the child's own starting stance— Rogers has stressed the developmental implications of an infant's imitative behavior (including that involved in emotional contagion) to the establishment of intersubjectivity, and the corresponding importance of "impairment in the ability to imitate another person's *movements*" (Rogers & Bennetto, 2000, p. 81, summarizing Rogers & Pennington's [1991] perspective, with emphasis added). So, too, in their more recent formulation, Rogers and Bennetto (2000) write:

> Social and communicative behaviors are largely motor behaviors, and thus generalized motor impairments have the potential of disrupting communication. . . . We are hypothesizing that a severe praxic and imitative deficit in an infant could markedly impair the physical coordinations involved in social exchanges. In so doing, the deficit would interfere with the establishment and maintenance of emotional connectedness between two people engaged in a typical social exchange. (pp. 84, 97)

Note that here the emphasis is on how praxic and motor–imitative deficits could affect emotional connectedness. Although this may indeed be an important part of the story, and even portray how identification may be undermined (and we think there are several ways in which this might occur), we anticipate that failures in identification will prove to be a major developmental *source* of dyspraxia. The reason is that our movements and actions are constantly shaped by our linkage with what lies behind the movements and actions of others. So, too, failures in emotional connectedness between children with autism and other people are part and parcel of the children's limited ability to identify with others. To return to Kanner's phrase, "affective contact" is an essential experiential component of the process by means of which the intersubjectively compelling and developmentally pivotal (and uniquely human) form of social engagement is achieved.

Is this proposal not encompassed by the suggestion by Rogers and Pennington (1991), that "the basis for autism lies in the deficient capacity to form or manipulate the particular (generally amodal) representations of self and others that underlie infant body imitation, affect mirroring and sharing, and awareness of other's subjective states" (p. 151)? We think this approach gets near to the heart of the matter, yet as Rogers has acknowledged (Rogers & Bennetto, 2000), difficulties with such a formulation remain. For example, children with autism do seem to recognize certain kinds of self-other correspondence, such as that required to register when they are being imitated. Moreover, on the identification view, forming and using representations of self and other are not the foundational processes. To be sure, the progressive development of such representations over the earliest years of life is a vitally important matter, and the thorny issue of whether representations underpin or result from the earliest forms of self–other connectedness and differentiation—and identification—is too complex (and too difficult) for us to address here. Yet what we need to stress is that through identification, one person not only resonates with another but also participates in the other's psychological orientation. Of course, this involves perception of and affective/conative responsiveness to the expressive behavior of another person. In addition, however, one individual is moved by and toward the stance of another. As we have stressed elsewhere, a relative lack of such psychological movement—as motivating, not merely motivated—might have profound implications for developing cognitive flexibility, acquiring concepts of mind, and adjusting to the pragmatics of language. Moreover, strictly speaking, one person identifies with what is expressed in and through another person's behavior, just as so-called emotion recognition entails perception of emotional meaning in facial and bodily gestures.

Therefore, whereas Rogers and her colleagues justifiably stress the developmental implications of a limited ability to imitate, we see the specific forms of imitative deficit manifest in autism as an expression of something else, and it is mainly the something else that is responsible for a range of serious developmental sequelae. A further difference between the two accounts occurs with respect to executive deficits, where we consider that a major source (rather than effect) of the children's difficulties in shifting points of view, reflecting on, planning, and controlling their own behavior and attitudes is their limited ability to identify with, and interiorize, others' attitudes to themselves (a theme common to the writings of both Vygotsky, 1962 and 1978, and Freud, 1924). We anticipate that the specificity of identification as entailing a quality of interpersonal engagement, and the specificity of its effects in a variety of domains within the syndrome of autism (including those of imitation and executive function), will account for many of the partial accomplishments that children with autism achieve in each of these domains. If all this is correct, it would mean that just as one cannot sideline the issue of intersubjectivity in any adequate account of the developmental psychopathology of autism, so too one cannot do without something like the concept of identification.

We should note that the kinds of divergence we have emphasized are not limited to comparisons between our account and that of Rogers (with whom our points of agreement are more marked than the differences). For example, Williams, Whiten, and Singh (2004) have published a recent, thoughtful review of the literature on imitation in autism, in which they suggest that stereotyped mimicking forms of imitation may derive from poorly developed integration of "vocal, affective, and motor expression in the imitation of an appropriate and possibly novel goal, identified through recognising others' intentions" (p. 296). We do not think the problem is one of recognizing intentions involved in goal-directed actions (Moore, Hobson, & Lee, 1997), and we are skeptical that integration of different expressions is the essential problem (although we do recognize the importance of coordinated perception and expression of feelings for human interpersonal engagement). In our account, the crux is the children's limitations in assuming another person's orientation as expressed through his or her behavior, whether this is in action, in attitude, or in communicative act. As we shall consider shortly, stereotyped, mimicking forms of imitation might well derive from copying without identification, and we think it is from failing to identify with others that the critical deficit in imitation derives. To repeat: Not all copying depends on identification, nor does the ability to register being copied. Moreover, not all identification is expressed in recognizably imitative acts, so the manifestations of failures in identification extend beyond the domain of imitation. Most important, the developmental sequelae range over a number of characteristic cognitive as well as socioemotional and motor abnormalities seen in autism.

As a final point for this discussion, we should refer to the clinical implications of our approach. The critical issue is how to foster the children's *movement* toward engaging with, and then being moved by, the psychological orientations of other people. There may be several ways to achieve this aim, and we acknowledge the potential value of imitating the child—although it remains to establish how far the effects of such intervention extend to facilitating the *kinds* of interpersonal engagement that promote intersubjective, emotionally patterned coordination, and cognitive as well as social perspective taking. A variety of clinical approaches that focus on social reciprocity, whether in imitation or social–affective routines (e.g., Dawson & Galpert, 1990; Rogers, Hall, Osaki, Reaven, & Herbison, 2002; Rogers, Herbison, Lewis, Pantone, & Reis, 1986; Wetherby & Prizant, 1999; Wieder & Greenspan, 2003), and especially those (e.g., Gutstein, in press; Gutstein & Sheely, 2002) that adjust predictability and novelty so that the child enters into movement with a social partner in order to cocreate and maintain coordinated states of interpersonal engagement, appear to have impressive potential in this respect.

Having highlighted some of critical theoretical issues, we turn to consider what kinds of self–other connection and differentiation are relatively intact among children with autism, and which are not.

Imitation without Identification: Echoing

An especially intriguing form of imitation is notable for its presence in the behavior of children with autism. This is how they echo the speech and sometimes the actions of others, something noted not only by clinicians such as Kanner (1943), Bosch (1970), Ricks and Wing (1975), and Blank, Gessner, and Esposito (1979), as well as by writers such as Fay (1973, 1979) or Brown and Whiten (2000) who have drawn on observational studies, but also by experimenters conducting research at the interface between cognitive and imitative abilities. In the late 1960s, for example, Hermelin and O'Connor (1970) administered tests of verbal memory to children with autism. On tests of immediate imitative recall, children with autism tended to echo the final parts of messages without regard for meaning. Such findings prompt us to seek the developmental sources of failure to ground memory and understanding in person- or language-anchored meanings.

From a social-developmental perspective, as several authors (e.g., Charney, 1981; Hobson, 1990; Kanner, 1943) have highlighted, much of what makes delayed echolalia or personal pronoun confusions idiosyncratic is anchorage of the communicative act in an original situation as experienced by the child but not shared with other people. It is in this respect that the phenomena reflect impairments in self–other differentiation. Instead of relating speech to another person's perspective, words or phrases become linked with the children's own egocentric take on what was happening at the time the utterances were heard, and what is happening when the child speaks. As Shapiro, Roberts, and Fish (1970) proposed, children with autism "incorporate but do not assimilate or digest; therefore they do not *identify* in the usual manner" (p. 564). While typically developing children use imitative responses involving structural change, something that entails taking the role of someone else and making this one's own, the echolalic speech of children with autism can often be characterized as comprising "unaltered reproductions" (Shapiro et al., 1970, p. 559).

Imitation (Sometimes) without Identification: Actions on Objects

A number of studies have established that children with autism are able to copy others' goal-directed actions on objects (e.g., Charman & Baron-Cohen, 1994; Ingersoll, Schreibman, & Tran, 2003; Morgan, Cutrer, Coplin, & Rodrigue, 1989; Stone, Ousley, & Littleford, 1997). On the other hand, there is evidence that, at least among very young children with autism, they have a reduced tendency to imitate even simple object-related actions (Charman et al., 1997; Rogers, Hepburn, Stackhouse, & Wehner, 2003). Interpreting a relative dearth of imitation by very young children with autism, Rogers and colleagues (2003) noted that the actions to be copied not only contradicted object affordances but also required the child—who had already been using the object in another way during a baseline condition—to shift to the adult's way of using the object. Such considerations are also relevant for understanding the children's difficulties in pantomiming actions in the absence of an object, or in using an object for novel purposes (Bartak, Rutter, & Cox, 1975; Curcio & Piserchia, 1978; Hammes & Langdell, 1981; Heimann, Ullstadius, Dahlgren, & Gillberg, 1992; Rogers, Bennetto, McEvoy, & Pennington, 1996).

There is a need to reconcile two alternative explanations for such observations. On the one hand, children with autism appear to have the ability to copy goal-directed actions, at least when these are relatively straightforward. On the other hand, they sometimes fail to do so. Is this simply a motivational issue? Perhaps that is the wrong question. It is not simply motivational, but yes, it is related to what the children are motivated to imitate. More important, it is related to *the way in which* children are motivated to imitate, the processes through which imitation occurs. In our view, one individual is drawn into identifying with, and therefore copying, someone else. Accordingly, the imitative profile of children with autism appears to reflect a subtle dissociation between a potential *ability to imitate*—the ability to read the intended goal-directed actions of someone else and, if prompted, to copy such actions—and a *disability in identifying*—a lesser inclination to attend to, become engaged with, and adjust one's orientation through someone else (although of course a person can also draw on identification when motivated to copy for other reasons). For the latter reason, there will be times when children with autism are not inclined to copy, even when they have the potential ability to do so, for they are not sufficiently involved with what the other person is doing or expressing; and this lack of identifying is the very same reason why they are (relatively) unable to achieve *certain* forms of imitating, even when they are motivated to do so. Identification involves us with another person in a particular way that "moves" us into the stance of the other, while remaining grounded in ourselves, and from a complementary perspective, it moves something of the other into ourselves, altering what we may become. The child with autism can still copy much of what someone else does by way of goal-directed action but may need to be specifically motivated to do so in other ways if he or she is not naturally prone to assume the other person's orientation.

The study by Rogers and colleagues (2003) yielded one further result consistent with this interpretation. Children's difficulty on tests of imitation was highly correlated with their limited tendency to initiate joint attention with a tester during the Early Social Communication Scales (ESCS; Mundy, Hogan, & Doehring, 1996) and their impaired social–communication scores on the Autism Diagnostic Observation Schedule—Generic (ADOS-G; Lord, Rutter, Dilavore, & Risi, 1999). Each of these measures provides an indication of children's involvement with the psychological orientation of someone else. It is precisely the nature and power of this involvement that reflects self–other engagement and, potentially at least, self–other role taking.

It may be appropriate to add one further perspective on the motivational aspect of this account. Based on an unanticipated observation that children with autism performed better when copying actions in which an acted-on toy produced sensory effects (Roeyers, Van Oost, & Bothuyne, 1998), Ingersoll and colleagues (2003) speculated that outcomes such as blinking lights or sounds can serve both as a nonsocial reward and as a goal for action. When compared with typically developing children, their participants with autism (mean age 37 months) were more likely to imitate actions on toys with strong sensory effects than in the condition in which the toys had no effects, and in this condition they also engaged in significantly less joint attention, directed less positive affect toward the tester, and made fewer social initiations. On the other hand, the groups were similar in directing positive affect toward the objects. Here we see correspondence between social versus nonsocial imitation, and social versus nonsocial affective engagement. These two aspects of social functioning are intimately related—perhaps through the single, affective–conative process of identification.

Action (Mostly) with Identification: Movement and Gesture

If it is the case that, in the course of moment-by-moment social interactions, typically developing children are not only perceiving but also identifying with the bodily expressed movements, actions, and gestures of others, and so being shaped by mutual engagement, the effects of a relative lack of such identificatory processes in children with autism will have negative implications for the development of coordination of movement, action, and gesture.

It is a relatively consistent finding from studies of imitation in children with autism that they display abnormalities in the ability to imitate facial, vocal, and gestural expressions, as well as meaningless movements (e.g., Dawson & Adams, 1984; DeMyer et al., 1972, 1974; Hertzig, Snow, & Sherman, 1989; Jones & Prior, 1985; Loveland et al., 1994; Ohta, 1987; Rogers et al., 1996, 2003; Smith & Bryson, 1994; but see Morgan et al., 1989). These convey expressive modes of relating rather than strategies of goal-directed action. Children with autism appear to be less responsive to such features of another person's actions (Hobson, 1995), and as Rogers (e.g., Rogers & Bennetto, 2000) has also discussed, this might be connected with a relative insensitivity to patterns of bodily configuration, rhythm, and flow that reveal something of a person's emotional quality or tone (see Stern, 1985). We believe that abnormalities in the movements and gestures of individuals with autism (e.g., manifest in ill-directed, limp farewell waves [Hobson & Lee, 1998] and in awkward posture and gait when walking) reveal something about actions unshaped by identification with what is expressed by others through their movements and gestures.

Yet it would be understandable if readers were to expect better reasons for invoking a concept of identification, with all the complexities this seems to entail, when more parsimonious explanations might serve for at least some of the phenomena we have been considering. In this regard, one observation appears to be especially telling. As several authors have noted (e.g., Barresi & Moore, 1996; Ohta, 1987; Smith & Bryson, 1998; Whiten, 2002; Whiten & Brown, 1998), children with autism sometimes appear to reproduce actions as seen when they watch a demonstrator, instead of reproducing what the demonstrator would have seen when acting. For example, Smith and Bryson (1998) described an error involving rotation of the hand by 180°, something that seemed to reflect a difficulty in translating the view of an action made by someone else into a matching action of the self. Barresi and Moore (1996) interpreted such phenomena in terms of a disorder of intermodal integration of first- and third-person information. Bråten (1998) expressed it differently, suggesting that children with autism observe from the outside but do not feel from the inside (i.e., participate in) the movements of the second person, and thus can only do what is seen from their own stance. Here is one form of imitation that might be especially revealing for the children's limited propensity to identify with the psychological stance of someone else. It is a phenomenon to which we shall shortly return.

Registering Self–Other Correspondences (without Identification?): Being Imitated

Several studies have reported how children with autism can show striking responsiveness to being imitated. They may become more socially engaged and interactive when an adult imitates their actions (Dawson & Adams, 1984; Dawson & Galpert, 1990; Nadel, Guérini, Pezé, & Rivet, 1999). For example, Nadel and colleagues (2000) introduced children to a setting in which the investigator initially sat immobile, more or less statue-like. Then the investigator came alive and mirrored the children's every move and expressive utterance or gesture. Finally, she returned to the still-face and still-body position. Following the period of imitative interaction, children with autism increased their social initiations toward the newly frozen investigator. A subsequent study by Esclaona, Field, Nadel, and Lundy (2002) replicated these results with younger children and established that highly contingent responsiveness yielded similar, albeit less striking, effects on the children's subsequent initiation of social contact. Note that during the imitative phase, it was not a case of the children *moving to* imitate another person—a cardinal feature of identification—but, rather, the other person moved to imitate the child. Although it was this that appeared to enhance the child's interest in the other person, Nadel (2002) cautioned that only in rare instances did children with autism test out whether the other person was intending to imitate them. She also noted that it remains questionable how far the children were able to engage in mutual, reciprocal exchanges with the turn taking and role switching these typically entail.

STUDIES IN IDENTIFICATION

We have tried to convey something of the nature and developmental significance of identification in typical development, and its significance for understanding the developmental psychopathology of autism. Now we attempt to fulfill a complementary aim: to indicate phenomena that are not only consistent with, but also require, something like the concept of identification for their explanation.

Style

In a methodologically novel study, Hobson and Lee (1999) tested matched groups of children with and without autism for their ability to imitate a person demonstrating four novel goal-directed actions on objects in two different styles. It is difficult to define what style means, but two actions may be distinuished according to the style with which they are executed, even when they have in common both a goal and a means to that goal. In the study by Hobson and Lee, goal-directed actions were executed in contrasting styles. For example, in one condition the demonstrator made a toy policeman-on-wheels move along by pressing down on its head *either* with his wrist cocked *or* with extended index and middle fingers. The results were as follows. The children with autism were perfectly able to copy the demonstrator's actions (e.g., in pressing down the policeman's head to make him move). On the other hand, they contrasted with control participants insofar as very few adopted the demonstrator's style of acting on the objects. Instead of adopting the wrist or two-finger approach to activating the toy, for example, most of them pressed down on the policeman's head with the palm of a hand. Here we stress a contrast between children's ability to observe and copy intended actions per se, relatively intact in autism, and the propensity to identify with and thereby imitate a *person's* expressive mode of relating to objects and events in the world.

The claim that children with autism are abnormal in identifying with someone else goes beyond the matter of copying bodily expressions, however. As we have seen, the concept of identification is one that entails a particular form of imitation through which an individual assumes the *stance* of the other. This means that actions and attitudes anchored in the other person's bodily located orientation toward the world become assimilated to the individual's own bodily located orientation. The most striking expression of this is when an individual imitates someone else's self-orientated action, so that the action becomes orientated to the individual's (rather than the copied person's) self.

This proved to be another feature that distinguished children with autism. For example, one condition involved the demonstrator holding a pipe rack against his own shoulder in order to strum it with a stick, either harshly or gently. Here a substantial majority of the control participants identified with the demonstrator and positioned the pipe rack against their own shoulders before strumming it. By contrast, most of the children with autism positioned it at a distance in front of them, on the table. Therefore, not only with respect to style but also with respect to self-orientation, the children with autism did not assume the manner with which the other person executed actions, even though they copied the actions per se.

It is noteworthy that in a recent review, Williams and colleagues (2004) commented on the significance of these reversal errors. On the other hand, somewhat curiously, they considered that this failure to identify with the tester and therefore adopt his self-orientation partially confounded the findings of a lesser propensity to imitate the style (i.e., harsh vs. gentle) of the actions. In fact, there was no confound here, because each type of error could and did occur alongside and independently of the other (as is the case in studies we cite later). Moreover, Williams and colleagues considered these reversal errors to support the theory of "self–other mapping" deficits of Rogers and Pennington (1991), but as we have argued, it is not clear that "mapping" is the critical deficiency here.

In subsequent studies, we have introduced systematic variation between the style and strategy/goal of an action (Hobson, Lee, & Meyer, 2003). Here we illustrate some of these investigations, for each of which we were able to establish good interrater reliability in judgments of videotaped actions by raters unaware of group constitution and the hypotheses underlying the studies.

First, we predicted that by turning style into an objective goal, children with autism would be able to copy the speed, rhythm, and configuration of the movements of actions—providing the movements were neither too *complex* nor *expressive* (two imprecise terms, but they will have to do for now). The reason for this qualification is that a person may enlist the process of identifying with someone else when it comes to imitating sophisticated or expressive gestures (how does a ballet dancer learn from his or her mentor?), and so here children with autism might face difficulty. We predicted relatively spared abilities among such participants, on the basis that once the goal of copying the style of the movements was clear, there would be no particular sensorimotor impediment to success. Note again: The requirement was to copy forms of movement-in-action, and this contrasts with conditions in which participants either do or do not assume the style with which a person happens to do something. In this *style-as-goal* condition, then, the task structure made it evident that the aim was to use the object in a particular way— something we anticipated our participants with autism would succeed in. An example was when the tester demonstrated turning gymnastic ribbons either in horizontal figure-8s or vertical spirals.

Second, we predicted that children with autism would show somewhat more difficulty when style was portrayed as the means to a goal. We called these *style-for-goal* conditions. Here the task was to accomplish a goal with the object, and a certain style of action was needed to ensure success. For example, it was necessary to pull a blob of blue-tack slowly if the goal was to stretch it—that is, the demonstrator's slow stretching effected the goal—whereas one needed to pull the blob apart forcefully, in order to break it in two. The point here is that once again, participants were motivated to notice and to copy a style of action because the style was part of a strategy of goal-directed action, a means to an end. They had reasons for imitating how the person did what she did, beyond the fact that this was simply the person's way of doing what she was doing.

Finally, we predicted that the groups would be most markedly different when style was a personal quality exhibited by the tester when carrying out the goal but seemingly bearing no relation to the goal itself. In our two *goal-with-style* conditions, therefore, style was presented as incidental to the goal. An example was when the tester threw a ball into a wastebin, either gently with an underhand toss or with a forceful overhand throw, where both strategies were equally successful.

Participants were carefully matched groups of 16 children with autism and 16 nonautistic children with learning difficulties. They ranged in age from 6 to 14 years, and had a mean verbal mental age of about 6 years. As part of our procedure, we established that the groups were similar in their ability and/or propensity to copy six simple goal-directed actions, on tasks yielding neither ceiling nor floor effects. Each of the objects we employed had a nonobvious affordance. These hidden possibilities constituted a potential outcome of action, but the outcome and the strategy required to achieve it were not evident until the child had seen the demonstration. For example, a small toy alien would sing a song, but only when both of its outstretched hands were pressed simultaneously. The groups were similar in that the children copied most of the newly revealed strategies to achieve the goals, approximately four of the six items.

When it came to performance on the critical conditions (and here all the children copied the simple actions), the profile of results for imitation of style was as predicted. Firstly, there was not a group difference on the two style-as-goal items. Several children in each group imitated style correctly on both occasions, and several in each group did not imitate style on either one. On the style-for-goal items, on the other hand, there was a significant but moderate group difference. For example, seven of the children in each group imitated style once, but only two in the control group compared with seven of those with autism failed to do so at all. Finally, on the two goal-with-style actions, children with autism were far less likely to imitate style. With the exception of two children, those in the comparison group all imitated style at least once, but most of the children with autism (13) did not imitate style at all.

Overall, although the mean score for imitation of actions was about four of six for both groups, and the mean score for imitating style was also approximately four of six for those in the comparison group, children with autism imitated style on only about two of the six items.

Self–Other Orientation

We also devised a fresh approach to investigating self–other orientation (Meyer & Hobson, 2004). We tested 32 children between the ages of 6 and 14 years, half with autism and half without autism but instead with learning difficulties or developmental delays. The children with and without autism were group-matched for chronological age, and language ability. Their verbal mental ages ranged between 2 and 13 years. We administered a test of visual–motor integration to ascertain that the groups were similar in their fine motor and visual–motor planning skills.

We met with each of the children in a quiet, familiar room in his or her school. The children were well acquainted with the tester. Our procedure began with the tester and child seated on carpet squares on the floor, situated on opposite ends of a testing mat, directly across from each other at a distance of approximately 20 inches. Ahead of time, we had placed two straight lines of blue tape stretching from one side to the other on the mat, 5 inches in front of the tester and the other at the same distance in front of the participant, leaving a 10-inch center area demarcated between the two lines of tape. The lines of tape were employed to standardize administration and allow for objective coding of the orientation of the actions.

There were four actions, each of which was presented in two different ways. For example, the experimenter picked up a small wheel with a metal handle (a castor from furniture) that had been placed in the middle of the testing mat and proceeded to roll it from one side of the mat to the other, *either* across the mat directly in front of herself (i.e., from left to right, neither away from or toward herself) *or*, leaning forward, across the front of the participant; another example was where she *either* lifted a blue box from its position in front of herself, placed it on top of a box positioned in front of the participant, and then returned it to the starting-point *or* lifted the box closest to the participant, placed that on top of the box nearest herself, then returned it to its original position. For each of the four conditions, children saw the investigator produce the action in one of two possible orientations—close to or toward herself, or close to or toward the child—on the first testing session and saw the alternative orientation for each condition in a second session on another day. After demonstrating each action, the examiner returned the object(s) to their original positions and instructed the child: "Now you." There was no explicit instruction to copy what the investigator had done.

The children's subsequent actions were scored as reflecting *identification* if the child copied the investigator's stance (i.e., the action in relation to self or other). For example, identification occurred when the children imitated the tester's close-to-self-orientation by rolling the wheel close to him- or herself (i.e., on the participant's side of his or her line of tape) or copied close-to-other-orientation by rolling the wheel close to the tester. In those cases in which the action was *not* characterized by identification with the other person's stance, we made a further categorization: Was it simply that the response was out of keeping with identification, and perhaps without specific orientation, or did it take the form of an exact replication of the action, so that it resulted in a second runthrough of the child's original view of what was done to the object(s)? In the latter case, we classified the response as being an instance of *geometric repetition* (akin to the reversal errors seen in studies of gesture imitation).

We draw attention to the fact that the actions in the study were designed to be relatively straightforward, although not immediately obvious. The only participants in either group who failed to copy all eight actions were one participant with autism and one child in the comparison group, each of whom copied all but one action. This established that the groups were similar in attentiveness, motivation, understanding the task, and basic copying abilities.

As we predicted, the children with autism were significantly less likely to imitate the self–other orientation of the actions. While half the children in the comparison group copied the self–other orientation of the actions on at least half of the eight trials, for example, only 3 of the 16 children with autism did so; and from a complementary perspective, 6 of the participants with autism imitated self–other orientation on fewer than two occasions, while only 1 participant in the comparison group did so as infrequently as this.

When we examined the children's responses according to the most prevalent category of response (i.e., whether they primarily responded with *identification* or with *geometric repetition*), there was no consistent orientation, half of the children (eight in each group) fell into this latter category and showed a lack of consistent orientation. Of the remaining eight children in the control group, *all* eight showed a predominant response of identifying with the investigator and adopting her self–other orientation relative to themselves. Therefore, not a single child in the comparison group used geometric repetition as a primary form of response. Of the remaining eight participants with autism, by contrast, five of the children showed a predominant response of geometric repetition and only three that of identification.

Thus, the response strategy of geometric repetition—that is, responding so that the physical movements and locations of the objects acted on were replicated—was predominant among some (albeit a minority) of the children with autism, but none of the children in the control group. This result is reminiscent of instances of pronoun reversal, mimicry, and echolalia reported in clinical accounts and early studies of autism and of sporadic instances of reversal errors in a number of recent studies on imitation (e.g., Smith & Bryson, 1998; Whiten & Brown, 1998). It might suggest that some of these children had a natural propensity to be object- or stimulus-bound in their focus of attention. In our view, it is more plausible that they had developed this mode of apprehending and/or dealing with the world because they relatively lacked an orientation toward other people's stance-in-acting. If the children were failing to identify with the tester (i.e., adopting her perspective and incorporating it in relation to the self), then geometric repetition represents an expectable approach to copying the action.

Identification and Intersubjectivity

The best picture of what identification *is*, is what identification achieves by way of interpersonal linkage, interpersonal differentiation, and intersubjective coordination and movement. It is to the final item in this list that we now turn. How does identification-in-imitating tie in with identification as a source of intersubjective linkage?

Here we draw on the program of research inspired especially by the work of Mundy and Sigman and their colleagues (Mundy, Kasari, & Sigman, 1989; Mundy & Sigman, 1989; Sigman, Mundy, Sherman, & Ungerer, 1986), as well as by others such as Loveland and Landry (1986), indicating that joint attention, and especially the initiation of joint attention, reflects something very basic about the impairments in intersubjective engagement that characterize autism. Sigman, Kasari, Kwon, and Yirmiya (1992) also demonstrated how young children with autism show markedly reduced social referencing. More recent investigations of ever younger groups of children with autism, either through direct study (e.g., Charman et al., 1997; Rogers et al., 2003) or through parental report (e.g., Wimpory, Hobson, Williams, & Nash, 2000), have established that abnormalities in joint attention, affective responsiveness, and imitation are early appearing in many of the children.

The question, then, is how these abnormalities are interrelated. One approach to this question is to consider what it means to share experiences (Hobson, 1989b). Joint attention *of a certain kind*, and social referencing of a certain kind, reflects moments in which one person shares experiences of the world with another (here we shall restrict the focus to triadic, person–person–world relations). True sharing involves movement toward and adoption of aspects of the other person's psychological stance vis-à-vis objects or events and coordination with one's own now-expanded subjective state. The important thing here is that one participates in the other person's state and maintains awareness of otherness in the person with whom one is sharing, while also being affectively involved from one's own standpoint. This is what identification is, and what identification achieves.

With this hypothesis in mind, we decided to investigate the role of joint attention in relation to the children's imitation of self–other orientation. Our inspiration came from a study involving young typically developing children and nonhuman primates in which a positive relation between joint attention skills and imitative learning had been reported for each of the groups. Carpenter, Tomasello, and Savage-Rumbaugh (1995) recoded videotapes of one of their earlier studies on imitation (Tomasello, Savage-Rumbaugh, & Kruger, 1993) on a second-by-second basis, with a special focus on participants' gaze patterns during the tasks. Compared with chimpanzees, the human children spent about twice as much time looking at the tester's face, but in both groups, joint attention (coordinating looks between the object and partner) was associated with the propensity to imitate the actions correctly. In their discussion, Carpenter and colleagues noted how some joint attention involves actual sharing of affect—that is, looks aimed at engaging the tester or assessing the tester's attitude toward the object—as opposed to checking, defined as monitoring the tester's attentional state. However, these authors opted for "an objective coding system" in which only direction of gaze was coded, and in their empirical approach they did not differentiate between the two types of look.

In the current investigation (Meyer & Hobson, 2006), we attempted to extend this work to children with autism and to test our hypothesis that specifically sharing looks (reflecting identification) would have a positive relation with the propensity to imitate self–other orientation. With this single prediction in mind, we took a closer look at the videotapes of self–other imitation in the study described previously. The demonstration and imitation sequences of the self–other orientation study were coded by an independent naive judge (reliable with a second rater) for (1) direction of gaze—to the tester, object, or away and (2) quality of joint attention looks—sharing, checking, or orientating to the speech or movement of the tester. Results were that children with autism spent less than half as much time looking at the tester and significantly more time looking at the objects, relative to children in the comparison group. This difference was not specific to a particular quality of joint attention look, as the pattern was similar for sharing, checking, and orienting looks. Furthermore, the percentage of time spent looking at the tester overall, as well as frequency of checking and orienting joint attention looks, were *not* related to imitation of self–other orientation in either group. By contrast, *sharing looks* were specifically and significantly associated with the children's propensity to imitate self–other orientation, both within and across the two groups.

These results complement the findings of Carpenter, Pennington, and Rogers (2002), who administered a battery of social-cognitive measures, including facial and manual imitation tasks, to young children with autism and comparison groups. These researchers also tracked whether or not, at any point, the children showed evidence of joint engagement, defined as a spontaneous look to the tester and back to the object. Whether or not the children with autism showed evidence of joint engagement (75% of the children with autism did so) was significantly associated with their performance on the imitation tasks, as well as many of the other social-cognitive measures. Results of the present study extend such findings (also Rogers et al., 2003) to reveal that a specific type of joint attention—namely, sharing—is directly related to the children's imitation of self–other orientation. If sharing looks are another manifestation of the propensity to be moved by (and often, to) others' subjective orientation, then this relationship should come as no surprise.

CONCLUSIONS

So we come full circle, to consider what is needed, psychologically speaking, to provide the essentials of sharing but at the same time to partition out an individual's experiences. Here, bodily expressed *and* experienced attitudes are of the essence. One needs to apprehend another person's subjective states *as* subjective states of the other, and one's own subjective states *as* subjective states of one's own. What is needed is, first, the process of identification, and second, circumstances that allow the process of identification to yield experiences of others' attitudes to shared objects and events, so that one may be moved to adopt and/or appreciate the attitudes of others. This second requirement may be undermined if children suffer extreme forms of deprivation in particular aspects of interpersonal relatedness, for example, through congenital blindness or the kinds of profound neglect that occurred in Romanian orphanages, which can predispose to autism or autistic-like clinical features (Fraiberg, 1977; Hobson, Lee, & Brown, 1999; Rutter et al., 1999).

The concept of identification, one most developed by psychoanalysts attempting to explain the way in which the mind (including the personality) grows by way of increasingly complex internalizations of patterns of self–other relatedness, is specifically concerned with how an individual not only resonates to the attitudes of others but also experiences those attitudes as separate from the self. Or, to put this differently, the individual infant, child, or adult experiences for him- or herself something of the attitude of the other as the other's, but also for him- or herself. He or she can make such attitudes more truly his or her own, by internalizing what is felt to come from without, and integrating these attitudes into his or her own repertoire.

The crux is that interpersonal engagement is especially powerful in shaping human development for this reason: Not only do we resonate with the bodily expressed attitudes of others, for example when we feel for others, but also we have this feeling *for others*, so that the feelings are both ours and theirs. More than this, we can be moved to the position/stance/attitude of another person, even before we can conceptualize the other person as another person. Indeed, our propensity to be moved in this way is the very grounding of our awareness of what other people are, that is, alternative centers of subjective life. A protracted developmental process that begins with this initial, partial, and unconceptualized linkage-cum-differentiation with others—a mode of relatedness apparent from the earliest months of life—ultimately yields fully articulated forms of self- and other-understanding in the later years of childhood (Hobson, 1993, 2004). In our view, it is from identification that advanced forms of self–other representation develop.

We do not suppose that that children with autism completely lack the propensity to identify with others, nor that they all share the same forms or degrees of limitation in this respect. First, clinical experience suggests that a number of children with autism have either some or perhaps intermittent ability to assume the orientation of others. And it is not a trivial observation that many children with autism acquire sophisticated language, feelings for and understanding of others, and so on. Second, therapeutic interventions that specifically scaffold interpersonal engagement and coordination appear to have real potential for fostering the kinds of interpersonal responsiveness and role taking that reflect the workings of identification. Third, if one takes seriously the lessons from blind and very severely socially deprived children, then it becomes clear that the developmental benefits of identification accrue only when the interpersonal engagement to which it gives rise are realized between a child and others. Congenital blindness is only one among a possible range of handicaps predisposing to difficulties in this regard. Yet having said all this, it is our hypothesis that a weakness in identifying with other people is a prime cause of the *kind* of social impairment that makes autism autism, which brings us to the final part of our account.

Earlier we alluded to the importance of social engagement for cognitive flexibility as well as social engagement and reciprocal coordination of attitudes. In our view of autism, a major part of the difficulties in symbolic and executive functioning arise as developmental sequelae to failures in identification. The children relatively lack experiences of being moved by others to adopt novel attitudes to shared objects and events. It is not merely that the kinds of metarepresentation required for (certain forms of) symbolic functioning, and the capacity to reflect on oneself and one's own thoughts, arise through identifying with others' attitudes to one's own attitudes. It is also the case that one needs to take a *variety* of attitudes to one's own impulses and intentions if one is to plan effectively. One needs to restrain oneself, to hold oneself from acting out of habit, to encourage oneself to look at things this way and then that. Without identification with the attitudes of others, all this is so much more difficult, if not impossible.

There is yet more to the story, for example, in the domains of personality and motor development, where patterns of relatedness on the one hand and bodily gestures and movements on the other are shaped by our constant, pervasive, almost unremitting identification with others' attitudes and expressive actions. To conclude this chapter, however, we return to imitation. To be sure, imitation is critical for our understanding of autism. But, primarily, we believe it is in that aspect of imitation we call identification that we approach the core of autism. We are a long way from having sufficient evidence to make the case, but here is what we anticipate for the future of research in our field: The tapestry of clinical features that we know as autism will unravel into the weft of the individual child's limited propensity to identify with others, and the warp of other people's difficulties in mutually identifying with the children, woven over the months and years of early human development.

ACKNOWLEDGMENTS

Research described in this chapter was funded by the Economic and Social Research Council (award reference R000239355), the Baily Thomas Charitable Foundation, and the Tavistock Clinic, London (with NHS R&D funding), and made possible by the involvement of staff, students and parents at Edith Borthwick School, Helen Allison School, Springhallow School, and Swiss Cottage School. We thank Dr. Tony Lee for helping to establish the foundations for this research. We completed the chapter while at the Center for Advanced Study in the Behavioral Sciences, Stanford University.

REFERENCES

Barresi, J., & Moore, C. (1996). Intentional relations and social understanding. *Behavioral and Brain Sciences, 19,* 107–154.

Bartak, L., Rutter, M., & Cox, A. (1975). A comparative study of infantile autism and specific developmental receptive language disorder: I. The children. *British Journal of Psychiatry, 126,* 127–145.

Blank, M., Gessner, M., & Esposito, A. (1979). Language without communication: A case study. *Journal of Child Language, 6,* 329–352.

Bosch, G. (1970). *Infantile autism.* New York: Springer-Verlag.

Bråten, S. (1998). Infant learning by altercentric participation: The reverse of egocentric observation in autism. In S. Bråten (Ed.), *Intersubjective communication and emotion in early ontogeny* (pp. 105–126). Cambridge, UK: Cambridge University Press.

Brown, J., & Whiten, A. (2000). Imitation, theory of mind and related activities in autism: An observational study of spontaneous behaviour in everyday contexts. *Autism, 4,* 185–204.

Carpenter, M., Pennington, B. F., & Rogers, S. J. (2002). Interrelations among social-cognitive skills in young children with autism. *Journal of Autism and Developmental Disorders, 32,* 91–106.

Carpenter, M., Tomasello, M., & Savage-Rumbaugh, S. (1995). Joint attention and imitative learning in children, chimpanzees, and enculturated chimpanzees. *Social Development, 4,* 217–237.

Charman, T., & Baron-Cohen, S. (1994). Another look at imitation in autism. *Development and Psychopathology, 6,* 403–413.

Charman, T., Swettenham, J., Baron-Cohen, S., Cox, A., Baird, G., & Drew, A. (1997). Infants with autism: An investigation of empathy, pretend play, joint attention, and imitation. *Developmental Psychology, 33,* 781–789.

Charney, R. (1981). Pronoun reversal errors in autistic children: Support for a social explanation. *British Journal of Disorders of Communication, 15,* 39–43.

Curcio, F., & Piserchia, E. A. (1978). Pantomimic representation in psychotic children. *Journal of Autism and Childhood Schizophrenia, 8,* 181–189.

Dawson, G., & Adams, A. (1984). Imitation and social responsiveness in autistic children. *Journal of Abnormal Child Psychology, 12,* 209–226.

Dawson, G., & Galpert, L. (1990). Mother's use of imitative play for facilitating social responsiveness in autistic children. *Journal of Abnormal Child Psychology, 12,* 209–226.

Dawson, G., & Lewy, A. (1989). Arousal, attention, and the socioemotional impairments of individuals with autism. In G. Dawson (Ed.), *Autism: Nature, diagnosis, and treatment* (pp. 49–74). New York: Guilford Press.

DeMyer, M. K., Alpern, D. G., Barton, S., DeMyer, W. E., Churchill, D. W., Hingtgen, J. N., et al. (1972). Imitation in autistic, early schizophrenic, and non-psychotic subnormal children. *Journal of Autism and Childhood Schizophrenia, 2,* 264–287.

DeMyer, M. K., Barton, S., Alpern, D. G., Kimberlin, C., Allen, J., Yang, E., & Steel, R. (1974). The measured intelligence of autistic children. *Journal of Autism and Childhood Schizophrenia, 4,* 42–60.

Esclaona, A., Field, T., Nadel, J., & Lundy, B. (2002). Brief report: Imitation effects on children with autism. *Journal of Autism and Developmental Disorders, 32,* 141–144.

Fay, W. H. (1973). On the echolalia of the blind and of the autistic child. *Journal of Speech and Hearing Disorders, 38,* 478–489.

Fay, W. H. (1979). Personal pronouns and the autistic child. *Journal of Autism and Developmental Disorders, 9,* 247–260.

Fein, D., Pennington, B., Markowitz, P., Braverman, M., & Waterhouse, L. (1986). Toward a neuropsychological model of infantile autism: Are the social deficits primary? *Journal of the American Academy of Child Psychiatry, 25,* 198–212.

Fraiberg, S. (1977). *Insights from the blind.* London: Souvenir.

Freud, S. (1924). A short account *of* psycho-analysis. In J. Strachey (Ed. & Trans.), *The standard edition of the complete psychological works of Sigmund Freud* (Vol. 19, pp. 191–209). London: Hogarth Press.

Gutstein, S. E. (in press). Preliminary evaluation of the Relationship Development Intervention program. *Journal of Autism and Developmental Disorders.*

Gutstein, S. E., & Sheely, R. K. (2002). *Relationship development intervention with young children: Social and emotional development activities for Asperger syndrome, autism, PDD, and NLD.* Philadelphia: Jessica Kingsley.

Hammes, J., & Langdell, T. (1981). Precursors of symbol formation and childhood autism. *Journal of Autism and Developmental Disorders, 11,* 331–346.

Heimann, M., Ullstadius, E., Dahlgren, S. O., & Gillberg, C. (1992). Imitation in autism: A preliminary research note. *Behavioural Neurology, 5,* 219–227.

Hermelin, B., & O'Connor, N. (1970). *Psychological experiments with autistic children.* Oxford, UK: Pergamon Press.

Hertzig, M. E., Snow, M. E., & Sherman, M. (1989). Affect and cognition in autism. *Journal of the American Academy of Child and Adolescent Psychiatry, 28,* 195–199.

Hobson, R. P. (1989a). Beyond cognition: A theory of autism. In G. Dawson (Ed.), *Autism: Nature, diagnosis, and treatment* (pp. 22–48). New York: Guilford Press.

Hobson, R. P. (1989b). On sharing experiences. *Development and Psychopathology, 1,* 197–203.

Hobson, R. P. (1990). On the origins of self and the case of autism. *Development and Psychopathology, 2,* 163–181.

Hobson, R. P. (1993). *Autism and the development of mind.* Hove, UK: Erlbaum.

Hobson, R. P. (1995). Apprehending attitudes and actions: Separable abilities in early development? Special Issue: Emotions in developmental psychopathology. *Development and Psychopathology, 7,* 171–182.

Hobson, R. P. (2004). *The cradle of thought.* New York: Oxford University Press.

Hobson, R. P., & Lee, A. (1998). Hello and goodbye: A study of social engagement in autism. *Journal of Autism and Developmental Disorders, 28,* 117–126.

Hobson, R. P., & Lee, A. (1999). Imitation and identification in autism. *Journal of Child Psychology and Psychiatry, 40,* 649–659.

Hobson, R. P., Lee, A., & Brown, R. (1999). Autism and congenital blindness. *Journal of Autism and Developmental Disorders, 29,* 45–56.

Hobson, R. P., Lee, A., & Meyer, J. (2003). *Identification in autism.* Paper presented at the biennial meeting of the Society for Research in Child Development, Tampa, FL.

Ingersoll, B., Schreibman, L., & Tran, Q. H. (2003). Effect of sensory feedback on immediate object imitation in children with autism. *Journal of Autism and Related Developmental Disabilities, 33,* 673–683.

Jones, V., & Prior, M. R. (1985). Motor imitation abilities and neurological signs in autistic children. *Journal of Autism and Developmental Disorders, 15,* 37–46.

Kanner, L. (1943). Autistic disturbances of affective contact. *Nervous Child, 2,* 217–250.

Lord, C., Rutter, M., Dilavore, P., & Risi, S. (1999). *Manual: Autism Diagnostic Observation Schedule.* Los Angeles: Western Psychological Services.

Loveland, K. A., & Landry, S. H. (1986). Joint attention and language in autism and developmental language delay. *Journal of Autism and Developmental Disorders, 16,* 335–349.

Loveland, K. A., Tunali-Kotoski, B., Pearson, D. A., Brelsford, K. A., Ortegon, J., & Chen, R. (1994). Imitation and expression of facial affect in autism. *Development and Psychopathology, 6,* 433–444.

Meltzoff, A., & Gopnik, A. (1994). The role of imitation in understanding persons and developing a theory of mind. In S. Baron-Cohen (Ed.), *Understanding other minds: Perspectives from autism* (pp. 335–366). London: Oxford University Press.

Meyer, J. A., & Hobson, R. P. (2004). Orientation in relation to self and other: The case of autism. *Interaction Studies, 5,* 221–244.

Meyer, J. A. & Hobson, R. P. (2005). *Identification: The missing link between joint attention and imitation?* Manuscript submitted for publication.

Moore, D., Hobson, R. P., & Lee, A. (1997). Components of person perception: An investigation with autistic, nonautistic retarded and normal children and adolescents. *British Journal of Developmental Psychology, 15,* 401–423.

Morgan, S. B., Cutrer, P. S., Coplin, J. W., & Rodrigue, J. R. (1989). Do autistic children differ from retarded and normal children in Piagetian sensorimotor functioning? *Journal of Child Psychology and Psychiatry and Allied Disciplines, 30,* 857–864.

Mundy, P., Hogan, M., & Doehring, P. (1996). *A preliminary manual for the Abridged Early Social Communication Scales.* Miami, FL: University of Miami.

Mundy, P., Kasari, C., & Sigman, M. (1992). Joint attention, affective sharing, and intersubjectivity. *Infant Behavior and Development, 15,* 377–381.

Mundy, P., & Sigman, P. (1989). Specifying the nature of the social impairment in autism. In G. Dawson (Ed.), *Autism: Nature, diagnosis, and treatment* (pp. 3–21). New York: Guilford Press.

Nadel, J. (2002). Imitation and imitation recognition: Functional use in preverbal infants and nonverbal children with autism. In A. N. Meltzoff & W. Prinz (Eds.), *The imitative mind: Development, evolution, and brain bases. Cambridge studies in cognitive perceptual development* (pp. 42–62). New York: Cambridge University Press.

Nadel, J., Croue, S., Mattlinger, M-J., Canet, P., Hudelot, C., Lecuyer, C., et al. (2000). Do children with autism have expectancies about the social behaviour of unfamiliar people? A pilot study using the still face paradigm. *Autism, 4,* 133–146.

Nadel, J., Guérini, C., Pezé, A., & Rivet, C. (1999). The evolving nature of imitation as a format for communication. In J. Nadel & G. Butterworth (Eds.), *Imitation in infancy* (pp. 209–234). Cambridge, UK: Cambridge University Press.

Ohta, M. (1987). Cognitive disorders of infantile autism: A study employing the WISC, spatial relationship conceptualisation, and gesture imitation. *Journal of Autism and Developmental Disorders, 17,* 45–62.

Ricks, D. M., & Wing, L. (1975). Language, communication, and the use of symbols in normal and autistic children. *Journal of Autism and Childhood Schizophrenia, 5,* 191–221.

Ritvo, S., & Provence, S. (1953). Form perception and imitation in some autistic children: Diagnostic findings and their contextual interpretation. *Psychoanalytic Study of the Child, 8,* 155–161.

Roeyers, H., Van Oost, P., & Bothuyne, S. (1998). Immediate imitation and joint attention in young children with autism. *Development and Psychopathology, 10,* 441–450.

Rogers, S. J. (1999). An examination of the imitation deficit in autism. In J. Nadel & G. Butterworth (Eds.), *Imitation in infancy* (pp. 254–283). Cambridge, UK: Cambridge University Press.

Rogers, S. J., & Bennetto, L. (2000). Intersubjectivity in autism: The roles of imitation and executive function. In A. M. Wetherby & B. M. Prizant (Eds.), *Autism spectrum disorders: A transactional developmental perspective* (Vol. 9, pp. 79–107). Baltimore: Brookes.

Rogers, S. J., Bennetto, L., McEvoy, R., & Pennington, B. F. (1996). Imitation and panto-
    mime in high-functioning adolescents with autism spectrum disorders. *Child Develop-
    ment*, 67, 2060–2073.
Rogers, S. J., Hall, T., Osaki, D., Reaven, J., & Herbison, J. (2002). The Denver model: A
    comprehensive, integrated educational approach to young children with autism and
    their families. In J. S. Handleman & S. L. Harris (Eds.), *Preschool education programs
    for children with autism* (2nd ed., 203–234). Austin, TX: Pro-Ed.
Rogers, S. J., Hepburn, S. L., Stackhouse, T., & Wehner, E. (2003). Imitation performance
    in toddlers with autism and those with other developmental disorders. *Journal of
    Child Psychology and Psychiatry*, 44, 763–781.
Rogers, S. J., Herbison, J., Lewis, H., Pantone, J., & Reis, K. (1986). An approach for
    enhancing the symbolic, communicative, and interpersonal functioning of young chil-
    dren with autism and severe emotional handicaps. *Journal of the Division of Early
    Childhood*, 10, 135–148.
Rogers, S. J., & Pennington, B. F. (1991). A theoretical approach to the deficits in infantile
    autism. *Development and Psychopathology*, 3, 137–162.
Rutter, M., Anderson-Wood, L., Beckett, C., Bredenkamp, D., Castle, J., Groothues, C., et
    al. (1999). Quasi-autistic patterns following severe early global privation. *Journal of
    Child Psychology and Psychiatry*, 40, 537–549.
Shapiro, T., Roberts, A., & Fish, B. (1970). Imitation and echoing. *Journal of the American
    Academy of Child Psychiatry*, 9, 421–439.
Sigman, M. D., Kasari, C., Kwon, J. H., & Yirmiya, N. (1992). Responses to the negative
    emotions of others by autistic, mentally retarded, and normal children. *Child Develop-
    ment*, 63, 796–807.
Sigman, M. D., Mundy, P., Sherman, T., & Ungerer, J. A. (1986). Social interactions of
    autistic, mentally retarded and normal children and their caregivers. *Journal of Child
    Psychology and Psychiatry*, 27, 647–656.
Smith, I. M., & Bryson, S. E. (1994). Imitation and action in autism: A critical review. *Psy-
    chological Bulletin*, 116, 259–273.
Smith, I. M., & Bryson, S. E. (1998). Gesture imitation in autism I: Nonsymbolic postures
    and sequences. *Cognitive Neuropsychology*, 15, 747–770.
Stern, D. N. (1985). *The interpersonal world of the infant.* New York: Basic Books.
Stone, W. L., Ousley, O. Y., & Littleford, C. D. (1997). Motor imitation in young children
    with autism: What's the object? *Journal of Abnormal Child Psychology*, 25, 475–485.
Tomasello, M., Savage-Rumbaugh, S., & Kruger, A. C. (1993). Imitative learning of actions
    on objects by children, chimpanzees, and enculturated chimpanzees. *Child Develop-
    ment*, 64, 1668–1705.
Vygotsky, L. S. (1962). *Thought and language* (E. Hanfmann & G. Vakar, Trans.). Cam-
    bridge, MA: MIT Press.
Vygotsky, L. S. (1978). Internalization of higher psychological functions. In M. Cole, V.
    John-Steiner, S. Scribner, & E. Souberman (Eds.), *Mind in society: The development of
    higher psychological processes* (pp. 52–57). Cambridge, MA: Harvard University
    Press.
Wetherby, A. M., & Prizant, B. M. (1999). Enhancing language and communication devel-
    opment in autism: Assessment and intervention guidelines. In D. B. Zager (Ed.),
    Autism: Identification, education, and treatment (2nd ed., pp. 141–174). Mahwah,
    NJ: Erlbaum.
Whiten, A. (2002). The imitator's representation of the imitated: Ape and child. In A. N.
    Meltzoff & W. Prinz (Eds.), *The imitative mind: Development, evolution, and brain
    bases* (pp. 98–121). New York: Cambridge University Press.
Whiten, A., & Brown, J. D. (1998). Imitation and the reading of other minds: Perspectives

from the study of autism, normal children and non-human primates. In S. Bråten (Ed.), *Intersubjective communication and emotion in early ontogeny* (pp. 260–280). Cambridge, UK: Cambridge University Press.

Wieder, S., & Greenspan, S. I. (2003). Climbing the symbolic ladder in the DIR model through floor time/interactive play. *Autism, 7,* 425–435.

Williams, J. H. G., Whiten, A., & Singh, T. (2004). A systematic review of action imitation in autistic spectrum disorder. *Journal of Autism and Developmental Disorders, 34,* 285–299.

Wimpory, D. C., Hobson, R. P., Williams, J. M. G., & Nash, S. (2000). Are infants with autism socially engaged? A controlled study of recent retrospective parental reports. *Journal of Autism and Developmental Disorders, 30,* 525–536.

PART II

EVOLUTIONARY AND NEURAL BASES OF IMITATION

CHAPTER 10

The Dissection of Imitation and Its "Cognitive Kin" in Comparative and Developmental Psychology

ANDREW WHITEN

As Rogers makes clear (Chapter 1, this volume), imitation has become a focus of intense recent research activity not only in relation to autism but across a very broad range of disciplines. These disciplines include developmental and comparative psychology, cognitive neuroscience, and robotics. The scope for researchers in any one of these disciplines to learn from work in the others is well illustrated by the recent compilations of Dautenhahn and Nehaniv (2002), Meltzoff and Prinz (2002), Frith and Wolpert (2003), and Hurley and Chater (2005). The comparative work within these enterprises now extends the study of imitation and its precursors to many species other than our own (Caldwell & Whiten, 2002; Galef & Heyes, 2004), creating the prospect of rich evolutionary and developmental models of how the capacity for imitation can get constructed and what its consequences for other aspects of social cognition may be.

Of particular relevance to this chapter, Rogers notes that evolutionary and comparative psychologists have devoted much effort to uncovering and classifying the intricate web of phenomena that appear to be imitation's "cognitive kin." These include a range of other processes whereby one individual's behavior may come to match another's in certain respects, but they also extend much more broadly to encompass such sociocognitive elements as components of theory of mind. The relevance of this work for developmental psychology was explicit in the title of a recent article by Want and Harris (2002), "How Do Children Ape? Applying Concepts from the Study of Nonhuman Primates to the Developmental Study of 'Imitation' in Children." In this paper, Want and Harris suggested that developmentalists have relied on a somewhat blinkered conception of what "imitation" entails, and that much might be learned by looking over the fence at the conceptual frameworks and methods of comparative researchers engaged in this and related topics. The first part of this chapter is intended to complement Want and Harris's important cross-disciplinary initiative with an account from within comparative psychology—rather more "from the horse's mouth," as it were (Whiten, Horner, Litchfield, & Marshall-Pescini, 2004). This is by no means to devalue Want and Harris's review, which offers a perceptive onlooker's perspective on what has been achieved in a sister discipline. But substantive cross-fertilization requires something more like an extended dialogue "over the fence," which I here aim to extend. Carpenter (Chapter 3, this volume) contributes in a complementary way.

However, comparative psychology's conceptual schemes for dissecting cognitive processes and the methods developed to achieve this in practice do not exhaust the relevance of the evolutionary perspective for the subject of this volume. Human imitation and the neurocognitive universe in which it is embedded are the products of an evolutionary process. The present-day architectures and developmental pathways underlying these abilities are accordingly likely to be more deeply understood if we can uncover the way in which they have been built up through evolutionary time, by modifications of their precursors. Comparative evolutionary psychologists are embarked on a mission to do this, principally through the "comparative method" applied to living species. The key underlying principle is that where a cognitive process is shared by a related group of animals, such as primates, its origins most likely lie in the ancestor common to that group. We can thus hope to gain an understanding of the evolutionary construction of a present-day process like human imitation by examining relevant abilities shared with species that had a common ancestry with ourselves at a succession of different points in the past, from chimpanzees (most closely related, with a common ancestor 5–7 million years ago) back to other taxa such as old-world monkeys (who shared ancestry with ourselves closer to 25–30 million years ago).

Surveying such comparisons, Whiten (1996; Whiten & Brown, 1999) and Suddendorf (1998, 1999) independently noted parallels between the clustering of such capacities as simple mindreading, pretense, and imitation during stages of human development and in our evolutionary past as reconstructed through comparative primatology. Encouraged by the convergences between these independently developed perspectives, we have joined forces to produce more comprehensive reviews of the relevant literatures from both developmental and evolutionary perspectives (Suddendorf & Whiten, 2001, 2003; Whiten & Suddendorf, in press). We concluded that current evidence does indeed support the existence of multiple parallels between clusterings of sociocognitive abilities in development and evolution, particularly in relation to the concept of "secondary representation" developed by Josef Perner

(1991). In the present context this may offer the prospect of novel insights into the place of imitation (and its cognitive kin) within developing or evolving primate sociocognitive systems. This work is accordingly outlined in the second part of this chapter, extending into a consideration of the role played by "mirror neurons" in primate brains.

DISSECTING IMITATION AND ITS COGNITIVE KIN

In their review "How Do Children Ape?," Want and Harris (2002) noted that "in studies of social learning in humans, any and all similarity between the actions of an observer and a model is often attributed to imitation without much further analysis. Thus, while developmental psychology has been very good at mapping out children's proclivity to replicate the actions of others, it has often said little about how they do so." (p. 2). They contrasted this with a "revolution" in comparative psychology, which in recent years has distinguished a plethora of processes through which an individual's actions can come to match (or, indeed, adaptively avoid matching) those of another individual. I refer to these here as imitation and its cognitive kin.

Want and Harris suggested that the discrepancy between the frameworks utilized in developmental and comparative psychology urgently requires bridging. They began this effort by first offering their interpretation of comparative psychology's dissection of these processes, then suggesting their own scheme for integrating these into a coherent classification.

Working within comparative psychology (and also frequently studying children's behavior in parallel learning experiments), I and my colleagues have recently revised and extended our own overall scheme for accommodating the theoretical and empirical advances of the last couple of decades of research in this area (Whiten et al., 2004). As one would hope, this maps quite well to Want and Harris's scheme, and to that of another influential group that combines comparative and developmental research (Call & Carpenter, 2002; see also Carpenter, Chapter 3, this volume), but it is more extensive in ways we think vital to capture all the distinctions that now need to be recognized. These are summarized in Figure 10.1 and explained, with illustrations, further below.

Evolving "Dissections" of Social Learning in Comparative Psychology: An Overview

To explicate the distinctions to be made, it will be helpful to précis some of the key historical developments in this work. Space constrains this to be brief in this chapter: For a fuller account, see Whiten and colleagues (2004) and Carpenter (Chapter 3, this volume).

Imitation has been studied by comparative psychologists for over a century (Whiten & Ham, 1992). For much of that time, a similar accusation to

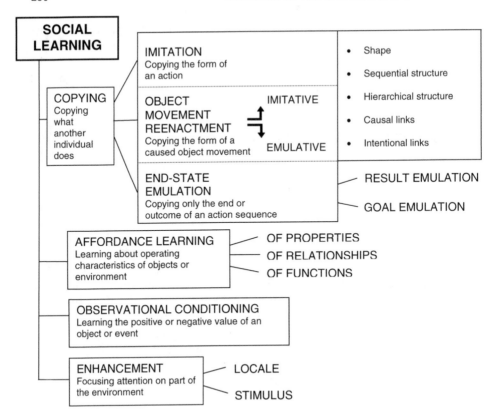

FIGURE 10.1. A taxonomy of social learning processes (after Whiten et al., 2004). This scheme represents a revision of that offered in Whiten and Ham (1992), that takes into account theoretical and empirical progress in the intervening period. In this scheme, different kinds of social learning process are discriminated, labeled, and partially defined (for further specification, see text). Categories are arranged so there is generally most potential for high-fidelity copying at the top (imitation) descending to enhancement at the bottom. Affordance learning may in principle be used to generate actions that vary in their degree of match to actions of the individual(s) observed. To the right of the "imitation" and "OMR" categories are listed a number of different aspects in relation to which matching to a model may occur: For example, hierarchical structure might be copied in relation to either imitation of bodily movements or OMR. The same is true for the spatiotemporal shape of actions, their sequential patterning, and causal and intentional aspects of the model's actions. Note that Whiten and Ham (1992) labeled all emulation *goal emulation*, whereas here, goal emulation is only a subcategory of emulation, for which a tighter specification is explained in the text.

that made by Want and Harris in relation to developmental psychology could often be leveled at comparative work too, insofar as imitation was too readily ascribed on the basis of evidence that social learning of some sort had occurred. When imitation *was* contrasted with other social learning processes, this was typically limited to "stimulus enhancement" (Spence, 1937), where the actions of a model merely drew the attention of an observer to an object or relevant parts of the task at hand (or alternatively to a location, sometimes distinguished as "locale enhancement"). In this circumstance, the observer may be more likely to end up acting in the same way as the model did than an individual who had no such observation opportunity, but this could occur through its own individual learning efforts rather than imitation. The match between observer and model could result from the model's approach simply being the most readily learned by the observer, once their attention to the model's focus had been "enhanced." Critical reviews of the comparative literature in the late 1980s and early 1990s suggested that many claims for imitation in nonhuman species had not satisfactorily ruled out a role for such apparently simpler forms of social learning (Galef, 1988; Visalberghi & Fragaszy, 1990; Whiten & Ham, 1992). Some doubted imitation had truly been identified in nonhuman species.

The dissection of social learning was significantly enriched following a study by Tomasello, Davis-DaSilva, Camak, and Bard (1987) on the acquisition of tool use in young chimpanzees, in which chimpanzees were shown to have benefited from watching an expert chimpanzee use a stick to retrieve out-of-reach food. They were more likely than nonobserving controls to use a stick for this purpose. However, they did not copy certain two-step tool-use tricks the model had developed to gain items trapped at the edge of the food tray. For this reason, Tomasello and colleagues concluded the chimpanzees were not truly imitating. However, the chimpanzees appeared to learn more than is usually implied by stimulus enhancement, for they differed from nonobserving controls not merely in handling the sticks but in applying them to the task. The authors suggested that the chimpanzees had learned about the stick's potential to *function as a tool* in the task at hand, and Tomasello (1990) later suggested that David Wood's (1989) concept of "emulation" would provide an apt term to describe this process. Wood had noted that "children not only attempt to impersonate others by imitating their actions but also try to emulate them by achieving similar ends or objectives" (p. 71), and he suggested that they might choose to do so by employing different behavioral means (so the similarity between observer and model would be limited to just the end results, or goals of what the model did) or similar means (which might thus appear to be imitative, but would not truly be so because the observer would not be directly copying the models' action).

In the ensuing period, others, as well as Tomasello himself, have used the term *emulation* in ways that have struck other authors as importantly different (e.g., Byrne, 1998; Custance, Whiten, & Fredman, 1999). This appears to have happened in part through some misunderstandings between authors, and differential usage of the term has certainly become a source of some confusion, even consternation, in the literature (see, e.g., the peer exchanges in Byrne & Russon, 1998; Want & Harris, 2002). However, my own view is that several of these different "senses" of emulation are actually worth distinguishing, both conceptually and of course empirically wherever possible, because they map real distinctions that may be significant in understanding social learning in normally and non-normally developing humans, as well as nonhuman animals. In the hope that the past period of confusion has perhaps been a necessary step toward "seeing the light" about how many varieties of social learning may coexist, three main senses of emulation are discriminated in the current taxonomy offered by Whiten and colleagues (2004; see Figure 10.1), which in turn represents an update of that set out in Whiten and Ham (1992). We shall examine some key categories distinguished in Figure 10.1 in turn, starting with the contrast between imitation and one of the senses of emulation—"object movement reenactment."

Imitation and Object Movement Reenactment

Tomasello (1998) concisely expressed one particular sense of emulation that may discriminate it from imitation: In emulation, individuals are "learning about the environment, not about behaviour" (p. 704). An illustration comes from our studies of social learning in which we allowed not only great apes but also young children to witness an expert "peeling" the defenses off an "artificial fruit" ("pin-apple"; Figure 10.2) in order to get at the prize inside. Each of several defenses can be removed in two alternative ways, and subjects in each experimental condition see just one of these, so the extent to which copying occurs is manifested in differences in the prevalence of the two alter-

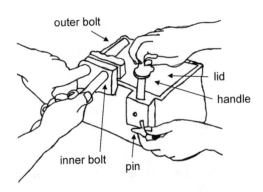

FIGURE 10.2. "Pin-apple" artificial fruit for experimental investigation of imitation. Actions illustrated are of poking through the outer bolt, pulling and twisting out the inner bolt, removing the pin, and pulling up the handle. Once all defenses are removed in these ways or others, the lid can be opened to gain access to an edible core.

native techniques in subjects' later attempts at the task. For example, the model either pulls the two bolts toward him with a twisting motion (twisting is in fact unnecessary, but provides another check on whether copying occurs) or uses a quite different technique, poking the bolts through and away using his finger. The extent to which such *differences* are copied can then be quantified.

We found evidence that normally developing children, chimpanzees, and gorillas showed varying degrees of statistically reliable matching to whichever alternative method they had seen (Stoinski, Wrate, Ure, & Whiten, 2001; Whiten, Custance, Gomez, Teixidor, & Bard, 1996). The children copied with the highest fidelity; the apes more patchily. However, others have questioned whether such results necessarily demonstrate "imitation" (Tomasello & Call, 1997), or instead "emulation" in the sense described earlier. Looked at in this way, the issue is essentially whether the subject was performing the bodily act he or she had seen (e.g., pulling and/or twisting) or was instead noting how the bolts moved (e.g., away from the manipulator, or in relation to the fruit itself) and recreating this.

The empirical problem here is that when the hands manipulate objects, the two learning possibilities may be inextricably confounded: If the action matched is *pulling out the bolts*, for example, the *bolts will move* in a corresponding way. However, perhaps fortuitously, our subjects have sometimes provided us with evidence that one or the other process is at work. In a study with capuchin monkeys, for example, Custance and colleagues (1999) found that subjects replicated the direction of movement of the bolts, but not the methods used: They might pull the bolts out of the back, for example, rather than poke them through as the model had done. Custance and colleagues thus named this particular brand of emulation *object movement reenactment* (OMR). Stoinksi and colleagues (2001) and Stoinksi and Whiten (2003) found a similar story in studies with gorillas and orangutans. By contrast, a study with chimpanzees and 2–4-year-old children did document matching at the level of actions (pulling and twisting vs. poking the bolts) (Whiten et al., 1996). The twisting in particular seemed unlikely to reflect OMR because the bolts themselves were covered by the hand, so that twisting of the hand was what was observable. More telling is a recent unpublished study with young wildborn Guinean chimpanzees. Those who watched the "poking" model had difficulty poking the bolts out, and so poked them back and forth repeatedly. Unlike the other nonhuman primates we tested, in doing this they clearly focused on replicating the action rather than the original direction of bolt movement.

However, it is a moot point whether the meaning of imitation should be restricted in this way, by "quarantining" off OMR as a separate category or whether the definition of imitation should be kept broad enough to *encompass* OMR (thus including *object movement imitation* as well as *bodily imitation*). We return to this issue later on. This broader sense of imitation is a prevalent one in developmental psychology, as Want and Harris (2002) implied, and the same appears true of clinical work. However, whichever

labels are applied, the essential distinction concerning copying of actions versus object movements may have particular relevance for autism. Reviewing
published studies of imitation deficits associated with autism spectrum disorder (ASD), Williams, Whiten, and Singh (2004) discerned a pattern suggesting
that deficits occur preferentially in imitation of bodily actions such as gestures, in comparison to those involving objects. We should thus recognize the
possibility that the latter capacity relies more on OMR, perhaps reflecting a
greater facility in analyzing object movements than the actions of other people.

Perhaps, then, teasing OMR apart from bodily imitation deserves more
attention. As noted previously, it may sometimes be possible to do so because
subjects' responses are fortuitously consistent with one process rather than the
other. However, those results suggest that the discrimination could be more
systematically pursued, by experimental designs involving four different conditions rather than two: *Different* actions can be used to create the *same*
object movement; and the *same* action can be used to create *different* object
movements. For example, with the bolts components of our pin-apple device,
the model could poke the bolts in one direction or the other (conditions 1 and
2), or pull them in one direction or the other (conditions 3 and 4).

A different experimental approach is the idea of the "ghost control"
(Heyes, Jaldow, Nokes, & Dawson, 1994), in which the subject sees the
manipulandum move without an agent involved. If this is sufficient to elicit a
matching response, OMR is implied. This has now been used with several
nonhuman species including rats (Heyes et al., 1994), pigeons (Klein &
Zentall, 2003), and (although involving a series of lit screens rather than
object movements as such) rhesus monkeys (Subiaul, Cantlon, Holloway, &
Terrace, 2004). Surprisingly, perhaps, this approach has only recently seeped
into developmental psychology—Thompson and Russell (2004), finding that
young children could learn as much from covertly motorized object movements as from equivalent movements performed by human models (and see
Huang, Heyes, & Charman, 2002, discussed further later).

While such potential discriminations between bodily imitation and OMR
may thus be illuminating, there is an important converse point to be made
about possible isomorphisms between the two. An observer may copy *the patterning of the model's actions* (bodily imitation) or *the patterning of the object
movements* (OMR) caused by the model. As Figure 10.1 indicates, such copying may involve the spatiotemporal shape of the movements (such as pulling
vs. poking), their sequencing, or their hierarchical structuring. In addition,
copies may in principle take into account causal or intentional links within the
observed sequence as a whole and use this analysis to selectively exclude or
include components of what is witnessed (Whiten, Horner, & Marshall-
Pescini, 2005). All these variables beg investigation, whether it is the bodily
actions, the object movements, or both that the observer is focusing on.

An example illustrating investigation of some of these distinctions has
employed a device we nicknamed the "keyway fruit" (Figure 10.3). This is

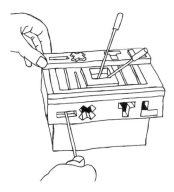

FIGURE 10.3. "Keyway" fruit for identifying imitation of hierarchical structure (after Whiten et al., 2005). A lid is held on an underlying box by four horizontal rods, that can be seen through the transparent lid. One way in which a model opens the fruit is by taking one of the handles from the central cup, stabbing it into a tablet held in a recess at the back of the lid, thus making a key, pushing this key into a correspondingly shaped slot at the front (illustrated here) to eject one of the rods, pulling out the rod thus protruding from the back of the box, and finally removing the key. A similar "column" of actions is performed for each of the shapes indicated (— X T L). In the alternative "row" method, all the handles are first stabbed into all the tablets, then all keys are placed in the appropriate locks, then all rods are pushed through and taken out, and finally all keys are removed. The two approaches thus include the same set of 16 actions, organized into two alternative hierarchical structures ("columns" vs. "rows").

essentially a box with a lid held in place by a row of four skewers passing through both box and lid. In each of the two conditions of the experiment, observers witness the same set of operations performed but organized into one of two different hierarchically structured patterns. In the "column" method, a handle is first wedged into a shaped tablet to form a "key," which is then inserted into a correspondingly shaped slot, pushing a skewer out a little; this is then pulled out and the key removed. This is repeated for each successive column of operations in turn. An alternative method demonstrated is a "row-wise" method, so-called because it involves making up all the keys in a row, then inserting a row of them, and completing the other operations along rows in similar fashion. Normally developing preschool children have been found to show quite high fidelity copying of whichever hierarchically structured format they see (Whiten, 2002a, 2002b), although they did not copy the specific sequence witnessed (they might proceed left to right along a row, for example, having observed the reverse). This study begs to be replicated in individuals with ASD, who might be expected to experience particular difficulties with it either because the task may require discerning the model's underlying hierarchical "plan" (a formulation that evokes mindreading connotations) and/or because it requires a certain level of executive functioning. Such an exploration is currently under way in collaboration with J. Williams and colleagues.

End-State Emulation

An alternative formulation of emulation was the original one emphasized by the developmental psychologist David Wood (1989) and later introduced into comparative psychology by Tomasello (1990; see also Tomasello et al., 1987). Wood (1989) suggested that "children attempt to impersonate others by imitating their actions but also try to emulate them by achieving similar ends or objectives" (p. 71). This sense of emulation thus contrasts not only with imitation but also with the copying of what may be an extensive sequence of environmental effects constituting OMR. However, there is still copying: It is just that the copying focuses only on an end result of what the model is doing, the observer going on to recreate this end result using his or her own means, different to that employed by the model.

Within this sense of emulation a further distinction has been made that may be particularly relevant for the case of autism: An observer might copy an *observable result* of what the model does ("result emulation"); or alternatively the observer may copy what he or she perceives to be the model's *goal* ("goal emulation"—see Figure 10.1). In many real-life cases, the latter may be indistinguishable from the former: It is just that the observer, if a natural mindreader, perceives a *result* obtained by the model as having been, simultaneously, his or her *goal*. In principle one could imagine species (and perhaps different stages of human development) in which only one of these options is available, or at least the favored perspective. Thus an organism might have no goal-recognition abilities yet be able to recognize desirable events caused by the model that it then seeks to re-create in its own way; alternatively, it might be natural for some organisms to prioritize goal recognition when observing the actions of others, including those they may learn from. Bekkering, Wohlschlager, and Gattis (2000; see also Gattis, Bekkering, & Wohlschlager, 2002; Gergely, Bekkering, & Király, 2002) have argued that this is the case for young, normally developing children.

Given difficulties with theory of mind in autism, such distinctions may prove profitable for investigation in ASD. Goal attribution, however, appears to be one of the more primitive elements of mindreading, for which there is increasing evidence in monkeys (Umiltà et al., 2001), apes (Call, Hare, Carpenter, & Tomasello, 2004) and human infants (Csibra, 2003; Gergeley, Nádasdy, Csibra, & Bíró, 1995). Individuals with ASD appear to perform relatively well in attributing goals and desires (Baron-Cohen, 1995; Harris, 1991). Nevertheless, whether goal emulation is compromised in ASD begs proper investigation.

As noted previously, the fact that result emulation and goal emulation may be typically confounded makes investigation far from straightforward. Two main approaches have been championed, principally from within the developmental literature itself, so they are discussed here only briefly. Readers are referred to Carpenter (Chapter 3, this volume) for a fuller treatment, particularly in relation to the first approach, which relies on the learner's ability to discriminate intended acts from accidents and has been studied particularly by Carpenter and her colleagues from both comparative and developmental perspectives (Carpenter, Akhtar, & Tomasello, 1998; see Carpenter, Chapter 3, this volume).

The second approach has been labeled "failed attempts." Pioneered by Meltzoff (1995), it involved the model failing to achieved an outcome he or she intended. Meltzoff showed that even 18-month-old infants would tend to infer and complete such outcomes when their turn came, rather than merely mimic the surface form of what the model had actually done. For example, when a model tried to drop a string of beads into a container but only managed to drape them over its lip, the infant would often go on to put them in the container, completing the model's intention. Similar ideas have been elaborated in a study of chimpanzee social learning by Myowa-Yamakoshi and Matsuzawa (2000), although with less clear-cut results. However, another recent study by Huang and colleagues (2002) sounded a note of warning about the "intentional" interpretation associated with this paradigm, for they found that similar results could be obtained in a condition in which infants were prevented from witnessing the model's attempts by an opaque barrier. Instead, infants were allowed to witness only the start and end states of the object movements involved, and in the experiment of Huang and colleagues this was sufficient to encourage them to "complete" the sequence. Huang and colleagues accordingly suggest that results of "failed attempts" studies may actually reflect the operation of other emulation processes, that in the present scheme (Figure 10.1) would perhaps map to (inferred) OMR. I suggest that an important potential variant on their interpretation is that infants approach such studies with significant real-world knowledge of canonical relationships between certain kinds of objects. To revisit the example cited previously, they know that an object like a string of beads half in a cup *means* "beads in cup": that is how the beads should canonically sit. This suggests that this paradigm may need to focus more on relatively *noncanonical* intended outcomes to tease out the central distinctions at stake, although this may raise a conundrum about how such intentions can actually be read in behavior when the outcomes are noncanonical!

Affordance Learning

The final sense of emulation to be dissected out is *affordance learning*. Tomasello, Kruger, and Ratner (1993) borrowed this term from ecological perception research to emphasize useful characteristics of the world revealed by a model's actions, that an observer could utilize in its own attempts on the task concerned. As Byrne (1998) noted, this might involve learning about a range of things that include object properties (such as the brittleness of a nutshell), relationships between objects (such as the way a lock holds down a lid), or functional properties (such as the capacity of a rake to bring a desirable object within reach). One could conceptualize this category as "learning that" rather than "learning how" (the latter covering all the other categories grouped under "copying" in Figure 10.1). One could also describe it as declarative or factual learning rather than procedural learning.

Again, there are two main ways in which these aspects of social learning have begun to be investigated. One focuses on information that is utilized not to copy the model but, on the contrary, to omit aspects of what has been witnessed. An example comes from a recent study by Horner and Whiten (2005) that compared young children and chimpanzees on an artificial tool-use task presented in one of two alternative experimental conditions. In one condition participants watched as a human model used a stick-tool to reveal a hole in the top of an opaque box (Figure 10.4) and then stabbed the stick into it three times. The model then opened a small door on the front of the box to reveal another hole, the mouth of a small tunnel into which they inserted the stick to retrieve a small reward object. The alternative condition was identical except that the box was transparent apart from the tunnel holding the reward. Our prediction was that in this condition it would be literally transparent that the first action in the top hole afforded no causal connection with the lower tunnel because it could be seen to be beating only on a false floor above the tunnel; accordingly this part of the model's performance might be omitted when the participant had his or her turn at the task. By contrast, the causal irrelevance of the action in the top hole would not be apparent in the case of the

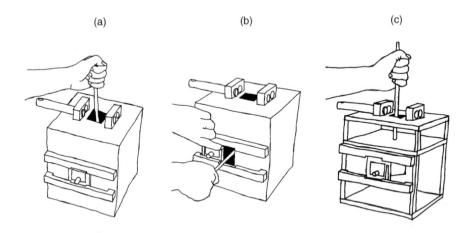

(a)   (b)   (c)

FIGURE 10.4. Testing for imitation/emulation switching (after Whiten et al., 2005; see Horner & Whiten, 2005). (a) Once the top bolt is moved out of the way, the stick is stabbed repeatedly into the top hole of the opaque box. (b) The bottom door is then opened (here, by sliding to the left) and the stick is used to fish out a reward from a tunnel. (c) When the transparent box is used, an observer can see that the stabbing action in the top hole is ineffectual, for it terminates on a transparent false ceiling above the reward location.

opaque box and we predicted that this group would be more likely to produce a more complete copy of the model that included this action.

The response of the young chimpanzees conformed to this prediction. They were significantly less likely to produce a full copy that included poking in the top slot when faced with the transparent version of the task, whether they experienced this first or only after working on the opaque box. Interestingly, if they worked on the transparent box first, they continued to omit the irrelevant act on transfer to the opaque box. This overall pattern of results suggests that the chimpanzees were indeed learning affordances—in this case, factual information concerning causal relations, that they learned in one condition (transparent box) and then applied in another (opaque box).

However, the 3- to 4-year-old children tested were not so discriminating! With a few exceptions they copied all parts of the task, with either box. This was true even when the experimenter left the room and allowed them to work on the task by themselves. Among several potential explanations for this intriguing contrast with the chimpanzee response, two are perhaps most promising and raise questions that could have relevance for the case of ASD. One explanation is simply that normally developing children are so much more strongly culturally oriented than chimpanzees that they are ready, at this age at least, to copy much of what human adults do even when the causal significance of their actions might appear suspect. If so, it could be instructive to test individuals with ASD on this task, or one that embodies its key principles, to see whether they are in fact more discriminating than the so overwhelmingly socially engaged normally developing children we studied.

A second explanation for our results hinges on the fact that the model repeated her whole approach three times before the child was allowed his or her first attempt. This may have offered a heightened signal that the actions in the top hole were intended—a factor that may have been less salient for the chimpanzees. This might explain why we found our child subjects so nondiscriminating, when others have found evidence of children selectively omitting parts of modeled behaviors that in certain circumstances are ineffective (Want & Harris, 2001). If so, this is another reason why one might predict a sample with ASD to be more discriminating in this kind of task than the normally developing children who copy so faithfully. Our present research seeks to tease out which explanation for our results should be favored, but whatever the answer, the foregoing logic suggests that comparative data for ASD could be worth collecting.

THE ARCHAIC FOUNDATIONS OF IMITATION AND THE SOCIAL MIND

Having considered imitation and its cognitive kin within the domain of social learning in some depth, we now turn to the relationship between imitation and more distant cognitive kin such as theory of mind (ToM). The human epigenetic system that builds such capacities through a complex developmental cascade is, like all biological systems, the result of a tortuous series of evolutionary edits made to ancestral forms. Successful modeling of this cognitive ancestry may eventually help us understand why development proceeds as it does, both in modal cases and when development takes non-normal pathways, such as in ASD.

Imitation, Mindreading, and Pretense in Apes

Whiten and Byrne (1991) noted Leslie's (1987) influential analysis of the roots of ToM in young children, which highlighted multiple isomorphisms between aspects of ToM and the pretend play that typically begins in a child's second year. Leslie had accordingly suggested that pretense signals the beginnings of those second-order mental processes that underwrite the development of ToM, and that the conjunction of deficits in both pretense and ToM in autism is consistent with this idea. Whiten and Byrne, relating this theory to a review of ape cognition, went on to hypothesize that phylogenetic parallels to these developmental linkages may exist in contrasts between cognition in the great apes and in other primates. Whiten and Byrne (1988) first reviewed evidence from their work on tactical deception in primates, suggesting that apes' deceptive repertoire is fueled by recognition of psychological states in others, notably their intentions and visual attention; they then examined scattered reports in the literature indicating an embryonic capacity for pretense in apes, not reported for other primates. Whiten and Byrne went on to suggest that other aspects of ape cognition, including imitation and mirror self-recognition, might be related to these distinctive abilities, possibly reflecting a fundamental elevation in representational capacities in the great apes. They predicted that, accordingly, imitation might be another domain suffering deficits in autism too.

In the same year, Rogers and Pennington (1991) published the first comprehensive review documenting consistent findings of imitation deficits in autism. They went on to offer a comprehensive developmental cascade model of the way in which disturbances in imitation, pretense, and ToM unfold in ASD.

Whiten (1996) built on all these studies in comparing further accumulating evidence for ontogenetic and evolutionary similarities in the clustering of manifestations of imitation, pretense, and mindreading, but now linked these with the concept of "secondary representation" that had in the meantime been elaborated by Perner (1991, a good year!). The essence of the notion of secondary representation, which avoids certain ambiguities and other difficulties in Leslie's earlier formulation of "metarepresentation," is the ability to entertain multiple cognitive models that may represent the same situation in different ways, including hypothetical versions. Independently, Suddendorf (1998, 1999) arrived at a similar perspective, and drawing some confidence from this we joined forces to complete a thorough review of both the developmental and comparative evidence for clustering of cognitive capacities consistent with secondary representation (Suddendorf & Whiten, 2001), which we have since updated (Suddendorf & Whiten, 2003; Whiten & Suddendorf, in press). This exercise extends the analysis to include not only pretense, mirror self-recognition, and early mindreading (i.e., representation of emotions, desires, intentions, seeing and attention, but not false belief) but also means–ends reasoning and the understanding of both hidden displacement of objects, and imitation. Note that although this list highlights important components of social cognition, it also includes nonsocial phenomena, as Leslie's (1987) original reference to pretense had done. Autism, too, of course, includes disturbances that span both social and nonsocial cognition such as pretense, that are linked theoretically in such formulations as those of Leslie and Perner described previously.

Recent years have seen extensive empirical contributions in these domains accumulate in both developmental and comparative research. Several influential authorities have adjusted their conclusions accordingly. How do recent comparative findings sit in relation to the ideas sketched earlier? There is, of course, insufficient space here to fully review the burgeoning corpus of relevant studies and readers are referred to the recent works cited above for details, complementing the summary that can be given here. We focus on three capacities particularly relevant to autism and the perspective of the present volume in particular: mindreading, pretense, and imitation.

Mindreading

The 1990s were characterized by a largely deflationary verdict on apes' capacity to discriminate psychological states in others. In particular, an extremely extensive and carefully conducted series of studies by Povinelli and Eddy (1996; Povinelli, 2000) showed a group of young chimpanzees to be remarkably undiscriminating in relation to psychological states presumed among the easiest to read—in particular, what a human interactant should be able to see or not see. The most thorough review of primate cognition (Tomasello & Call, 1997) concurred that "there is no solid evidence that nonhuman primates understand the intentionality or mental states of others . . . a healthy agnosticism, or even skepticism, would seem to be the wisest position" (pp. 340–341).

Other studies such as those of Byrne and Whiten (1992) and Gomez (1996) offered contrary data but were outweighed by the greater mass of negative findings. However, recent data collected by some of the leading "skeptics" themselves has led them to a revised view (Tomasello, Call, & Hare, 2003). In particular, a series of experiments involving chimpanzees competing with other chimpanzees over access to food resources have provided converging evidence that these apes take into account what others can and cannot see (Hare, Call, Agnetta, & Tomasello, 2000; Hare, Call, & Tomasello, 2001) and other studies offer evidence of recognition of intent (Call, Hare, Carpenter, & Tomasello, in press). The results of these experimental studies thus now square well with Whiten and Byrne's earlier interpretations of observational data on deceptive interactions among wild apes. Parallel studies with monkeys failed to find similar appreciation of the significance of "seeing" (Hare, Addessi, Call, Tomasello, & Visalberghi, 2003).

Pretense

Pretense is inherently more difficult to subject to experimentation. In nonhuman primates the evidence typically comes from observations of spontaneous behavior, and appears to be limited to the great apes. In the most recent review, Whiten and Suddendorf (in press) tabulate 12 significant sources of such observations scattered in the literature, concerning chimpanzees, gorillas, and orangutans. The most convincing cases are those in which the ape conforms to the demanding criterion set by Leslie (1987), of adjusting its apparent pretend behavior to local circumstances in a way that appears "logical." Whiten and Suddendorf illustrated this by reference to the actions of the home-reared chimpanzee Viki (Hayes, 1951), who was described as dragging along an imaginary pull-toy (as with real pull-toys she played with) and acting through the implications of tangling the string around a knob; but we were forced to lament that no video records exist to inspire confidence in the textual descriptions published. At the recent 20th Congress of the International Primatological Society, however, Matsuzawa (2004) showed remarkable video records of precisely these qualities in the actions of a young chimpanzee who at first played directly with some building blocks, dragging clutches of them across a smooth floor. In the episode in question, this chimpanzee then began to repeat exactly this behavior but with the actual blocks apparently deliberately left to one side. He performed the same actions as before, as if continuing to juggle along several (nonexistent) blocks, even shepherded these *around* a real block that was in his path.

Such actions represent rudimentary and fleeting evidence of pretense at best, but the descriptions that have steadily accumulated in the literature are remarkable for their distribution, occurring only in apes. Such actions are most noticeable in apes operating on novel human artifacts like the pull-toy and building bricks mentioned earlier, but such actions have not been described in monkeys reared in similar environments. Pretense therefore appears to co-occur with the beginnings of mindreading in a subset of primates: the great apes.

Imitation

Whiten and Byrne (1991) had suggested that imitation may fit this pattern, for at that time there was doubt that imitation occurred in species other than the apes (Visalberghi & Fragaszy, 1990; Whiten & Ham, 1992). The theoretical basis for the prediction was discussed in some depth by Whiten (1996) and its essence lay at the heart of Rogers and Pennington's (1991) proposal that imitation may be the earliest reflection of the difficulties in appreciating the cognitive perspective of others that characterize the later phases of autism: Essentially, imitation shares with mindreading a translation process that can be glossed as being able, cognitively, to "stand in the other's shoes." More formally, Rogers and Pennington described the fundamental underlying process as "the formation/coordination of specific self–other representations" (p. 152).

However, as Whiten (1996) already acknowledged, a few studies had begun to suggest that some forms of imitation are more widespread in the animal kingdom (in mammals and birds, at least) and in any case, imitation appears in human infancy well before the middle of the child's second year, when pretense and early mindreading begin to be noticeable (see Rogers, Chapter 1, this volume, for an overview). Rogers and Pennington (1991) acknowledged this, identifying imitation as perhaps the first public manifestation of impaired "self–other representations," and Meltzoff and Gopnik (1993) similarly proposed that early imitation has properties that could make it crucial in the building of more sophisticated forms of these representations, en route to ToM. In recent years, an impressive range of experimental studies demonstrating imitation in animals other than apes has been published. Perhaps most striking is the evidence from species of birds whose brains are minuscule compared with those of apes. These studies have used a rigorous "two-action" approach, in which observer animals watch only one of two alternative models, to demonstrate such effects as matching the body part a conspecific model used to operate the same device (beak vs. foot to operate a treadle, in pigeons: Zentall, Sutton, & Sherburne, 1996), or using the bill in one of two different demonstrated ways to remove a stopper (pick and discard vs. poke in, in budgerigars: Heyes & Saggerson, 2002). Reviewing the bird studies, Zentall (2004) can now cite evidence for a number of phenomena beyond the basic existence of imitation, including a preference to copy a model's responses that lead to a reward, and deferred imitation (over a half hour) as well as emulation of the OMR kind (demonstrated using a "ghost" control procedure).

Taken together, this growing body of findings suggests not that it is mistaken to posit a foundational role for imitation in the emergence of mindreading, pretense, and related cognitive capacities but, rather, that some quite sophisticated forms of self–other mapping are more widespread in the animal kingdom than was known even a decade ago (the discovery of mirror neurons in monkeys is a different, but perhaps related illustration of this essential point, discussed further below). Simple forms of imitation exist in infancy without the accompaniment of ToM and pretense, but they are posited to form the foundation for these more sophisticated abilities; in a similar fashion, it can be suggested that imitation exists in many animals without the accompaniment of ToM and pretense, while in apes it may form a foundation on which precisely these abilities are constructed.

In addition, more rarefied kinds of imitative phenomenon may remain unique to great apes (or, at least, not occur in other primates) and may be linked to the capacity for secondary representation posited to underlie the other abilities reviewed previously. Perhaps the most obvious of these is the recognition of the imitative process itself. Whiten (2000) noted that only great apes (and dolphins, that like apes, have also been shown to recognize themselves in mirrors) have so far proved capable of learning the "Do-as-I-do game," performing novel imitative acts to match those of a model who requests "Do this!" and suggesting the grasp of a concept of imitation. Similarly, Neilsen, Collier-Baker, Davis, and Suddendorf (2004) have provided the first evidence that chimpanzees can recognize when others are imitating them. Other candidates for special ape abilities discussed by Whiten and colleagues (2004) include copying of acts with marked variety, novelty, or structural complexity, which might make distinctive demands on self–other representational processes, and sensitivity to context, such as causal efficacy.

The overall profile of imitation and its "cognitive kin" in great apes accordingly suggests that several basic components of the developmental architecture posited in Rogers and Pennington's cascade model for human development had begun to evolve in our common ancestor with chimpanzees and possibly the other apes. These may in turn explain the unprecedented cultural variation now documented in wild chimpanzees and orangutans (van Schaik et al., 2003; Whiten, 2005; Whiten et al., 1999). It is these cognitive capacities that were reshaped and elaborated on to make the ontogeny of human social cognition what it is today, including affordances for alternative developmental routes that occur in conditions such as ASD.

MONKEYS, MIRROR NEURONS, AND IMITATION

Mirror neurons, discovered by the "Parma group" (Gallese, Fadiga, Fogassi, & Rizzolatti, 1996; Rizzolatti, Fadiga, Gallese, & Fogassi, 1996) have been shown to fire both when a monkey executes a certain action, such as a precision grasp of an object, and also when the monkey merely watches another individual perform a similar action. In the latter case, the output from the neuron is inhibited. More recently, neurons that mirror mouth actions have also been found (Ferrari, Gallese, Rizzolatti, & Fogassi, 2004). We can thus start to envisage a kind of "homunculus" in the brain, somewhat like the sensory and motor ones we have long been familiar with, but in this case effectively a sensorimotor homunculus, perhaps better thought of a marionette, that covertly "imitates" the actions of any individual its owner watches.

When we ask what the function of such a mirror-neuron (MN) system may be, an obvious first thought would thus be that it provides machinery for imitation. Yet paradoxically, MN activation in macaque cortex has not been associated with imitation, and indeed a view has developed that little or no evidence exists for imitation in monkeys generally (Visalberghi & Fragaszy,

1990; Whiten & Ham, 1992). The Parma group have therefore suggested that instead the MN system allows the monkey to "make sense" of other's actions, in particular to recognize their goals, through forming a motor representation in the self of what it would be like to do what the other is doing. In humans, they suggest that this system has been coopted to permit both imitation (Iacoboni et al., 2001; Rizzolatti, Fadiga, Fogassi, & Gallese, 2002) and a mindreading-by-simulation capacity (Gallese & Goldman, 1998). Williams, Whiten, Suddendorf, and Perrett (2001) further suggested that damage to the MN system may accordingly offer an explanation for several of the characteristics of autism (see Williams & Waiter, Chapter 15, this volume).

I want to sound a note of caution about the Parma group's rejection of imitation, in favor of primitive mindreading, as the explanation for the role of MNs in the monkey brain. Such a step may have been premature. It appears to have been much influenced by Visalberghi and Fragaszy's (1990) review, which emphasized the lack of evidence for imitation in monkeys. However, it is important to recognize that there is much more to social learning than imitation. This is already indicated in Figure 10.1, but in addition it should be remembered that Figure 10.1 does not include a whole category that Whiten and Ham (1992, Figure 1) described as social influence, including such phenomena as contagion, in which actions relatively routine in an animal's repertoire are elicited by similar actions in companions.

In monkeys there may not be much sign of imitation in Thorpe's (1963) strict sense of copying a "novel or otherwise improbable" act, but as in many other taxa of animals there is much more evidence of some kind of social learning, and these cases seem just the kind of phenomena in which MNs could play a crucial role. Some instances are in fact labeled *imitation* on the basis of criteria other than those emphasized by Thorpe. For example, a study by Voelkl and Huber (2000) showed that marmosets that watched a model using their mouth to open a food canister rather than their hand were themselves more likely to use their mouth than their hand, unlike a second group that watched a model use a manual technique. Because this could not be explained by any kind of emulative process concerning the canister, this paper was titled "True Imitation in Marmosets." Caldwell and Whiten (2004) identified a similar effect in a study of marmosets working on a small artificial fruit. From what we know of the properties of MNs, it seems highly plausible they could play an important role in how the brains of these monkeys would code what they see the model do.

Other social learning effects have been logged in macaques, although I know of no studies on the species used in the MN studies. Japanese macaques have of course produced the most famous evidence for social learning, and although the renowned case of sweet-potato washing does not necessarily demonstrate imitation and is even suspect as social learning (Galef, 1990), the spread of other behavior patterns such as stone-handling (Huffman, 1996) appear explicable only through social learning. A very different kind of evidence comes from a recent experiment that showed rhesus macaques could learn by observation the correct sequence of four target images to press, even though the location of these changed in each trial (Subiaul et al., 2004). The authors showed through a kind of ghost control that it is essential the demonstrator monkey is seen to be touching the images, and although the manual response itself (touching) did not itself need to be learned, they suggest that motor coding through MNs could facilitate the copying their subjects evidenced, which they described as cognitive imitation.

If my speculation that MNs have a functional role in such monkey social learning phenomena proves correct, then the hypothesized human linkages between MNs, imitation, and ToM likely has a longer and more continuous evolutionary ancestry than presently conceived. A role for MNs in social learning, possibly even in some simple imitative phenomena of the kind sketched previously, would likely have existed in our ancient ancestors shared with the monkeys. More recently, in our common ancestor with the great apes, these phenomena would have become linked to fuller expressions of imitation, operating within a suite of other social learning processes (Figure 10.1) and simple forms of mindreading and perhaps pretense. It is these that would in turn have been elaborated into the present human social mind, along with the particular distortions to which it is vulnerable, such as autism.

As has been apparent in this chapter, the comparative studies that begin to outline this picture have benefited much from the approaches generated in developmental psychology. This chapter has endeavored to make it more of a two-way street, in the spirit advocated by Want and Harris (2002). It is to be hoped that further rewards will be garnered through continued interdisciplinary engagement between the research efforts of developmental and evolutionary psychologists.

REFERENCES

Baron-Cohen, S. (1995). *Mindblindness: An essay on autism and theory of mind*. Cambridge, MA: MIT Press.
Bekkering, H., Wohlschlager, A., & Gattis, M. (2000). Imitation of gestures in children is goal-directed. *Quarterly Journal of Experimental Psychology A, 53*, 153–164.
Byrne, R. W. (1998). Commentary on Boesch, C. & Tomasello, M. Chimpanzee and human culture. *Current Anthropology, 39*, 604–605.
Byrne, R. W., & Russon, A. E. (1998). Learning by imitation: A hierarchical approach. *Behavioral and Brain Sciences, 21*, 667–721.
Byrne, R. W., & Whiten, A. (1992). Cognitive evolution in primates: Evidence from tactical deception. *Man, 27*, 609–627.
Caldwell, C., & Whiten, A. (2002). Evolutionary perspectives on imitation: Is a comparative psychology of social learning possible? *Animal Cognition, 5*, 193–208.
Caldwell, C. A., & Whiten, A. (2004), Testing for social learning and imitation in common marmosets, *Callithrix jacchus*, using an "artificial fruit." *Animal Cognition, 7*, 77–85.
Call, J., & Carpenter, M. (2002). Three sources of information in social learning. In K. Dautenhahn & C. L. Nehaniv (Eds.), *Imitation in animals and artifacts* (pp. 211–228). Cambridge, MA: MIT Press.

Call, J., Hare, B. H., Carpenter, M., & Tomasello, M. (2004). "Unwilling" versus "unable": Chimpanzees' understanding of human intentional actions. *Developmental Science, 7,* 488–498.

Carpenter, M., Akhtar, N., & Tomasello, M. (1998). Fourteen through 18-month-old infants differentially imitate intentional and accidental actions. *Infant Behavior and Development, 21,* 315–330.

Custance, D. M., Whiten, A., & Fredman, T. (1999). Social learning of artificial fruit processing in capuchin monkeys (*Cebus apella*). *Journal of Comparative Psychology, 113,* 13–23.

Csibra, G. (2003). Teleological and referential understanding of action in infancy. *Philosophical Transactions of the Royal Society of London, B, Biological Sciences, 358,* 447–458.

Dautenhahn, K., & Nehaniv, C. L. (Eds.). (2002). *Imitation in animals and artifacts.* Cambridge, MA: MIT Press.

Ferrari, P. F., Gallese, V., Rizzolatti, G., & Fogassi, L. (2003). Mirror neurons responding to the observation of ingestive and communicative mouth actions in the monkey ventral premotor cortex. *European Journal of Neuroscience, 17,* 1703–1714.

Frith, C. D., & Wolpert, D. M. (Eds.). (2003). *Decoding, imitating and influencing the actions of others: The mechanisms of social interaction.* Oxford, UK: Oxford University Press.

Galef, B. G., Jr. (1988). Imitation in animals: History, definition, and interpretation of data from the psychological laboratory. In T. R. Zentall & B. G. Galef, Jr. (Eds.), *Social learning: Psychological and biological perspectives* (pp. 3–28). Hillsdale, NJ: Erlbaum.

Galef, B. G., Jr. (1990). Traditions in animals: Field observations and laboratory analyses. In M. Bekoff & D. Jamieson (Eds.), *Interpretation and explanation in the study of animal behaviour* (pp. 74–95). Boulder, CO: Westview Press.

Galef, B. G., Jr., & Heyes, C. M. (Eds.). (2004). Social learning and imitation [Special issue]. *Learning and Behavior, 32*(1).

Gallese., V., Fadiga, L., Fogassi, L., & Rizzolatti, G. (1996). Action recognition in the premotor cortex. *Brain, 119,* 593–609.

Gallese, V., & Goldman, A. (1998). Mirror neurons and the simulation theory of mindreading. *Trends in Cognitive Sciences, 2,* 493–501.

Gattis, M., Bekkering, H., & Wohlschlager, A. (2002). Goal-directed imitation. In A. Meltzoff & W. Prinz (Eds.), *The imitative mind* (pp. 183–205). Cambridge, UK: Cambridge University Press.

Gergeley, G., Bekkering, H., & Király, I. (2002). Rational imitation in preverbal infants. *Nature, 415,* 755.

Gergeley, G., Nádasdy, Z., Csibra, G., & Bíró, S. (1995). Taking the intentional stance at 12 months of age. *Cognition, 56,* 165–193.

Gomez, J.-C. (1996). Nonhuman primate theories of (nonhuman primate) minds: Some issues concerning the origins of mindreading. In P. Carruthers & P. K. Smith (Eds.), *Theories of theories of mind* (pp. 330–343). Cambridge, UK: Cambridge University Press.

Hare, B., Addessi, E., Call, J., Tomasello, M., & Visalberghi, E. (2003). Do capuchin monkeys, *Cebus apella*, know what conspecifics do and do not see? *Animal Behaviour, 65,* 131–142.

Hare, B., Call, J., Agnetta, B., & Tomasello, M. (2000). Chimpanzees know what conspecifics do and do not see. *Animal Behaviour, 59,* 771–785.

Hare, B., Call, J., & Tomasello, M. (2001). Do chimpanzees know what conspecifics know? *Animal Behaviour, 61,* 139–151.

Harris, P. (1991). The work of the imagination. In A. Whiten (Ed.), *Natural theories of mind: Evolution, development, and simulation of everyday mindreading* (pp. 283–304). Oxford, UK: Basil Blackwell.

Hayes, C. (1951). *The ape in our house.* New York: Harper.

Heyes, C. M., Jaldow, E., Nokes, T., & Dawson, G. R. (1994). Imitation in rats: The role of demonstrator action. *Behavioral Processes, 32,* 173–182.

Heyes, C. M., & Saggerson, A. (2002). Testing for imitative and nonimitative social learning in the budgerigar using a two-object/two-action test. *Animal Behaviour, 64,* 851–859.

Horner, V. K., & Whiten, A. (2005). Causal knowledge and imitation/emulation switching in chimpanzees (*Pan troglodytes*) and children. *Animal Cognition, 8,* 164–181.

Huang, C.-T., Heyes, C., & Charman, T. (2002). Infants' behavioral reenactment of "failed attempts": Exploring the roles of emulation learning, stimulus enhancement, and understanding of intentions. *Developmental Psychology, 38*(5), 840–855.

Huffman, M. A. (1996). Acquisition of innovative cultural behaviours in nonhuman primates: A case study of stone handling, a socially transmitted behaviour in Japanese macaques. In C. M. Heyes & B. G. Galef, Jr. (Eds.), *Social learning in animals: The roots of culture* (pp. 267–289). London: Academic Press.

Hurley, S., & Chater, N. (2005). *Perspectives on imitation: From mirror neurons to memes.* Boston: MIT Press.

Iacoboni, M., Woods, R. P., Brass, M., Bekkering, H., Mazziotta, J. C., & Rizzolatti, G. (1999). Cortical mechanisms of human imitation. *Science, 286,* 2526–2528.

Klein, E. D., & Zentall, T. R. (2003). Imitation and affordance learning by pigeons (*Columbia livia*). *Journal of Comparative Psychology, 117,* 414–419.

Leslie, A. M. (1987). Pretense and representation in infancy: The origins of "theory of mind." *Psychological Review, 94,* 412–426.

Matsuzawa, T. (2004, August). *The chimpanzee's mind: A synthesis of field and laboratory studies.* Plenary paper delivered at the 20th Congress of the International Primatological Society, Turin, Italy.

Meltzoff, A., & Prinz, W. (2002). *The imitative mind: Development, evolution and brain bases.* Cambridge, UK: Cambridge University Press.

Meltzoff, A. N. (1995). Understanding the intentions of others: Re-enactment of intended acts by 18-month-old children. *Developmental Psychology, 31,* 1–16.

Meltzoff, A. N., & Gopnik, A. (1993). The role of imitation in understanding persons and developing a theory of mind. In S. Baron-Cohen, H. Tager-Flusberg, & D. J. Cohen (Eds.), *Understanding other minds: Perspectives from autism* (pp. 335–366). Oxford, UK: Oxford University Press.

Myowa-Yamakoshi, M., & Matsuzawa, T. (2000). Imitation of intentional manipulatory actions in chimpanzees (*Pan troglodytes*). *Journal of Comparative Psychology, 114*(4), 381–391.

Neilsen, M., Collier-Baker, E., Davis, J., & Suddendorf, T. (2005). Imitation recognition in a captive chimpanzee (*Pan troglodytes*). *Animal Cognition, 8,* 31–36.

Perner, J. (1991). *Understanding the representational mind.* Cambridge, MA: MIT Press.

Povinelli, D. J. (2000). *Folk physics for apes.* Oxford, UK: Oxford University Press.

Povinelli, D. J., & Eddy, T. J. (1996). What young chimpanzees know about seeing. *Monographs of the Society for Research in Child Development, 61*(2).

Rizzolatti, G., Fadiga, L., Fogassi, L., & Gallese, V. (2002). From mirror neurones to imitation: Facts and speculations. In A. N. Meltzoff & W. Prinz (Eds.), *The imitative mind* (pp. 247–266). Cambridge, UK: Cambridge University Press.

Rizzolatti, G., Fadiga, L., Gallese, V., & Fogassi, L. (1996). Premotor cortex and the recognition of motor actions. *Brain Research: Cognitive Brain Research, 3,* 131–141.

Rogers, S. J., & Pennington, B. F. (1991). A theoretical approach to the deficits in infantile autism. *Developmental Psychopathology, 3,* 137–162.

Spence, K. W. (1937). Experimental studies of social learning and higher mental processes in infra-human primates. *Psychological Bulletin, 34*, 806–850.

Stoinski, T. S., & Whiten, A. (2003). Social learning by orangutans (*Pongo pygmaeus*) in a simulated food processing task. *Journal of Comparative Psychology, 117*, 272–282.

Stoinski, T. S., Wrate, J. L., Ure, N., & Whiten, A. (2001). Imitative learning by captive western lowland gorillas *(Gorilla gorilla gorilla)* in a simulated food-processing task. *Journal of Comparative Psychology, 115*, 272–281.

Subiaul, F., Cantlon, J. F., Holloway, R. L., & Terrace, H. S. (2004). Cognitive imitation in rhesus macaques. *Science, 305*, 407–410.

Suddendorf, T. (1998). Simpler for evolution: Secondary representation in apes, children, and ancestors. *Behavioral and Brain Science, 21*, 131.

Suddendorf, T. (1999). The rise of the metamind. In M. C. Corballis & S. E. G. Lea (Eds.), *The descent of mind: Psychological perspectives on hominid evolution* (pp. 218–260). London: Oxford University Press.

Suddendorf, T., & Whiten, A. (2001). Mental evolution and development: Evidence for secondary representation in children, great apes and other animals. *Psychological Bulletin, 127*, 629–650.

Suddendorf, T., & Whiten, A. (2003). Reinterpreting the psychology of apes. In K. Sterelny & J. Fitness (Eds.), *From mating to mentality: Evaluating evolutionary psychology* (pp. 173–196). New York: Psychology Press.

Thompson, D. E., & Russell, J. (2004). The ghost condition: Imitation versus emulation in young children's observational learning. *Developmental Psychology, 40*, 882–889.

Thorpe, W. H. (1963). *Learning and instinct in animals*. London: Methuen.

Tomasello, M. (1990). Cultural transmission in the tool use and communicatory signalling of chimpanzees? In S. Parker & K. Gibson (Eds.), *Language and intelligence in monkeys and apes: Comparative developmental perspectives* (pp. 274–311). Cambridge, UK: Cambridge University Press.

Tomasello, M. (1998). Emulation learning and cultural learning. *Behavioural and Brain Sciences, 21*, 703–704.

Tomasello, M., & Call, J. (1997). *Primate cognition*. New York: Oxford University Press.

Tomasello, M., Call, J., & Hare, B. (2003). Chimpanzees understand psychological states— The question is which ones and to what extent. *Trends in Cognitive Sciences, 7*, 153–156.

Tomasello, M., Davis-Dasilva, M., Camak, L., & Bard, K. (1987). Observational learning of tool-use by young chimpanzees. *Human Evolution, 2*, 175–183.

Tomasello, M., Kruger, A. C., & Ratner, H. H. (1993). Cultural learning. *Behavioral and Brain Sciences, 16*, 495–552.

Umiltà, M. A., Kohler, E., Gallese, V., Fogassi, L., Fadiga, L., Keysers, C., et al. (2001). I know what you are doing: A neurophysiological study. *Neuron, 31*, 155–165.

van Schaik, C. P., Ancrenaz, M., Borgen, G., Galdikas, B., Knott, C. D., Singleton, I., et al. (2003). Orangutan cultures and the evolution of material culture. *Science, 299*, 102–105.

Visalberghi, E., & Fragaszy, D. (1990). Do monkeys ape? In S. Parker & K. Gibson (Eds.), *Language and intelligence in monkeys and apes: Comparative developmental perspectives* (pp. 247–273). Cambridge, UK: Cambridge University Press.

Voelkl, B., & Huber, L. (2000). True imitation in marmosets. *Animal Behaviour, 60*, 195–202.

Want, S. C., & Harris P. L. (2001). Learning from other people's mistakes: Causal understanding in learning to use a tool. *Child Development, 72*, 431–443.

Want, S. C., & Harris, P. L. (2002). How do children ape? Applying concepts from the study of non-human primates to the developmental study of "imitation" in children. *Developmental Science, 5*, 1–13.

Whiten, A. (1996). Imitation, pretence and mindreading: Secondary representation in comparative primatology and developmental psychology? In A. W. Russon, K. A. Bard, & S. T. Parker (Eds.), *Reaching into thought: The minds of the great apes* (pp. 300–324). Cambridge, UK: Cambridge University Press.

Whiten, A. (2000). Primate culture and social learning. *Cognitive Science, 24,* 477–508.

Whiten, A. (2002a). Imitation of sequential and hierarchical structure in action: Experimental studies with children and chimpanzees. In K. Dautenhahn & C. L. Nehaniv (Eds.), *Imitation in animals and artifacts* (pp. 191–209). Cambridge, MA: MIT Press.

Whiten, A. (2002b). The imitator's representations of the imitated. In A. Meltzoff & W. Prinz (Eds.), *The imitative mind* (pp. 98–121). Cambridge, UK: Cambridge University Press.

Whiten, A. (2005). The second inheritance system of chimpanzees and humans. *Nature, 437,* 52–55.

Whiten, A., & Brown, J. D. (1999). Imitation and the reading of other minds: Perspectives from the study of autism, normal children and non-human primates. In S. Bråten (Ed.), *Intersubjective communication and emotion in early ontogeny* (pp. 260–280). Cambridge, UK: Cambridge University Press.

Whiten, A., & Byrne, R. W. (1988). Tactical deception in primates. *Behavioral and Brain Sciences, 11,* 233–273.

Whiten, A., & Byrne, R. W. (1991). The emergence of metarepresentation in human ontogeny and primate phylogeny. In A. Whiten (Ed.), *Natural theories of mind: Evolution, development and simulation of everyday mindreading* (pp. 267–281). Oxford, UK: Basil Blackwell.

Whiten, A., Custance, D. M., Gomez, J.-C., Teixidor, P., & Bard, K. A. (1996). Imitative learning of artificial fruit processing in children (*Homo sapiens*) and chimpanzees (*Pan troglodytes*). *Journal of Comparative Psychology, 110,* 3–14.

Whiten, A., Goodall, J., McGrew, W. C., Nishida, T., Reynolds, V., Sugiyama, Y., et al. (1999). Cultures in chimpanzees. *Nature, 399,* 682–685.

Whiten, A., & Ham, R. (1992). On the nature and evolution of imitation in the animal kingdom: Reappraisal of a century of research. In P. J. B. Slater, J. S. Rosenblatt, C. Beer, & M. Milinski (Eds.), *Advances in the study of behaviour* (Vol. 21, pp. 239–283). New York: Academic Press.

Whiten, A., Horner, V., Litchfield, C., & Marshall-Pescini, S. (2004). How do apes ape? *Learning and Behaviour, 32,* 36–52.

Whiten, A., Horner, V., & Marshall-Pescini, S. (2005). Selective imitation in child and chimpanzee: A window on the construal of others' actions. In S. Hurley & N. Chater (Eds.), *Perspectives on imitation: From mirror neurons to memes* (pp. 263–283). Cambridge, MA: MIT Press.

Whiten, A., & Suddendorf, T. (in press). Great ape cognition and the evolutionary roots of human imagination. *Proceedings of the British Academy.*

Williams, J. H. G., Whiten, A., & Singh, T. (2004). A systematic review of action imitation in autistic spectrum disorder. *Journal of Autism and Developmental Disorders, 34,* 285–299.

Williams, J. H. G., Whiten, A., Suddendorf, T., & Perrett, D. I. (2001). Imitation, mirror neurons and autism. *Neuroscience and Biobehavioral Reviews, 25,* 287–295.

Wood, D. (1989). Social interaction as tutoring. In M. H. Bornstein & J. S. Bruner (Eds.), *Interaction in human development* (pp. 59–80). Hillsdale, NJ: Erlbaum.

Zentall, T. R. (2004). Action imitation in birds. *Learning and Behavior, 32,* 14–23.

Zentall, T. R., Sutton, J. E., & Sherburne, L. M. (1996). True imitative learning in pigeons. *Psychological Science, 7*(6), 343–346.

CHAPTER 11

A Cognitive Neuroscience View of Imitation

JEAN DECETY

In recent years, there has been a great upsurge in the neurophysiological investigations of imitation, particularly because new neuroimaging methods have become available to look at the anatomical areas involved in the perception–action coupling under diverse sophisticated paradigms. In addition, the discovery of mirror neurons in the monkey has provided a physiological model for the basic mechanism of perception–action coupling that is involved in imitation and action understanding.

The chapter begins by defining imitation. Then it reviews the neural mechanism for perception–action coupling and its link with motor representations both in monkeys and in humans. This coupling mechanism explains motor priming and social facilitation. Next, neuroimaging studies of imitation are discussed with a special section on imitation and emotion processing. It is then argued that executive inhibition is an important component of imitation. Neuroimaging research concerning reciprocal imitation and the sense of agency are presented. Finally, I discuss some important questions for future direction, notably whether brain systems involved in representing goal-directed action are distinct from the brain regions associated with mentalizing.

One critical aspect of functional imaging research is that data do not make much sense if they are not framed within a cognitive model of imitation leading to specific predictions about its neural implementation. Thus, a first requirement is to use a clear definition of what imitation is and what functions it subserves. Indeed, there are a variety of behaviors that have been indistinctively categorized under imitation. Yet, do flocks of birds acting together, people in conversation that synchronize their speech rate and body mannerisms, ballet dancers performing in unison, or an individual learning fencing account for the same phenomena? Are these different behaviors mediated by the same mechanism?

All theorists of human imitation acknowledge that it is an incredibly powerful way to learn skills and develop a sense of self, an important form of communication, a milestone in the development of intentional communication and more generally social interaction (e.g., Meltzoff & Gopnik, 1993; Nadel, Guérini, Pezé, & Rivet, 1999; Rogers, 1999). Despite the fact that there are many definitions and disagreements over what is imitation, most scholars agree that it is a natural mechanism that involves perception and action coupling for mapping one's own behavior onto the behavior observed in others, and that it serves an adaptive function. Indeed, imitation is a powerful mechanism for individual learning, which gives a level of flexibility that does not require the genetic predisposition to match the nature of the environment in which the individual will have to survive (Zentall, 2003). However, such a minimal definition of imitation is not sufficient to fully account for its role in human social development, if one appreciates that imitation allows individuals to ascribe internal experience to both themselves and others (Mitchell, 1993), is a mechanism for developing theory of mind (Meltzoff & Gopnik, 1993), a precursor for empathy (Trevarthen, 1979), or a critical means to develop awareness of self-other coordination (Rogers, 1999). In addition, in humans, imitation is likely to depend on the motivation of the observer to attend to the behavior of the model.

In this chapter, rather than considering imitation as a simple matching mechanism, it is viewed as a molar construct, which includes different subcomponents such as perception–action coupling, visual attention, short-term memory, body schema, mental state attribution, and agency. These components rely on distributed network connectivity as demonstrated by a number of brain imaging studies that are discussed here. Each component of the network computes a different aspect of imitative behavior, and together the network orchestrates the task. The role of neuroscience is to help to identify the mechanisms responsible for imitation and decipher the contribution of each of its components. However, the various forms of imitation—ranging from copying a movement after seeing it done to reproducing an action intentionally offline—may well constitute a continuum from simple acts to complex ones, from unconscious mimicry to intentional reproduction, as well as from familiar actions to novel actions. This view of imitation is compatible with the idea of a hierarchy of mechanisms. Table 11.1 summarizes a number of apparently competitive theories of imitation and how these theories can be associated to specific brain mechanisms.

A first glance shows that there are more similarities than differences between these theories. In fact major disagreements seem to arise from the level (or definition) of imitation that is being used (e.g., simple vs. complex actions, immediate vs. differed imitation). But again, one may view these various behaviors on a continuum that ranges from response facilitation (i.e., the automatic tendency to reproduce an observed movement) to learning a new behavior that is not present in the motor repertoire. It will be argued that the basic neural mechanism that unifies this variety of phenomena relies on the

TABLE 11.1. Different Theoretical Accounts of Imitation, and Their Putative Neural Underpinnings

- Byrne and Russon (1998) distinguish two processes involved in imitation: (1) the action level that allows one to copy actions following the surface form, and (2) the program level that allows one to copy the hierarchical organization of a complex action and ultimately learn new behavior. The system of mirror neurons may provide the neural basis for the former process.

- The direct mapping approach states that the motor system is activated by the perception of an action performed by another individual (Butterworth, 1993). Evidence from mirror neurons in the premotor cortex and parietal cortex seems sufficient to account for that theory.

- The active intermodal matching (AIM) model states that infants code human acts within an innate supramodal system that unifies observation and execution of motor acts (Meltzoff & Moore, 1997). Such a system may be similar to the notion of body schema. The posterior parietal cortex would then be of critical importance for this theory.

- The kinesthetic–visual matching requires some kinesthetic involvement in visual experiences of bodies, including one's own and those of others (Mitchell, 1993). The left parietal cortex is a key neural component of that theory.

- The goal-directed theory suggests that children first decompose observed actions and then reproduce them according to a hierarchy of goals (Bekkering, Wohlschläger, & Gattis, (2000). This theory requires the mirror system and executive functions (attention, action parsing, working memory), and thus would predict prefrontal cortex participation in imitation.

- The associative sequence learning (ASL) suggests that imitation is experience based and consists of a set of bidirectional excitatory links between sensory and motor representations of movement units (Heyes, 2001). This theory is compatible with the mirror neuron account but also requires nonspecific imitation mechanisms that regulate intentional action. These mechanisms are likely to be subserved by the prefrontal cortex.

- Rogers and Pennington (1991) proposed that two macrocomponents are implicated in imitation: (1) cross-modal representation processes extract patterns of similarity between self and other, and (2) executive functions. Prefrontal cortex in conjunction with the parietal cortex are crucial neural systems for this theory.

Note. This list is not intended to be exhaustive but aims at showing the similarities and the differences between these different theories.

direct perception–action coupling mechanism, also called the mirror system. Such a system provides a key foundation for the building of imitative and mindreading competencies. However, additional computational mechanisms are necessary to account for their full maturation.

PERCEPTION–ACTION COUPLING AND MOTOR REPRESENTATIONS

Imitation requires that one maps one's own behavior onto the behavior observed in another individual. Such a mapping between the demonstrator and the imitator is the functional bedrock of any form of social learning, copying, or mimicry and supposes a correspondence between two agents. It also necessitates a coupling mechanism between perception and action. In fact, perception and action cycles constitute the fundamental base of the nervous system. These processes are functionally intertwined: Perception is a means to action and action is a means to perception. Indeed, the vertebrate brain has evolved for governing motor activity with the basic function to transform sensory patterns into patterns of motor coordination (Sperry, 1952). The metaphor of "affordance" was coined to account for the direct link between perception and action (Gibson, 1966). Such affordances are the possibilities for use, intervention, and action offered by the local environment to a specific type of embodied agent. For example, a human perceives a garbage can as "affording trashing," but the affordances presented by a garbage can to a raccoon would be radically different. Then Shepard (1984) argued that as a result of biological evolution and individual learning, the organism is, at any given moment, tuned to resonate to the incoming patterns that correspond to the invariants that are significant for it. These patterns, according to Shepard have become most deeply internalized (i.e., represented), and even in the complete absence of external information, the system can be excited entirely from within (e.g., while imagining). Thus, unlike Gibson, Shepard makes explicit reference to internal representation, and makes it possible to articulate the notion of resonance with that of motor representations.

In addition, humans actively seek information about themselves and others. This latter aspect is compatible with contemporary theory of motor representations, which stresses the autonomy of the individual with respect to the external milieu and views his or her actions as a consequence of triggering by the environment or as a consequence of an internal process (Jeannerod, 1994). The concept of motor representations of action designate both the mental content related to the goal or the consequences of a given action and the covert neural operations that are supposed to occur before an action begins. There is no ontological reason to consider these two levels of description (i.e., mental and neural) as separate, and least of all independent from one another.

Today, the common coding theory claims parity between perception and action. Its core assumption is that actions are coded in terms of the perceivable effects (i.e., the distal perceptual events) they should generate (Prinz, 1997). This theory states that perception of an action should activate action representations to the degree that the perceived and the represented action are similar (see Knoblich & Flach, 2003, for empirical evidence).

The discovery of "mirror neurons" in the ventral premotor cortex (F5 region) of the macaque monkey that fire both when it carries out a goal-directed action and when it observes the same action performed by another individual (Rizzolatti, Fadiga, Gallese, & Fogassi, 1996) provided the first convincing physiological evidence for a direct matching between action perception and action representation. More recently, it was found that a subset of these mirror neurons also respond when the final part of an action, crucial in triggering the response when the action is seen entirely, is hidden, and can only be inferred (Umilta et al., 2001). Therefore, specific neurons in this region respond to the representation of an action rather than to the action itself. Ongoing work by this laboratory extended this idea by showing that some neurons display mirror properties between motor and other modalities such as audition (Kohler et al., 2002). This demonstrates that single neurons are concerned with some actions regardless of the modality through which a given action is inferred (i.e., it is the consequence of the action that is represented). Such neurons are not restricted to the premotor cortex but have also been recorded in other areas of the brain, notably in the posterior parietal cortex (area PF) in relation to actions performed with objects (Gallese, Fogassi, Fadiga, & Rizzolatti, 2002). In a recent study, Raos, Evangeliou, and Savaki (2004) used the quantitative [^{14}C]deoxyglucose method (a quantitative autoradiographic method used to map very precisely the spatial distribution of metabolic activity) in monkeys that either grasped three-dimensional objects or observed the same movements executed by humans. They found that the forelimb regions of the primary motor cortex (MI) and the primary somatosensory (SI) cortex were significantly activated in both cases. This study provides strong evidence for use of MI representations during the observation of actions by demonstrating that the observation of an action is represented in the primary motor and somatosensory cortices as is its execution. It also indicates that in terms of neural correlates, recognizing a motor behavior is like executing the same behavior, requiring the involvement of a distributed system encompassing not only the premotor but also the primary motor cortex. These findings support the direct-matching hypothesis that holds that one understands actions when one maps the visual representation of the perceived action onto one's own motor representation of the same action.

Another cortical region that contains neurons responding to the observation of actions performed by others is located in the superior temporal sulcus (STS). In the macaque monkey, Perrett and colleagues (1989) have found that there are neurons in the superior part of the STS that are sensitive to the sight of static and dynamic information about the body. The majority of these cells are selective for one perspective view and are considered to provide viewer-centered descriptions. For some cells in the lower bank of STS the responses to body movements are related to the object or to the goal of the movements. Movements effective in eliciting neuron responses in this region include walking, turning the head, bending the torso, and moving the arms. A small set of STS neurons discharge also during the observation of goal-directed hand movements (Perrett, Mistlin, Harries, & Chitty, 1990). Moreover, a population of cells, located in the anterior part of the STS respond selectively to the sight of reaching, but only when the agent performing the action is seen attending to the target position of the reaching (Jellema et al., 2000). In addition, the responses of a subset of these cells are modulated by the direction of attention (indicated by head and body posture of the agent performing the action). This combined analysis of direction of attention and body movements supports the detection of intentional actions.

It is noteworthy that unlike F5 neurons, STS neurons do not appear to be endowed with motor properties. It was suggested that the "action detecting" system in STS provides an initial "pictorial" description of the action that would then feed to the F5 motor vocabulary, where it would acquire a meaning for the individual and also activate circuits comprising mirror neurons, which can, in principle, reproduce the perceived action (Rizzolatti, Fogassi, & Gallese, 2001). The two areas, STS and F5, are not directly connected, but both of them are linked to the parietal lobule area, which projects to the premotor cortex (see Figure 11.1 for corresponding areas in the human brain).

Evidence for a matching system between perception and action in humans continues to accumulate. For instance, it was found that when individuals observe a block-stacking task, the coordination between their gaze and the actor's hand is predictive of the next action, rather than reactive to their last movement, and is highly similar to the gaze–hand coordination when they perform the task themselves (Flanagan & Johansson, 2003). These results indicate, in accordance with the common coding theory, that during action observation subjects implement eye motor programs directed by motor representations of manual actions.

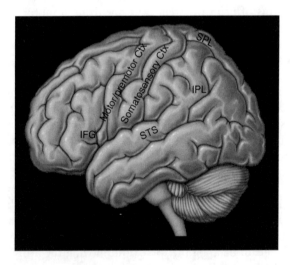

FIGURE 11.1. A lateral view of a human left hemisphere. IFG, inferior frontal gyrus; STS, superior temporal sulcus; IPL, inferior parietal lobule (Brodmann's areas 39 and 40); SPL, superior parietal lobule (Brodmann's areas 5 and 7). Note that the IFG corresponds to the ventral premotor cortex in monkeys in which area F5 is located. The premotor cortex has a central role in the selection of movements. Neurons in the posterior portion of the STS are triggered by the sight of actions performed by others. The SPL is involved in coding space and in directing spatial attention in relation to the control of body movements. The left IPL mediates motor representations, and the right IPL is critical for the sense of agency.

The activation pattern in the premotor cortex elicited by the observation of actions performed by another individual follows its somatotopic organization. Watching mouth, foot, and hand actions elicits different sites in the premotor and superior parietal cortices, which would be normally involved in the actual execution of the observed actions (Buccino et al., 2001). In another domain it has been found that speech listening is associated with an increase of motor-evoked potentials (MEP) recorded from the listeners' tongue muscles when the presented words strongly involve tongue movements when uttered (Fadiga, Craighero, Buccino, & Rizzolatti, 2002; Watkins, Strafella, & Paus, 2003). In another recent study, participants were asked to observe, imagine or imitate hand actions while transcranial magnetic stimulation (TMS) was delivered over their hand motor area of the left hemisphere (Clark, Tremblay, & St.-Marie, 2003). TMS generates magnetic field impulses, which stimulate underlying neurons in a focused volume and allow one to measure peripheral responses such as latencies and amplitudes. While the condition of imitation was the one to produce the greatest MEP, recorded in muscles of the dominant hand, there is significant response in both the observation and imagery conditions (Figure 11.2).

This perception–action matching system offers a parsimonious explanation of how we understand the actions of others, by a direct mapping of the visual representation of the observed action into our motor representation of the same action (Blakemore & Decety, 2001). This direct translation of perceived actions in others into motor output in oneself constitutes a shared rep-

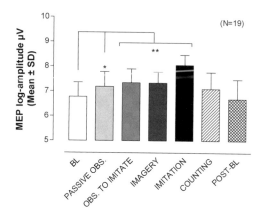

FIGURE 11.2. Comparison of the mean changes in motor evoked potentials log—amplitude in a group of participants during various experimental conditions including passive observation, observation to imitate, mental imagery, and imitation of hand actions. BL, baseline. From Clark, Tremblay, and St. Marie (2003). Copyright 2003 by Pergamon Press. Reprinted by permission.

resentational framework for self and other actions at both computational and neural levels (Decety & Sommerville, 2003). Furthermore, the fact that perception is itself tangled up with specific possibilities of action raises the idea that internal representations the mind uses to guide actions are best understood as action- and context-specific control structures rather than as passive recapitulations of external reality (Clark, 2001).

FROM MOTOR PRIMING TO SOCIAL FACILITATION

One consequence of the functional equivalence between perception and action is that watching an action performed by another person facilitates the later reproduction of that action in oneself. For instance, a series of psychophysics studies demonstrated that when subjects are asked to produce gestures on cue, the response is quicker when stimulus and response gestures matched than when they were incongruent (Sturmer, Aschersleben, & Prinz, 2000). The response was also faster when subjects are asked to produce the response under imitative cueing than under symbolic cueing conditions (e.g., when shown a certain color). These findings also cast some light into "social facilitation," which accounts for the demonstration that the presence of other people can affect individual performance.

A series of experiments on spatial compatibility, based on reaction time, demonstrated that actions at the disposal of another agent are represented and have impact on one's own actions, even when the task at hand does not require taking the actions of another person into account (Sebanz, Knoblich, & Prinz, 2003). The authors used a spatial compatibility task distributed among two people so that each participant had control of one of two responses. Subjects were asked to press a key in response to a cue (e.g., color of a visual stimulus) while an irrelevant cue was simultaneously presented. The speed with which subjects produced the desired response was influenced by the direction of the arrow (irrelevant cue), a finding that can be explained if subjects were representing the actions of the other as if they were their own. These results show that one's own actions and others' actions are represented and planned in a functionally equivalent way. This mechanism also accounts for response facilitation (i.e., the automatic tendency to reproduce an observed movement, known as mimicry) (see Moody & McIntosh, Chapter 4, this volume) a type of imitative response. It is important to note that this behavior does not imply an understanding of the meaning of the imitated action (e.g., laughing and yawning). Copying the behavior of conspecifics (social learning) depends on the relative automaticity of some forms of imitation. It has an adaptive advantage for communication and social interaction (Chartrand & Bargh, 1999).

Another consequence of this perception–action matching mechanism is that stimuli that can be tied to the representation of one's own body should be more imitable than those that cannot be mapped. In one experiment, Castiello, Lusher, Mari, Edwards, and Humphreys (2002) explored the nature and specificity of motor priming by examining behavioral responses to actions produced by a robotic arm versus that produced by a human arm. They showed a priming advantage for the latter. A cerebral correlate of this effect seems to involve the premotor cortex and the right parietal cortex. Perani and colleagues (2001) reported greater activity in these regions when participants observed grasping movements executed by a human hand than when the same actions were performed by a virtual hand. Subsequent work by Castiello (2003) showed priming effects even when the kinematics of a model are not available and suggests that the motor intention of conspecifics can be inferred from their gaze. In a follow-up functional magnetic resonance imaging (fMRI) study, the same group demonstrated selective activation of the left premotor cortex when participants observed a human model performing grasping actions (Tai, Scherfler, Brooks, Sawamoto, & Castiello, 2004). This activation was not evident for the observation of similar actions performed by a robot.

A further argument in favor of the common mechanism for observed and executed action is provided by the study of Kilner, Paulignan, and Blakemore (2003) that showed interference effect, in the form of increased variance of movement, when subjects execute a movement while simultaneously observing someone else executing an incongruent movement. This interference occurred only when the incongruent movements were executed by another human agent, and not when they were performed by a robotic arm.

Another compelling demonstration of the involvement of motor representation in the perception of bodily movements is provided by studies making use of the phenomenon of apparent motion. Stevens, Fonlupt, Shiffrar, and Decety (2000) adapted the apparent motion paradigm, originally developed by Shiffrar and Freyd (1990), to present participants in the scanner with a human model in different positions. Depending on the activation conditions, the subjects were shown either possible or impossible biomechanical paths of apparent motion. The left primary motor cortex and parietal lobule in both hemispheres were found to be selectively activated when the subjects perceived possible paths of human movement (performed with a right limb). No activation in these areas was detected during conditions of impossible biomechanical movement paths.

Altogether these findings provide strong evidence that one represents one's own action and other's actions according to a similar neural and cognitive framework and fit neatly with the idea that we implicitly use our own motor representations system as a model to perceive and understand others. In addition, these data are consistent with developmental research, which has shown that our tendency to imitate reflects a consistent differentiation of animate and inanimate objects. For instance, a study indicates that young infants of ages 5–8 weeks imitate tongue protrusion openings of a human model but not when this gesture is performed by an object (Legerstee, 1991).

IMITATION: FROM SIMPLE ACTS TO COMPLEX ACTIONS

Given the growing evidence for the direct perception–action coupling in the premotor/motor and posterior parietal cortices during action observation, it is likely that such a mechanism is at play during imitation. This direct mapping would at least partly account for the inborn ability to match seen movements of others with felt movements of their own (Meltzoff & Moore, 1977).

Some first evidence for the involvement of the mirror system during imitation of simple finger movements comes from an fMRI study conducted by Iacoboni and colleagues (1999). In that study, individuals were tested in two conditions: observation only and observation–execution. In the former condition, subjects were shown a moving finger, a cross on a stationary finger, or a cross on an empty background. The instruction was to observe the stimuli. In the observation–execution condition, the same stimuli were presented, but this time the instruction was to lift the right finger, as fast as possible, in response to them. The results showed that the activity was stronger during imitation trials than during the other motor trials in four areas: the left pars opercularis of the inferior frontal gyrus (which is considered to be homologue to F5 in the monkey), the right anterior parietal region, the right parietal operculum, and the right STS region.

A series of neuroimaging studies demonstrated that the intention to imitate has a top-down effect on the brain regions involved in the observation of actions. In the scanner, participants were instructed to carefully watch pantomimed actions performed by a human model either for later recognition or for imitation (Decety et al., 1997; Grèzes, Costes, & Decety, 1998). When conditions of observation of action were contrasted with a baseline condition, in which static postures were shown, increased activity was detected in the premotor cortex at the level of the upper limb representation, the inferior frontal gyrus (Broca's area), the posterior STS, and the parietal cortex. When subjects observed actions for later imitation, as compared with passive observation of the same actions, a specific hemodynamic increase was detected in the supplementary motor area (SMA), the middle frontal gyrus, the premotor cortex, and the superior and inferior parietal cortices in both hemispheres (Plate 11.1). A different pattern of brain activation was found when subjects were observing the actions for recognition. In that case, the parahippocampal gyrus in the temporal lobe was chiefly activated. Thus the intention to imitate triggers additional information processing of executive functions that are necessary to hold in working memory the actions perceived, and also inhibitory mechanism to refrain imitating during the scanning.

Using magnetoencephalography (MEG), Nishitani and Hari (2000) investigated the cortical temporal dynamics of action representation during execution, online imitation, and observation of righthand reaching movements that ended with a precision pinch of the tip of a manipulandum. During execution, the left inferior frontal cortex was activated first (peak around 250 milliseconds [ms] before the pinching); this activation was followed within 100–200 ms by activation in the left primary motor area and 150–250 ms later. During imitation and observation, the sequence was otherwise similar, but it started from the left occipital cortex. Activation was always strongest during action imitation. Only the occipital activation was detected when the subject observed the experimenter reaching his hand without pinching.

In a second study, neuromagnetic measures were taken in participants who observed still pictures of lip forms, online imitated them, or made similar forms in a self-paced manner (Nishitani & Hari, 2002). In all conditions and in both hemispheres, cortical activation progressed in 20–70 ms steps from the occipital cortex to the superior temporal region (where the strongest activation took place), the inferior parietal lobule, and the inferior frontal lobe (Broca's area), and finally, 50–140 ms later, to the primary motor cortex (see Figure 11.3). The signals of Broca's area and motor cortex were significantly stronger during imitation than other conditions. These results demonstrate that still pictures, only implying motion, can activate the human mirror neuron system in a well-defined temporal order.

In one recent study, Williams and colleagues (2006) compared a group of autistic individual to a control group in an imitation task (finger movements). Both groups performed the task well. In comparison with healthy subjects, they found reduced hemodynamic activity in brain areas involved in movement analysis (visual cortex, temporoparietal cortex) and integration of this

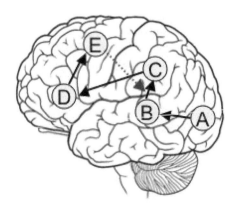

FIGURE 11.3. Schematic representation of the neural regions that constitute the basic neural architecture of imitation. (A) Visual cortex; (B) posterior STS; (C) rostral sector of the inferior parietal lobule; (D) inferior frontal gyrus; (E) motor cortex. The solid arrows indicate the assumed order of cortical activation measured by MEG (Nishitani & Hari, 2002). The dashed arrow represents the putative efferent copies of motor commands, which are used to predict the sensory consequences of the planned imitative behavior (see Decety, Chaminade, Grèzes, & Meltzoff, 2002; Iacoboni et al., 2001).

information into body knowledge (parietal cortex), action production, and mental state attribution (medial prefrontal cortex). Interestingly, this study did not reproduce the activation in Broca's region in the control group (see Table 11.2). The authors argued that the STS and inferior parietal cortex serve a self–other matching function between observed and executed actions by matching the intentions; it recognizes two different actions as similar even if they are achieved differently.

As described by Whiten (Chapter 10, this volume), action reproductions involving goals and means are dissociable (as seen in emulation) and therefore may partly tap distinct neural processes. Support for this hypothesis comes from a neuroimaging study that examined the neural instantiation of processing the goal and the means in an imitation paradigm (Chaminade, Meltzoff, & Decety, 2002). In this experiment, participants observed a human agent (only his hand and forearm were visible) building Duplo block constructions, and they were asked to observe and imitate either (1) the whole action performed by the experimenter (means and goal), (2) the goal only (end state of the object manipulation), or (3) the means only (the gesture without the last position). Partially overlapping clusters of activation were found in the right dorsolateral prefrontal cortex and in the cerebellum when subjects imitated either the goal or the means, suggesting that these regions are involved in processing both aspects of the action. Moreover, specific activity was detected in the medial prefrontal cortex during the imitation of the means, whereas imitating the goal was associated with increased activity in the left premotor cortex (see Figure 11.4).

These findings support the idea that the means and the goal of imitation partially rely on dissociable circuits. Interestingly, the medial prefrontal region activation during imitation of the means indicates that observing the means used by another individual prompts the observer to construct/infer the goal toward which this human agent is aiming. This region is known to play a critical role in inferring others' intentions and is consistently involved in mentalizing (i.e., the ability to understand that human actions are governed by mental states such as beliefs, desires, and intentions) (Frith & Frith, 2003). An alternative and complementary interpretation of the implication of the medial prefrontal cortex is based on the hypothesis that it contributes to goal achievement by three processes: goal-based action selection, rapid action evaluation, and discrimination of the early steps from the final steps toward the goal (Matsumoto & Tanaka, 2004). This latter aspect is present in conditions of imitation of the means without knowing the final position of the action made by the model.

In a recent fMRI study, Buccino and colleagues (2004) addressed the issue of imitation of a new skill. Musically naïve individuals were scanned during four conditions: (1) observation of guitar chords played by a guitarist, (2) a pause following model observation, (3) execution of the observed chords, and (4) rest. The results showed that the basic circuit underlying imitation learning consists of the inferior parietal lobule and the posterior of the

TABLE 11.2. Questions for Future Directions

Neuroimaging data help to answer fundamental questions about the mechanisms subserving imitation. However, their interpretation in relating structure to function should be done with caution. It is difficult to derive the computational function of an area without taking into account its extrinsic and intrinsic connectivity, the distribution of receptor types, and the information processing of the intrinsic neurons. Such information is generally lacking. In addition, a set of cortical areas may be active in a wide range of functions from action perception to theory of mind, but across those functions the networks in which they participate may be quite different (Cacioppo et al., 2003). In the domain of imitation, a number of specific questions need to be elucidated, including but not limited to:

- What is the role of Broca's region in action–perception coupling and imitation? While there is no dispute that in the monkey, neurons in F5 region code the goal of action and are involved in action understanding (Rizzolatti & Craigero, 2004), findings appear more diverse in humans. For instance, it has been demonstrated that the perception of auditory or visually presented temporal patterns involves area 44 (Schubotz & von Cramon, 2000), and that attention to the timing property of three consecutively presented visual objects (i.e., small circles) activates that region too (Schubotz & von Cramon, 2001). Broca's area participates in delayed execution and as such in movement preparation (Makuuchi, 2005). A recent fMRI experiment suggests that the left inferior frontal gyrus serves as a mechanism for general selection beyond that in semantic retrieval (Zhang, Feng, Fox, Gao, & Tan, 2004). It should, however, be noted that Broca's region contains motor representation of hand and mouth movements. It is thus logical to detect its activation in observation and imitation of hand and speech (e.g., Iacoboni et al., 2001).

- The posterior portion of the temporal cortex is an important component in a circuit involved in social cognition, which, through direct and indirect connections, receives input both from the ventral and the dorsal visual streams, the amygdala, the orbitofrontal cortex, and the prefrontal cortices. It seems that this region can be subdivided into different areas (in the right hemisphere), which may play distinct roles in the detection of agency and the representation of intentional actions (Saxe, Xiao, Kovacsc, Perrett, & Kanwisher, 2004).

- Which circuit mediates forward modeling? Activation of the superior parietal cortex, present when participants are instructed to observe action to imitate (e.g., Grèzes et al., 1998), may reflect backward projections of sensory copies of intended actions. A similar mechanism is thought to take place in the parietal operculum (Blakemore, Frith, & Wolpert, 1999), and in the STS (Iacoboni et al., 2001). The cerebellum is also considered to instantiate forward and inverse models (Wolpert, Miall, & Kawato, 1998).

- How is the motor resonance system functionally linked (and which anatomical pathways are involved) with theory of mind processes? Neuroimaging studies have revealed a system with three components: the medial prefrontal cortex, temporal poles, and posterior STS. This latter region is also found in action observation and thus may play a special role in linking the two systems. Importantly, the posterior STS has direct connections with the medial prefrontal cortex. Frith and Frith (2003) have proposed that this area is involved in detecting the behavior of agents, and analyzing the goals and outcomes of this behavior.

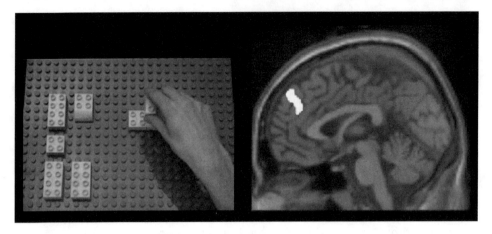

FIGURE 11.4. When participants observe, in order to imitate, another human agent building a Duplo construction (on the right) and when the goal of his actions is hidden, selective activation of the right medial prefrontal cortex was detected. This region is acknowledged to play a critical role in theory of mind. From Chaminade, Meltzoff, and Decety (2002). Copyright 2002 by Academic Press. Adapted by permission.

inferior frontal gyrus plus the adjacent premotor cortex (mirror neuron circuit). This circuit, known to be involved in action understanding, starts to be active during the observation of the guitar chords. During pause, the middle frontal gyrus (area 46) in addition to the structures involved in motor preparation (dorsal premotor cortex, superior parietal lobule, rostral mesial areas) also become active. The authors proposed that during learning of new motor patterns by imitation, the observed actions are decomposed into elementary motor acts that activate, via mirror mechanism, the corresponding motor representations in the parietal and ventral premotor cortices and in the inferior frontal gyrus. Once these motor representations are activated, they are recombined, according to the observed model by the prefrontal cortex with Brodmann's area 46 playing a fundamental orchestrating role.

IMITATION AND EMOTION PROCESSING

The perception–action coupling mechanism may also apply (at least partly) to emotion processing. In this vein, the perception of facial expression of emotions (e.g., disgust) activates the neural mechanisms that are responsible for the generation of emotions. Such a system prompts the observer to resonate with the state of another individual, with the observer activating the motor representations and associated autonomic and somatic responses that stem from the observed target (i.e., a sort of inverse mapping) (Adolphs, 2002). This is the facial feedback hypothesis as described by Moody and McIntosh

(Chapter 4, this volume). For example, while watching someone smile, the observer activates the same facial muscles involved in producing a smile at a subthreshold level, which creates the corresponding feeling of happiness in the observer. There is evidence for this mechanism in the recognition of emotion from facial expression. For instance, viewing facial expressions triggers expressions on one's own face, even in the absence of conscious recognition of the stimulus (e.g., Wallbott, 1991).

Making a facial expression generates changes in the autonomic nervous system and is associated with feeling the corresponding emotion). In a series of experiments, Levenson, Ekman, and Friesen (1990) instructed participants to produce facial configurations for anger, disgust, fear, happiness, sadness, and surprise while heart rate, skin conductance, finger temperature, and somatic activity were monitored. The authors found that such a voluntary facial activity produces significant levels of subjective experience of the associated emotions, as well as specific and reliable autonomic measures. In another study, Ekman and Davidson (1993) demonstrated similar patterns of electro-encephalographic activity for spontaneous and voluntary forms of smiling. Recently, an fMRI experiment confirmed these results by showing that when participants are required to observe or to imitate facial expressions of various emotions, increased neurodynamic activity is detected in the STS, the anterior insula, and the amygdala, as well as areas of the premotor cortex correspond-ing to the facial representation (Carr, Iacoboni, Dubeau, Mazziotta, & Lenzi, 2003). In another study, participants were scanned while watching movies of facial expressions (smile or frown) and hand movements (move index or mid-dle finger). The participants watched the movies under three different condi-tions: passive viewing, active imitation, and an active motor control. The authors found evidence for a common cortical imitation circuit for both face and hand imitation, consisting of Broca's area, bilateral dorsal and ventral premotor areas, right superior temporal sulcus, supplementary motor area, posterior temporo-occipital cortex, and cerebellar areas. For faces, passive viewing led to significant activation in the right ventral premotor area, whereas imitation produced bilateral activation (Leslie, Johnson-Frey, & Grafton, 2004).

The direct link between perception and action mediates the phenomenon of emotional contagion, defined as "the tendency to automatically mimic and synchronize facial expressions, vocalizations, postures, and movements with those of another person and consequently to converge emotionally" (Hatfield, Caccioppo, & Rapson, 1994). For instance, disgust is a strong negative emo-tion that, like fear, carries important survival cues for the self but also for the other who learns to avoid the ingestion of toxic aliments just by observing another conspecific's reaction. Phillips and colleagues (1997) have shown that normal volunteers presented with both strong and mild expressions of disgust activated anterior insular cortex but not the amygdala, and that strong disgust also activated structures linked to a limbic cortico–striatal–thalamic circuit. Another fMRI study extended these findings by showing that similar brain networks were involved in both the recognition (watching video clips of facial expression) and the experience (inhaling odorants) of disgust (Wicker et al., 2003). The authors found that observing facial expressions and feeling disgust activated the same sites in the anterior insula and anterior cingulate cortex.

The capacity to copy facial expressions of others appears to originate in the prewired direct mapping between visually perceived faces of others and the motor system of the observer. This motor activity can drive the matching emotional response. Such a primitive sympathetic response, which is often subliminal, constitutes one important process involved in emotion sharing. However, while this mechanism may be necessary, it does not seem to be sufficient to support empathy (i.e., an affective response that stems from the perception and the understanding of another emotional state without confusion between self and other). It has been argued that without self–other awareness, executive function, and emotion regulation processing, there is no true empathy (see Decety & Jackson, 2004).

THE ROLE OF INHIBITION

If one accepts that imitation is, to some degree, a prepotent response tendency such as in mimicry, it is, however, not an adaptive behavior in many everyday situations. Why then do we not imitate every behavior we encounter? One possible explanation is that most of the time, the mere observation activates motor representations at a subthreshold level, enough to lead to motor priming, as demonstrated by behavioral studies (e.g., Brass, Bekkering, Wohlschläger, & Prinz, 2000), but not sufficiently to elicit the overt behavior. Another explanation is that a component of executive control, cognitive inhibition, is at play. Substantial evidence for the inhibitory role of the prefrontal cortex has been reported in patients with large, bifrontal damage from degenerative and diverse mass lesions, who exhibit unsuppressed imitation or utilization behavior (e.g., Lhermitte, Pillon, & Serdaru, 1986). These authors proposed that prefrontal cortex damage resulted in the loss of inhibitory control, a deficit in response inhibition. Consequently, the parietal lobe was released to engage whatever came within its perceptual sights, leading to a behavioral pattern of environmental dependency. However, neither the parietal association nor prefrontal cortices have direct projections to primary motor cortex or spinal cord. Access is dependent on premotor structures including the rostral region of the SMA in the mesial aspects of the superior frontal gyrus. Neuroimaging studies have pointed to a trend for medial premotor cortex dominance in internally guided action and the lateral premotor cortex in externally guided action (Schubotz & von Cramon, 2003). In terms of proposed lesion effects, medial premotor damage causes impairment of endogenously driven motor control, effecting a "release" of exogenously driven premotor system responses to perceived objects. The loss of internally driven and inhibitory control may underlie what patients describe as feeling compelled to use objects (i.e., utilization behavior). This refinement of frontal–parietal mechanisms opens up new ways for not only interrelating diverse motor release deficits and motor control mechanisms but also for considering the subcortical–cortical and cortico–cortical neural networks subserving self-regulation and how humans balance internally driven and externally activated motor behaviors in order to achieve goals (Eslinger, 2002).

In that context, it is interesting to note that in healthy individuals, the right frontopolar cortex is reliably activated when they watched actions for later imitation (Decety et al., 1997; Grèzes et al., 1998), but not when they observed these actions for later recognition. Furthermore, this prefrontal activation was detected only for those actions that were in the motor repertoire of the subjects (e.g., meaningful actions) but not for meaningless actions. Moreover, when meaningless actions were learned by the participants a few days before the positron emission tomography (PET) exam, and thus became familiar, the frontopolar cortex was then engaged during observation with the intent to imitate (Grèzes, Costes, & Decety, 1999). Consistent with this view, Brass, Zysset, and von Cramon (2001) carried out an fMRI study to investigate the cortical mechanisms underlying the inhibition of imitative responses. Their experiment employed a simple response task in which subjects were instructed to execute predefined finger movements (tapping or lifting of the index finger) in response to an observed congruent or incongruent finger movement (tapping or lifting). The comparison of the hemodynamic response during incongruent versus congruent trials revealed strong activation in the dorsolateral prefrontal cortex (middle frontal gyrus) and activation in the right frontopolar cortex. These results support the assumption of prefrontal involvement in response inhibition and extend this assumption to a "new" class of prepotent responses, namely, to imitative actions.

It is important to note that the prefrontal cortex, which appears to exert its functions mostly through inhibition, is not fully mature immediately after birth. While cytoarchitecture reaches full development before birth in human, the myelination of prefrontal connective fibers extends long after birth, until adolescence (Fuster, 1997). This lack of inhibition, or mild inhibition at the beginning of childhood, confers developmental benefits through imitation. Then, inhibitory mechanisms progressively develop, in parallel to cognitive abilities for which inhibition is a requisite. Without executive functions (including attention, self-regulation, and inhibition), one would be driven by impulsive acts or automatic responses to physiological needs or environmental stimuli.

RECIPROCAL IMITATION AND THE SENSE OF AGENCY

Imitation in human beings is not restricted to mimicry or learning new skills. We also recognize when others are imitating us. Reciprocal imitation is an essential part of communicative exchanges and plays an important role in developing shared feelings and shared motivational states with others (e.g., Hobson, 1989). Moreover, there is good evidence that reciprocal imitation plays a constitutive role in the early development of an implicit sense of self as a social agent (Rochat, 1999). The ability to recognize oneself as the agent of an action, thought, or desire (the sense of agency) is crucial for attributing a behavior to its proper agent and plays a pivotal role in the development of cognition. The distinction between self-generated actions and actions produced by others is a key function for self-recognition. Such tracking or monitoring mechanism is crucial in social interaction in general and in reciprocal imitation in particular.

A number of functional imaging studies have pointed out the involvement of the right inferior parietal lobule in the process of attribution of an action to its proper agent. Such a process has been associated with specific increased activity in the right inferior parietal lobe. For instance, Farrer and Frith (2002) instructed participants to use a joystick to drive a circle along a T-shaped path. They were told that the circle would be driven either by themselves or by the experimenter. In the former case subjects were requested to drive the circle, to be aware that they drove the circle, and thus to mentally attribute the action seen on the screen to themselves. In the latter case they were also requested to perform the task, but they were aware that action seen on the screen was driven by the experimenter. The results showed that being aware of causing an action was associated with activation in the anterior insula, whereas being aware of not causing the action and attributing it to another person was associated with activation in the right inferior parietal cortex.

One functional imaging study explored the extent to which being imitated and imitating the other relies on similar or distinct underlying neural mechanisms (e.g., Chaminade & Decety, 2002). In that study, participants were scanned while they imitated an experimenter performing constructions with small objects and while the experimenter imitated them (Decety, Chaminade, Grèzes, & Meltzoff, 2002). Results showed that a network of regions were commonly involved in the two reciprocal imitation conditions in comparison to a baseline condition (self-action). This network included the inferior frontal gyrus, left inferior parietal lobule, the superior frontal gyrus, the STS, the pre-SMA, and the right medial frontal cortex. In the condition in which participants imitated the other, increased activity was detected in the left inferior parietal cortex. This result is consistent with neuropsychological observations (e.g., Halsband et al., 2001), as well as functional imaging studies that have pointed out the systematic implication of the left parietal cortex in imitation (e.g., Chaminade, Meltzoff, & Decety, 2005; Makuuchi, in press; Tanaka & Inui, 2002; Williams et al., 2006). When participants' actions were imitated, additional activity was detected in the right inferior parietal cortex (see Plate 11.2).

The right inferior parietal lobule in reciprocal imitation can be explained with regard to its role in agency. Making agency judgments about who has performed an action is likely to be made on the basis of central representations coded in allocentric coordinates (Jeannerod, 1999). A common coding system of this kind is needed when being imitated by the other, because it is not possible to represent the actions of others in the egocentric coordinates used for generating our own actions. There is strong physiological evidence that the inferior parietal cortex implements this kind of remapping process that would be needed to generate representations of body movements in allocentric coordinates.

Interestingly, the mechanism that accounts for the correct attribution of actions and thoughts to their respective agents is also involved when one mentally simulates actions for oneself or for another individual. Ruby and Decety (2001) instructed participants to imagine actions either from the first-person perspective (self) or from the third-person perspective (other). First-person perspective was associated with specific increase in the left parietal lobule. By contrast, the third-person perspective resulted in activation in the right inferior parietal lobule.

Further evidence for the role of the right inferior parietal cortex in the sense of agency is provided by neuropsychological studies in humans. For instance, Blanke, Ortigue, Landis, and Seeck (2002) have shown that direct cortical stimulation of this region in neurological patients induced out-of-body experience (i.e., the experience of dissociation of self from the body). While the left parietal region is involved in somatic experience in relation to action, the right region seems to also be involved in somatic experience but related to awareness. It is also associated with body knowledge and self-awareness, and its lesion can produce a variety of body representation-related disorders such as anosognosia, asomatognosia, or somatoparaphrenia (Berlucchi & Aglioti, 1997).

CONCLUSION

Taken together, the neurophysiological data reviewed in this chapter suggest that the basic circuit underlying imitation coincides with that which is active during action observation. This direct mapping of the observed action and its motor representation is mediated in the premotor cortex and the posterior parietal cortex. Such a mechanism (when not inhibited) is sufficient to explain motor mimicry and social facilitation. A similar mechanism is involved in emotion contagion, which is considered as an important precursor to the development of empathy. Thus, this basic mechanism accounts for continuity between all sorts of imitation. However, additional cognitive and neural mechanisms are required to fully account for human imitative capabilities, which extend beyond a simple motor resonance between self and other. For instance, the right inferior parietal cortex, in conjunction with the prefrontal cortex, play a critical role in the sense of agency and self–other correspondence. This is very important given the link between imitation, theory of mind ability, and empathy (see Rogers, 1999). The fact that children represent the behavior of others in a psychological framework involving goals and intended acts, instead of purely physical movements or motions, and that they are capable of rational imitation, constitutes compelling demonstrations for such a functional link. Hence, some complex forms of imitation are also dependent on the attribution of intentions for which the medial prefrontal cortex and posterior temporal cortex (at the junction with the parietal cortex) are essential. Such a view is consistent with the idea that imitation is a precursor to full theory of mind, but the two capacities are not totally overlapping (Meltzoff & Decety, 2003; Rogers & Pennington, 1991; Williams, Whiten, Suddendorf, & Perrett, 2001) and may thus be implemented by different systems.

Future research is needed to elucidate the functional relation between the mirror system, executive functions, and mentalizing process and how they can be fragmented into subcomponents with their respective neural implementation (see Table 11.2 on page 263).

In addition, the identification of a network of brain regions involved in imitation does not fully inform us which areas (or nodes) are critical for the imitation function. Neuroimaging findings must therefore be complemented by lesion studies in neurological patients to better understand the computational role of each area within the network. Finally, functional neuroimaging studies with people who are impaired in imitation, such as those affected by autistic spectrum disorders are also desirable to cast some light on the neural and cognitive mechanisms that subserve imitation (see Williams & Waiter, Chapter 15, this volume).

REFERENCES

Adolphs, R. (2002). Recognizing emotion from facial expressions: Psychological and neurological mechanisms. *Behavioral and Cognitive Neuroscience Reviews, 1*, 21–62.

Bekkering, H., Wohlschläger, A., & Gattis, M. (2000). Imitation of gestures in children is goal-directed. *Quarterly Journal of Experimental Psychology, 53*, 153–164.

Berlucchi, G., & Aglioti, S. (1997) The body in the brain: Neural bases of corporeal awareness. *Trends in Neuroscience, 20*, 560–564.

Blakemore, S. J., & Decety, J. (2001). From the perception of action to the understanding of intention. *Nature Reviews Neuroscience, 2*, 561–567.

Blakemore, S. J., Frith, C. D., & Wolpert, D. M. (1999). Spatiotemporal prediction modulates the perception of self-produced stimuli. *Journal of Cognitive Neuroscience, 11*, 551–559.

Blanke, O., Ortigue, S., Landis, T., & Seeck, M. (2002). Stimulating illusory own-body perceptions: The part of the brain that can induce out-of-body experiences has been located. *Nature, 419*, 269.

Brass, M., Bekkering, H., Wohlschläger, A., & Prinz, W. (2000). Compatibility between observed and executed finger movements: Comparing symbolic, spatial, and imitative cues. *Brain and Cognition, 44*, 124–143.

Brass, M., Zysset, S., & von Cramon, Y. (2001). The inhibition of imitative response tendencies. *NeuroImage, 14*, 1416–1423.

Buccino, G., Binkofski, F., Fink, G. R., Fadiga, L., Fogassi, L., Gallese, V., et al. (2001). Action observation activates premotor and parietal areas in a somatotopic manner: An fMRI study. *European Journal of Neuroscience, 13*, 400–404.

Buccino, G., Vogt, S., Ritzi, A., Fink, G. R., Zilles, K., Freund, H. J., & Rizzolatti, G. (2004). Neural circuits underlying imitation learning of hand actions: An event-related fMRI study. *Neuron, 42*, 323–334.

Butterworth, G. E. (1993). Dynamic approaches to infant perception and action. In L. B. Smith & E. Thelen (Eds.), *A dynamic systems approach to development: Applications* (pp. 171–187). Cambridge, MA: MIT Press.

Byrne, R. W., & Russon, A. E. (1998). Learning by imitation: A hierarchical approach. *Behavioral and Brain Sciences, 21*, 667–709.

Cacioppo, J. T., Berntson, G. G., Lorig, T. S., Norris, C. J., Rickett, E., & Nusbaum, H. (2003). Just because you're imaging the brain doesn't mean you can stop using your head: A primer set of first principles. *Journal of Personality and Social Psychology, 85*, 650–661.

Carr, L., Iacoboni, M., Dubeau, M. C., Mazziotta, J. C., & Lenzi, G. L. (2003). Neural mechanisms of empathy in humans: A relay from neural systems for imitation to limbic areas. *Proceedings of National Academy of Sciences USA, 100*, 5497–5502.

Castiello, U. (2003). Understanding others' people actions: Intention and attention. *Journal of Experimental Psychology: Human Perception and Performance, 29*, 416–430.

Castiello, U., Lusher, D., Mari, M., Edwards, M., & Humphreys, G.W. (2002). Observing a human or a robotic hand grasping an object: Differential motor priming effects. In W. Prinz & B. Hommel (Eds.), *Common mechanisms in perception and action* (pp. 315–333). New York: Oxford University Press.

Chaminade, T., & Decety, J. (2002). Leader or follower?: Involvement of the inferior parietal lobule in agency. *Neuroreport, 13*, 3669–3674.

Chaminade, T., Meltzoff, A. N., & Decety, J. (2002). Does the end justify the means? A PET exploration of the mechanisms involved in human imitation. *NeuroImage, 12*, 318–328.

Chaminade, T., Meltzoff, A. N., & Decety, J. (2005). An fMRI study of imitation: Action representation and body schema. *Neuropsychologia, 43*, 115–127.

Chartrand, T. L., & Bargh, J. A. (1999). The chameleon effect: The perception–behavior link and social interaction. *Journal of Personality and Social Psychology, 71*, 464–478.

Clark, A. (2001). *Being there*. Cambridge, MA: MIT Press.

Clark, S., Tremblay, F., & St.-Marie, D. (2003). Differential modulation of the corticospinal excitability during observation, mental imagery and imitation of hand actions. *Neuropsychologia, 42*, 105–112.

Decety, J., Chaminade, T., Grèzes, J., & Meltzoff, A. N. (2002). A PET exploration of the neural mechanisms involved in reciprocal imitation. *NeuroImage, 15*, 265–272.

Decety, J., Grèzes, J., Costes, N., Perani, D., Jeannerod, M., Procyk, E., et al. (1997). Brain activity during observation of action. Influence of action content and subject's strategy. *Brain, 120*, 1763–1777.

Decety, J., & Jackson, P. L. (2004). The functional architecture of human empathy. *Behavioral and Cognitive Neuroscience Reviews, 3*(2), 71–100.

Decety, J., & Sommerville, J. A. (2003). Shared representations between self and others: A social cognitive neuroscience view. *Trends in Cognitive Science, 7*, 527–533.

Ekman, P., & Davidson, R. J. (1993). Voluntary smiling changes regional brain activity. *Psychological Science, 4*, 342–345.

Eslinger, P. J. (2002). The anatomic basis of utilization behavior: A shift from frontal-parietal to intra-frontal mechanisms. *Cortex, 38*, 273–276.

Fadiga, L., Craighero, L., Buccino, G., & Rizzolatti, G. (2002). Speech listening specifically modulates the excitability of tongue muscles: A TMS study. *European Journal of Neuroscience, 15*, 399–402.

Farrer, C., & Frith, C. D. (2002). Experiencing oneself vs. another person as being the cause of an action: The neural correlates of the experience of agency. *NeuroImage, 15*, 596–603.

Flanagan, J. R., & Johansson, R. S. (2003). Actions plans used in action observation. *Nature, 424,* 769–771.

Frith, U., & Frith, C. D. (2003). Development and neurophysiology of mentalizing. In, C. D. Frith & D. Wolpert (Eds.), *The neuroscience of social interaction* (pp. 45–75). New York: Oxford University Press.

Fuster, J. M. (1997). *The prefrontal cortex.* Philadelphia: Lippincott, Raven.

Gallese, V., Fogassi, L., Fadiga, L., & Rizzolatti, G. (2002). Action representation and the inferior parietal lobule. In W. Prinz & B. Hommel (Eds.), *Attention and performance* (Vol. 19, pp. 247–266). New York: Oxford University Press.

Gibson, J. J. (1966). *The senses considered as perceptual systems.* Boston: Houghton-Mifflin.

Grèzes, J., Costes, N., & Decety, J. (1998). Top-down effect of the perception of human biological motion: A PET investigation. *Cognitive Neuropsychiatry, 15,* 553–582.

Grèzes, J., Costes, N., & Decety, J. (1999). The effect of learning on the neural networks engaged by the perception of meaningless actions. *Brain, 122,* 1875–1887.

Halsband, U., Schmitt, J., Weyers, M., Binkofski, F., Grutzner, G., & Freund, H. J. (2001). Recognition and imitation of pantomimed motor acts after unilateral parietal and premotor lesions: A perspective on apraxia. *Neuropsychologia, 39,* 200–216.

Hatfield, E., Caccioppo, J. T., & Rapson, R. L. (1994). *Emotional contagion.* Cambridge, UK: Cambridge University Press.

Heyes, C. (2001). Causes and consequences of imitation. *Trends in Cognitive Sciences, 5,* 253–261.

Hobson, R. P. (1989). On sharing experiences. *Development and Psychopathology, 1,* 197–203.

Iacoboni, M., Koski, L., Brass, M., Bekkering, H., Woods, R. P., Dubeau, M. C., et al. (2001). Reafferent copies of imitated action in the right superior temporal cortex. *Proceedings of the National Academy of Sciences USA, 98,* 13995–13999.

Iacoboni, M., Woods, R. P., Brass, M., Bekkering, H., Mazziotta, J. C., & Rizzolatti, G. (1999). Cortical mechanisms of human imitation. *Science, 286,* 2526–2528.

Jeannerod, M. (1994). The representing brain. Neural correlates of motor intention and imagery. *Behavioral and Brain Sciences, 17,* 187–245.

Jeannerod, M. (1999). To act or not to act: Perspectives on the representation of actions. *Quarterly Journal of Experimental Psychology, 52A, 1–29.*

Kilner, J. M., Paulignan, Y., & Blakemore, S. J. (2003). An interference effect of observed biological movement on action. *Current Biology, 13,* 522–525.

Knoblich, G., & Flach, R. (2003). Action identity: Evidence from self-recognition, prediction, and coordination. *Consciousness and Cognition, 12,* 620–632.

Kohler, E., Keysers, C., Umilta, M. A., Fogassi, L., Gallese, V., & Rizzolatti, G. (2002). Hearing sounds, understanding actions: Action representation in mirror neurons. *Science, 297,* 846–848.

Legerstee, M. (1991). The role of person and object in eliciting early imitation. *Journal of Experimental Child Psychology, 51,* 423–433.

Leslie, K. R., Johnson-Frey, S. H., & Grafton, S. T. (2004). Functional imaging of face and hand imitation: Towards a motor theory of empathy. *NeuroImage, 21,* 601–607.

Levenson, R. W., Ekman, P., & Friesen, W. V. (1990). Voluntary facial action generates emotion-specific autonomic nervous system activity. *Psychophysiology, 27,* 363–384.

Lhermitte, F., Pillon, B., & Serdaru, M. (1986). Human autonomy and the frontal lobes. Part I: Imitation and utilization behavior: A neuropsychological study of 75 patients. *Annals of Neurology, 19,* 326–34.

Makuuchi, M. (2005). Is Broca's area crucial for imitation. *Cerebral Cortex, 15,* 563–570.

Matsumoto, K., & Tanaka, K. (2004). The role of the medial prefrontal cortex in achieving goals. *Current Opinion in Neurobiology, 14,* 1–8.

Meltzoff, A. N., & Decety, J. (2003). What imitation tells us about social cognition: A rapprochement between developmental psychology and cognitive neuroscience. *Philosophical Transactions of the Royal Society of London, B, Biological Sciences, 358,* 491–500.

Meltzoff, A. N., & Gopnik, A. (1993). The role of imitation in understanding persons and developing a theory of mind. In S. Baron-Cohen, H. Tager-Flusberg, & D. J. Cohen (Eds.), *Understanding other minds: Perspective from autism* (pp. 335–366). Oxford, UK: Oxford University Press.

Meltzoff, A. N., & Moore, M. K. (1977). Imitation of facial and manual gestures by human neonates. *Science, 198,* 75–78.

Meltzoff, A. N., & Moore, M. K. (1997). Explaining facial imitation: A theoretical model. *Early Development and Parenting, 6,* 179–192.

Mitchell, R. W. (1993). Mental models of mirror-self recognition: Two theories. *New Ideas in Psychology, 11,* 295–325.

Nadel, J., Guérini, C., Pezé, A., & Rivet, C. (1999). The evolving nature of imitation as a format for communication. In J. Nadel & G. Butterworth (Eds.), *Imitation in infancy* (pp. 209–234). Cambridge, UK: Cambridge University Press.

Nishitani, N., & Hari, R. (2000). Temporal dynamics of cortical representation for action. *Proceedings of the National Academy of Sciences USA, 97,* 913–18.

Nishitani, N., & Hari, R. (2002). Viewing lip forms: Cortical dynamics. *Neuron, 36,* 1211–1220.

Perani, D., Fazio, F., Borghese, N. A., Tettamanti, M., Ferrari, S., Decety, J., & Gilardi, M. C. (2001). Different brain correlates for watching real and virtual hand actions. *NeuroImage, 14,* 749–758.

Perrett, D. I., Harries, M. H., Bevan, R., Thomas, S., Benson, P. J., Mistlin, A. J., et al. (1989). Frameworks of analysis for the neural representation of animate objects and action. *Journal of Experimental Biology, 146,* 87–114.

Perrett, D. I., Mistlin, A. J., Harries, M. H., & Chitty, A. J. (1990). Understanding the visual appearance and consequences of hand actions. In M. A. Goodale (Ed.), *Vision and action: The control of grasping* (pp. 163–180). Norwood, NJ: Ablex.

Phillips, M. L., Young, A. W., Senior, C., Brammer, M., Andrew, C., Calder, A. J., et al. (1997). A specific neural substrate for perceiving facial expressions of disgust. *Nature, 389,* 495–498.

Prinz, W. (1997). Perception and action planning. *European Journal of Cognitive Psychology, 9,* 129–154.

Raos, V., Evangeliou, M. N., & Savaki, H. E. (2004). Observation of action: Grasping with the mind's hand. *NeuroImage, 23,* 193–201.

Rizzolatti, G., & Craighero, L. (2004). The mirror-neuron system. *Annual Review of Neuroscience, 27,* 169–192.

Rizzolatti, G., Fadiga, L., Gallese, V., & Fogassi, L. (1996). Premotor cortex and the recognition of motor actions. *Brain Research: Cognitive Brain Research, 3,* 131–141.

Rizzolatti, G., Fogassi, L., & Gallese, V. (2001). Neurophysiological mechanisms underlying the understanding and imitation of action. *Nature Reviews Neuroscience, 2,* 661–670.

Rochat, P. (1999). *Early social cognition: Understanding others in the first months of life.* Mahawah, NJ: Erlbaum.

Rogers, S. J. (1999). An examination of the imitation deficit in autism. In J. Nadel & G. Butterworth (Eds.), *Imitation in infancy* (pp. 254–283). Cambridge, UK: Cambridge University Press.

Rogers, S. J., & Pennington, B. F. (1991). A theoretical approach to the deficits in infantile autism. *Development and Psychopathology, 3,* 137–162.

Saxe, R., Xiao, D. K., Kovacsc, G., Perrett, D. I., & Kanwisher, N. (2004). A region of right posterior superior temporal sulcus responds to observed intentional actions. *Neuropsychologia, 42*, 1435–1446.

Schubotz, R. I., & von Cramon, Y. (2000). Time perception and motor timing: a common cortical and subcortical basis revealed by fMRI. *NeuroImage, 11*, 1–12.

Schubotz, R. I., & von Cramon, Y. (2001). Functional organization of the lateral premotor cortex: fMRI reveals different regions activated by anticipation of objects properties, location and speed. *Cognitive Brain Research, 11*, 97–112.

Schubotz, R. I., & von Cramon, Y. (2003). Functional-anatomical concepts for human premotor cortex: evidence from fMRI and PET studies. *NeuroImage, 20*, S120–S131.

Sebanz, N., Knoblich, G., & Prinz, W. (2003). Representing others' actions: Just like one's own? *Cognition, 88*, B11–B21.

Shepard, R. N. (1984). Ecological constraints on internal representation: Resonant kinematics of perceiving, imagining, thinking, and dreaming. *Psychological Review, 91*, 417–447.

Shiffrar, M., & Freyd, J. J. (1990). Apparent motion of the human body. *Psychological Science, 1*, 257–264.

Sperry, R. W. (1952). Neurology and the mind–body problem. *American Scientist, 40*, 291–312.

Stevens, J. A., Fonlupt, P., Shiffrar, M. A., & Decety, J. (2000). New aspects of motion perception: Selective neural encoding of apparent human movements. *Neuroreport, 11*, 109–115.

Sturmer, B., Ascherleben, G., & Prinz, W. (2000). Correspondence effects with manual gestures and postures: A study of imitation. *Journal of Experimental Psychology Human Perception and Performance, 26*, 1746–1759.

Tai, Y. F., Scherfler, C., Brooks, D. J., Sawamoto, N., & Castiello, U. (2003). The human premotor cortex is mirror only for biological actions. *Current Biology, 14*, 117–120.

Tanaka, S., & Inui, T. (2002). Cortical involvement for action imitation of hand/arm postures versus finger configurations: An fMRI study. *Neuroreport, 13*, 1599–1560.

Trevarthen, C. (1979). Communication and cooperation in early infancy. In M. Bullowa (Ed.), *Before speech: The beginning of human communication* (pp. 321–347). London: Cambridge University Press.

Umilta, M. A., Kohler, E., Gallese, V., Fogassi, L., Fadiga, L., Keysers, C., & Rizzolatti, G. (2001). I know what your are doing: A neurophysiological study. *Neuron, 32*, 91–101.

Wallbott, H. G. (1991). Recognition of emotion from facial expression via imitation? Some indirect evidence for an old theory. *British Journal Social Psychology, 30*, 207–219.

Watkins, K. E., Strafella, A. P., & Paus, T. (2003). Seeing and hearing speech excites the motor system involved in speech production. *Neuropsychologia, 41*, 989–994.

Wicker, B., Keysers, C., Plailly, J., Royet, J. P., Gallese, V., & Rizzolatti, G. (2003). Both of us disgusted in my insula: The common neural basis of seeing and feeling disgust. *Neuron, 40*, 655–664.

Williams, J. H. G., Waiter, G. D., Gilchrist, A., Perrett, D. I., Murray, A. D., & Whiten, A. (2006). Neural mechanisms of imitation and "mirror neuron" functioning in autistic spectrum disorder. *Neuropsychologia, 44*, 610–621.

Williams, J. H. G., Whiten, A., Suddendorf, T., & Perrett, D. I. (2001). Imitation, mirror neurons and autism. *Neuroscience and Behavioral Reviews, 25*, 287–295.

Wolpert, D. M., Miall, R. C., & Kawato, M. (1998). Internal models in the cerebellum. *Trends in Cognitive Sciences, 2*, 338–347.

Zhang, J. X., Feng, C. M., Fox, P. T., Gao, J. H., & Tan, L. H. (2004). Is left inferior frontal gyrus a general mechanism for selection? *NeuroImage, 23*, 281–287.

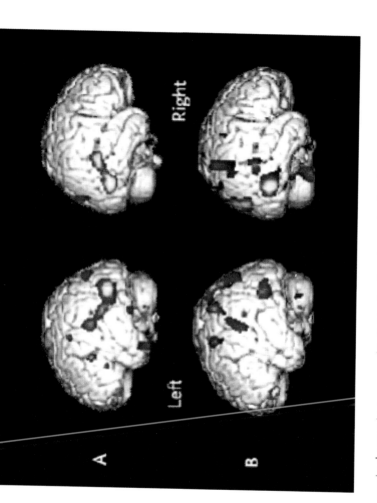

Left   Right

A

B

PLATE 11.1. Neurohemodynamic changes in a group of individuals who observed videoclips depicting meaningful right upper limb pantomimes executed by a human model with no specific task (A), and during the observation of similar stimuli with the intention to imitate them at the end of the scanning session (B). These two conditions are contrasted with the observation of static hand postures. Regions in which significant activation occurred during the perception of actions (Condition A) include the premotor cortex, Broca's area, STS, and left parietal cortex. The intention to imitate (Condition B) is associated with increase of hemodynamic activity in the supplementary motor area, the right premotor, and right parietal cortex. From Grèzes, Costes, and Decety (1998). Copyright 1998 by Psychology Press. Adapted by permission.

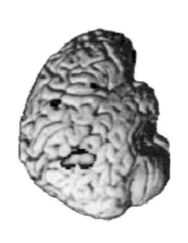

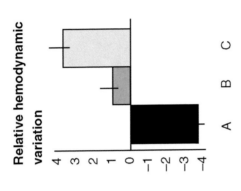

Relative hemodynamic variation

A B C

PLATE 11.2. Right inferior parietal lobule activation at the junction of the temporal cortex superimposed on a rendered MRI. In this study, participants were scanned during a variety of object-directed actions with small objects, including self-action (A), imitation of actions performed by an experimenter (B), and observation of their actions being imitated by the experimenter (C). Note the dramatic increase in this region in this latter condition. This region plays a pivotal role in the sense of agency. From Decety, Chaminade, Grèzes, and Meltzoff (2002). Copyright 2002 by Academic Press. Adapted by permission.

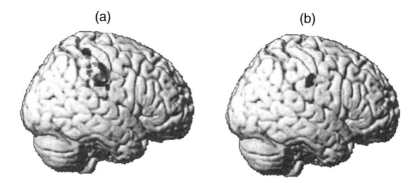

PLATE 15.1. Imitation versus [average of spatial cue execution + symbolic cue execution] masked to include frontal and parietal regions only. Random-effects analysis, threshold at $p < .001$ uncorrected. (a) Controls; (b) group with ASD.

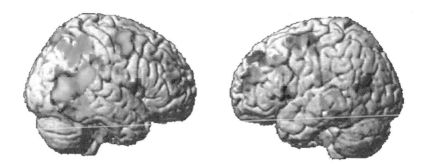

PLATE 15.2. Results of the two main contrasts rendered onto a single, semi-transparent, standard three-dimensional structural MRI image. Activation related to joint attention versus rest is in red; that due to non-joint attention versus rest is in green. Overlap is in yellow. Threshold at $p < .001$ uncorrected.

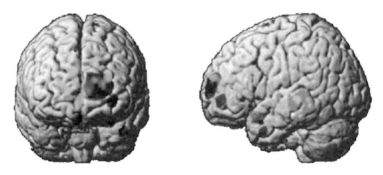

PLATE 15.3. Results of two separate studies rendered onto a single three-dimensional standard structural MRI image. Areas where activation during joint attention is greater than during non-joint attention in this study are in green. Areas involving a separate group of individuals from Waiter et al. (2004), where gray matter volume in ASD was increased relative to controls, are in red. Areas of overlap are yellow.

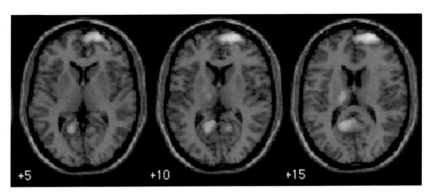

PLATE 15.4. Sagittal sections of the brain showing areas of gray matter increase in ventral temporal cortex, left superior frontal gyrus, and right temporoparietal regions particularly. The blue area shows decrease in thalamic gray matter volume. The left side of the figure represents the right side of the brain.

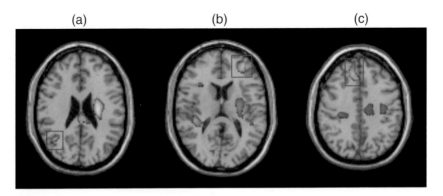

PLATE 15.5. Sagittal sections of the brain showing reduced white matter volume in ASD compared to controls. (a) Left middle temporal; (b) right middle frontal; (c) left superior frontal regions. The left side of the figure represents the left side of the brain.

PART III

IMITATION IN AUTISM AND OTHER CLINICAL GROUPS
Biobehavioral Findings and Clinical Implications

CHAPTER 12

Imitation in Autism
Findings and Controversies

SALLY J. ROGERS
JUSTIN H. G. WILLIAMS

The lack of natural, spontaneous imitative and interpersonally coordinated movements one observes when interacting with people with autism is striking. Yet, this aspect of autism is often camouflaged by the overall lack of social and emotional reciprocity and interpersonal engagement that is fundamental to autism. To what extent these two areas of difficulty may be related is a question that has barely been addressed in autism research to date.

The possibility that primary problems in imitating others could be a significant contributor to the social and learning deficits in autism was first suggested over 25 years ago, by Marian DeMyer (DeMyer et al., 1972) in the first comparative study of imitation in autism. Accumulating evidence of imitative deficits in autism was documented in an important research review (Prior, 1979) but ignored in cognitive theories of autism through the next decade. The lack of attention to imitation in the autism world is somewhat surprising, given the emphasis that major figures in psychology had placed on the roles of imitation, both immediate and deferred, in child development, among them Piaget (1962), Baldwin (1906), Skinner (1957), and Bandura (Bandura, Ross, & Ross, 1963). The landmark early imitation studies of Meltzoff and colleagues (Meltzoff & Moore, 1977, 1989) during the late 1970s and 1980s might have stimulated interest in imitation as a contender in the search for primary neuropsychological deficits in autism. However, the reorientation of autism theorists to the social aspects of autism (Fein, Pennington, Markowitz, Braverman, & Waterhouse, 1986) and the exciting new findings of Baron-Cohen, Frith, and colleagues (Baron-Cohen, Leslie, & Frith, 1985) focused attention on theory of mind and related, more mature capacities as a primary explanation for the cognitive aspects of autism.

However, at the same time, papers began to appear that documented autism-specific developmental abnormalities in social cognitive skills that developed years before theory of mind. This pioneering work, led by Marian Sigman and a succession of graduate students and postdoctoral fellows, including Judy Ungerer, Peter Mundy, Connie Kasari, and Nurit Yirmiya, documented autism-related abnormalities in joint attention behavior, dyadic emotional responsivity, imitation, and symbolic play in preschool children (Kasari, Sigman, Mundy, & Yirmiya, 1990; Mundy, Sigman, Ungerer, & Sherman, 1987; Sigman & Ungerer, 1984; Ungerer & Sigman, 1987; Yirmiya, Kasari, Sigman, & Mundy, 1989). This work helped refocus the field to look for markers of autism that developed much earlier than theory of other minds.

In 1991, Rogers and Pennington suggested a developmental model of autism in which early cascading social–communicative impairments might stem from early deficits in motor imitation, affecting emotional mirroring and sharing and impeding growing awareness of the other as a subjective psyche. Such a cascade, they suggested, would severely affect the development of joint attention, verbal and nonverbal communication, and symbolic play. Furthermore, they suggested a brain–behavior link, hypothesizing that prefrontal cortex might play an important role in performance of motor imitation, and in autism-related difficulties, both in intentional imitation and in other executive acts.

Arguments for considering imitation as one possible primary deficit in autism must address four issues both in the theories and in empirical studies. First, if imitation is a building block of typical social development and a primary influence in autism symptoms, there should be supportive evidence of these interrelationships across time and across developmental acquisitions, in both typical development and autism. Second, studies of behavioral differences in autism need to consider the many levels or relations between a behavioral act and a neurobiological starting state difference. Third, imitation is not one behavior. Rather, there are a variety of different behaviors or skills that may be involved, as described in a taxonomy of matching behaviors developed by comparative psychologists that needs to infiltrate autism imitation research (Want & Harris, 2002). Finally, imitative deficits documented in lab studies need to be reconciled with imitative phenomena such as echolalia and imitative acts reported by parents and observed by clinicians. Understanding imitative performance in autism will require that we can explain the general imitative deficit while accounting for imitative performances.

To address these topics, we (1) review the evidence for a central imitation deficit in autism, (2) review existing theories that seek to explain the imitation problems and their supportive evidence, (3) integrate autism findings into comparative psychology's taxonomy of "imitative" behaviors, (4) examine evidence of brain–behavior relations regarding imitation in autism, and (5) direct attention to questions that need additional research.

FINDINGS FROM CONTROLLED STUDIES OF IMITATION IN AUTISM

We draw from the most recent and comprehensive review of imitation research in autism covering literature to 2002 (Williams, Whiten, & Singh, 2004), as well as the most recent findings from the empirical literature. The Williams and colleagues (2004) article provided the field with an exhaustive review that identified 124 articles concerning autism and imitation and reviewed in depth 21 controlled studies of hand or body movement imitations in autism that had been published up to March 2002. The review paper first considered the overriding question, "Is there an imitative deficit in autism?" Of the 21 studies, two found no group differences in an adequately designed study. Two more that reported no group differences were confounded by ceiling effects. Three studies did not report the statistical tests necessary for answering this question. The remaining 14 studies reported an autism-specific deficit, generally at very high levels of significance even though the groups were small. Thus, 14 of 16 methodologically adequate studies have reported an autism-specific deficit in imitation of body or hand movements. Furthermore, Williams and colleagues pooled the findings from these studies involving 281 subjects with autism spectrum disorders, using the Logit method, resulting in a combined p value of $p = .00005$ ($n = 248$ subjects, $t = -4.260$, 89 df).

Next, the authors considered whether the imitative deficit might be due to a secondary cause. They examined studies in which comparison groups had other clinical conditions, including undifferentiated mental retardation, Down syndrome, language impairment, and developmental dyspraxia. Each of these studies found significantly greater impairment in the group with autism than in the other clinical group. The authors concluded that there was widespread evidence of a specific impairment in imitation in autism.

Studies That Have Occurred Since 2002

Eight controlled studies of imitative performance, not previously reviewed and published since the Williams and colleagues (2004) review, are briefly reviewed here.

Bernabei, Penton, Fabrizi, Camaioni, and Perucchini (2003) compared a large group of 46 preschoolers with autism and very severe intellectual impairments to 45 age-mates with similar intellectual impairments on the Užgiris–Hunt scales (Užgiris & Hunt, 1975). The children with autism were significantly more mature than comparisons on the four object-oriented scales: object permanence, means–end, causality, and spatial relations. Intragroup examination of scores revealed an autism-specific deficit in the imitation subscales compared to the object-oriented subscales. The group with intellectual disability showed similar level of performance on all the scales (with lower performance on vocal imitation) and strong intercorrelations across the areas. In contrast, the group with autism demonstrated a statistically significant weakness in imitation (with equivalent performance on gestural and verbal imitation) compared to their other scores. Furthermore, in the autism group, vocal imitation did not correlate with any other performance. Thus, the group with autism showed a relative weakness in imitation and a lack of overall integration of skills across the object and social (imitative) domains compared to the contrast group.

Ingersoll, Schreibman, and Tran (2003) examined the performance of 15 young children with autism, ages 23–53 months, and 14 typical toddlers, ages 16–32 months. This study examined imitative performance under varying object conditions. Three pairs of novel simple objects were carefully constructed. Each afforded a simple and familiar sensorimotor action, with half the objects provided visual and auditory sensory stimuli when the children carried out the action in imitation of the adult. Between-group performance did not differ significantly in either condition on these simple actions, though ceiling effects and very familiar acts may have masked underlying imitative differences. However, unlike the comparison group, children with autism showed a significant deficit in their imitative performance in the nonsensory feedback condition compared to the sensory condition. The authors interpreted the findings as demonstrating that imitating other people is intrinsically motivating to children who do not have autism but is less so for children with autism.

Avikainen, Wohlschlager, and Hari (2003) compared the performance of eight adults with Asperger syndrome or high-functioning autism and typical IQ with eight typically functioning adults on a simple object imitation task. In the task, the subject sat across from the experimenter. In front of each adult were two cups of different colors, with a magic marker between the cups. The model picked up the marker with one of two grip patterns (ulnar or radial) and inserted it into one of the two cups. The subject was told to either imitate the model as if the model was a mirror image or to imitate the model with the same-sided hand, which necessitated crossing the body to carry out the task. The typical group demonstrated an advantage in the mirroring condition as seen in fewer errors in all three target behaviors (hand, cup, grip) across the 80 trials. However, the group with autism showed no such advantage and differed from the typical group only in this condition, particularly in errors made involving hand choice or grip position. Given the very small group sizes and the huge error rates from these high-functioning adults (15–20%) on hand choice and cup choice, a replication with a larger sample will be extremely helpful for interpreting these findings.

Meyer and Hobson (2004) examined a particular aspect of imitation: self–other orientation (identification) in a study of 16 older children with autism and moderate mental retardation, and 16 comparison children matched on age and IQ. There were four object-oriented tasks like rolling a wheel and stacking objects. A line in front of the child and in front of the experimenter, who sat on the floor facing the child, marked each person's "personal space." Each task was demonstrated once in the child's "space" and again in the adult's "space." After each model, the child was given the toy and encouraged to imitate. The children with autism made significantly fewer responses that modeled the self–other orientation to the object than did the comparison subjects. The patterns of relationships across groups also differed, with the delayed children demonstrating significant correlations between IQ and placement patterns that were absent in autism. This finding is consistent with data from several other studies demonstrating an autism-specific difficulty in correctly imitating the orientation of an action in relation to the model's body (e.g., Avikainen et al., 2003; Ohta, 1987; Smith & Bryson, 1998). Meyer and Hobson (2004) interpret this as a failure of identification and draw parallels between performance on this task and ability to understand others' perspectives and to mentally shift from one perspective to another. These authors are drawing attention to and replicating a very interesting phenomenon in autism imitation that needs to be studied and explained.

Rogers, Hepburn, and Stackhouse (2003) examined the performance of 24 2-year-olds with autism, compared to well-matched samples of children with fragile X ($n = 18$), other delays ($n = 20$) and typical development ($n = 15$) on three types of imitative tasks: gestural, oral–facial, and novel object imitations. The study was designed to examine (1) profiles of imitative performance across groups and (2) relations between imitative performance, other aspects of the autism phenotype, and tasks of skilled motor planning and execution. Significant relationships were found across the three types of imitation tasks, indicating a general imitative skill underlying all tasks. Children with autism showed a deficit in imitation in relation to both comparison groups, with the most deficient performances on the oral–facial and, surprisingly, the object-oriented tasks and their imitative performance correlated strongly with severity of autism symptoms. There was also a significant relation with initiation of joint attention behavior, and with language development. However, contrary to hypotheses, there was no autism-specific deficit on the motor planning/execution tasks, nor did performance on those tasks relate to imitative performance for the children with autism. Interestingly, the imitative performance of children with fragile X syndrome was strongly related to the presence and severity of their autism symptoms.

Bennetto (1999) examined five components of imitation in high-functioning children with autism ($n = 19$), compared to children with developmental dyslexia ($n = 19$) matched on age and verbal IQ. Specific tasks and within-subject experiments assessed basic motor functioning, body schema, dynamic spatiotemporal representation, memory, and motor execution of nonmeaningful hand and arm gestures. Consistent with previous research, participants with autism demonstrated overall worse imitation skill. Further analyses revealed a specific pattern of impairment characterized by difficulty with the kinesthetic aspects of postures and movements, particularly during complex sequences. Participants with autism also demonstrated impairments in basic motor skills, which appeared to account for some, but not all of their imitation deficits. Participants with autism did not differ from comparison participants on body schema, spatiotemporal representation, or memory, suggesting that their imitation deficits were not secondary to problems in these areas.

McIntosh, Reichmann-Decker, Winkielman, and Wilbarger (in press) reported a psychophysiological study of automatic facial imitation, or mimicry, carried out with 14 high-functioning adolescents or adults with autism spectrum disorders and 14 typically developing age- and vocabulary-matched comparison subjects. Subjects viewed photos of eight happy and eight angry photos in two conditions: observation only and intentional imitation. Electromyographic recordings from brow and check muscles revealed an autism-specific impairment in specificity of the automatically mimicked emotion but no group difference in the intentional condition (though the response measured was muscle activation, not accuracy of imitation or normalcy of the expression).

Finally, Scambler and colleagues (in press) reported a study of automatic facial imitation involving affective expressions in 26 2-year-olds with autism, 24 children with other delays, and 15 children with typical development to four different emotional expressions of adults occurring in naturalistic displays (fear, joy, disgust, and distress). Microanalytic scoring techniques were used to rate intensity, hedonic tone, and latency of child response. Children with autism demonstrated fewer episodes of matching responses than did the comparison groups, and when there were matching responses, the intensity of their emotional expressions were much less intense, or more muted, than the two comparison groups.

Thus, consistent with a large number of previously reviewed studies, eight recent controlled studies of imitation demonstrate autism-specific difficulties in subject groups ranging from toddlers and severely disabled preschool children to adults with Asperger syndrome. The evidence continues to support the existence of a central deficit in motor imitation in autism. In addition to impairments in intentional imitations, we have two reports of impairments in automatic imitative responses as well. However, describing a problem does not explain it. What accounts for the imitative problems in autism? We next consider the major theories accounting for the imitative deficit in autism, and the existing support for those theories. We begin by briefly mentioning theories that have been suggested in the past but can be rejected based on the current body of evidence.

EXPLANATORY THEORIES OF IMITATION PROBLEMS IN AUTISM

Explanations for the imitation deficits in autism fall into five main areas: problems in representing the target action, problems executing the target action, problems with attention to the target action, problems with cross-modal integration of perceptual information, and problems with the motivation for producing the target action. We review each in turn here.

Impairments in Representation of the Target Act

The well-known difficulties that children with autism display in symbolic play and in language development have led many to hypothesize autism-specific problems in forming and manipulating representations. Several different kinds of representational problems have been suggested to underlie imitation difficulties, including problems with the symbolic nature of some of the tasks, problems representing the motor movements involved, problems representing one's body, and problems in coordinating representations between self and other. Each of these is discussed in turn.

Symbolic Representations

Earlier theories of imitation problems in autism focused on the more symbolic aspects of representations and the links between pantomime, imitation, and symbolic play (Curcio, 1978). Linking these skills together is supported both by cognitive theories of child development and by clinical studies of patients with apraxia (Heilman, 1979). However, several studies specifically tested this hypothesis and found no supportive evidence. As reviewed in Williams and colleagues (2004), two groups found that symbolic content improved the imitative performance of children with autism (Rogers, Bennetto, McEvoy, & Pennington, 1996; Stone, Ousley, & Littleford, 1997) and others have found no impairment related to symbolic representation (Smith & Bryson, 1998). Thus, no support has been found for a symbolic representation as the source of the imitative deficit.

Motor Representations

Another aspect of representation that might be involved, however, involves motor representational capacity. Three studies have specifically examined whether people with autism form accurate representations of the target movements and hold them on line in working memory for sufficient periods to act on them (Bennetto, 1999; Rogers et al., 1996, Smith & Bryson 1998). Bennetto's (1999) work is particularly informative here. Children's ability to discriminate correct from incorrect video models, with variable time delays, was carefully examined, with no evidence of autism-specific problems. No autism-specific differences in the ability to form mental representations of movements and hold them on line have been identified thus far, and thus this hypothesis lacks support.

Self-Representation

A further motor concept that arises has to do with representation of one's own body. There is a clinical hypothesis that children with autism lack appropriate awareness of their own bodies. Two studies provide some data on this.

Bennetto (1999) used a neuropsychological task specifically focused on representation of one's own body (Semmes, Weinstein, Ghent, & Teuber, 1963). There were no autism-specific group differences on accuracy of identifying points on one's body related to those on a two-dimensional model, compared to a carefully matched clinical group of children. However, this task is concerned primarily with self-concept of static locations rather than ability to represent dynamic changes in limb positions in relation to one another. A recent electroencephalography (EEG) study of response to self-generated versus other's generated movements did not detect any difference in mu wave suppression between the autism group and comparison group in response to self-generated hand movements (Oberman et al., 2005) Thus, we currently lack data that support this hypothesis.

Self–Other Representation or Mapping

Two theories have been put forward concerning difficulties with coordinating representations of self and other: the self–other mapping theory and the identification theory.

The self–other mapping hypothesis arose in 1991 by Rogers and Pennington, who suggested that an imitation deficit involving seeing "the other as a template of the self," or self–other mapping of representations, might be a primary behavioral/neuropsychological deficit in autism. Williams, Whiten, Suddendorf, and Perrett (2001) expanded on this idea, suggesting that mirror neurons could provide a neural mechanism underlying such a deficit. Several papers published in the last few years have used methods to examine self–other mapping.

Avikainen and colleagues (2003) isolated a phenomenon that had been previously reported but never before directly examined in various autism imitation studies—problems with direct mirroring of the model (other groups that have also identified this problem include Bennetto, 1999; Meyer & Hobson, 2004; Ohta, 1987; Smith & Bryson, 1998). The specificity of the imitation problem in these studies allows us to consider a very fundamental problem involving neuron systems that allow for direct mapping of specific movements between humans. At least in animal research, neurons involved in perceiving and executing action appear to have this level of specificity. Jellema, Baker, Oram, and Perrett (2002) report that, in the macaque, neurons in superior temporal sulcus (STS) are quite specific in their response to movements of individual body parts: mouth, eyes, head, legs, and so on, and specific in their response to specific actions: walking, climbing, crouching, etc. They suggest that different cell populations appear equipped to break down complex motor acts into their basic components, both in detection and in performance. Examination of mirror neuron activation in autism has begun and is summarized in the section on brain–behavior relations. At the current time, this hypothesis is still considered viable, with initial support from both brain imaging and neuropsychological studies.

Identification Theory

Hobson (Hobson & Meyer, Chapter 9, this volume) offers a contrasting interpretation that appears to challenge the self–other mapping perspective, suggesting that "identification" is the key deficit in autism. These two concepts appear quite similar; however, there are subtle but distinct differences. Identification refers to individuals recognizing aspects of themselves that are the same within other individuals. In contrast, mapping refers to establishing correspondences rather than sameness.

In development, the origin of these two processes might be very different. Correspondence starts from an assumption that two individuals are separate but bear some resemblances. The concept of self–other mapping appears to involve capacities seen in young infants' abilities to detect correspondences among stimuli, even across sensory modalities, and precedes infants' capacities for identification, which appear to require development of more advanced representational abilities. Identification may develop from earlier capacities to detect self–other similarities and mappings, but identification is unlikely to be a prerequisite for self–other mapping.

To summarize, hypotheses concerning autism-specific difficulties in representation of target actions lack empirical support. Hypotheses concerning autism-specific difficulties with representation of one's own body have just begun to be studied and thus can neither be accepted or refuted at this point. There is evidence from a number of studies to support difficulties in *coordinating* representations of self and other's movements, and this is a promising area for further investigation.

Motor Execution Problems

The suggestion that the imitation deficit in autism could reflect a neurologically based difficulty with producing the movements per se was first suggested by Damasio and Maurer (1978). There is a body of evidence (see Dewey & Bottos, Chapter 17, this volume, for a review) that documents abnormal movements, muscle tone, and balance in persons with autism compared to those with other conditions or with typical development.

Several methodological approaches have been used to test the hypothesis that difficulties with motor imitation may be due to more fundamental difficulties in producing precise and well-coordinated movements. One approach uses clinical comparison groups who are also known to have motor production problems. Many autism imitation studies have used clinical comparison groups (for examples, see Rogers et al., 1996; Sigman & Ungerer, 1984; Stone et al., 1997). In each of these studies, a comparison group of participants with another clinical condition (usually intellectual handicap) has been matched to the experimental group with autism in terms of age and IQ functioning, with occasional matching for motor development as well.

The findings from these studies are somewhat inconsistent and reflect the nature of the groups being studied. When high-functioning subjects with autism are used, and are compared to typically developing controls, autism-specific motor deficits are generally found. However, when lower-functioning and younger subjects are examined and are compared to subjects with equivalent levels of mental retardation, then autism specific motor differences are not necessarily found. Several groups have demonstrated that toddlers and preschoolers with autism demonstrate fine motor skills that are no more impaired than the clinical comparisons (e.g., Rogers et al., 2003; Stone et al., 1997). However, a legitimate criticism of this approach is that the children with autism may have a type of motor difficulty more severe than comparison children that is not being adequately measured or adequately controlled for in the design.

A second methodological approach has involved choosing a comparison group with known motor impairment, like developmental coordination disorder, and matching it to the autism group on motor measures. If the children with autism demonstrate poorer imitation performance than controls, a motor impairment hypothesis cannot really account for the findings. This approach has been followed in only one study (Green et al., 2002). These authors found imitation performance among individuals with autism spectrum disorder (ASD) to be worse than those with developmental coordination disorder.

A third methodological approach has involved measuring children's motor performance directly on tasks that tap motor coordination and examining the relations between the motor performance and imitative productions. This approach has been used by several different experimental groups (Bennetto, 1999; Rogers et al., 2003; Smith & Bryson, 1998) all of whom demonstrated that the diagnosis of autism continued to be related to imitation performance, even after the variance associated with motor performance was removed. A statistical point to note is that partial correlations and multiple regressions assume that the confounding variable has an equal effect on the variance of each group. However, at least some groups report that imitation has a different relationship with motor skills in autism than it does in control groups (see Rogers et al., 2003). Therefore, the approach of controlling for variance in motor ability may not fully address this concern. To summarize, the few studies that have addressed this hypothesis suggest that while motor impairment affects imitation performance, it does not fully account for the autism imitation deficit. This is an area in which much more research is needed.

Difficulties with Attentional Flexibility

Many structured imitation batteries require multiple shifts in visual attention, even in single-action stimuli, which require shifts from the model's face to an object and then to the model's body. Children with autism have been shown to have difficulties with attentional flexibility (Ozonoff, Strayer, McMahon,

& Filloux, 1994) and may have unusual attentional foci during social interaction tasks (Klin, Jones, Schultz, Volkmar, & Cohen, 2002).

Given the well-known lack of typical eye contact and attention to others, imitation studies need to determine whether they have the visual attention of their subjects. While a few studies have tried to examine this concept (e.g., Rogers et al., 2003), ensuring that a subject is attending does not guarantee that the subject is looking at the relevant aspects of the movement. As eye-tracking studies of autism are teaching us (Klin et al., 2002), visual attention may be focused on something other than the critical stimulus, even with attentive subjects. It will be quite important for future studies to monitor gaze within imitation studies in order to provide better information on orienting, visual attention, and gaze shifts during imitation tasks.

The relationship between visual attention and imitation in autism is likely to be complex. As discussed elsewhere (see Williams & Waiter, Chapter 15; Decety, Chapter 11; Mon-Williams, Chapter 14, this volume), visual attention and motor activity are usually tightly coordinated. It is quite possible that eye movement patterns can be shaped by repeated experiences of visual tracking of complex, goal-directed action sequences. Thus, repeated practice in joint attention and imitative exchanges may "train" the infant's attentional processes and foster attentional flexibility (Williams et al., 2001, 2006). This idea is supported by evidence from both McEvoy, Rogers, and Pennington (1993) and Griffith, Pennington, Wehner, and Rogers (1999), who found significant relationships between executive function and joint attention in young children with autism.

Cross-Modal Processing Abilities

Imitation requires that one coordinate visual–spatial information input from the partner's movements with proprioceptive and kinesthetic output regarding one's own body and thus rests on cross-modal information processing abilities. We lack a body of solid empirical information on the integrity of cross-modal processing in autism. Two recent studies have examined this problem in relation to imitation. As described previously, Bennetto's (1999) study found no differences on a task requiring a very similar kind of cross-modal transfer, from visual stimuli involving a two-dimensional representation of a body onto the child's own body. Williams, Massaro, Peel, Bosseler, and Suddendorf (2004) recently examined speech reading in children with autism, in which no deficits in cross-modal processing were documented. However, at this point, we do not have the data needed to accept or reject this theory.

Motivational Factors

Imitation deficits may be an epiphenomenon of a more general social disinterest in autism. This has been a popular way of discussing, or perhaps dismissing, the imitative findings in autism. The line of reasoning is this: People with autism are less interested in other people than comparison groups, and thus look at them less, are less motivated to do what other people do, less motivated to cooperate with experimenters, and for all these reasons have less practice in imitating others, resulting in poorer performance on experimental batteries. This view has been described most recently by Trevarthen and Aitken (2001; see also Dawson et al., 2002; Zelazo, 2001).

Ingersoll and colleagues (2003) highlighted motivational aspects by manipulating object effects during imitation tasks. While this study provides an important reminder that motivational factors must be considered in every autism imitation study, other studies appear to indicate that the social motivation factor alone cannot account for the imitation performance deficit in autism. For example, a motivational problem would predict equally poor performance on easy and difficult imitation tasks (Williams, Massaro, et al., 2004). Yet the body of studies has consistently demonstrated differential performance patterns in autism based on task difficulty. Children with autism have been found to perform adequately on very simple imitative tasks (Charman & Baron-Cohen, 1994). Indeed, one study (Libby, Powell, Messer, & Jordan, 1997) found the children with autism to be less negative about performing imitations than comparisons. Even with very young children, Rogers and colleagues (2003) reported no differences between 2-year-olds with autism and two other developmentally matched groups on cooperative, contingent acts in response to a model. Another characteristic that may differentially affect motivation is the intentional nature of the task. Studies of automatic imitative processes (e.g., McIntosh et al., in press; Scambler et al., in press; Yirmiya et al., 1989) are probably not as dependent on motivation as tasks involving intentional gestural imitation. Thus, although the motivation question needs to be asked and considered in each study, it is also an area that can be addressed to some extent at the level of task design (including using methods to tap automatic processes and to enhance motivation) and examined in the analyses.

Another argument against the motivational hypothesis is that it suggests an experiential deficit accruing over time. Fewer imitative experiences day by day will over time result in increasing disparity of experience and lack of equivalent amount of practice in the wide range of skills that young children learn via imitation (Williams, Massaro, et al., 2004). An example would be poor ball-throwing skills because of reduced practice in reciprocal play (Hoon & Reiss, 1992). This leads to the hypothesis that very young children with autism should show less experiential imitative deficit, and that progressively older groups should show progressively larger deficits. However, imitation studies in autism find significant group differences at the earliest ages even when carefully controlled for visual attention and cooperative responses to the examiner (Charman et al., 1997; Kalmanson, 1987; Rogers et al., 2003; Sigman & Ungerer, 1984).

A final problem with the motivation hypothesis is that it assumes that imitation is a unitary, intentional phenomenon that results in some positive interpersonal (and intrinsic) reward. Yet, different types of imitative behavior (to be discussed further later) lead to different consequences. Automatic imitation, or mimicry, is considered to be an unintentional behavior that occurs outside awareness, a relatively hard-wired phenomenon. Imitation used in the apprenticeship function involves intentional motivated acts to learn or accomplish a motivated skill, as in imitating someone's acts that open a candy box. The reward is in the accomplishment of a personal goal, and there is no basis for hypothesizing an autism-specific deficit in this type of motivation. The third type of imitation, intentional imitation of another's behavior in a social–communicative exchange like infant–parent games, could be considered less intrinsically rewarding for children with autism than others. However, the studies of response to being imitated conducted by Dawson and Galpert (1990) and Escalona, Field, Nadel, and Lundy (2002) have clearly demonstrated that children with autism enjoy being imitated, seek to continue the experience when it ends, and respond with increased imitation. The social imitative experience appears intrinsically rewarding to the children in these studies. Thus, while the motivational hypothesis needs to be considered, the construct of "motivation" itself seems too general to be very helpful in understanding autism-specific imitation difficulties. Much more precise hypotheses are needed.

To conclude this section, evidence supports theories regarding the contribution of both motor and motivational deficits in autism to imitative performance, but neither of these appears to fully account for autism-specific differences. Two aspects of representation of movement appear to be differentially affected: self–other orientation and affective quality of gestures. The evidence of specific difficulties with orientation of a movement in relation to the partner's body has been cited previously. Examination of "style," or affective quality of acts involving manual movements, has thus far only been reported by Hobson and colleagues. These aspects of "style" may well reflect affectively related automatic imitation, or mimicry, of body movements. Abnormal mimicry in autism is currently being reported. Studies of facial mimicry also demonstrate autism-specific deficits in affective mirroring of facial expressions (McIntosh et al., in press; Scambler et al., in press; Yirmiya et al., 1989).

The social variables involving attention to the model, experience and practice with imitation, and motivation to perform are critical variables and in some ways get to the heart of autism. Motivation to perform tasks needs to be addressed and examined in individual studies. Focus of attention needs to be examined with more sophisticated methods than have thus far been used. Experiential history is a very real consideration and may indicate the need for a training study or study in which groups are already matched on capacity to imitate movements precisely, to examine the role of additional processes affecting imitative performances. It does not appear at this time that the imitation deficit in autism is reducible to one simple deficient process. Imitating another is a complex act with many degrees of freedom; currently the evidence suggests multiple affected subcomponents.

LESSONS LEARNED FROM COMPARATIVE PSYCHOLOGY: THE VARIETY OF WAYS THAT SOCIAL MODELS CAN INFLUENCE BEHAVIOR

One of the many contributions that the comparative psychologists have made to imitation research has been their careful dissection of the different kinds of "matching" behaviors. While researchers studying humans tend to use the generic term *imitation* to refer to any kind of matching behavior, comparative psychologists have differentiated at least five different kinds of matching behaviors that occur between conspecifics. As Want and Harris (2002) suggested, child researchers would be wise to learn these finer distinctions (as described by Whiten, Chapter 10, this volume). This careful taxonomy of copying behavior has been extremely helpful to the animal researchers who study social learning. What might we gain by applying this careful taxonomy of matching behavior to the autism imitation literature?

Mimicry and the Transmission of Affect

In the human literature, the term *mimicry* refers to automatic, (nonintentional) matching behaviors, particularly involving facial, postural, and gestural movements that occur rapidly and outside of awareness. The occurrence of mimicry in typically developing adults is well established in the social psychology literature; see Moody and McIntosh (Chapter 4, this volume) for a review. It can involve simple movements, as well as emotionally salient stimuli. The best-known examples are social smiling and yawning. Mimicry is closely related to emotional contagion, whereby the perception of another's expression of emotion elicits the same emotion in the observer (Hatfield et al., 1999).

There are only three controlled studies of mimicry in the published autism literature, all focusing on facial mimicry of emotional expressions. Two of the studies examined children's responses to experimenter's discrete emotion expressions. Both studies reported a deficient mimicry response (Scambler et al., in press; Sigman, Kasari, Kwon, & Yirmiya, 1992). The third controlled study examined the response of high-functioning adults to emotional displays delivered on a computer screen and measured using electromyography (EMG; MacIntosh et al., in press; see Moody & MacIntosh, Chapter 4, for a description). All three report autism-specific deficits in mimicry. In addition, tasks like Hobson's form versus function task (Hobson & Lee, 1999) can likely be included in this group. This study reported a large autism-specific deficit in mimicking the dynamic style of an object-directed action in two independent samples of people with autism.

These findings from four independent studies are exciting and provocative. A deficit in automatic mirroring of others' emotional behavior could have significant effects on social–emotional behavior, especially reciprocity and emotion expression via facial display and gesture. Mimicry is an important area for further study in autism, at both the behavioral and the brain levels.

Emulation

Emulation refers to completing an observed goal-directed task by achieving the modeled end state, but not necessarily modeling the specific behaviors used to achieve the goal state. Whiten further distinguishes between goal emulation and result emulation. In result, or end, emulation the end state is copied. In goal emulation, the individual copies what he or she considers to be the goal of the actor. Although there have not been studies in autism that specifically target result emulation, goal emulation has been investigated in several studies using Meltzoff's (1995) failed intentions task. The paradigm examines whether young children with autism can complete simple means–end tasks in both a modeled and in a disrupted, or failed, condition, in comparison to developmentally matched typical and/or clinical groups. Performance of the intended act in the failed condition demonstrates goal emulation.

Two published studies have demonstrated that the majority of children with autism complete the target task in the imitated condition (though in some of the studies they performed significantly fewer of these tasks than the comparison subject group), as well as in the failed condition (Aldridge, Stone, Sweeney, & Bower, 2000; Carpenter, Pennington, & Rogers, 2001). In addition, several other studies have demonstrated lack of autism-specific differences in imitation tasks involving familiar and functional means–end acts on objects, like the Hobson studies. Thus, there does not seem to be evidence of autism-specific problems in goal emulation in the literature. It could be that intact goal emulation underlies many of the successful object imitation performances in autism involving simple (and usually familiar) acts.

Object Movement Reenactment or Intentional, Means–End Imitation

As discussed in depth by Whiten (Chapter 10, this volume) the distinction between emulation and imitation may be a fine one, as copying the action (imitation) and copying the effects of the action (emulation) may be indistinguishable. For example, Tomasello and colleagues (Nagell, Olguin, & Tomasello, 1993) used a rake task, in which subjects (toddlers and chimpanzees) observed an adult use a rake to retrieve an object in a box. In one condition the rake was turned prong-side down, and in the other condition, prong-side up—a less efficient way to use a rake to retrieve an object. This kind of task nicely separates copying means and copying goals but does not mean that participants were imitating means–end behavior. They could simply be re-creating the rake position and action. One might then ask if participants copied the overhand or underhand grip, but such a distinction is unlikely to be relevant to the action outcome. Whiten advocates introduction of the term *object movement reenactment* (OMR) to clarify the situation.

The number of papers reporting relative strengths in OMR compared to gestural or facial imitations might lead us to suspect that children with autism can carry out these tasks adequately. However, a study by Rogers and colleagues (2003) raises questions about this assumption, while also presenting a challenge to Whiten's classification. This study presented copying tasks to young children that required them to perform simple acts on objects, but the actions were novel in relation to the objects. They involved operating a squeak toy with the elbow, inverting a toy car and patting the underbody, and banging duplos together rather than stacking them. The car inversion, compression of the squeak toy, and duplo manipulation were clearly OMRs. Surprisingly, the children with autism demonstrated as impaired performance on these tasks as on the gestural or facial tasks. This recollects the Hammes and Langdell (1981) findings where the children would not imitate drinking from the teapot.

These findings suggest that the difficulty of bodily imitation in autism may indeed occur in object tasks as well, although the use of familiar or conventional acts or acts that are well-supported by the affordances of the object may mask this difficulty. An alternative interpretation is that OMR skills may be usually intact in autism but are susceptible to interference when they differ to those previously learned to be associated with the object being used. A methodological issue to note here is that identifying such problems requires a scoring system sensitive to the precision of the imitation: posture, the limbs used, directionality of the movement, timing of the action, orientation in space, and so on. While this level of coding may seem overly detailed, the precision of an imitation may have important effects in natural social interactions, in that a smoothly executed automatic mirroring movement may be so synchronous as to go almost unnoticed in an interaction, but rather "felt" as a natural social response, whereas an uncoordinated, poorly timed, or poorly reproduced movement may stand out as "odd" (see Stern, 1985, for a similar concept).

Gestural or Body-Level Imitation

How should intentional gestural acts be classified? Many of the autism imitation studies, perhaps the majority, have asked subjects to copy manual or bodily postures and movements and oral and/or facial movements or expressions. This kind of imitation differs from tasks in the mimicry paradigms in that in the intentional tasks, imitation is explicitly instructed and the resulting behavior is thus intentional rather than automatic. Response to instructed imitation is not typically part of the classification system used in the comparative studies, and yet it occurs in humans in a very regular basis. In older children and adults it is frequent in learning situations, as in sports or dance lessons, learning musical instruments, and so on. In infancy and early childhood this kind of imitation is seen in parent–infant interaction games, and in toddlers and preschoolers in songs and chants involving finger or body movements, in imitation of actions on toys and outdoors in play.

As reported here, virtually every autism study involving gestural imitations, except for the work of Beadle-Brown and Whiten (2004), has reported autism-specific differences, and this includes studies that tap the full range of age groups and severity levels. Although most of the work has involved hand and body movements, those that include oral–facial movements also report autism-specific deficits. Again, a sensitive coding system is necessary to fully capture problems with this area. Clearly, persons with autism have great difficulties with this type of imitative behavior.

To conclude, the application of the comparative psychology classification system helps identify the nature of the imitative problems in autism with somewhat greater precision. The difficulty does not appear to involve understanding the intention of the model for the action, particularly involving objects. The imitative difficulty appears to center on mirroring of others' body movements, both automatic and intentional. To what extent these are independent is unknown. Although Rogers and colleagues (1996, 2003) demonstrated strong correlations across different types of simple intentional imitation tasks, Stone and colleagues (1997) revealed the opposite, and most studies of imitation have not provided the needed analyses. In terms of brain function, some neural mechanisms involved during imitation of purposeful use of objects may be independent of those involved in mimicry or in intentional bodily imitation. We need integrated studies involving behavioral science and neuroscience to help us drill down more deeply into the nature of these different types of imitative behavior.

BRAIN–BEHAVIOR RELATIONS INVOLVED IN IMITATION

The complex capacity for interpersonal imitation seen in human beings implies specific brain mechanisms evolved to support such capacities. How and why has such evolution occurred? This question was addressed early on by Bruner (1972), who observed the contributions of tool use, imitation, and play to cognitive development in humans. Byrne and Whiten (1988) argued that a selective advantage evolved from being able to manage and use information inherent to social complexity, and this advantage resulted in massive expansion of cerebral cortex over a period of about 2 million years. They consider three different social abilities—cooperation, deception, and imitation—as particularly important forces behind these evolutionary changes. Merlin Donald (1991) suggested four main epochs in social evolution of humans, with imitation, or mimesis, playing a fundamental role in the third epoch, in which occurs the evolution of social–communicative behavior specific to our species. Drawing from the neurological and neuropsychological studies available at that time, he hypothesized a model of brain evolution of multiple structures with increasingly specialized roles in imitative behavior, which would require integration of multiple brain regions across both hemispheres.

Discovery of Mirror Neurons

In 1992, reports from single-cell physiological studies of monkeys demonstrated the first evidence of neurons with the property of firing both during observation and during execution of an action (di Pellegrino, Fadiga, Fogassi, Gallese, & Rizzolatti, 1992). These were dubbed "mirror neurons" and provided the first direct evidence of perception–action coupling at the level of a single neuron. This extremely important discovery stimulated a burst of brain-based studies involving imitation in humans. While these neurons were first identified in animals without the capacity for intentional imitation, the locus of these neurons in the monkey homolog to Broca's area allowed hypotheses for the role of mirror neurons in language, imitation, and other crucial human social–communicative abilities, suggested earlier by Donald, to develop rapidly (Rizzolatti & Arbib, 1998). Mirror neurons were quickly seen as a potential mechanism that might explain both imitative deficits and the greater social–communicative deficits associated with autism, particularly as a starting-state mechanism responsible for a slowly accruing series of social deficits (Williams et al., 2001). This discovery stimulated a wave of theorizing about potential roles of mirror neurons in human development and evolution (Rizzolatti & Arbib, 1998; Williams et al., 2001) and neuroimaging studies of brain responses to imitative tasks, both in typical development and in autism.

Neuroimaging Studies of Imitation in Typically Developing Subjects

Increasingly, perspectives on brain functioning do not see action and perception as served by separate apparatus. Rather, cortical functioning tends to be dependent on connectivity between brain areas. The "mirror neuron" discovery is important as one of the earlier experimental findings in accord with this perspective. Areas of visual cortex have now been identified that are sensitive to motor input (Astafiev, Stanley, Shulman, & Corbetta, 2004), and spatial attention appears to be dependent upon parietofrontal connectivity (Gaffan, 2005; Thiebaut de Schotten et al., 2005).

The neural substrate of imitation is reviewed by Decety (Chapter 11, this volume). To summarize very briefly, inferior and superior aspects of parietal lobe are likely to be important in relating visual aspects of movement to codings of actions derived from proprioceptive input. In addition, frontal brain areas are likely to be important in inhibiting and commissioning imitation. The STS is likely to be important in assigning intention to observed action (Jellema et al., 2000). Keysers and Perrett (2004) suggest that in forming connectivity with inferior frontal lobe through the observation of self-generated action, the STS plays a vital role in developing the mapping of visual to self-codings that are required for the mirror neuron network and imitation. The insula is also a potentially important area that may be involved in more affectively laden imitation (Gallese, Keysers, & Rizzolatti, 2004).

The distinction between ventral and dorsal stream processing (Milner & Goodale, 1995) has also attracted interest recently, as researchers study basic visual processing in autism. In essence, the ventral stream has high sensitivity to spatial variance but a lower sensitivity to changes in temporal dynamics. It is thought to be associated with processing static visual content and processes information along ventral temporal cortex. The dorsal stream processes visual information that changes rapidly with time, along the dorsal stream involving mirror neurons in parietal lobe. Some authors argue that autism could be a dorsal stream problem (Milne et al., 2002; Spencer et al. 2000). The dichotomy is of interest to imitation research in understanding which aspects utilize these different streams and how they might relate to one another.

Neuroimaging Studies of Imitation in Autism

As reviewed in Williams and Waiter (Chapter 15, this volume), studies are beginning to explore relationships between imitative abilities and neural systems in autism. Nishitani, Avikainen, and Hari (2004) reported a magneto-encephalography (MEG) study of subjects with Asperger syndrome (AS) observing and imitating oral–facial movements from still photos (see Williams & Waiter, Chapter 15, for a more detailed description of this study). Compared to typical adult control subjects, those with AS demonstrated decreased activation of Broca's area during imitation, but no differences in STS activation implying that the AS difference in brain response was specific to the imitation condition and was not seen during observation.

Williams and colleagues (in press) utilized a functional magnetic resonance imaging (fMRI)–imitation protocol involving the Iacaboni and colleagues (1999) isolated finger movement task in a study of ASD and typical controls. They demonstrated several areas of autism-specific differences. One involved decreased activation of the mirror neuron (MN) regions of the right inferior parietal lobe in ASD during both the observation and imitation phases of the experiment. The authors suggest that this may represent problems with the parietal mirror neuron system involving a generalized poor proprioceptive input to self-generated movements, regardless of the stimulus, in ASD. A second very important finding involved decreased left amygdala activation during the imitation condition in ASD. Amygdala activation has not before been identified in fMRI–imitation studies. Williams and colleagues interpret this finding as possibly reflecting a different, and lessened, emotional experience associated with imitation in ASD. This hypothesis has direct connections to Dawson and colleagues' (2004) recent suggestion that deficient social behavior in early autism is due to lack of typical positive affective feedback—

the intrinsic reinforcement system, as well as to various studies reporting amygdala differences in autism (Abell et al., 1999; Bauman & Kemper, 1998). Finally, the lack of activation in the posterior aspect of STS in the ASD group during imitation but not observation (in the face of the opposite occurring in controls) was particularly interesting given that subjects with autism also show decreased responses is this same area of STS during mental state tasks (Castelli, Frith, Happe, & Frith, 2002).

Oberman and colleagues (2005) reported a pilot EEG study of mu wave suppression, which has been demonstrated to be correlated with MN activity. A group of high-functioning persons with autism observed videos of several stimuli, including a hand movement, and were asked to imitate the movement. The subjects demonstrated lack of mu wave suppression during imitation but not during observation, suggesting lack of activation of the MN system during imitation (which they performed adequately).

The final neuroimaging study of autism and imitation to be discussed here was recently published by Dapretto and colleagues (2006). This group reported a fMRI study of 10 high-functioning children with ASD and 10 typically developing comparison children, matched by age and IQ. The stimuli involved pictures of five different emotional expressions, which the participants either imitated or passively viewed in the scanner. Half of the group subsequently repeated the experiment outside the scanner on an eye tracker, with no differences in fixation times to faces. Precision of imitation was not measured, although judges did not rate the emotional expressions of the two groups differently. The group with ASD demonstrated many activations similar to controls, but did not demonstrate activity in the mirror neuron area of pars opercularis during both imitation and observation. During imitation, the typically developing group showed significantly greater activation in insula and amygdaloid areas than the ASD group, who showed greater parietal and visual association activation. Furthermore, Dapretto and colleagues found significant negative correlations between the intensity of social symptoms specific to autism and activity in pars opercularis, insula, and limbic structures, insula and social symptoms specific to autism, even with IQ controlled. Furthermore, there was adequate monitoring of visual fixations to ensure that this difference was not due to looking patterns. These findings suggested that children with autism use some different neural strategies during both imitation and observation of emotion faces, and this probably results in less felt emotion for them. This is the most convincing study yet that ties autism to MN system differences.

Although it is seductive to attribute many aspects of the autism profile to MN deficiency (Theoret et al., 2005; Williams et al., 2001), and although the evidence currently supports the hypothesis that the MN network functions abnormally in autism, experimental tests of this hypothesis need to consider some important issues. The most important of these is that MN function has been demonstrated at a single cell level in monkeys and not humans. Yet, the functions that are being ascribed to MNs such as theory of mind, language, and imitation are only found in humans. MN circuitry in monkeys appears to assist with understanding others' actions, and perhaps with intention reading (Fogassi et al., 2005; Perrett et al., 1989). Two different research groups have used simple intention reading tasks with children with autism, and neither has reported a deficit in their response (Aldridge et al., 2000; Carpenter et al., 2001). These tasks, which should elicit MN activation, have not shown any autism-specific impairment.

A second issue for an MN hypothesis for autism has to do with a biological model for a MN deficit. Imagining some type of specific impairment of the mirror neurons at the core of autism is difficult given that the mirror neurons are unique only in their functions and not in their structure, location, development, and migration (V. Gallese, personal communication, April 2005; Petrides, Cadoret, & Mackey, 2005). Williams and colleagues (in press) suggested an alternative mechanism. The left anterior frontal lobe (serving what has been classified here as an MN function) is normally characterized by an unusually high level of pruning appropriate to its serving an integrative function. One biological function that could theoretically result in an impaired MN function would be an impaired neuronal pruning mechanism. An alternative suggestion is a general problem with connectivity, and general connectivity problems have been suggested in autism (Just, Cherkassky, Keller, & Minshew, 2004). However, a general connectivity theory better addresses problems that require higher-order skills than early skills like simple gestural imitation. In addition, and as discussed by Williams and Waiter (Chapter 15, this volume) there is poor evidence for a general connectivity impairment in ASD.

Therefore, although we have some tentative evidence in support of the MN hypothesis of autism offered by Williams and colleagues (2001), the function and neural substrate of the MN system is now being recognized as much more sophisticated than was previously imagined. As the fMRI studies have demonstrated, there are many brain responses to imitation tasks, and many ways in which autism-related imitation differences might be reflected in brain responses. Given current models of brain development and the crucial role of experience in developing expertise, we assume that neural responses to imitative tasks reflect learning and practice histories, as well as possible starting-state differences. The early mirroring seen in young infants suggests that there is a starting-state mechanism present and active at the time of birth. However, given the interactive differences that children with autism experience, we should be cautious about assuming a starting-state difference in infants with autism as the explanation for either the behavioral or the brain activation differences related to imitation studies. Prospective studies of infants who go on to develop autism will help us understand the interactions among starting-state capacities and developmental histories. Such studies are currently ongoing in several different countries.

To conclude, the aforementioned studies demonstrate our growing knowledge of the neuroscience of imitation. As expected, given the behavioral evidence of imitation problems in autism, the initial neuroimaging studies of autism report differences in neural activity during imitation tasks in subjects with ASDs, and the Williams and colleagues (2006) study suggests that the differences do not involve one particular structure but, rather, appear widely distributed. Imitation involves the coordination of multisensory information with the execution of motor acts, automaticity of responses, the interpretation of self and others' behavior, and affective responses that may well influence frequency of response through differences in intrinsic emotional reward systems. What is emerging is a complex picture of neurology of imitation. Although there is tremendous emphasis at the moment on mirror neurons in Broca's area as the "site" of imitation and other kinds of self–other relations, their role in human ontogeny is still completely unknown. If, as Donald (1991) hypothesized, the whole cortical expansion was driven by the selective advantages conferred by being able to copy, communicate, and read actions, one would expect that imitation would be a property more of the whole cortex than of an individual area.

INTEGRATING CURRENT RESEARCH
ON DEVELOPMENT OF IMITATION AND AUTISM

A long time ago, we suggested that the core social difficulty in autism involved the coordination of self–other schemas, at a bodily sense as well as a psychological sense. We suggested that impaired imitation early in autism might be the initial reflection of this difficulty and might also contribute to difficulties coordinating other kinds of self–other schemas (Rogers & Pennington, 1991). Having reviewed all the published studies to date, there is very strong evidence of autism-specific impairments in imitation of model's gestures, oral–facial movements, and actions on objects in participants ranging in age from 2 to adulthood and across the intellectual range of autism, as well as the severity range of autism and its milder variants. Imitation is not absent in autism but, rather, less frequent and less precise than in other groups.

Are imitative deficits related to other core features of autism? Several papers have examined concurrent relations. Imitative ability correlated strongly with the presence and severity of autism symptoms in very young children with autism (Rogers et al., 2003). Early imitation has demonstrated relations with language development (for which imitation is a strong predictor, in both typically developing children and those with autism; Charman & Baron-Cohen, 2003; Rogers et al., 2003; Stone & Yoder, 2001 and reviewed by Charman, Chapter 5, this volume). Only one study has examined relations between imitation, dyadic responsivity, and joint attention behavior in autism, reporting significant and moderately strong relations for children with autism (Rogers et al., 2003). In the only study to examine it, intentional imitation was not correlated with unintentional, or automatic, imitation (mimicry) of emotional expressions (Scambler et al., in press). Treatment studies have begun to demonstrate collateral effects of imitation abilities on children with autism: increased social engagement with others, language skills (Wert & Neisworth, 2003), social initiations (Nikopoulos & Keenan, 2003), social initiations (Nikopoulos & Kennan, 2003), and generalized effects of imitation training (Garfinkle & Schwartz, 2002). Thus, while studies of concurrent relations support the hypothesis that imitation has links to other core features of autism, the prospective longitudinal studies of typical and atypical development from early infancy through the preschool years needed to test this model have not yet been published.

Do imitative deficits in autism precede development of other autism symptoms? Zwaigenbaum and colleagues (2005) have provided the first lab-based evidence of imitation problems in infants prior to diagnosis of autism. In a large study of the early development of infant siblings of children with autism, he and his colleagues followed 65 infant siblings from 6 to 24 months. Nineteen children presented with symptoms corresponding to an ASD at 24 months. Imitation items (along with several other indicators of social impairment) administered at 12 months predicted these 19 children at a p value of .003. This is the first direct lab evidence that imitation impairments exist in infants prior to the time the full syndrome emerges.

The imitation deficit associated with autism does not appear to be due primarily to motor dexterity though motor maturity and coordination contribute to poor-quality performances. Neither have imitation problems in autism been linked yet primarily to poor motivation to perform, though this has not been well studied and it is an extremely important variable to manage well in task design and procedures. The focus of attention during imitation tasks has been examined by a few: No abnormalities have yet been identified.

The types of imitative difficulties found, particularly involving self–other perspectives, body part orientations, and role reversals, provide support for autism-specific difficulties in forming and coordinating, or mapping representations of self and other—as originally proposed by Rogers and Pennington (1991) and later expanded by Williams and colleagues (2001). Self–other mapping in imitation tasks relies on connectivity across the entire brain, from visual to motor cortex and from right to left hemisphere. Therefore, to the extent to which autism involves white matter connectivity, skills that require widespread connectivity, like self–other mapping, are likely to be strongly affected. Several studies have described brain processes involved in imitative tasks, and the few comparative studies of autism document autism-specific differences in brain activation patterns during imitative tasks. White matter deficits of the type documented in autism by Piven, Bailey, Ranson, and Arndt (1997) and replicated by Hardan, Minshew, and Keshavan (2000) and Waiter and colleagues (2004) should have greatest impact on behavioral functions that depend on cortical integration between the most spatially disparate structures, like imitation. More than any other developmental or neuropsychological impairment in autism, imitation appears to meet the primary deficit criteria of specificity, universality, precedence, and persistence (Pennington & Ozonoff, 1991).

In typical development, reciprocal mirroring between parent and infant appear to form an important part of the repertoire of reciprocal social interactions. These appear pleasurable to both partners, and we assume that repeated experiences of imitating and being imitated strengthen the infant's neural connections involved in self–other mappings through repetition and positive affect and lead to increased frequency across early childhood (the Hebbian model of MN learning described by Keysers & Perrett, 2004). Both automatic and intentional imitative processes appear in the first year of life, and the relations between them are unknown. Several starting-state conditions are at play: a capacity to produce some early motor imitations (which demonstrates starting-state neural coordination of perception–action circuitry), partners who imitate the infant and provide models for imitation, infant discrimination of reciprocal imitations, and positive affect experienced during reciprocal imitations.

Impairment in any one or more of these conditions may interfere with the development of coordinated and reciprocal motoric and affective interaction patterns, resulting in infrequent social imitations, lack of enjoyment in imitative exchanges, lack of expectation for reciprocity, and thus lack of practice and lack of developing automaticity. Similarities among infants who will develop autism, infants with blindness, infants with extreme deprivation, and infants of depressed mothers, similarities involving affective neutrality and decreases in contingent responsiveness, may mark the early difficulties in this general domain, even though the derailing variable differs for each group. Given the pleasure children with autism show during episodes of being imitated, and the apparent reinforcement value therein, being imitated provides positive experiences for them (Dawson & Galpert, 1990; Escalona et al., 2002; Harris, Handleman, & Fong, 1987). Lack of reinforcement does not appear to be a viable hypothesis concerning imitative deficits in autism.

For infants who will develop autism, developing cognitive and motor abilities support successful interactions with objects. Their interest and knowledge about objects develop, and they learn means–end relations and observe and comprehend others' intentions on objects, which we assume involves MN activation. Their ability to understand others' acts may well support the development of intentional imitation of interesting actions on objects. However, the neurobiology of autism impedes the development of imitation as a source of social communication and affects automatic mimicry processes as well. The final picture in autism would be of a capacity for intentional imitation of object skills, though lacking in precision (due to lack of practice, motor difficulties, and/or other causes), combined with a large deficit in automatic mimicry of other's facial, vocal, postural, gestural, and other expressive behaviors in appropriate social interactions. Altered neural responses to imitative stimuli may reflect lack of practice and lack of expertise, primary neural differences, and/or recruitment to other functional circuits. However, the evidence suggests that in autism, the capacity for more typical imitative responses is present, as seen in imitations of acts on objects, echolalia, occasional echopraxia, video copying, and the capacity of some young children with autism to acquire much more typical imitative skills through treatment.

We continue to suggest that the "cause" of the imitation problem in autism lies in abnormal functioning of neural processes that entrain us to each other and result in coordination of bodily movements and actions, and later, entrainment of affective and social cognitive processes. This failure of entrainment, neurally and behaviorally, is core to the symptoms of autism. This could result from a deficient capacity to automatically map others' actions onto the self and produce imitative responses. Evidence seems more supportive of impairments in these areas than in detecting mirroring responses of the other. Longitudinal studies of imitative development from birth through the second year, in both typical and atypical development, are desperately needed. A great deal of developmental theorizing about the role of imitation in development, including our own, has been built on very little longitudinal data. We need to follow Heimann and Ullstadius's (1999) lead and put early imitation theories to the test.

ADDITIONAL TOPICS FOR RESEARCH AND RESOLUTION

Delay versus Deficit

Throughout this chapter we have addressed questions in need of further research. There is one other issue that needs to be resolved. Much discussion has hinged on the distinction between a *delay* in imitative development and a *deficit* in imitative ability in autism. Several studies have demonstrated specific imitative impairments in high-functioning adults (Avikainen et al., 2003; Rogers et al., 1996). Identification of unusual patterns of imitative performance in autism in relation to delayed groups also supports a deviance model, as seen problems with oral–motor impairments in Rogers and colleagues (2003), and with self-orientated movements in Smith and Bryson (1998), Avikainen and colleagues (2003), and Meyer and Hobson (2004), among others. However, the issue may well involve the semantics of the term *delay*. Although an immature performance in children may be considered a delay, adult differences, even when they reflect immaturities, are typically not referred to as delays. At some point, delay becomes deviance. Examination of the developmental sequences and trajectories of intentional and automatic imitation in early autism would help distinguish between delayed and deviant patterns of development.

IQ and Imitation

IQ is often significantly correlated with imitative ability, and imitation skills have been found to predict to later IQ in the very few longitudinal studies that have been reported, as reviewed by Hepburn and Stone (Chapter 13, this volume). However, interpretation of this relationship is not straightforward. Given that an IQ score reflects a person's past learning rate, imitation may be an important determinant of IQ performance. If imitation ability is the powerful early learning tool that theorists suggest, then lack of imitative experiences would result in a diminished repertoire of skills and abilities and reflected in lower IQ scores. The nature of the relation between imitation and IQ score is not yet known, and experimenters should be cautious about statistically controlling for IQ in analyses, because they may be controlling for the very variable that they wish to study.

More Precise Conceptualization and Coding of Imitative Tasks

The range of tasks being used in autism imitation studies raises many questions. The comparative psychologists have given clinical researchers a taxonomy for tightening definitions and choice of tasks, and using such distinctions will help communication across studies. In terms of tasks, some of the imitative tasks used in the scanner (simple finger raising) are so simple that they barely seem to tap imitative phenomena. Is such a simple task really parallel to imitating a sequence of meaningless actions, or to automatic responses to natural emotional expressions of others? The "messiness" of the actions used in autism imitation studies makes it difficult to extract core difficulties, particularly given evidence that brain responses vary specifically and differentially to stimuli involving different body parts. Finally, most imitative tasks have multiple degrees of freedom involved, including body position, limb position, and movement dynamics, among others. Detailed coding systems that examine errors provide much more information about the nature of the performance than pass–fail systems.

Response to Being Imitated

We need greater understanding of people with autism's awareness of being imitated, which has begun to be examined by Nadel and her colleagues, Nielsen (Nielsen, Suddendorf, & Dissanayake, Chapter 7, this volume) and Decety (Chapter 11, this volume) but few others. Escalona and colleagues (2002) have developed further Dawson's early finding that children with autism responded differentially to being imitated (Dawson & Galpert, 1990; Harris et al., 1987), responding with attention to contingency but with approach and touch after being imitated. Sensitivity to being imitated brings to mind initial hypotheses concerning contingency raised early by Dawson and Lewy (1989) and more recently by Gergely and Watson (1999). Response to being imitated suggests awareness of self and other in important ways. It would be interesting to examine response to imitation in light of the self–other orientation problems highlighted by Meyer and Hobson (2004). To what extent children with autism demonstrate a typical or atypical response to others' imitations of them is unknown, and this represents a very fruitful area for further investigation.

Echolalia and Echopraxia in Autism

Finally, we have very little information about the phenomena of echolalia and echopraxia, whether in autism or in other neurological disorders, and their relation to other types of imitative behavior. Decety (Chapter 11, this volume) has provided an intriguing theory concerning both phenomena, and we need both behavioral and imaging studies to help us understand the nature of these responses compared to other types of intentional and automatic imitative responses.

Treatment of Imitation Difficulties

One aspect of the general research agenda for autism focuses on developing more effective treatments for autism, and as such, imitation provides us with a potentially important tool. Intervention studies have demonstrated that imitation skills are quite responsive to contingencies and teaching (as are other early deficits in autism, including language, joint attention, and play skills, to name a few). If the developmental theories of imitation in autism continue to be supported by increasing evidence, then early development of imitative capacity in very young children with autism may have a marked effect on outcomes (see Sallows & Graupner, 2005, for positive evidence). The extent to which interventions that develop improved intentional imitation also result in more normalized automatic imitation is completely unexplored but of potentially great importance.

We have raised a number of areas in which further research is clearly needed. The importance of imitation problems in the ontogeny of the syndrome is unknown, and the question awaits research on starting-state imitation, examination of imitative responses during the period of symptom onset, in both regressed and early onset cases, and the role of various types of imitation in other aspects of both typical and atypical social development. However, 15 years of imitation research in autism have provided strong support for the centrality and pervasiveness of the difficulties that people with autism have in coordinating self with other at the bodily level as well as the psychological level.

ACKNOWLEDGMENTS

Sally J. Rogers's work was partially supported by Grant No. U19 HD35468 from the National Institute of Child Health and Human Development and Grant Nos. R21 MH0673631, R01 MH068398, and R01 MH068232 from the National Institutes of Health. Debra Galik's assistance with manuscript preparation is gratefully acknowledged. Dr. Williams's work was supported by grants from the Health Foundation and the National Alliance for Autism Research.

REFERENCES

Abell, F., Krams, M., Ashburner, J., Passingham, R., Friston, K., Frackowiak, R., et al. (1999).The neuroanatomy of autism: A voxel-based whole brain analysis of structural scans. *Neuroreport, 10,* 1647–1651.

Aldridge, M. A., Stone, K. R., Sweeney, M. H., & Bower, T. G. R. (2000). Preverbal children with autism understand intentions of others. *Developmental Science, 3,* 294–301.

Astafiev, S. V., Stanley, C. M., Shulman, G. L., & Corbetta, M. (2004). Extrastriate body area in human occipital cortex responds to the performance of motor actions. *Nature Neuroscience, 7,* 542–548.

Avikainen, S., Wohlschlager, A., & Hari, R. (2003). Impaired mirror-image imitation in Asperger and high-functioning autistic subjects. *Current Biology, 13,* 339–341.

Baldwin, J. M. (1906). Social and ethical interpretations in mental development. New York: Macmillan.

Bandura, A., Ross, D., & Ross, S. A. (1963). Vicarious reinforcement and imitative learning. *Journal of Abnormal and Social Psychology, 67,* 601–607.

Baron-Cohen, S., Leslie, A. M., & Frith, U. (1985). Does the autistic child have a "theory of mind"? *Cognition, 21,* 37–46.

Bauman, M. L., & Kemper, T. L. (1998). Histoanatomic observations of the brain in early infantile autism. *Neurology, 35,* 866–874.

Beadle-Brown, J., & Whiten, A. (2004). Elicited imitation in children and adults with autism: Is there a deficit? *Journal of Intellectual and Development Disability, 29,* 147–163.

Bennetto, L. (1999). A componental approach of imitation and movement deficits in autism. *Dissertation Abstracts International, 60*(2B), 0819.

Bernabei, P., Penton, G., Fabrizi, P., Camaioni, L., & Perucchini, P. (2003). Profiles of sensorimotor development in children with autism and with developmental delay. *Perceptual and Motor Skills, 96,* 1107–1116.

Bruner, J. (1972). Nature and uses of immaturity. *American Psychologist, 27,* 687–708.

Buccino, G., Binkofski, F., Fink, G. R., Fadiga, L., Fogassi, L., Gallese, V., et al. (2001). Action observation activates premotor and parietal areas in a somatotopic manner: An fMRI study. *European Journal of Neuroscience, 13,* 400–404.

Byrne, R. W., & Whiten, A. (1988). Tactical deception of familiar individuals in baboons. In R. W. Bryne & A. Whiten (Eds.), *Machiavellian intelligence: Social expertise and the evolution of intellect in monkeys, apes, and human* (pp. 205–210). Oxford, UK: Clarendon.

Carpenter, M., Pennington, B. F., & Rogers, S. J. (2001). Understanding of others' intentions in children with autism. *Journal of Autism and Developmental Disorders, 31,* 589–599.

Castelli, F., Frith, C., Happe, F., & Frith, U. (2002). Autism, Asperger syndrome and brain mechanisms for the attribution of mental states to animated shapes. *Brain, 125*(Pt. 8), 1839–1849.

Charman, T., & Baron-Cohen, S. (1994). Another look at imitation in autism. *Development and Psychopathology, 6,* 403–413.

Charman, T., Baron-Cohen, S., Swettenham, J., Baird, G., Drew, A., & Cox, A. (2003). Predicting language outcome in infants with autism and pervasive developmental disorder. *International Journal of Language and Communication Disorders, 38,* 265–285.

Charman, T., Swettenham, J., Baron-Cohen, S., Cox, A., Baird, G., & Drew, A. (1997). Infants with autism: An investigation of empathy, pretend play, joint attention, and imitation. *Developmental Psychology, 33,* 781–789.

Curcio, F. (1978). Sensorimotor functioning and communication in mute autistic children. *Journal of Autism and Childhood Schizophrenia, 8,* 281–292.

Damasio, A. R., & Maurer, R. G. (1978). A neurological model for childhood autism. *Archives of Neurology, 35,* 777–786.

Dapretto, M., Davies, M. S., Pfiefer, J. H., Scott, A. A., Sigman, M., Bookheimer, S. Y., & Iacoboni, M. (2006). Understanding emotions in others: Mirror neuron dysfunction in children with autism spectrum disorders. *Nature Neuroscience, 9*(1), 28–30.

Dawson, G., & Galpert, L. (1990). Mothers' use of imitative play for facilitating social responsiveness and toy play in young autistic children. *Development and Psychopathology, 2,* 151–162.

Dawson, G., & Lewy, A. (1989). Arousal, attention, and the socio-emotional impairments of individuals with autism. In G. Dawson (Ed.), *Autism: Nature, diagnosis, and treatment* (pp. 49–74). New York: Guilford Press.

Dawson, G., Munson, J., Estes, A., Osterling, J., McPartland, J., Toth, K., et al. (2002). Neurocognitive function and joint attention ability in young children with autism spectrum disorder versus developmental delay. *Child Development, 73,* 345–358.

Dawson, G., Toth, K., Abbott, R., Osterling, J., Munson, J., & Liaw, J. (2004). Defining the early social attention impairments in autism: Social orienting, joint attention, and responses to emotions. *Developmental Psychology, 40*(2), 271–283.

DeMyer, M. K., Alpern, G. D., Barton, S., DeMyer, W. E., Churchill, D. W., Hingtgen, J. N., et al. (1972). Imitation in autistic, early schizophrenic, and nonpsychotic subnormal children. *Journal of Autism and Childhood Schizophrenia, 2,* 264–287.

di Pellegrino, G., Fadiga, L., Fogassi, L., Gallese, V., & Rizzolatti, G. (1992). Understanding motor events: A neurophysiological study. *Experimental Brain Research, 91,* 176–180.

Donald, M. (1991). *Origins of the modern mind.* Cambridge, UK: Harvard University Press.

Escalona, A., Field, T., Nadel, J., & Lundy, B. (2002). Brief report: Imitation effects on children with autism. *Journal of Autism and Developmental Disorders, 32,* 141–146.

Fein, D., Pennington, B. F., Markowitz, P., Braverman, M., & Waterhouse, L. (1986). Toward a neuropsychological model of infantile autism: Are the social deficits primary? *Journal of the American Academy of Child and Adolescent Psychiatry, 25,* 198–212.

Fogassi, L., Ferrari, P. F., Geseriech, B., Rozzi, S., Chersi, F., & Rizzolatti, G. (2005). Parietal lobe: From action organization to intention understanding. *Science, 308,* 661–7667.

Gaffan, D. (2005). Widespread cortical networks underlie memory and attention. *Science, 309,* 2172–2173.

Gallese, V., Keysers, C., & Rizzolatti, G. (2004). A unifying view of the basis of social cognition. *Trends in Cognitive Sciences, 8,* 396–403.

Garfinkle, A. N., & Schwartz, I. S. (2002). Peer imitation: Increasing social interactions in children with autism and other developmental disabilities in inclusive preschool classrooms. *Topics in Early Childhood Special Education, 22,* 26–38.

Gergely, G., & Watson, J. S. (1999). Early socio-emotional development: Contingency perception and the social-biofeedback model. In P. Rochat (Ed.), *Early social cognition: Understanding others in the first months of life* (pp. 101–136). Mahwah, NJ: Erlbaum.

Green, D., Baird, G., Barnett, A. L., Henderson, L., Huber, J., & Henderson, S. E. (2002). The severity and nature of motor impairment in Asperger's syndrome: A comparison with specific developmental disorder of motor function. *Journal of Child Psychology and Psychiatry and Allied Disciplines, 43,* 655–668.

Griffith, E. M., Pennington, B. F., Wehner, E. A., & Rogers, S. J. (1999). Executive functions in young children with autism. *Child Development, 70,* 817–832.

Hammes, J. G., & Langdell, T. (1981). Precursors of symbol formation and childhood autism. *Journal of Autism and Developmental Disorders, 11,* 331–346.

Hardan, A. Y., Minshew, N. J., & Keshavan, M. S. (2000). Corpus callosum size in autism. *Neurology, 55,* 1033–1036.

Harris, S. L., Handleman, J. S., & Fong, P. L. (1987). Imitation of self-stimulation: Impact on the autistic child's behavior and affect. *Child and Family Behavior Therapy, 9,* 1–21.

Hatfield, E., Cacioppo, J. T., & Rapson, R. L. (1994). *Emotion contagion.* New York: Cambridge University Press.

Heilman, K. M. (1979). Apraxia. In K. M. Heilman & E. Valenstein (Eds.), *Clinical neuropsychology* (pp. 159–185). New York: Oxford University Press.

Heimann, M., & Ullstadius, E. (1999). Neonatal imitation and imitation among children with autism and Down's syndrome. In J. Nadel & G. Butterworth (Eds.), *Imitation in infancy* (pp. 235–253). Cambridge, UK: Cambridge University Press.

Hobson, R. P., & Lee, A. (1999). Imitation and identification in autism. *Journal of Child Psychology and Psychiatry, 40,* 649–660.

Hoon, A. H., & Reiss, A. L. (1992). The mesial-temporal lobe and autism: Case report and review. *Developmental Medicine and Child Neurology, 34,* 252–265.

Iacoboni, M., Woods, R. P., Brass, M., Bekkering, H., Mazziotta, J. C., & Rizzolatti, G. (1999). Cortical mechanisms of human imitation. *Science, 286,* 2526–2528.

Ingersoll, B., Schreibman, L., & Tran, Q. H. (2003). Effect of sensory feedback on immediate object imitation in children with autism. *Journal of Autism and Developmental Disorders, 33,* 673–683.

Jellema, T., Baker, C. I., Oram, M. W., & Perrett, D. I. (2002). Cell populations in the banks of the superior temporal sulcus of the macaque and imitation. In A. N. Meltzoff & W. Prinz (Eds.), *The imitative mind: Development, evolution, and brain bases* (pp. 267–290). Cambridge, UK: Cambridge University Press.

Just, M. A., Cherkassky, V. L., Keller, T. A., & Minshew, N. J. (2004). Cortical activation and synchronization during sentence comprehension in high-functioning autism: Evidence of underconnectivity. *Brain, 127*(Pt. 8), 1811–1821.

Kalmanson, B. (1987). Infant–parent psychotherapy with an autistic toddler. *Infant Mental Health Journal, 8,* 382–396.

Kasari, C., Sigman, M., Mundy, P., & Yirmiya, N. (1990). Affective sharing in the context of joint attention interactions of normal, autistic, and mentally retarded children. *Journal of Autism and Developmental Disorders, 20,* 87–100.

Keysers, C., & Perrett, D. I. (2004). Demystifying social cognition: A Hebbian perspective. *Trends in Cognitive Sciences, 8,* 501–507.

Klin, A., Jones, W., Schultz, R., Volkmar, F., & Cohen, D. (2002). Visual fixation patterns during viewing of naturalistic social situations as predictors of social competence in individuals with autism. *Archives of General Psychiatry, 59,* 809–816.

Libby, S., Powell, S., Messer, D., & Jordan, R. (1997). Imitation of pretend play-acts by children with autism and Down syndrome. *Journal of Autism and Developmental Disorders, 27,* 365–383.

McEvoy, R. E., Rogers, S. J., & Pennington, B. F. (1993). Executive function and social communication deficits in young autistic children. *Journal of Child Psychology and Psychiatry, 34*, 563–578.

McIntosh, D. N., Reichmann-Decker, A., Winkielman, P., & Wilbarger, J. L. (in press). When the social mirror breaks: Deficits in automatic, but not voluntary mimicry of emotional facial expressions in autism. *Developmental Science.*

Meltzoff, A., & Moore, M. K. (1977). Imitation of facial and manual gestures by human neonates. *Science, 198*, 75–78.

Meltzoff, A. N. (1995). Understanding the intentions of others: Re-enactment of intended acts by 18-month-old children. *Developmental Psychology, 31*, 838–850.

Meltzoff, A. N., & Moore, M. K. (1989). Imitation in newborn infants: Exploring the range of gestures imitated and the underlying mechanisms. *Developmental Psychology, 25*, 954–962.

Meyer, J., & Hobson, R. P. (2004). Orientation in relation to self and other; the case of autism. *Interaction Studies, 5*, 221–244.

Milne, E. Swettenham, J. Hansen, P., Campbell, R., Jeffries, H., & Plaisted, K. (2002). High motion coherence thresholds in children with autism. *Journal of Child Psychology and Psychiatry, 43*, 255–263.

Milner, A. D., & Goodale, M. A. (1995). *The visual brain in action.* Oxford, UK: Oxford University Press.

Mundy, P., Sigman, M., Ungerer, J., & Sherman, T. (1987). Nonverbal communication and play correlates of language development in autistic children. *Journal of Autism and Developmental Disorders, 17*, 349–364.

Nagell, K., Olguin, R. S., & Tomasello, M. (1993). Processes of social learning in the tool use of chimpanzees (Pan troglodytes) and human children (*Homo sapiens*). *Journal of Comparative Psychology, 107*, 174–186.

Nikopoulos, C. K., & Keenan, M. (2003). Promoting social initiation in children with autism using video modeling. *Behavioral Interventions, 18*, 87–108.

Nishitani, N., Avikainen, S., & Hari, R. (2004). Abnormal imitation-related cortical activation sequences in Asperger's syndrome. *Annals of Neurology, 55*, 558–562.

Oberman, L. M., Hubbard, E. M., McCleery, J. P., Altschuler, E. L., Ramachandran, V. S., & Pineda, J. A. (2005). EEG evidence for mirror neuron dysfunction in autism spectrum disorders. *Cognitive Brain Research, 24*, 190–198.

Ohta, M. (1987). Cognitive disorders of infantile autism: A study employing the WISC, spatial relationships, conceptualization, and gestural imitation. *Journal of Autism and Developmental Disorders, 17*, 45–62.

Ozonoff, S., Strayer, D. L., McMahon, W. M., & Filloux, F. (1994). Executive function abilities in autism and Tourette syndrome: An information processing approach. *Journal of Child Psychology and Psychiatry, 35*, 1015–1032.

Pennington, B. F., & Ozonoff, S. (1991). A neuroscientific perspective on continuity and discontinuity in developmental psychopathology. In D. Cicchetti & S. L. Toth (Eds.), *Rochester Symposium on Developmental Psychopathology, Volume 3: Models and integrations.* Rochester, NY: University of Rochester Press.

Perrett, D. I., Harries, M. H., Bevan, R., Thomas, S. Benson, P. J., Chitty, A. J., et al. (1989). Frameworks of analysis for the neural representation of animate objects and actions. *Journal of Exploratory Biology, 146*, 87–113.

Petrides, M., Cadoret, G., & Mackey, S. (2005). Orofacial somatomotor responses in the macaque monkey homologue of Broca's area. *Nature, 435*, 1235–1238.

Piaget, J. (1962). *Play, dreams, and imitation in childhood.* New York: Norton.

Piven, J., Bailey, J., Ranson, B. J., & Arndt, S. (1997). An MRI study of the corpus callosum in autism. *American Journal of Psychiatry, 154*(8), 1051–1056.

Prior, M. (1979). Cognitive abilities and disabilities in infantile autism: A review. *Journal of Abnormal Child Psychology, 7,* 357–380.

Rizzolatti, G., & Arbib, M. A. (1998). Language within our grasp. *Trends in Neuroscience, 21,* 188–194.

Rogers, S. J., Bennetto, L., McEvoy, R., & Pennington, B. F. (1996). Imitation and pantomime in high functioning adolescents with autism spectrum disorders. *Child Development, 6,* 2060–2073.

Rogers, S. J., Hepburn, S. L., & Stackhouse, T. (2003). Imitation performance in toddlers with autism and those with other developmental disorders. *Journal of Child Psychology and Psychiatry and Allied Disciplines, 44,* 763–781.

Rogers, S. J., & Pennington, B. F. (1991). A theoretical approach to the deficits in infantile autism. *Development and Psychopathology, 3,* 137–162.

Sallows, G. O., & Graupner, T. D. (2005). Intensive behavioral treatment for children with autism: Four-year outcome and predictors. *American Journal on Mental Retardation, 110,* 417–438.

Scambler, D. J., Hepburn, S., Rutherford, M. D., Wehner, E., & Rogers, S. J. (in press). Emotional responsivity in children with autism children with other developmental disabilities, and children with typical developments. *Journal of Autism and Developmental Disorders.*

Semmes, J., Weinstein, S., Ghent, L., & Teuber, H. L. (1963). Correlates of impaired orientation in personal and extra personal space. *Brain, 86,* 747–772.

Sigman, M., & Ungerer, J. (1984). Cognitive and language skills in autistic, mentally retarded, and normal children. *Developmental Psychology, 20,* 293–302.

Sigman, M. D., Kasari, C., Kwon, J. H., & Yirmiya, N. (1992). Responses to the negative emotions of others by autistic, mentally retarded, and normal children. *Child Development, 63,* 796–807.

Skinner, B. F. (1957). *Verbal behavior.* Englewood Cliffs, NJ: Prentice Hall.

Smith, I. M., & Bryson, S. E. (1998). Gesture imitation in autism I: Nonsymbolic postures and sequences. *Cognitive Neuropsychology, 15,* 747–770.

Spencer, J., O'Brien, J., Riggs, K., Braddick, O., Atkinson, J., & Wattam-Bell, J. (2000). Motion processing in autism: Evidence for a dorsal stream deficiency. *Neuroreport, 11*(12), 2765–2767.

Stern, D. N. (1985). *The interpersonal world of the human infant.* New York: Basic Books.

Stone, W. L., Ousley, O. Y., & Littleford, C. D. (1997). Motor imitation in young children with autism: What's the object? *Journal of Abnormal Child Psychology, 25,* 475–485.

Stone, W. L., & Yoder, P. J. (2001). Predicting spoken language level in children with autism spectrum disorders. *Autism, 5,* 341–361.

Theoret, H., Halligan, E., Kobayashi, M., Fregni, F., Tager-Flusberg, H., & Pascual-Leone, A. (2005). Impaired motor facilitation during action observation in individuals with autism spectrum disorder. *Current Biology, 15,* R84.

Thiebaut de Schotten, M., Urbanski, M., Duffau, H., Volle, E., Levy, R., Dubois, B., & Bartolomeo, P. (2005). Direct evidence for a parietal–frontal pathway subserving spatial awareness in humans. *Science, 309,* 2226–2228.

Trevarthen, C., & Aitken, K. J. (2001). Infant intersubjectivity: Research, theory, and clinical applications. *Journal of Child Psychology and Child Psychiatry, 42,* 3–48.

Ungerer, J. A., & Sigman, M. D. (1987). Categorization skills and receptive language development in autistic children. *Journal of Autism and Developmental Disorders, 17,* 3–16.

Užgiris, I. C., & Hunt, J. M. (1975). *Assessment in infancy: Ordinal scales of psychological assessment.* Urbana: University of Illinois Press.

Waiter, G. D., Williams, J. H. G., Murray, A. D., Gilchrist, A., Perrett, D. I., & Whiten, A. (2004). Structural white matter deficits in high-functioning individuals with autism spectrum disorder: A voxel-based investigation. *NeuroImage, 22*(2), 619–625.

Want, S. C., & Harris, P. L. (2002). How do children ape? Applying concepts from the study of non-human primates to the developmental study of "imitation" in children. *Developmental Science, 5*, 1–41.

Wert, B. Y., & Neisworth, J. T. (2003). Effects of video self-modeling on spontaneous requesting in children with autism. *Journal of Positive Behavior Interventions, 5*, 30–35.

Williams, J. H. G., Massaro, D.W., Peel, N. J., Bosseler, A., & Suddendorf, T. (2004). Visual–auditory integration during speech imitation in autism. *Research in Developmental Disabilities, 25*, 559–575.

Williams, J. H. G., Waiter, G. D., Gilchrist, A., Perrett, D. I., Murray, A. D., & Whiten, A. (2006). Neural mechanisms of imitation and "mirror neuron" functioning in autistic spectrum disorder. *Neuropsychologia, 44*, 610–621.

Williams, J. H. G., Whiten, A., & Singh, T. (2004). A systematic review of action imitation in autistic spectrum disorder. *Journal of Autism and Developmental Disorders, 34*, 285–299.

Williams, J. H. G., Whiten, A., Suddendorf, T., & Perrett, D. I. (2001). Imitation, mirror neurons and autism. *Neuroscience and Biobehavioral Reviews, 25*, 287–295.

Yirmiya, N., Kasari, C., Sigman, M., & Mundy, P. (1989). Facial expressions of affect in autistic, mentally retarded and normal children. *Journal of Child Psychology and Psychiatry, 30*, 725–735.

Zelazo, P. R. (2001). A developmental perspective on early autism: Affective, behavioral, and cognitive factors. In J. A. Burack, T. Charman, N. Yirmiya, & P. R. Zelazo (Eds.), *The development of autism: Perspectives from theory and research* (pp. 39–60). Mahwah, NJ: Erlbaum.

Zwaigenbaum, L., Bryson, S., Rogers, T., Roberts, W., Brian, J., & Szatmari, P. (2005). Behavioral manifestations of autism in the first year of life. *International Journal of Developmental Neuroscience, 23*, 143–152.

CHAPTER 13

Longitudinal Research on Motor Imitation in Autism

SUSAN L. HEPBURN
WENDY L. STONE

Motor imitation is a pivotal social cognitive process that results from—and contributes to—a host of developmental accomplishments. The act of imitation involves social, motivational, perceptual, motor, cognitive, and representational components. At the most basic level, an imitator must be not only capable of observing the actions of another person but also motivated to do so. He or she must have the representational skills to translate the observed behavior into an action plan, as well as the motor capabilities for carrying out the plan.

Considering the underlying social components and cross-modal complexities inherent in the process of imitation, it is not surprising that individuals with autism would have difficulties in this developmental domain. Over the past 30 years, research comparing the imitation skills of individuals with autism to comparison samples matched on chronological age, mental age, and/or language abilities has consistently revealed impaired imitation abilities in the groups with autism. There is now substantial evidence that the imitation deficit in autism emerges early, is specifically impaired relative to children with other developmental disabilities, and is evident at different ages (Meltzoff & Prinz, 2002; Nadel & Butterworth, 1999; Williams, Whiten, & Singh, 2004). Perhaps the most remarkable aspect of these consistent findings is the fact that they were obtained by studies that have differed markedly in the manner in which imitation was conceptualized and measured.

While group comparison studies have clearly demonstrated the existence of an imitation deficit in autism, it is only through longitudinal research that we will be able to fully understand the causes and consequences of this impairment for individuals with autism. Longitudinal research on imitation in individuals with autism has the potential to shed light not only on the developmental

changes in imitation abilities that occur over time but also on the skills and processes underlying the development of imitation, and on the effects that individual differences in imitation ability may have on development in other domains.

The need for a dynamic approach to the study of symptom development
in autism and other developmental disorders has been acknowledged by several authors (Burack, Charman, Yirmiya, & Zelazo, 2001; Oliver, Johnson,
Karmiloff-Smith, & Pennington, 2000). Burack and colleagues (2001) have
emphasized the importance of longitudinal studies of behavior development in
autism that examine the *rate* (i.e., timing of emergence of specific skills or deficits); *structure* (i.e., characteristic developmental progression of specific
skills); *concurrent processes* (i.e., interrelationships among skills); and *developmental precursors* (i.e., specific skills that are necessary and/or sufficient for
the development of others). Such studies would increase our understanding
of developmental sequences, reciprocal influences between developmental
domains, discontinuities in development, and directionality of influence.

This chapter reviews the longitudinal research that has been conducted
on motor imitation skills in individuals with autism. We describe studies that
have provided information about the developmental changes in imitation that
occur over time, as well as studies that have contributed to our knowledge of
the developmental precursors and developmental sequelae of imitation development and deficits. The emphasis of this chapter is on studies employing longitudinal designs. However, research using cross-sectional methods and comparing single-age samples are also included to the extent that they illuminate
developmental trends. Differences between imitation development in autism
and in comparison samples (especially those with typical development) are
highlighted. Following are some of the specific questions guiding this review:

- How do imitation abilities change over time for individuals with
  autism? Does the nature of the imitation deficit change with development?
- What types of prerequisite skills or behaviors underlie the ability to
  imitate in individuals with autism? To what extent do early disorders
  in social, representational, and motor skills contribute to the imitation
  deficit?
- How do imitation skills in young children affect the subsequent development of social, emotional, communication, and language skills?
  What role does an early emerging imitation deficit have on the developing phenotype of autism?

DEVELOPMENTAL COURSE OF IMITATION

This section reviews our knowledge about the course of development of imitation skills in children with autism. We begin with an overview of imitation
development in normative samples and then turn to studies of imitation devel-

opment in children with autism. The primary question to be addressed in this section is how different types of imitation change over time in children with autism.

Imitation Development in Typically Developing Children

Nichols (2005) provides an elegant history of imitation research in children with typical development. She suggests that although early developmental theorists wrote extensively about the importance of imitation in development (Piaget, 1945/1962; Vygotsky, 1978), few empirical studies have been conducted on the development of imitation skills across time, particularly from the neonatal period to toddlerhood.

Longitudinal research with typically developing infants suggests a developmental progression in imitation ability that is characterized by an overall increase in the amount and diversity of actions that are imitated across the first year of life, with some discontinuity in the types of actions that are imitated at different ages (Heimann & Ullstadius, 1999; Kugiumutzakis, 1999). Heimann and Ullstadius (1999) studied the development of elicited imitation of simple motor actions and facial movements across the first year of life and found that neonatal imitation was not related to imitation at 12 months. In contrast, correlations between imitation at 3 months and 12 months were found. Correlations among specific behaviors indicated that tongue protrusion at 3 months was correlated with vocal imitation at 12 months, and mouth opening at 3 months was correlated with actions on objects at 12 months.

Through cross-sectional studies, other researchers have demonstrated that imitation skills increase dramatically between 9 and 12 months of age (Abravenel, Leven-Goldschmidt, & Stevenson, 1976). Nadel (Chapter 6, this volume) describes the developmental trajectory of peer imitation skills in typically developing children as discontinuous, with improving skills from 12 months onward with peak performance at 30 months and a decline in spontaneous imitation of actions between 42 and 46 months. She links this decline with the emergence of language, which reduces the need to rely on imitation skills as a primary communication system.

Imitation research with typically developing children has also revealed developmental trends in the emergence of *different types* of imitation skills. Guided in large part by Piagetian theory, studies have examined the type of actions (e.g., familiar/novel and visible/invisible) that children are able to imitate at different ages. True to prediction, the age of emergence of imitation skills in typical development appears to vary according to the type of imitation studied (Užgiris, 1999). In general, simple, familiar actions are imitated earliest, followed by the development of more complex and novel imitated actions (Masur & Ritz, 1984; McCabe & Užgiris, 1983; Piaget, 1945/1962). The absence or presence of visible feedback also affects gestural imitation within the first year of life (Masur, 1993), with imitation of visible gestures emerging at approximately 6 months and imitation of invisible gestures (e.g., head shake) emerging around 1 year (Kaye & Marcus, 1981; Masur & Ritz, 1984).

Other dimensions of imitation acts have also been studied. Two- to 3-week-old infants have been shown to imitate facial movements (Meltzoff & Moore, 1977), 6-month-olds begin to imitate simple hand movements (Meltzoff & Moore, 1999; Vinter, 1986), and gestural imitations improve between 6 and 9 months (Barr, Dowden, & Hayne, 1996; Heimann & Meltzoff, 1996; Meltzoff, 1988). Imitative actions on objects have been shown to emerge between 6 and 9 months (Meltzoff, 1988; Piaget, 1952) and develop through the first 2 years of life (Abravenel et al., 1976; Killen & Užgiris, 1981; Masur, 1993; Pawlby, 1977; Rogdon & Kurdek, 1977). Infants up to 20 months old are more likely to imitate actions on objects than to imitate gestural acts (Abravenel et al., 1976; Masur & Ritz, 1984; Rogdon & Kurdek, 1977; Snow, 1989). Similarly, infants up to 17 months are more likely to imitate meaningful, as opposed to nonmeaningful, actions (Killen & Užgiris, 1981; Masur & Ritz, 1984; McCabe & Užgiris, 1983). By 22 months, most infants are imitating both meaningful and nonmeaningful actions (Killen & Užgiris, 1981; McCabe & Užgiris, 1983). Imitation of sequences of actions emerges later in toddlerhood (McCall, Parke, & Kavanaugh, 1977).

In summary, the imitation skills of typically developing children increase across development in terms of the complexity and novelty of acts imitated, as well as the precision of the imitation act (Nichols, 2005; Užgiris, 1999). The results of imitation research with typically developing children are important for several reasons: (1) they illuminate the developmental nature of imitation ability; (2) they suggest specific ages at which the emergence of different types of imitation might be expected; and (3) they provide a framework for considering different dimensions of imitation tasks. Table 13.1 presents some of the dimensions studied. As we shall see, imitation research in autism has only recently begun to take a developmental approach that acknowledges the impact of specific dimensions of the imitation task on the performance of young children.

TABLE 13.1. Dimensions of Motor Imitation Tasks Used with Typically Developing Children

Dimension	Examples
Type of motoric response	• Manual–gestural • Oral–facial • Body movements • Actions with objects
Complexity of motor demands	• Single-step actions versus sequential actions
Availability of visual feedback	• Visible actions versus invisible actions
Degree of novelty	• Familiar–conventional actions versus unfamiliar–unconventional actions

Imitation Development in Children with Autism

At present, only two longitudinal investigations of imitation development in children with autism have been published. Stone, Ousley, and Littleford (1997) used the Motor Imitation Scale (MIS) to compare the performance of 2-year-old children with autism to that of children with developmental delay and children with typical development who were matched on mental age and expressive language. Two types of single-step imitation were assessed by the MIS: imitation of body movements and imitation of actions with objects. Longitudinal data on the MIS at age 2 and age 3 were collected for the children with autism only. Results revealed significant improvement over time for both body imitation and imitation of actions with objects, suggesting that the ability to imitate simple, single-step actions increases with age in children with autism.

Two other findings from this study warrant attention. First, this study provided evidence that *body and object imitation represent independent dimensions*. These two MIS scores were not correlated at age 2 or age 3 in the group with autism. Moreover, the two types of imitation demonstrated different patterns of correlations with other developmental skills. Object imitation was correlated with play skills, whereas body imitation was correlated with expressive vocabulary. Second, results of this study suggest that *imitation of single-step actions may be delayed, rather than disordered*, in children with autism. The children with autism demonstrated a similar pattern of performance on body versus object imitation tasks relative to both comparison groups: All three groups obtained lower scores on body imitation than on object imitation. Furthermore, the MIS scores of the children with autism obtained at age 3 were comparable to those obtained by the children with developmental delay at age 2. Taken together, these findings suggest that the acquisition of simple imitation skills in children with autism lags behind but does not differ qualitatively from, that of developmentally matched comparison children.

Additional information about the developmental course of imitation is available from an independent sample of 35 children with diagnoses of either autism (n = 24) or pervasive developmental disorder not otherwise specified (n = 11) who were assessed with the MIS at ages 2, 3, and 4 (Stone, 2004). Results from this longitudinal sample suggested a dissociation in the pattern of growth between object and body imitation. Increases in object imitation between ages 2 and 4 were linear, reflecting a constant rate of growth over the 2-year period. In contrast, improvements in body imitation were nonlinear, with more change observed between the ages of 2 and 3 than between the ages of 3 and 4 (see Figure 13.1).

The Heimann and Ullstadius (1999) study mentioned previously also included a sample of five children with autism at two time points. The children were seen initially at a mean age of 4 (median age = 54 months, range = 39–62 months, mental age range = 25–51 months) and were evaluated again at approximately 6 years old. A reference group of three 4-year-old children

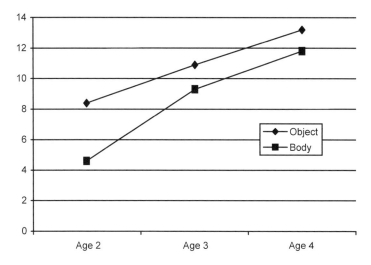

FIGURE 13.1. Changes in imitation from ages 2 to 4 years.

with typical development was also included. All the children with autism improved in imitation skills over time for all types of imitation studied; however, individual child gains were difficult to predict. Relative to the typically developing peers, children with autism demonstrated deficits in imitating simple motor gestures, facial movements, and symbolic actions. Heimann and Ullstadius commented that the imitation improvements observed may have been related to an increased motivation to imitate over time.

Not only is there a dearth of longitudinal studies of imitation in autism, but few cross-sectional studies have been conducted examining imitation skills at different ages. An alternative approach toward understanding the development of different types of imitation in autism, then, is to compare the results of studies that have focused on specific age groups. Most research on imitation has been conducted with young children, but the few studies that have included adolescents and adults have proven to be quite informative in this regard.

Nature of Imitation Deficits in Young Children with Autism

As indicated previously, even single-step imitation tasks prove difficult for young children with autism, though improvement from age 2 to age 3 has been observed (Stone et al., 1997). Further confirmation of improvement in simple imitation tasks comes from studies that have used infant imitation tasks with 7–11-year-olds with autism (whose mental ages fell within 3–5 years); these studies have failed to find impaired performance in the samples with autism relative to controls (Charman & Baron-Cohen, 1994; Morgan, Cutrer, Coplin, & Rodrigue, 1989).

Some studies with young children with autism have assessed dimensions of imitation that parallel those studied with typically developing children. Recall that children with typical development up to about 20 months of age are more likely to imitate object actions than gestures (Abravenel et al., 1976; Masur & Ritz, 1984; Rogdon & Kurdek, 1977; Snow, 1989). This pattern has been found in children with autism as old as 3 years (Stone et al., 1997) and 6 years (DeMyer et al., 1972). Along similar lines, imitation of familiar actions is more common than imitation of unfamiliar actions in typically developing children up to 12 months (Abravenel et al., 1976; Masur & Ritz, 1984; McCabe & Užgiris, 1983; Piaget, 1945/1962). A similar pattern was observed in children with autism as old as 6 years (Dawson & Adams, 1984). These results suggest not only that the pattern of performance of children with autism on these imitation dimensions is similar to that of developmentally younger children but also that the children with autism perform at levels below their own developmental age on these tasks.

Other studies of young children with autism have employed imitation tasks that vary on dimensions that are more specifically related to the learning style and deficits of autism. For example, Ingersoll, Schreibman, and Tran (2003) examined the effect of sensory feedback on object imitation in a group of 2–4-year-olds with autism as compared to a mental age-matched group of typically developing children (1–2 years old). Results revealed improved performance on the toys that provided visual and auditory feedback (compared to those providing no sensory feedback) for the children with autism only. This observation is particularly interesting in light of their finding that both groups of children showed a preference for interacting with the sensory toys during a free-play period.

A study by Stone and colleagues (2004) examined the performance of 2- and 3-year-olds with autism on imitation tasks that varied according to the degree of structure provided. Highly structured tasks were those that were conducted at a table and involved the presentation of materials one at a time. Low-structure imitation tasks were presented during play interactions on the floor, among a variety of toys. Results revealed superior performance in the high-structure condition relative to the low-structure condition. This study also found improvements in imitation over a 6-month period.

In summary, several interesting findings have emerged regarding the development of imitation in young children with autism. First, it appears that early deficits in simple, single-step imitation improve with age. Second, it seems that the specific nature of the imitation task may affect the performance of children with autism to a greater degree than children with typical development. Relative to typically developing children, those with autism show differential performance on different types of imitation tasks for more extended periods and also demonstrate improved performance on imitation tasks that have a sensory component. These results highlight the importance that the type of imitation task may play in the performance of children with autism and have several implications for research designs.

One important implication is the need for studies to carefully consider multiple dimensions when constructing imitation tasks and interpreting findings. As Ingersoll and colleagues (2003) point out, children with autism may not be driven to participate in imitation activities for the social interaction component that may motivate typically developing children. In contrast, the characteristics of the specific task and contextual variables may affect motivation and performance levels (Ingersoll et al., 2003; Stone et al., 2004). If this is the case, it may be very difficult to draw conclusions about imitation abilities in children with autism from studies that have employed different types of tasks to assess the construct of imitation.

On the other hand, these results also point to an important direction for future imitation research in samples of children with autism. The systematic study of performance on different types of imitation tasks has the potential not only to illuminate the systems that are driving imitation performance but also to contribute to our understanding of the mechanisms that children with autism use to learn and to navigate their social environments. Table 13.2 presents a list of different dimensions of the measurement *context* (as opposed to the types of imitation *tasks* that are presented in Table 13.1) that may be important to consider in assessing imitation in children with autism.

Nature of Imitation Deficits in Older Individuals with Autism

There are far fewer imitation studies that have included adolescents and/or adults. The studies that exist suggest that deficits in imitation in older samples may reflect difficulty with more complex actions (Rogers, 1999; Rogers, Bennetto, McEvoy, & Pennington, 1996) or differences in "attitude" or "style" of imitation rather then impairments in imitation of basic motoric actions (Hobson & Lee, 1999).

Rogers and colleagues (1996) studied imitation and pantomime abilities in 17 adolescents with high-functioning autism, as compared to 15 adolescents with various developmental disorders. Participants ranged in age from

TABLE 13.2. Dimensions of Measurement Contexts Used in Assessment of Motor Imitation

Dimension	Examples
Setting	• Clinic/lab versus natural environment
Imitative model	• Adult versus peer • Live versus videotape
Response type	• Spontaneous versus prompted
Type of reward	• Intrinsic (e.g., mastery and pride) • Extrinsic (e.g., tangible and sensory) • Social
Scoring approach	• Quantitative (e.g., accuracy) • Qualitative (e.g., fluency)

11 to 21 years and had Verbal IQ scores above 69. Three types of imitation tasks were presented: those involving hand movements, face movements, and pantomime tasks (i.e., pretending to complete an action with and without an object, such as brushing hair). Each type of task included items involving single actions, sequences, meaningful actions, and nonmeaningful actions. Control tasks for motor ability and memory skills were also included in the battery. Adolescents with autism were significantly more impaired than the comparison sample on all three types of imitation tasks, with pantomine tasks and tasks involving nonmeaningful or sequential actions presenting the greatest challenge. Neither motor ability nor memory abilities influenced task performance. There were no significant differences between the groups on imitating single hand actions (meaningful or not), single meaningful facial actions, or pantomime of single actions with the objects present.

Hobson and Lee (1999) compared the performance of 16 adolescents with autism to 16 adolescents with mild mental retardation on an imitation battery and examined their proficiency in copying the specific motor acts, as well as the qualitative or stylistic aspects (e.g., "harsh" or "gentle") of the imitative behavior. Participants in the two groups were roughly matched on chronological age (9 –18 years) and verbal ability (4–7 years). Imitation tasks were all goal-directed, novel actions involving objects. The adolescents with autism demonstrated no impairments in the imitation of specific motoric acts (immediate or delayed) but did differ in style from the model significantly more often than the participants in the comparison group. Specifically, 11 of 16 participants with autism failed to imitate style for *any* of the tasks, whereas none of the comparison participants showed this pattern. Thirteen of 16 comparison participants imitated style on at least two of three tasks; however, only one participant with autism imitated style more than once. In addition, participants with autism were more likely to make errors of orientation while imitating; they did not take the perspective of their observer but, rather, oriented the actions to themselves. Hobson and Lee interpreted these results as indicating difficulties with the differentiation of self and other and suggested that the imitation deficit in autism reflects a core difficulty in intersubjectivity.

In summary, fewer studies of developmental change in imitation ability have been conducted in samples with autism relative to samples with typical development. There has been less attention to overall changes in abilities over time, as well as to changes in performance on different types of imitation tasks. Nevertheless, the results of research reviewed in this section suggest that: (1) imitation impairments in individuals with autism are present at least through adolescence; and (2) the nature of the deficit changes over time. While the ability to imitate simple, single-step imitation improves, difficulties imitating more complex or sequential actions and more subtle and stylistic aspects of the modeled act become more apparent with advancing age. In addition, there is emerging evidence for differential performance on different types of imitation tasks (e.g., those with and without sensory components) and in different imitation contexts (e.g., high vs. low levels of structure) that needs to be considered in designing and interpreting imitation studies with children with autism. Moreover, the systematic study of performance on different types of imitation tasks is highly recommended as a productive strategy for understanding how imitation develops, progresses, and relates to other developmental skills and accomplishments.

DEVELOPMENTAL PRECURSORS OF IMITATION

It is clear that numerous competencies and skills are involved in the process of imitation. Smith and Bryson (1994) described the need to identify the developmental prerequisites of imitation in autism, suggesting that problems in imitation in autism are secondary to problems in other domains of functioning. Candidate component skills include visual attention, cross-modal transfer, motor production, memory for manipulation of representations, activation of motor act, representation of body schema, formulation of motor plan, holding representation in working memory, initiating a motor plan, and monitoring and correcting the plan (see also Rogers, 1999).

Yando, Seitz, and Zigler (1978) proposed a two-factor theory of imitation in which social/motivational factors and cognitive/motor factors interact to influence the development of imitation skills. Rogers (1999) also described the relative contributions of social–affective and cognitive components of imitation skills. She suggested that as children with autism grow up they learn to use imitation as a cognitive strategy, without the benefit of the affective enrichment. Interactions between impairments in the affective and cognitive components of imitation may help to explain the variability in the skills across time, between diagnostic groups, across age levels, and even within children. Empirical exploration of the relative importance of social/motivational versus cognitive/motor skills in the development of imitation skills in autism could be quite informative, both for developmental theory and for identifying targets for early intervention. Table 13.3 outlines some of the component skills that have been proposed to underlie imitation ability. As we will see, all require further study to identify the role they may play in the developmental of imitation in individuals with autism.

Given the sparseness of longitudinal studies of imitation in children with autism, it should not be surprising that there is even less information about the *predictors* of motor imitation development. One interesting line of research began with a longitudinal study of the development of social cognitive skills in typically developing infants. Carpenter, Nagell, and Tomasello (1998) followed infants from 9 to 15 months and found that social communication skills (e.g., joint attention and attention following) preceded the development of imitation skills in this sample. These results shed some light on potential developmental precursors of imitation in typical development by providing data to suggest that imitation ability has a foundation in early social communication development.

Two research groups used a similar approach to examine developmental sequences in children with autism. Both employed cross-sectional rather than

TABLE 13.3. Proposed Components Underlying the Motor Imitation Deficit in Autism

Underlying component	Source
Affective functioning—imitation impairments stem from a core deficit in emotional attunement with others.	Hobson (1986, 1993); Rogers (1999)
Motor/praxis—imitation impairments are secondary to motor planning difficulties.	Rogers & Pennington (1991); Rogers et al. (2003); Smith & Bryson (1994)
Social overarousal—imitation impairments stem from overstimulation, which leads to social avoidance.	Dawson (1991)
Mental representations—imitation impairments are secondary to problems in information processing.	Ohta (1987); Rogers & Pennington (1991); Smith & Bryson (1994); Stone et al. (1997)
Social motivation—imitation impairments reflect decreased social interest and motivation.	Whiten & Brown (1999); Zelazo, Burack, Boseovski, Jacques, & Frye (2001)

longitudinal designs and examined patterns of development in each skill area for individual children. Carpenter, Pennington, and Rogers (2002) studied group of 3- and 4-year-olds with a diagnosis of either autism or developmental delay. Results revealed that the children with developmental delay demonstrated a developmental progression that was similar to that seen in Carpenter and colleagues' (1998) study (i.e., social communication skills preceded imitation skills). However, the pattern for children with autism was quite different, in that imitation *preceded* (rather than followed) the development of social–communication skills. Turner and colleagues (2003) replicated these results in a different sample of 4-year-olds with autism and also extended the finding to younger ages by observing that the same pattern was observed in the children with autism at 2 years of age. Taken together, these findings suggest that imitation development may have social origins for children with typical development, but not for children with autism.

One study of children with autism examined predictors of improvement in imitation skills between the ages of 2 and 3 (Turner, Pozdol, & Stone, 2002). Imitation was measured using the Screening Tool for Autism in Two-Year-Olds (STAT) (Stone, Coonrod, & Ousley, 2000). Three predictors were examined: age 2 cognitive standard score, age 2 expressive language score, and the number of intervention hours received between age 2 and 3. Results revealed that children's cognitive score was the only predictor of gains in imitation after controlling for age 2 imitation.

Several research groups have examined the *concurrent* relations between imitation and other developmental skills. Although directionality of influence cannot be inferred from these correlational studies, the results do provide us with insight into skills associated with imitation that can be incorporated into future longitudinal studies addressing precursors (or sequelae) of imitation in children with autism.

Concurrent relations between imitation ability and *social skills* have been examined by several research groups. Nadel, Guérini, Pezé, and Rivet (1999) studied imitative behavior in eight dyads of school-age children in which a child with autism was paired with a child with typical development. Strong correlations were found between imitation behaviors and positive (non-imitative) social behaviors, such as seeking proximity and accepting or offering toys. Two studies have examined the effect of *being* imitated on the social behavior of preschool-age children with autism. Results revealed that being imitated was associated concurrently with increased social behaviors, including eye contact, social orienting, social responsiveness, and social initiations (Dawson & Adams, 1984; Tiegerman & Primavera, 1981). Dawson and Adams (1984) suggested that imitating the actions of young children with autism provides a developmentally appropriate opportunity to establish social reciprocity and a sense of mutual connectedness, which is usually effortless for typically developing children.

Ingersoll and colleagues (2003) coded socially oriented and object-oriented behaviors that occurred while children were imitating. Results revealed that children with autism initiated fewer social behaviors (e.g., coordinated joint attention, directing positive affect, and social initiations) during imitation than did typically developing children. No group differences in object-oriented behaviors during imitation were observed. These results are consistent with other observations of decreased initiation of joint attention and shared positive affect in children with autism (e.g., Kasari, Sigman, Yirmiya, & Mundy, 1993; Roeyers, Van Oost, & Bothuyne, 1998) Unfortunately, the relation between children's imitation proficiency and their social behavior was not examined in this study.

Concurrent relations between imitation and *language* have also been found. Sigman and Ungerer (1984) found correlations between elicited object and body imitation and concurrent measures of receptive language in preschoolers with autism. Stone and colleagues (1997) found a concurrent association between body imitation and expressive language in 2-year-old children with autism. Similarly, Rogers, Hepburn, Stackhouse, and Wehner (2003) found that imitation of body gestures was correlated with expressive language ability at the age of 2–3 years.

Rogers and Pennington (1991) suggested that imitation and *executive function skills* may be related, a theory that has been tested by several groups to date. In a sample of preschool-age children with autism, Dawson, Meltzoff, Osterling, and Rinaldi (1998) obtained significant correlations between simple object, facial, and body imitation tasks and tasks involving cognitive flexibility and set shifting (i.e., infant executive function tasks). However, these findings were not replicated by Smith and Bryson (1994), or Bennetto (1999) who did not find relations between object and body imitation and executive function abilities. These studies differed from the previous studies in their inclusion of older, higher-functioning persons with autism.

A recent study sought to determine whether different developmental skills were associated with different types of motor imitation tasks (McDuffie et al., in press). Different patterns of correlations were found for the different tasks in a sample of 2 and 3 year olds with autism. Performance on a structured imitation task was associated with attention following, performance on an observational learning imitation task was associated with both fine motor skills and attention following, and performance on an interactive imitation task was associated with social reciprocity. These results were obtained after controlling for the effect of general cognitive level. Thus it appears that social communicative skills as well as motor skills are related to performance on different types of imitation tasks. Interestingly, Rogers and colleagues (2003) did not find an association between motor skills and imitation for their group of 2–3-year-old children with autism on structured tasks of simple acts with body, acts with objects, and oral–motor acts. Overall developmental level accounted for most of the variance in imitation ability. These findings again highlight the fact that all imitation tasks are not equal, and different tasks may entail different demands in terms of social, cognitive, and motor skills. However, at this point we know very little about the direction of these relations, and the extent to which specific skills might be necessary or sufficient for the development of imitation in autism. The studies by Carpenter and colleagues (1998, 2002) and Turner and colleagues (2002) are perhaps most intriguing in their suggestion of the possibility that imitation may be less driven by social interest for children with autism relative to children with typical development.

DEVELOPMENTAL SEQUELAE OF IMITATION

Imitation has been conceptualized and described as a pivotal skill for early learning and is considered to play an important role in the development in social, cognitive, and language domains, particularly during infancy and early childhood (Nadel, 2002). In the social domain, imitative exchanges are thought to provide the context for early parent–infant interactions, thus helping to establish the foundations of social reciprocity and spontaneous, back-and-forth interactions (Meltzoff & Moore, 1999; Užgiris, 1981). Imitative exchanges also provide opportunities for infants to develop a sense of identity of self and other, which may lead to the development of empathy and perspective taking (Meltzoff & Moore, 1994, 1999). Meltzoff and Gopnik (1993) proposed that early imitation is fundamental for the development of understanding of other's beliefs, attitudes, and intentions. Barresi and Moore (1996) further emphasize that imitative exchanges in infancy are particularly important for building an understanding of others' intentions, which is a precursor to later development of higher-level social–cognitive abilities, such as theory of mind.

In the language domain, imitation is described as contributing to verbal and nonverbal communicative development. Nadel (2002) conceptualizes imitation as a transitory communication system—an essential "initial step" in sharing information with others. Piaget (1945/1962) proposed that early imitation was a precursor to the development of symbolic representations, which, in turn, lead to advances in language and communication. In the cognitive domain, imitation is thought to function as a reliable and efficient problem-solving strategy, enabling the developing infant to rapidly acquire new skills (Užgiris, 1981; Yando et al., 1978). It also provides a context in which children learn about the world and other people, which leads to the ability to form mental representations and develop abstract thought (Piaget, 1945/1962; Smith & Bryson, 1994; Vygotsky, 1978).

Given the hypothesized importance of imitation to development in other key areas, it is surprising that more research has not been conducted to study specific predictive relations. How do individual differences in imitation impact on specific developmental accomplishments at different ages? Are the consequences of early deficits in imitation remediable, or are there lasting sequelae of these early disruptions? Is there a critical period for imitation development, after which time developmental pathways are forever shifted?

Most of the empirical research that has been conducted in this area has focused on the contribution of imitation to language development. A relation between early motor imitation skills and later language has been found in several studies of children with typical development (Bates, Benigni, Bretherton, Camaioni, & Volterra, 1979; Bloom, Hood, & Lightbown, 1974; Snow, 1981, 1989). In addition, the Carpenter and colleagues (1998) study observed that imitation was one of the foundational skills for the development of referential language in their typically developing infants.

Several longitudinal studies with children with autism have suggested a predictive relation between imitation skills and later language. Stone and colleagues (1997) found that imitation skills at age 2 were predictive of expressive language ability at age 3. Stone and Yoder (2001) followed a different set of 35 children with autism spectrum disorders (25 with autism, 11 with pervasive developmental disorder, not otherwise specified) from age 2 to age 4 and measured several child and environmental variables that were considered to be potential predictors of a composite measure of expressive language. Child variables included play skills, motor imitation (assessed by the MIS), and joint attention skills at age 2, and environmental variables included socioeconomic level and the number of hours of speech/language therapy children received between the ages of 2 and 3 years. After controlling for children's initial language levels, the only significant predictors of expressive language at age 4 were age 2 imitation skills and speech–language therapy; stronger motor imitation skills at age 2 and more speech–language therapy between age 2 and 3 were associated with better language at age 4.

Charman and colleagues (2003) also conducted a longitudinal study of predictors of language development. Imitation (actions on objects and body within a structured paradigm), joint attention, and play were measured in infants with autism at 20 months of age, and follow-up assessments of language ability and autism symptom severity were conducted at a mean age of 42 months. Language abilities at the follow-up evaluation were associated with children's earlier motor imitation and joint attention skills, again supporting a predictive relation between imitation and later language. In addition, the Carpenter and colleagues (2002) and Turner and colleagues (2005) studies, though not longitudinal, replicated the pattern found for typical infants by Carpenter and colleagues (1998), in that imitation was found to precede referential language in 2- and 4-year olds with autism.

Despite these fairly consistent findings of a longitudinal relation between imitation and language development in children with autism, a great deal of additional work is needed to understand this phenomenon more fully. For example, future longitudinal research can explore questions about the extent to which imitation is necessary and/or sufficient for the development of language and the nature of the reciprocal relations between imitation and language at different ages and developmental levels. This information will serve not only to improve our understanding of the developing phenotype of autism but also to inform our ability to develop sophisticated and targeted intervention programs for (1) remediating early deficits and (2) minimizing the impact of early deficits on later development and functioning.

CONCLUDING COMMENTS

Although there is ample evidence of an autism-specific deficit in imitation, few longitudinal studies examining the natural history, developmental precursors, or developmental sequelae of imitation in persons with autism have been undertaken. Prospective longitudinal studies will provide important information concerning the timing of emergence of the imitation deficit, the changing nature of the deficit over time, the prerequisite skills underlying imitation development, and the consequences of an imitation deficit for development of key social and communication skills.

Recent methodological and conceptual advances have the potential to lead to significant improvements in the design of longitudinal studies of children with autism. Advances in the early identification of autism have enabled us to study children at very young ages, often before 36 months. Moreover, recognition of the extended behavioral phenotype and genetic vulnerabilities has led to the possibility of assessing imitation skills in very young infant siblings of children with autism (Bryson, Rogers, & Fombonne, 2003). Imitation tasks and batteries for various age groups have been developed and are well described (Charman et al., 1997; Rogers et al., 2003; Stone et al., 1997). In addition, there has been increased attention to specific characteristics, demands, and contexts inherent to different types of imitation tasks, and to the impact that these factors can have on the performance of children with autism. Ideally, this increased awareness will be used to design future studies in which individual dimensions of tasks (e.g., interpersonal context, complexity, and type of reward) are manipulated systematically to disentangle the influences of social, cognitive, and motor skills on performance.

Mervis and Robinson (1999) have advocated for a model of longitudinal analysis that involves the collection of multiple measures on each child, the generation of individual profiles of skills and deficits, and the systematic comparison of individual profiles across groups. They emphasize that intra-individual analysis of a broad range of imitation skills would constitute an important improvement over previous work that has relied primarily on cross-group comparisons. Longitudinal studies of different types of imitation (e.g., object and gestural) in different diagnostic groups (e.g., autism, Down syndrome, and fragile X syndrome) would provide important insight about whether imitation in autism develops in a phenotypic-specific way. Understanding the natural history of imitation skills in autism will contribute to our understanding of the etiology and evolution of symptoms over time, as well as help to focus our intervention efforts on the most relevant, well-timed, and developmentally appropriate goals.

REFERENCES

Abravanel, E., Levan-Goldschmidt, E., & Stevenson, M. B. (1976). Action imitation: The early phase of infancy. *Child Development, 47,* 1032–1044.

Barr, R., Dowden, A., & Hayne, H. (1996). Developmental changes in deferred imitation by 6- to 24-month-old infants. *Infant Behavior and Development, 19,* 159–170.

Barresi, J., & Moore, C. (1996). Intentional relations and social understanding. *Behavioral and Brain Sciences, 19,* 107–154.

Bates, E., Benigni, L., Bretherton, I., Camaioni, L., & Volterra, V. (1979). *The emergence of symbols: Cognition and communication in infancy.* New York: Academic Press.

Bennetto, L. (1999). A componential approach to imitation in autism. *Dissertation Abstracts International, 60*(2-B), 0819.

Bloom, L., Hood, L., & Lightbown, P. (1974). Imitation in language development: If, when and why. *Cognitive Psychology, 76,* 380–420.

Burack, J. A., Charman, T., Yirmiya, N., & Zelazo, P. R. (2001). Development and autism: Messages from developmental psychopathology. In J. A. Burack, T. Charman, N. Yirmiya, & P. R. Zelazo (Eds.), *The development of autism: Perspectives from theory and research.* Mahwah, NJ: Erlbaum.

Carpenter, M., Nagell, K., & Tomasello, M. (1998). Social cognition, joint attention, and communicative competence from 9 to 15 months of age. *Monographs of the Society for Research in Child Development, 63*(4).

Carpenter, M., Pennington, B. F., & Rogers, S.J. (2002). Interrelations among social-cognitive skills in young children with autism. *Journal of Autism and Developmental Disorders, 32,* 91–106.

Charman, T., & Baron-Cohen, S. (1994). Another look at imitation in autism. *Development and Psychopathology, 6,* 403–413.

Charman, T., Swettenham, J., Baron-Cohen, S., Baird, G., Drew, A., & Cox, A. (2003). Predicting language outcomes in infants with autism and pervasive developmental disorder. *International Journal of Language and Communication Disorders, 38,* 265–285.

Charman, T., Swettenham, J., Baron-Cohen, S., Cox, A., Baird, G., & Drew, A. (1997). Infants with autism: An investigation of empathy, pretend play, joint attention, and imitation. *Developmental Psychology, 33*(5), 781–789.

Dawson, G. (1991). A psychobiology perspective on the early socio-emotional development of children with autism. In D. Cicchetti & S. Toth (Eds.), *Rochester symposium on developmental psychopathology* (Vol. 3, pp. 207–234). Rochester, NY: University of Rochester Press.

Dawson, G., & Adams, A. (1984). Imitation and social responsiveness in autistic children. *Journal of Abnormal Child Psychology, 12,* 209–226.

Dawson, G., Meltzoff, A. N., Osterling, J., & Rinaldi, J. (1998). Neuropsychological correlates of early symptoms of autism. *Child Development, 29,* 1276–1285.

DeMyer, M. K., Alpern, G. D., Barton, S., DeMyer, W. E., Churchill, D. W., Hingtgen, J. N., et al. (1972). Imitation in autistic, early schizophrenic, and nonpsychotic subnormal children. *Journal of Autism and Childhood Schizophrenia, 2,* 264–287.

Hammes, J. G. W., & Langdell, T. (1981). Precursors of symbol formation and childhood autism. *Journal of Autism and Developmental Disorders, 11,* 331–346.

Heimann, M., & Meltzoff, A. (1996). Deferred imitation in 9- and 14-month-old infants: A longitudinal study of a Swedish sample. *British Journal of Developmental Psychology, 14,* 55–64.

Heimann, M., & Ullstadius, E. (1999). Neonatal imitation and imitation among children with autism and Down's syndrome. In J. Nadel & G. Butterworth (Eds.), *Imitation in infancy* (pp. 235–253). Cambridge, UK: Cambridge University Press.

Hertzig, M., Snow, M., & Sherman, M. (1989). Affect and cognition in autism. *Journal of the American Academy of Child and Adolescent Psychiatry, 28,* 195–199.

Hobson, R. P. (1986). The autistic child's appraisal of expressions of emotions: A further study. *Journal of Child Psychology and Psychiatry, 27,* 321–342.

Hobson, R. P. (1993). *Autism and the development of mind.* Hove, UK: Erlbaum.

Hobson, R. P., & Lee, A. (1999). Imitation and identification in autism. *Journal of Child Psychology and Psychiatry, 40,* 649–659.

Ingersoll, B., Schreibman, L., & Tran, Q. H. (2003). Effect of sensory feedback on immediate object imitation in children with autism. *Journal of Autism and Developmental Disorders, 33*(6), 673–683.

Kasari, C., Sigman, M., Yirmiya, N., & Mundy, P. (1993). Affective development and communication in young children with autism. In A. Kaiser & D. B. Gray (Eds.), *Enhancing children's communication: Research foundations for intervention* (pp. 201–222). Baltimore: Brookes.

Kaye, K., & Marcus, J. (1981). Infant imitation: The sensory–motor agenda. *Developmental Psychology, 17,* 258–265.

Killen, M., & Užgiris, I. C. (1981). Imitation of actions with objects: The role of social meaning. *Journal of Genetic Psychology, 138,* 219–229.

Kugiumutzakis, G. (1999). Genesis and development of early infant mimesis to facial and vocal models. In J. Nadel & G. Butterworth (Eds.), *Imitation in infancy* (pp. 36–59). Cambridge, UK: Cambridge University Press.

Masur, E. F. (1993). Transitions in representational ability: Infants' verbal, vocal, and action imitation during the second year. *Merrill-Palmer Quarterly, 39,* 437–456.

Masur, E. F., & Ritz, E. G. (1984). Patterns of gestural, vocal, and verbal imitation performance in infancy. *Merrill-Palmer Quarterly, 30,* 369–392.

McCabe, M., & Užgiris, I. C. (1983). Effects of model and action on imitation performance in infancy. *Merrill-Palmer Quarterly, 30,* 69–82.

McCall, R., Parke, R., & Kavanaugh, R. (1977). Imitation of live and televised models by children one to three years of age. *Monographs of the Society for Research in Child Development, 42*(5, Serial No. 173).

McDuffie, A., Turner, L., Stone, W., Toder, P., Wolery, M., & Ulman, T. (in press). Developmental correlates of different types of motor imitation in young children. *Autism.*

Meltzoff, A. N. (1988). Infant imitation and memory: Nine-month-olds in immediate and deferred tests. *Child Development, 59,* 217–225.

Meltzoff, A. N., & Gopnik, A. (1993). The role of imitation in understanding persons and developing a theory of mind. In S. Baron-Cohen, H. Flusberg & D. J. Cohen (Eds.),

Understanding other minds: Perspectives from autism (pp. 335–366). Oxford, UK: Oxford University Press.

Meltzoff, A., & Moore, M. K. (1977). Imitation of facial and manual gestures by human neonates. *Science, 198,* 75–78.

Meltzoff, A. N., & Moore, M. K. (1994). Imitation, memory, and the representation of persons. *Infant Behavior and Development, 17,* 83–99.

Meltzoff, A. N., & Moore, M. K. (1999). Persons and representation: Why infant imitation is important for theories of human development. In J. Nadel & G. Butterworth (Eds.), *Imitation in infancy* (pp. 9–35). Cambridge, UK: Cambridge University Press.

Meltzoff, A. N., & Prinz, W. (2002). *The imitative mind: Development, evolution, and brain bases.* Cambridge, UK: Cambridge University Press.

Mervis, C. B., & Robinson, B. F. (1999). Methodological issues in cross-syndrome comparisons: Matching procedures, sensitivity (Se) and specificity (Sp.) *Monographs of the Society for Research in Child Development, 64,* 115–130.

Morgan, S., Cutrer, P., Coplin, J., & Rodrigue, J. (1989). Do autistic children differ from retarded and normal children in Piagetian sensorimotor functioning? *Journal of Child Psychology and Psychiatry, 30,* 857–864.

Nadel, J. (2002). Imitation and imitation recognition: Functional use in preverbal infants and nonverbal children with autism. In A. N. Meltzoff & W. Prinz (Eds.), *The imitative mind: Development, evolution, and brain bases* (pp. 42–62). Cambridge, UK: Cambridge University Press.

Nadel, J., & Butterworth, G. (1999). *Imitation in infancy.* Cambridge, UK: Cambridge University Press.

Nadel, J., Guérini, C., Pezé, A., & Rivet, C. (1999). The evolving nature of imitation as a format for communication. In J. Nadel & G. Butterworth (Eds.), *Imitation in infancy* (pp. 209–234). Cambridge, UK: Cambridge University Press.

Nichols, S. L. (2005). *Information processing abilities and parent-child interaction: Prediction of imitative ability in the first year.* Unpublished doctoral dissertation, Dalhousie University, Halifax, NS, Canada.

Ohta, M. (1987). Cognitive disorders of infantile autism: A study employing the WISC, spatial relationship conceptualization and gesture imitations. *Journal of Autism and Developmental Disorders, 17,* 45–62.

Oliver, A., Johnson, M. H., Karmiloff-Smith, A., & Pennington, B. F. (2000). Deviations in the emergence of representations: A neuroconstructivist framework for analyzing developmental disorders. *Developmental Science, 3*(1), 1–23.

Pawlby, S. J. (1977). Imitative interaction. In H. R. Schaffer (Ed.), *Studies in mother–infant interaction* (pp. 203–224). New York: Academic Press.

Piaget, J. (1952). *The origins of intelligence in children.* New York: International Universities Press.

Piaget, J. (1962). *Play, dreams, and imitation.* New York: Norton. (Original work published 1945)

Rodgon, M. M., & Kurdek, L. A. (1977). Vocal and gestural imitation in 9-, 14-, and 20-month-old children. *Journal of Genetic Psychology, 131,* 115–123.

Roeyers, H., Van Oost, P., & Bothuyne, S. (1998). Immediate imitation and joint attention in children with autism. *Development and Psychopathology, 10*(3), 441–450.

Rogers, S. J. (1999). An examination of the imitation deficit in autism. In J. Nadel & G. Butterworth (Eds.), *Imitation in infancy* (pp. 254–283). Cambridge, UK: Cambridge University Press.

Rogers, S. J., Bennetto, L., McEvoy, R., & Pennington, B. F. (1996). Imitation and pantomime in high-functioning adolescents with autism spectrum disorders. *Child Development, 67,* 2060–2073.

Rogers, S. J., Hepburn, S. L., Stackhouse, T., & Wehner, E. (2003). Imitation performance in toddlers with autism and those with other developmental disorders. *Journal of Child Psychology and Psychiatry and Allied Disciplines, 44*, 763–781.

Rogers, S. J., & Pennington, B. F. (1991). A theoretical approach to the deficits in infantile autism. *Development and Psychopathology, 3*, 137–162.

Sigman, M., & Ungerer, J. (1984). Cognitive and language skills in autistic, mentally retarded, and normal children. *Developmental Psychology, 20*, 293–302.

Smith, I., & Bryson, S. (1994). Imitation and action in autism: A critical review. *Psychological Bulletin, 116*, 259–273.

Snow, C. E. (1981). The uses of imitation. *Journal of Child Language, 8*, 205–212.

Snow, C. E. (1989). Imitativeness: A trait or a skill? In G. E. Speidel & K. E. Nelson (Eds.), *The many faces of imitation in language learning* (pp. 73–90). New York: Springer-Verlag.

Stone, W. L. (2004). [Imitation performance across time]. Unpublished raw data, Vanderbilt University.

Stone, W. L. Coonrod, E. E., & Ousley, O. Y. (2000). Brief report: Screening Tool for Autism in Two-Year-Olds (STAT): Development and preliminary data. *Journal of Autism and Developmental Disorders, 30*(6), 607–612.

Stone, W. L., Ousley, O. Y., & Littleford, C. (1997). Motor imitation in young children with autism: What's the object? *Journal of Abnormal Child Psychology, 25*, 475–485.

Stone, W. L., Ulman, T., Swanson, A., McMahon, C., Turner, L., Yoder, P. J., et al. (2004, May). *Abilities underlying motor imitation in high vs. low structure settings.* Poster session presented at the International Meeting for Autism Research, Sacramento, CA.

Stone, W. L., & Yoder, P. J. (2001). Predicting spoken language level in children with autism spectrum disorders. *Autism, 5*, 341–361.

Turner, L., McDuffie, A., Stone, W., Yoder, P., Ulman, T., & Wolery, M. (2005, April). *Developmental correlates of different types of motor imitation tasks in young children with ASD.* Paper presented at the biannual meeting of the Society for Research on Child Development, Atlanta, GA.

Turner, L., Pozdol, S., & Stone, W. L. (2002). *Changes in social-communicative skills from age 2 to age 3 in children with autism.* Poster presented at the International Meeting for Autism Research, Orlando, FL.

Užgiris, I. C. (1981). Two functions of imitation during infancy. *International Journal of Behavioral Development, 4*, 1–12.

Užgiris, I. C. (1999). Imitation as activity: Its developmental aspects. In J. Nadel & G. Butterworth (Eds.), *Imitation in infancy* (pp. 186–206). Cambridge, UK: Cambridge University Press.

Vinter, A. (1986). The role of movement in eliciting early imitations. *Child Development, 57*, 66–71.

Vygotsky, L. S. (1978). *Mind in society: The development of higher psychological processes.* Cambridge, MA: Harvard University Press.

Whiten, A., & Brown, J. (1999). Imitation and the reading of other minds: Perspectives from the study of autism, normal children and non-human primates. In S. Bräten (Ed.), *Intersubjective communication and emotion in ontogeny: A sourcebook* (pp. 260–280). Cambridge, UK: Cambridge University Press.

Williams, J., Whiten, A., & Singh, T. (2004). A systematic review of action imitation in autistic spectrum disorder. *Journal of Autism and Developmental Disorders, 34*, 285–299.

Yando, R., Seitz, V., & Zigler, E. (1978). *Imitation: A developmental perspective.* Hillsdale, NJ: Erlbaum.

Zelazo, P. D., Burack, J. A., Boseovski, J. J., Jacques, S., & Frye, D. (2001). A cognitive complexity and control framework for the study of autism. In J. Burack, T. Charman, N. Yirmiya, & P. R. Zelazo (Eds.), *The development of autism: Perspectives from theory and research* (pp. 195–217). Mahwah, NJ: Erlbaum.

CHAPTER 14

Measuring the Development of Motor-Control Processes in Neurodevelopmental Disorders

MARK MON-WILLIAMS
JAMES R. TRESILIAN

The purpose of this chapter is to consider imitation and autism spectrum disorders (ASD) from the context of research into skilled movement. We suggest that studies investigating "imitation" must identify the level of representation required for success in the imitation task. We provide an overview of techniques for measuring skilled movement (using aiming and prehension movements as an example) and highlight the value of kinematic measurement techniques for precise quantification of imitation behavior. We discuss a study indicating that movement control per se is not necessarily impaired in ASD and speculate on why imitation deficits might lie at the heart of autism.

THE HIERARCHICAL AND MODULAR ORGANIZATION OF MOTOR CONTROL

Imitation requires the perception of another's behavior and the production of the appropriate action. Thus, issues related to motor control are central to understanding tasks requiring imitation. The purpose of this chapter is to provide a framework for considering how the human nervous system produces skilled motor action. We hope to demonstrate that movement production involves at least three hierarchical levels of representation. Moreover, we anticipate that identifying these different levels of representation will be of use when considering what aspects of movement might be copied in imitative tasks.

An accepted principle in motor control is that the processes of skilled motor action production are organized as a hierarchical series of representations. The details of motor execution start with an abstract representational level in which only the goal of the action is specified and are then progressively determined through a series of ever more concrete levels, ultimately reaching a lowest level that specifies the commands to the individual muscles involved in performance (e.g., Hogan, Bizzi, Mussa-Ivaldi, & Flash, 1987; Saltzman, 1979). Although the number and content of sensorimotor representations in the hierarchy is unresolved, most theorists today agree on at least three representational levels (see, e.g., Feldman & Levin, 1995; Hogan et al., 1987; Latash, 1993; Saltzman & Kelso, 1987): (1) an abstract, effector-independent representation of the goal outcome; (2) a representation of how the "working point(s)" move(s) to achieve the goal outcome; and (3) a representation of how the system of effectors (e.g., joint angles and muscles) behaves to move the working point(s) in the manner defined at level 2. We use the term *muscle–joint–angle* when referring to (3). The term *effector* refers to an anatomical feature (e.g., the right hand) so that an effector-independent representation means that the representation is independent of whether (e.g.) the right or left hand carries out the action. A common example used to illustrate an effector-independent (goal) representation is the action of signing one's name. It is a matter of common observation that the end product (the canonical shape of the signature) is remarkably similar whether one signs one's name with the right or left hand or clenches the writing implement in the teeth. The handwriting example does not provide compelling evidence for the existence of effector-independent representations but serves as a useful illustration.

A second basic principle of motor control is that skilled motor action production is organized in a modular fashion. That is, different actions are associated with specific production mechanisms: motor programs (Woodworth, 1898), motor schema (Arbib, 1981, 1989, 2005; Piaget, 1969), or motor pattern generators (e.g., Houk, Singh, Fisher, & Barto, 1990). We use the latter term and abbreviate it to MPG. MPGs can be lower-order (i.e., be responsible for fundamental actions) or higher-order (production mechanisms for more complex skills) and we consider later how higher-order MPGs might be constructed from their lower-order counterparts.

To be able to skillfully perform an action (e.g., mouth opening, finger tapping, and knot tying) one must possess the appropriate MPG. Each MPG is organized hierarchically as outlined in the previous paragraphs and must exist as a modular entity. Modularity follows from the ability to perform only one action at any given time without interference from other actions (the difficulty in simultaneously rubbing one's stomach and patting one's head is often used as an example of interference), which implies that each MPG can be activated independently of any other (selective activation). It is important to emphasize that MPGs represent *functional* modularity, with an MPG producing a specific action, such as moving the tip of the finger from one location to another. This kind of functional modularity does not necessarily involve anatomical modularity or localization—different MPGs may share the same neural substrates, make use of common computational resources, and be distributed across multiple levels of the central nervous system.

To execute an action whose production is governed by an MPG, at least three things are necessary: (1) the MPG must be selectively activated; (2) how the working point needs to move to achieve the goal in the current conditions must be determined; (3) the effectors to be used (limbs, joints and muscles) must be specified. The latter two of these are processes of motor preparation (e.g., Rosenbaum, 1980); the second normally involves using perceptual (typically visual) information to determine the required motion. For example, to reach and poke an object the tip of the prodding digit (the working point) must move toward the object, demanding information about the distance, direction, and size of the object: information a person acquires through vision.

Activation of an MPG can occur in at least two ways: voluntary (willed) activation and perceptual activation. The former occurs when we make a voluntary decision to do something, from which execution of the action follows. The latter can occur when the physical object of an action is perceived: for example, perceiving an apple activates the MPGs associated with actions that can be performed on apples (see, e.g., Arbib, 1989, for discussion). Perceptual activation will usually be insufficient to lead to behavioral execution in neurologically intact individuals—exceptions are involuntary stimulus-elicited behaviors (reflexes) such as orienting and startle reactions. The range of exceptions expands to behaviors usually classed as voluntary in people with certain types of frontal lobe damage who show a compulsion to act on objects when they see them, a phenomenon known as *utilization behavior* (Lhermitte, 1983). For example, seeing a comb may involuntarily elicit hair-combing behavior in the patient with frontal lobe damage. In this respect, utilization behavior resembles simple reflex behavior: the response follows the stimulus in an automatic, involuntary way. Normally, the intact brain is able to prevent perceptual activation from being sufficient to elicit behaviors in the absence of a voluntary intent to act. This suggests that performance of an action not only involves activation of the MPG associated with that action but also inhibition of concurrently active MPGs that could compete for control of behavior (e.g., Gallistel, 1980). As Tipper, Howard, and Houghton (1998) observe, "Paradoxically, the best definition of voluntary action is those actions that can be suppressed" (p. 1385).

It is clear that sensory processes (perceptions) play important roles in motor control. Perception can activate MPGs eliciting certain actions and provide the information required to fit the behavior to the circumstances of execution (motor preparation). These roles are in addition to the part perception plays in correcting errors and adjusting for unanticipated disturbances (feedback control). These perceptual processes may include all the different sensory modalities, but in this chapter we restrict our attention to vision. We consider how visual signals are transformed into signals for the control of movement (visual–motor transformations) both when interacting with objects and when interacting with other people.

Skill Refinement

According to the outline of motor organization just presented, performing an individual action in one's repertoire is to activate, prepare, and "run" an MPG. An MPG can be acquired through relevant experience (motor learning), or it may develop independently of experience (innate). Examples of innate MPGs include the mechanisms of certain stimulus-elicited behaviors such as withdrawal, startle, and orienting reflexes and the neural mechanisms of loco-motor pattern generation involved in tasks such as walking, crawling, and running (Gallistel, 1981). Innate MPGs may provide the basic building blocks of behavior on which more complex skills are built. The presence of innate MPGs may be an important precursor to development, but it is through learn-ing that the majority of human skills are acquired and refined. Motor learning can lead either to an improvement of the skill with which an already acquired action can be performed or to the acquisition of the ability to perform a new action such as tying shoelaces. We consider first the enhancement of an already acquired skill. The refinement of an existing skill can be considered a process that occurs within a particular MPG (and/or within shared resources used by that MPG) and may depend on trial-and-error practice (learning that is constrained and channeled by physiological and anatomical factors).

It is useful to consider recent theoretical accounts of motor control when considering learning processes. Modern theories of motor control suggest that the human nervous system must use "internal models" to either predict the consequences of motor commands or to determine the commands required to produce a desired movement. In support of these theories, there has been overwhelming support for the presence of internal models. For example, Flanagan and Wing (1997) have shown that individuals precisely modulate their grip force as they raise and lower an object in a time frame that is too short to allow for feedback correction—suggesting that the system can pre-cisely predict the movement-induced load (which is a function of the move-ment of the arm and the object held in the hand). Two types of internal mod-els are postulated. The *forward model* describes the relationship between the input and the output of any motor system. A forward model predicts the future state of the hand (or eye) given its present state and the commands being sent. Forward models allow the system to make predictions (necessary in pursuit eye movements, the regulation of grip forces etc.). The *inverse model* inverts the system and provides the command that will cause a desired change in state. We can think of inverse models as *controllers*. According to the scheme just outlined, skilled individuals have built up internal models (controllers and forward models) that represent specific movements. Wolpert, Ghahramani, and Flanagan (2001) have suggested that there are multiple paired forward and inverse models, with each module (controller and forward model) suitable for only a small set of contexts.

It should be noted that the existence of internal models is not sufficient to ensure that movements remain accurate and precise. The problem is that the system is open to the influence of noise (perceptual noise, errors in motor commands, etc.) and must continually calibrate itself. In situations in which the system is denied information that can drive calibration, movements rapidly become inaccurate and imprecise. Nevertheless, the presence of information for calibration will allow the system to achieve stable movement patterns. It follows that the skilled individual must continually refine his or her behavior in order to maintain performance level. Thus, trial-and-error learning is an essential component of even well-established "everyday" skills.

Figure 14.1 provides a schematic of the postulated processes involved in the learning of movement skills. A selected (desired) movement trajectory is produced through an inverse model that generates the motor command appropriate for the necessary state change. This "feedforward" motor command is sent to the appropriate effector to produce the movement. A feedback loop provides the system with the ability to compare the desired trajectory with the actual trajectory and a feedback controller allows the system to correct any errors. The feedback motor command can then be used to update the inverse model in order to ensure that it produces a feedforward motor command with the greatest possible accuracy. The updating of the inverse model is the process through which the system refines skilled movement through trial and error (practice).

Skill Acquisition

The refinement of existing skills is an important component of motor learning, but the vast majority of human skills are acquired from new. This raises the question of how new skills are acquired? The acquisition of a new capability is not well understood in general but in some cases involves assembling a number of existing MPGs into a combined structure that can produce the movement patterns needed to execute the new behavior. This is known to occur when a number of individual actions need to be executed in a specific ordered sequence in order to achieve an overall goal outcome (reviewed by

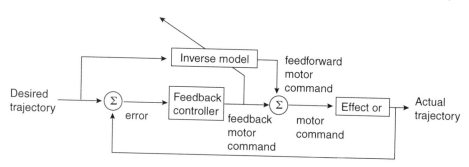

FIGURE 14.1. An adaptation of a model indicating the processes involved in the learning of motor skills (see Wolpert, Ghahramani, & Flanagan, 2001; Wolpert, Miall, & Kawato, 1998).

Schmidt & Lee, 1999). An example is learning to change gears in a motor vehicle with a manual transmission. The learner driver must execute a series of individual actions in the required order: remove the foot from the accelerator pedal, push in the clutch pedal, move the gear-stick into the required position, slowly release the clutch pedal, reapply the foot to the accelerator. The complete novice executes each of these as a separate action and executes the required sequence by remembering the correct order and then performing the separate actions in this order. This is highly attention demanding and constitutes the initial or "cognitive" stage in the three-stage description of motor learning first explicitly identified by Paul Fitts (see Schmidt & Lee, 1999). This is followed by the "associative" phase and the "autonomous" phase.

The associative phase occurs with the repeated performance of a sequence of actions (i.e., practicing). Performance becomes less cognitively demanding and more automatic in the sense that it becomes resistant to interference from concurrently executed tasks (e.g., Schneider & Fisk, 1983). Second, performance becomes quicker and acquires a characteristic rhythmic structure (stereotypical relative timing of component actions). These changes are associated with the elimination of time delays between one component action and the next; indeed, one component in a sequence may come to start before the previous one is complete. For example, it has been found that skilled typists frequently start moving the finger that will make the next key stroke before the previous stroke has been completed (Dennerlein, Mote, & Rempel, 1998). Thus, practice results in the acquisition of the ability to execute the action sequence automatically as a kind of higher-order unit with a coordinated pattern that is characterized in some cases by a consistent relative timing of its components. This *associative stage* of motor learning involves assembling existing MPGs into a unitary grouping (Schmidt & Lee, 1999) and the grouping could be considered a new, higher-order MPG. Once this process has been completed, the third stage of learning is reached (the *autonomous stage*). If the result of the first two stages is the construction of a new, higher-order MPG from existing MPGs, the result of practice during the autonomous stage is the refinement of the skill and the autonomy of performance mentioned earlier.

Observational Learning

Observational learning is likely to play a role in both the refinement of an MPG and in the process of creating higher-order MPGs from lower-order actions. An MPG can be refined by observing someone else perform the same skill, both in terms of action content and the contexts in which it is applied. Observational learning can also assist in the process of assembling previously learned skills together into a single skill—that is, bringing existing MPGs (lower-order) into a combined structure (a higher-order MPG). To learn the action sequence involved in doing something like changing gears, one must first determine the sequence required to achieve the overall goal. Easy solutions are to have someone tell you (instruction) or to watch someone else doing it (observation). Instruction typically involves listing the actions that need to be performed in the required order (a recipe); these actions are specified by their goals and not by the movements that might be made to achieve them. Therefore, an instruction to "push in the clutch pedal" is unlikely to be presented as a description of the movements of the joints or muscles of the leg required to achieve this action.

It is reasonable to assume that learning through observation will also depend primarily on representing the goal of the movement rather than representing the joint or muscle movements used to achieve the action. Whiten and Ham (1992) drew a distinction between imitation that involves copying both form and content of action and emulation whereby only the outcome is copied (for further discussion, see Whiten, Chapter 10, this volume). Goal-level "emulation" is a potentially important component of observational learning and many primates appear to possess this ability (Whiten, Chapter 10). Copying at the goal level (emulation) is useful if the observer already knows how to perform the actions observed (possesses the appropriate MPGs). In this case, observing another individual perform can help the observer learn what can be done in a particular situation (e.g., that it is safe to do something) or with a particular object (e.g., that footballs are for kicking). In addition, and as considered earlier, observation of a sequence of actions that combine to achieve an overall goal can provide the learner with information about the sequence needed to achieve that goal.

Nevertheless, observation of performance potentially provides more information than instruction because not only can the sequence of required outcomes (subgoals) be observed, but the movements produced in achieving these outcomes can also be studied. Observation of a person performing a task could, therefore, influence the motor learning process at more than one level of the control hierarchy. We have already seen that observation can inform the learner about the sequence of subgoals needed to achieve an overall goal (information at the abstract, goal level). Observation can also provide information about the form of the movements required to achieve a particular goal and therefore assist an individual in skill acquisition (through copying at the "movement level" rather than an abstract goal level).

It is possible to distinguish two types of copying at the movement level—"muscle–joint–angle" copying and "working point" copying. Copying muscle–joint–angle movements is typically an extremely difficult task. A large number of natural actions involve motion at more than one joint; for example, reaching out to grasp something involves motion at the shoulder, elbow, wrist, and fingers—as many as 17 different joints. Visually attending to all these motions in the very short time available (typically about half a second for a reach to grasp movement) is beyond the capability of the human visual system and so, at the very least, repeated observation would be needed. Furthermore, the movements a person makes to achieve the same outcome are never the same on two different occasions and may differ dramatically.

Indeed, different joint movements will be required to perform the same action in different circumstances. Thus, not only is copying joint movements very difficult, but it is often not particularly useful. Rather, copying movement at the working point level is more achievable: To copy the working point requires direction of attention to only the most pivotal limb movement required to execute an action. It therefore enables copying the action as well as its effects without making unreasonable attentional demands.

An Imitation Hierarchy

Goal-level copying requires that the observer be able to activate those MPGs that are observed when others perform. In the simplest case, observing a single action would activate the MPG for that action. Activation of an MPG at the goal level of representation would then occur either as the result of a decision to perform the associated action or as a result of observing while someone else performs that action. The existence of a neural system that responds in this way is demonstrated by the discovery of "mirror neurons" in primate frontal and parietal cortex (see Rizzolatti & Craighero, 2004, for a review) that facilitates production of a particular action in the context of its observation and potentially assists observers in developing associations with actions as they are represented in their own MPGs. Monkeys appear to be capable of observational learning—association of a particular behavior with particular contexts or objects, while more sophisticated observational learning of action sequences leading to an overall goal outcome appears to be shown only by great apes and humans (though see Whiten, Chapter 10, this volume). Evidently, possession of mirror neurons is not sufficient for more complex forms of observational learning, though this neural network may be an important component of the systems underlying these abilities.

The advantage of representing another's movement at the working-point level is that one can obtain information regarding not only the goal of the action but the movements that facilitate achievement of that goal. To copy the form of a movement, the observer's attention needs to be directed to the location of the actor's "working point(s)." The fact that humans can imitate an action where there is no clear goal (e.g., twirling a finger in a series of abstract shapes) provides evidence that humans are capable of copying movement at a working-point level. It seems plausible (and perhaps even probable) that humans exploit their ability to copy movement at a working-point level when acquiring and refining certain complex movement patterns (i.e., this information plays an important role in human learning), although unambiguous evidence for this notion is sparse.

We have already highlighted the difficulties of muscle–joint–angle copying. We suggest, therefore, that it is probable that muscle–joint–angle copying plays a limited role in a large number of learning contexts. Our suggestion does not imply that observation and copying of whole body movement is not important for a number of skills. Indeed, it must be the case that skills such as fly fishing require a novice to copy the movement of various effectors (though trial-and-error learning via repeated practice is probably required once the basic form of the movement has been learned). We would argue, however, that in tasks such as fly fishing, the learner must identify (or be informed about) the critical working points and copy the movement at that level. It follows that skills become increasingly hard to copy as the number of critical working points increases. Thus, copying the movement of an index finger is relatively straightforward if the movement of the wrist and elbow is not critical. If the copying task requires the elbow and wrist to move concomitantly with the finger in a particular manner, then imitation is that much harder because (1) attention needs to be paid to three times as many working points and (2) more constraints exist on how the finger movement can be achieved.

Our suggestion is that the complexities of muscle–joint–angle copying probably results in a limited role for this type of observational learning. Nevertheless, it is reasonable to assume that muscle–joint–angle copying must be important when interacting with other people. Gestures and facial expressions are likely to be difficult to represent meaningfully at an abstract goal level or in terms of the movement of simple working point(s) in the initial stages of learning. A system that could somehow capture a representation of gestural posture and facial expression would allow, for example, an observer to learn a given facial expression or a particular postural configuration. We suggest that gestural and facial MPGs are refined at least partially through copying at a muscle–joint–angle level and this refinement begins at a very early stage in childhood development. In our opinion, the ability to copy at this level is restricted to humans and represents the pinnacle of imitative behavior. Evidence for this behavior can be found in the everyday observation of humans (even babies) imitating facial expressions and copying the essence of complex social "gesture" cues. The ability to copy at this level might be due to specific processes responsible for perceiving another's actions or may simply represent a general superiority in the attention capabilities of the human visual system.

In summary, there are two levels that can be distinguished in copying at the movement level: a working point and muscle–joint–angle level of representation. It is probable that working-point copying plays a role in observational learning and may guide the development of complex skills (e.g., learning a backhand slice in tennis). In contrast, the complexities of muscle–joint–angle copying mean that it probably plays a limited role in the motor learning processes. Nevertheless, we know that humans can copy gestures and facial expressions and this ability may be employed in processes of social skill development. It seems reasonable to imagine that muscle–joint–angle copying might underpin systems of social communication and ultimately provide a system that facilitates self–other mapping. This does not mean that copying at other levels is not important for self–other mapping and it is probable that skilled social communication relies on copying at all levels.

We suggest that imitation becomes increasingly difficult as tasks move from an abstract level of representation through the working-point level to the muscle–joint–angle representation. Moreover, even within a given level of representation, tasks will be of disparate difficulty. Thus, copying a movement where only two working points are critical is easier than imitating a movement where the relative motion of four working points must be copied for task success. This consideration leads to the conclusion that it is possible to quantify the imitation difficulty of different tasks and to explore the point (level of representation and level of complexity within a representation) at which imitation breaks down.

THE ASSESSMENT OF NEURODEVELOPMENTAL DISORDER

Neurodevelopmental Disorder

Disruption to the different aspects of motor skill acquisition is likely to have differential clinical consequences. For example, people with a specific deficit in action production might be expected to show signs of poor motor coordination. Likewise, people with deficits confined to the system responsible for learning action sequences would be expected to have reasonable motor coordination (the MPG networks are intact) but show poor performance when learning a complex sequence of steps. Finally, people with deficiencies in imitation might show impaired social communication (as discussed throughout this book). Naturally, the clinical picture is unlikely to be so straightforward, but deficits at these different levels may map onto different clinical disorders. There is likely to be high levels of interaction between these different systems so that disruption to any one network will have deleterious consequences for the other networks. It follows that children with neurodevelopmental problems are likely to have a range of different problems but with clusters of core difficulties in specific domains. A symptom cluster that maps onto the motor deficit is constituted by developmental coordination disorder (DCD). DCD occurs in a significant proportion of children, who present with impaired body/eye coordination and show poor acquisition of motor skills. DCD can be defined as a specific problem with coordinative tasks despite normal IQ and no evidence of neurological, biochemical, or physical abnormalities (American Psychiatric Association, 1994). In common with most childhood disorders, estimates of prevalence vary, but it is reasonable to consider approximately 5% of the childhood population as having DCD (Henderson & Sugden, 1992). Within this population there may be a subgroup of children who map onto the second level with specific impairment in action–organization. These children are described as "dyspraxic" (see Dewey & Bottos, Chapter 17, this volume). Dyspraxia is considered similar to *apraxia*, a term used for a neurological disorder characterized by a loss of the ability to carry out complex movements (e.g., dressing and speech) and gestures, despite having the desire and the physical ability to perform them. The existence of dyspraxia provides support for our notions, but a detailed consideration of this condition is not in the scope of this chapter and we do not consider issues relating specifically to this population. Finally, deficits in imitation may map onto children with ASD. We provide some evidence later that children with ASD may have reasonable movement skills. It also appears that some children with ASD are able to follow a complex action sequence as data exist, suggesting that children with autism are able to repeat a complex sequence of actions in order to achieve a goal (J. Williams & A. Whiten, personal communication, January 2005). It is plausible that the problems with social interaction experienced by people with ASD stem from deficits in the ability to copy at the movement level and we will consider this further.

Development and Disruption of Imitation

Gestural communication requires a complex of visual–motor skills and executive function that requires perception of and attention to relevant behavior, inhibition of inappropriate responses (such as automatic mimicry), and commission of appropriate reactions. These interacting processes must be intensively practiced over childhood, as discussed extensively elsewhere in this book, often in the context of dyadic exchanges and imitation. Therefore, a failure to engage socially is likely to have consequences for neurodevelopment. We would suggest that a lack of social engagement will affect normal learning processes and hinder the development of MPGs.

In turn, a failure to develop MPGs may have serious consequences for perception, as an inability to produce an action may cause difficulties in perceptions related to that action. For example, Japanese speakers find it difficult to enunciate the letter "r" and these problems of production have been associated with a difficulty in aurally distinguishing the sound of this letter (e.g., Miyawaki et al., 1975). It follows that an initial deficit in perceiving or attending to relevant behaviors might create a negative feedback loop where MPGs do not develop optimally creating additional "perceptual" problems, further hindering refinement of the associated MPGs.

If our conjecture is correct, it is likely that deficits in observational learning will have an impact at the earliest stages of neonatal development. One of the earliest motor skills refined in human babies is the ability to direct gaze toward objects of interest (involving coordination of the head and eyes). Eye movements can be considered either conjugate (including saccadic and pursuit movements) or disconjugate (vergence eye movements). It appears that both conjugate and disconjugate movements represent innate MPGs, but early eye movements are relatively crude and require refinement through experience over childhood. It is probable that trial-and-error learning plays a major role in the refinement of these MPGs, but this learning process could be assisted by observational copying (following the head and eye movements of a parent).

The ability to direct gaze is of central importance because humans need to foveate objects in order to interact skillfully with them. Thus, one of the most fundamental MPGs is the ability to direct gaze to an object of interest. We have argued within this chapter that complex skills are underpinned by lower-order ("fundamental") MPGs. It can be seen, therefore, that eye movement control is essential to a large number of human motor skills. For example, Riek, Tresilian, Mon-Williams, Coppard, and Carson (2003) reported that bimanual movements (moving the right and left hand together) consist of the nervous system orchestrating a number of separate actions using different effectors in an efficient manner. A detailed inspection of the movement kinematics in adults carrying out a bimanual task revealed a synchronous and sequential pattern of hand and eye movements that was organized with military precision (Riek et al., 2003). It follows that the ability to control gaze is an important precursor to the full development of manual control. It is entirely possible that simple eye and hand movements can develop through trial-and-error learning mechanisms, but it seems reasonable to assume that observation of another's behavior would assist learning in terms of both action content and application contexts. Moreover, observational learning would allow children to learn the more complex patterns of eye–hand coordination necessary for a wide range of skills acquired over childhood.

The implication of our conclusions is that deficits in observational learning would hinder the development of MPGs in the developing child. A failure or delay in acquiring and refining MPGs will have serious consequences, as the absence of a fundamental "building block" of behavior will hinder the development of more complex skills. For example, a neonatal failure to observe and copy eye and head movements will obstruct the development of this fundamental skill and may affect subsequent eye–hand coordination. A failure to observe and copy movement does not prevent a skill (e.g., prehension) being acquired through trial-and-error learning, but it may produce inefficient learning processes. Moreover, a deficit in attending to and copying eye and head movements might have additional consequences for the developing child. The primary means of directing attention in humans is through overt attention (i.e., foveating an object of interest). Observational learning of eye and head movements can play a pedagogical role in selecting objects of interest, following another person's attention (as indexed by gaze angle) and shifting attention appropriately within an environmental context. As we have discussed earlier, deficits in these mechanisms will further hamper the development of MPGs, producing a vicious circle of neurodevelopmental problems (problems that can be observed at a later developmental stage through deficits in clinical tasks involving imitation).

MOVEMENT MEASUREMENT

Assessment

Methods of studying movement control (including imitation) fall on a spectrum from subjective observation through quantitative measures of performance. Subjective observation relies on an observer scoring the quality of the movement and determining whether it achieved a given goal (with or without some form of interobserver reliability assessment). These types of rating have been the mainstay of experimental approaches to imitation research. To provide greater consistency, some methods of movement evaluation rely on standardized tests of movement ability that allow for objective measurement. In these tests (such as the Movement Assessment Battery for Children [MABC] Henderson & Sugden, 1992, described below), movement skills are indexed relative to some criterion (typically, time taken to perform a given task). For example, a child is timed while threading a number of beads on a thread. These tests are useful tools for determining whether an individual falls within or without an age-appropriate level of performance on a particular task. The limitation of such tests is that they provide no indication of *how* someone carried out the task or why a task caused particular difficulties for an individual. Thus, the "gold standard" in movement measurement is a complete descriptive breakdown of the observable kinematic variables associated with task performance.

We provide a brief consideration of objective and kinematic methods used in evaluating children's goal-directed behavior. We provide a description of a standardized test of movement control (the MABC) employed in a number of studies investigating motor skills and discuss some of the kinematic measures that can be used to provide a complete descriptive breakdown of goal-directed behavior in arm movements. The reason for selecting these particular tests and movements will become apparent when we discuss a study of motor control in children with ASD.

A Standardized Battery

The MABC (Henderson & Sugden, 1992) is widely accepted as the de facto gold standard for assessing motor competence in children. This consists of a checklist section and a performance component. The checklist details a range of "normal activities," which are individually scored on a 4-point scale to provide an overall performance score. The checklist is a useful adjunct to the performance section and provides information on whether a child's motor difficulties are increased when the child and/or the environment move (Sugden & Sugden, 1992). The performance section evaluates motor ability in three areas: manual dexterity, ball skills, and balance (static and dynamic). Performance in these three areas is assessed using two separate functional tasks (the actual tasks depend on the child's age), with each task providing a score between 0 and 5. At the end of the test the total score (the sum of the different task scores) is compared with normative data expressed in percentile rankings. The MABC is designed to evaluate motor performance in children age 4 years and above. Diagnosis of extreme disability is relatively straightforward in reasonably young children, but variability of motor function means that a diagnosis of DCD is very difficult in children below the age of 4 years. The appeal of the MABC, rather than a test aimed purely at manual control, is that a child's postural, manipulative, and interceptive skills are assessed, creating a specific profile of a child's coordination difficulties. Children may therefore be subtyped on the basis of whether difficulties with manual control coexist with problems in other motor domains or whether they represent a topographically delineated disorder. The MABC has been designed so that a gross impairment of manual control can, by itself, result in a diagnosis of DCD.

Modular Decomposition

The use of a general assessment battery can provide a common frame of reference between studies but has limited capacity to determine why performance is deficient, or appraise what aspects of functioning have contributed to a decrement in performance. One way of addressing this goal might appear to be the adoption of a process-oriented approach. In a process-oriented approach, research is focused on examining the integrity of postulated basic processes that contribute to functional skills (e.g., response inhibition). The major weakness with this approach is that these processes may be merely diffuse hypotheses as to the nature of the problem, and even if we accept the validity of a specific process, the research hinges on finding a definitive and exclusive test of that process. Unfortunately, many of the major elements of skilled behavior are often required in tests that purport to measure a specific process and it is very difficult to design tests that achieve domain specificity and to extrapolate from findings of poor performance on a test that purports to measure one process when so many others are likely to be involved.

One approach that might prove profitable in exploring complex skill acquisition may be to break the task down into a number of subtasks and consider each as a separate module. Typical examples are the modules of *transport-grasp* coordination and *grip-force* modulation, each of which can be performed and studied in isolation but which are merged in the act of picking up a glass of water. This statement may seem to converge on the process approach, but the important difference is that it avoids theoretical presuppositions. If a child fails to grasp an object, it is a simple act of decomposition to determine whether this was due to an error of limb positioning or an error of grasp timing. Hence it is possible to identify modular areas such as trajectory formation and fingertip control that are the building blocks of a specific skill, without slipping toward hypothetical processes. An approach that decomposes complex tasks into modular components has the advantage that intervention can be directed at those areas that most restrict performance for an individual child. We would not deny that there will be "processes" at the root of an individual's problem, which undermine their abilities. We would, however, argue that moving from a general diagnosis to appraising hypothesized underlying processes is too great a step without first decomposing the contributory factors in skilled behavior. Our proposal is that a distinction must be made between *processes* that may underpin control and *modules* that must be implicated.

Quantifying Action Execution

Recent advances in technology mean that there are well-established techniques that allow one to explore in detail how a movement unfolds in time. These techniques allow for objective quantification of movement skills and provide the experimenter with a tool for examining different aspects of goal directed actions. We consider some of the measures that can be used to provide a complete description of goal-oriented action and that could be potentially applied to the study of imitation in children with and without neurodevelopmental disorders. For example, one of the key skills that must be required in imitation is the ability to generate skilled movement. Thus, one reason why children with ASD could perform poorly on tasks requiring imitation is because they have fundamental problems in movement control. To assess this notion, it is necessary to investigate that "module"—in other words, it is useful to study goal-directed action in ASD.

Aiming Movements

One of the simple ways to measure movement production is through reaction time. Reaction time simply describes the length of time between the appearance of an imperative stimulus to move and the commencement of movement (reflecting the time taken to perceive the stimulus and prepare the movement). Reaction time (RT) is often used in studies of cognitive performance but is also usefully measured when goal-directed action is studied. Individual differences influence how quickly an individual reacts, and RT is susceptible to sex (males show faster RT), age (RT decreases over childhood but increases in later years) and numerous physiological factors (see Schmidt & Lee, 1999). The value of RT as a measure lies in the fact that regardless of an individual's baseline RT, reaction time changes lawfully as the nature of the task alters. Simple reaction times to imperative stimuli are well known to be altered in attention-deficit/hyperactivity disorder (e.g., Sergeant, Geurts, & Oosterlaan, 2002) and DCD (Mon-Williams, Tresilian, Coppard, Bell, & Carson, 2005) but are not impaired in ASD (e.g., Senju, Tojo, Dairoku, & Hasegawa, 2004).

Reaction times can be informative but obviously provide a limited picture of goal-directed behavior. It therefore makes sense to explore how movements unfold over time. Some of the most straightforward actions to investigate are aiming movements (e.g., moving the tip of the index finger from a starting position to a target location). A large number of studies have investigated human performance in aiming tasks. The performance of such tasks is often described in terms regarding the thing being moved—the "working point" (partly because of the theoretical notion that it is this point that is the focus of control). This raises the question of how the nervous system plans the trajectory (spatial path and temporal movement characteristics) of the working point. A number of investigators have explored the path followed in aiming tasks restricted to a horizontal plane. The initial conclusion was that hand paths are straight and this was used to support theoretical accounts of movement control. Similar straight paths are found in completely unconstrained movements (e.g., moving from one location in free space to another). Subsequent studies modified this conclusion by showing that paths generated in some regions of the workspace are characterized by smoothly varying curvature. Three explanations were provided for the observed curvature under the assumption that the system was trying to produce a straight path: (1) imprecise control (Flash & Hogan, 1985); (2) visual distortion (Wolpert,

Ghahramani, & Jordan, 1994); (3) neuromuscular interference (Flash, 1987). More recently Osu, Uno, Koike, and Kawato (1997) showed that despite the observed curvature, participants produce straight paths when explicitly instructed to do so, indicating that in some situations the human nervous system deliberately plans a curved path (often advantageous for a number of reasons including the circumvention of unwanted frictional forces).

The important point about the different paths shown in aiming movements is that they are highly stereotypical across and within participants. Thus, unconstrained and movements restricted to a horizontal plane are typically straight and these straight paths are found across all participants. We have found that the curvature of the path observed under different task constraints is also stereotypical across and within participants. If participants make movements of their fingertip from one location on a tabletop to another location (otherwise unconstrained), their hand lifts upwards to a maximum height before descending to the target. We have found that the maximum height occurs approximately halfway through the movement (i.e., the path is approximately parabolic) and the height scales with reach distance (Loftus, Murphy, McKenna, & Mon-Williams, 2004; Loftus, Servos, Goodale, Mendarozqueta, & Mon-Williams, 2004). These parabolic paths are found under a wide range of conditions across all participants regardless of the effector used to generate the movement (as predicted form an abstract representation of aiming movements).

Investigations into aiming movements have found that not only are the spatial paths stereotypical but so are the temporal characteristics. The position of the working point is normally recorded over time, and then this signal is mathematically differentiated to provide a tangential speed profile. The speed profile allows one to determine the beginning and end of the movement with the movement time being the difference between these two measures. The speed profiles tend to have a stereotypical "bell shape" where the maximum speed is reached approximately halfway through the movement. It is widely considered that adjustments to the movement occur in the deceleration phase of the movement and increasing the accuracy demands of the task results in a leftward skew of the profile (i.e., a longer deceleration phase occurs). Moreover, the time taken to move can be reliably determined for an individual by the size of the target and its distance from the finger. The different kinematic landmarks, including movement time, allow reliable quantification of the whole movement. Once again, aiming movements have been shown to be slow in DCD (Mon-Williams et al., in press) but, as discussed below, are normal in ASD.

Prehension

Aiming movements provide a simple tool for exploring goal-directed actions, but it is informative to study more complex movements. Prehension describes reach-to-grasp movements. Performance typically involves coordinated movements of the fingers, wrist, arm, and shoulder. In the early parts of this chapter, we argued that new, higher-order MPGs can be created by grouping

MPGs. One possible example of such a higher-order MPG might be provided by the precontact phase of prehension (see later) where the MPG of grasp formation and digit aiming are merged into the single reach-to-grasp action. Prehension behavior appears within the first year of a human baby's life and can be considered a unitary action in adulthood. Nevertheless, it is possible to describe the movement in terms of its constituent components. Movement and force production in prehension have been widely studied in adults and methods of data collection and analysis have been firmly established in the literature. Two phases may be identified in the execution of prehension tasks: the *precontact phase* (prior to object contact) and the *grip-and-lift phase* (following object contact). The precontact phase can be considered to have two functionally distinct components that are executed concurrently in a coordinated fashion (Haggard & Wing, 1991; Paulignan, Jeannerod, MacKenzie, & Marteniuk, 1991; Paulignan, MacKenzie, Marteniuk, & Jeannerod, 1991): the transport component and the grasp component. The *transport component* describes the arm movements that place the hand into a position where it can grasp an object. This phase is constrained by both the distance of an object and its size and by the context in which the prehension act is performed. The transport phase is also dependent on the coupling that exists between the body and the hand (e.g., the relationship between the shoulder, elbow, and hand). The *grasp component* describes the preshaping of the fingers and thumb into a grasp configuration. The intrinsic characteristics of the object, such as its size, shape, weight, and surface texture affect both the planning and execution of the grasp component of prehension. Skilled performance involves coordination of the concurrently executed transport and grasp components and their mutual adaptation to task variables (task goal, presence or absence of visual feedback, object distance, size, shape, weight, and surface characteristics). Such adaptations have been found to be highly robust and replicable in healthy adults (Jakobson & Goodale, 1991; Marteniuk, Leavitt, MacKenzie, & Athenes, 1990; Wallace & Weeks, 1988; Wier, MacKenzie, Marteniuk, & Cargoe, 1991; Weir, MacKenzie, Marteniuk, Cargoe, & Frazer, 1991; Wing, Turton, & Fraser, 1986) and reflect the invariant structure of sensori-motor organization in prehension (i.e., the underlying movement structure that remains the same despite variations in the conditions of execution). Perturbation experiments have demonstrated that the nervous system attempts to preserve this structure when environmental conditions are altered during execution (Castiello, Bennett, & Stelmach, 1993; Haggard & Wing, 1995; Paulignan, Jeannerod, et al., 1991; Paulignan, MacKenzie, et al., 1991).

PREHENSION IN AUTISM SPECTRUM DISORDERS

Early and more recent descriptions of ASD (Asperger, 1944; Wing, 1981) include symptoms of "clumsiness." The *International Classification of Diseases* (World Health Organization, 1992) stated with respect to Asperger syndrome: "It is common for them to be markedly clumsy." Standardized tests of motor function support clinical observations that movement problems exist in ASD (Green et al., 2002; Manjiviona & Prior, 1995; Miyahara et al., 1997). Green and colleagues (2002) reported that catching skills were particularly impaired in ASD. Nevertheless, these observations do not establish if an intrinsic motor difficulty exists or if established difficulties with social interaction lead to poor performance. We recently used a prehension task and an interceptive timing task to determine if motor deficits, per se, exist in children with ASD (Livingstone, Williams, & Mon-Williams, 2004). Performance in our tasks was compared with a conventional measure of skill (i.e., the MABC).

The major question of interest within the study was whether there were any reliable differences between groups of children of different ages and a group of children with ASD. A between-group analysis of variance (ANOVA) revealed no group effect on any of the kinematic variables in our unimanual reaching-to-grasp or in our interceptive timing task. These included reaction times, movement times, and time to grasp. The difficulty with carrying out between-group statistical analyses is that the tests assume homogeneity within groups. This assumption is probably not merited in the case of ASD where clear differences exist in the clinical manifestation of the disorder. To circumvent this limitation, the measures from each individual participant were compared with the group of children in the control population but no individual child fell below the range of scores achieved by the control children. Therefore, analysis of the results for individual children led to the same conclusions as the analyses carried out at a group level—namely, there was no evidence of a motor deficit common to the children diagnosed with ASD.

One might question whether the tasks were too easy for the children such that they all performed at a ceiling level. Nonetheless, these results did reflect a range of performance, and increasing difficulty manifested reduced performance in prehension, with increased movement times when the grasping size of the object was reduced or the nonpreferred hand was used. This pattern of results was consistent across all children whether or not they were affected by ASD. Thus, our findings suggest that the same response to changes in task difficulty observed previously in adults (e.g., Tresilian, Stelmach, & Adler, 1997) also exist similarly in children with and without ASD. There are two further reasons why it seems unlikely our tasks were too insensitive to detect the underlying performance difficulties experienced by the children with ASD. First, these kinematic measures are sensitive indicators of motor deficits in conditions such as developmental coordination disorder (Mon-Williams et al., in press), where almost all children show impaired performance as indexed by variables such as movement time. Second, the experimental tasks employed are *a priori* more demanding of motor skill than some of the tasks of the MABC on which these children performed so poorly. Indeed, a striking feature of the results from this study was the contrast between the motor performance measured within the laboratory and the motor performance measured by the standardized test of movement. The children with ASD in this study were also reported to have poor movement skills by clinicians, parents, and teachers (although interestingly these observations were often accompanied by reports of the children excelling at computer games). There are at least two possible explanations for the discrepancy between the different measures of motor performance in our study.

One possibility is that motor performance is sensitive to social context in a wide range of tasks. As discussed previously, many motor skills develop through imitation in a social context, and if this is missing it is likely to have an impact on the development of complex motor skills. Motor skills such as ball catching may be learned through (and subsequently depend upon) the monitoring and interpretation of another's actions. In contrast, the laboratory tasks we explored could be refined through trial-and-error learning and might be less influenced by observation (hence a deficit in observational learning might have minimal impact upon these tasks). In addition, social contexts are more variable than laboratory testing situations and the MABC is likely to require a greater flexibility in performance than the laboratory tasks (as the content changes to a greater extent more frequently).

One previous study examined prehension performance in ASD. Mari, Castiello, Marks, Marraffa, and Prior (2003) suggested that both quantitative and qualitative differences might be observed in children with ASD of low IQ (despite clumsiness being more traditionally associated with Asperger syndrome). Mari and colleagues reported that the grasp formation phase of prehension occurred some time (802 milliseconds) after the onset of the transport phase in an ASD population with IQ below 80. Examination of the results from all the children included in our study showed no evidence of qualitative differences in the pattern of movement, with the onset of grasp formation occurring in close temporal proximity to the onset of the transport phase. Thus, qualitatively different prehension and interception patterns are not inevitable and do not seem to be a core feature of ASD (even with individual children who have a British Picture Vocabulary Scale < 79).

It is possible at this moment in time to forward the hypothesis that "pure" motor deficits are not a core feature of ASD (although children with ASD may perform poorly on movement tasks because of other factors). The strength of this hypothesis lies in the relative ease with which it may be disproved—any evidence of a "pure" motor deficit within a majority of children with ASD in nonsocial contexts would suffice. These findings may have important implications for educational practice. Children with ASD may appear to lack sporting and athletic prowess, but their disengagement from physical activity may have long-term adverse impact on their health and deprive them of engagement in activities that they could find pleasurable and rewarding. Our findings suggest that children with ASD might be encouraged into physical activities that are less demanding on social skills or imitation, and which are more repetitive, such as cycling, running, or swimming. In addition, participation in such sports through clubs could encourage social engagement at a level that children with ASD find manageable. The other side of this coin is that the lack of evidence for core motor deficits does not make the movement impairment evident in the social context any less real. Rather, careful thought might be given to its origins before remedial measures are suggested.

In conclusion, the results from our recent study were somewhat surprising. The children who participated in our study were all assumed to have some form of central motor deficit, with the aim of the study being to try and identify the nature of the deficit using standardized kinematic measures on well-described motor tasks. Instead, the ASD population's performance was indistinguishable from that shown by control children. The marked disparity between the performance levels indexed by a detailed investigation of the movement and the level indicated by standardized movement tests was of particular note. This contrast raises the possibility that any movement problems observed in ASD might reflect other aspects of movement skill rather than a deficit in motor production per se. The challenge to the research community is to devise means of circumventing potential confounds within tests in order to obtain distinguish between domains of impairment in ASD.

CONCLUSIONS

In this chapter, we have considered the hierarchical and modular control of movement. This consideration led to the identification of three levels of representation: an abstract goal level, a working-point movement level, and a muscle–joint–angle movement level. We argued that imitation within humans can occur at all three levels but becomes increasingly difficult as one moves from copying at the abstract goal level to copying at the level of the muscle–joint–angle. We suggested that social communication probably involves processes of copying at the working-point and muscle–joint–angle movement level and that disruption to these processes might produce the type of problems experienced by people with autism. It follows that a fruitful line of investigation in autism research would be to study imitation at different representational levels. One prediction from our consideration is that children with ASD will be relatively unimpaired in copying at the abstract goal level but show increasing difficulty as this becomes impossible (e.g., imitating meaningless gestures or facial expressions). We note there is empirical support for this prediction (Williams, Whiten, & Singh, 2004). Our conclusions are broadly consistent with existing accounts of imitation deficits lying at the heart of autism. We suggested that progress in understanding neurodevelopmental deficit requires a process of modular decomposition—the identification of components that must underpin those skills that cause difficulty to an individual. We attempted to demonstrate the advantage of using well-established kinematic measures to provide an insight into the control of actions such as imitation. We reported the results of an experiment that explored the "module" of movement production (a module that must be involved in imitation). Our findings suggest that a deficit in motor production is not a necessary feature of ASD. These findings indicate that perceptual processing of human movement (another essential module within imitation behavior) might be the stumbling block causing imitation deficits within the ASD population.

REFERENCES

American Psychiatry Association. (1994). *Diagnostic and statistical manual of mental disorders* (4th ed.). Washington, DC: Author.

Arbib, M. A. (1981). Visuomotor coordination: From neural nets to schema theory. *Cognition and Brain Theory*, 4, 23–39.

Arbib, M. A. (1989). *The metaphorical brain 2: Neural networks and beyond.* New York: Wiley Interscience.

Arbib, M. A. (2005). From monkey-like action recognition to human language: An evolutionary framework for neurolinguistics. *Behavioral and Brain Sciences*, 28, 105–124.

Asperger, H. (1944). Die "Autistischen Psychopathen" im Kindesalter [Autistic psychopathy in childhood]. *Archiv fur Psychiatrie und Nervenkrankheiten*, 117, 76–136.

Castiello, U., Bennett, K. M. B., & Stelmach, G. E. (1993). Reach to grasp: The natural response to a perturbation of object size. *Experimental Brain Research*, 94, 165–178.

Dennerlein, J. T., Mote, C. D., Jr., & Rempel, D. (1998). Control strategies for finger movement during touch typing: The role of the extrinsic muscles during a keystroke. *Experimental Brain Research*, 121, 1–6.

Feldman, A. G., & Levin, M. F. (1995). Positional frames of reference in motor control. The origin and use. *Behavioral and Brain Sciences*, 18, 723–806.

Flanagan, J. R., & Wing, A. M. (1997). The role of internal models in motor learning and control: Evidence from grip force adjustments during movements of hand-held loads. *Journal of Neuroscience*, 17, 1519–1528.

Flash, T. (1987). The control of hand equilibrium trajectories in multi-joint arm movements. *Biological Cybernetics*, 57, 257–274.

Flash, T., & Hogan, N. (1985). The coordination of arm movements: An experimentally confirmed mathematical model. *Journal of Neuroscience*, 5(7), 1688–1703.

Gallistel, C. R. (1980). The organization of action: A new synthesis. *Behavioral and Brain Sciences*, 4, 609–650.

Green, D., Baird, G., Barnett, A. L., Henderson, L., Huber, J., & Henderson, S. E. (2002). The severity and nature of motor impairment in Asperger's syndrome: A comparison with specific developmental disorder of motor function. *Journal of Child Psychology and Psychiatry and Allied Disciplines*, 43, 655–668.

Haggard, P., & Wing, A. M. (1991). Remote responses to perturbation in human prehension. *Neuroscience Letters*, 122, 103–108.

Haggard, P., & Wing, A. M. (1995). Coordinated responses following mechanical perturbation of the arm during prehension. *Experimental Brain Research*, 102, 483–494.

Henderson, S. E., & Sugden, D. A. (1992). *Movement Assessment Battery for Children.* London: Psychological Corporation.

Hogan, N., Bizzi, E., Mussa-Ivaldi, F. A., & Flash, T. (1987). Controlling multijoint motor behaviour. *Exercise and Sports Science Reviews*, 15, 153–190.

Houk, J. C., Singh, S. P., Fisher, C., & & Barto, A. G. (1990). An adaptive network inspired by the anatomy and physiology of the cerebellum. In T. Milner, R. S. Sutton, & P. J. Werbos (Eds.), *Neural networks for control* (pp. 301–348). Cambridge MA: MIT Press.

Jakobson, L. S., & Goodale, M. A. (1991). Factors affecting higher-order movement planning: A kinematic analysis of human prehension. *Experimental Brain Research*, *86*, 199–208.

Latash, M. L. (1993). *Control of human movement*. London: Human Kinetics.

Lhermitte, F. (1983). "Utilization behaviour" and its relation to lesions of the frontal lobes. *Brain*, *106*, 237–255.

Loftus, A., Murphy, S., McKenna, I., & Mon-Williams, M. (2004). Reduced fields of view are neither necessary nor sufficient for distance underestimation but reduce precision and may cause calibration problems. *Experimental Brain Research*, *158*, 328–335.

Loftus, A., Servos, P., Goodale, M. A., Mendarozqueta, N., & Mon-Williams, M. (2004). When two eyes are better than one in prehension: Monocular viewing and end-point variance. *Experimental Brain Research*, *158*, 317–327.

Manjiviona, J., & Prior, M. (1995). Comparison of Asperger syndrome and high-functioning autistic children on a test of motor impairment. *Journal of Autism and Developmental Disorders*, *25*, 23–39.

Mari, M., Castiello, U., Marks, D., Marraffa, C., & Prior, M. (2003). The reach-to-grasp movement in children with autism spectrum disorder. *Philosophical Transactions of the Royal Society of London, B*, *358*, 393–403.

Marteniuk, R. G., Leavitt, J. L., MacKenzie, C. L., & Athenes, S. (1990). Functional relationships between grasp and transport components in a comprehension task. *Human Movement Science*, *9*, 149–176.

Miyahara, M., Tsujii, M., Hori, M., Nakanishi, K., Kageyama, H., & Sugiyama, T. (1997). Brief report: Motor incoordination in children with Asperger syndrome and learning disabilities. *Journal of Autism and Developmental Disorders*, *27*, 595–603.

Miyawaki, K., Strange, W., Verbrugge, R., Liberman, A. M., Jenkins, J. J., & Fujimura, O. (1975). An effect of linguistic experience: The discrimination of [r] and [l] by native speakers of Japanese and English. *Perception and Psychophysics*, *18*, 331–340.

Mon-Williams, M., Tresilian, J. R., Coppard, V., Bell, V., & Carson, R. C. (2005). The preparation of reach-to-grasp movements in adults, children and children with developmental coordination disorder. *Quarterly Journal of Experimental Psychology*, *58*, 1153–1344.

Osu, R., Uno, Y., Koike, Y., & Kawato, M. (1997). Possible explanations for trajectory curvature in multijoint arm movements. *Journal of Experimental Psychology: Human Perception and Performance*, *23*, 890–913.

Paulignan, Y., Jeannerod, M., MacKenzie, C., & Marteniuk, R. (1991). Selective perturbation of visual input during prehension movements. 2. The effects of changing object size. *Experimental Brain Research*, *87*, 407–420.

Paulignan, Y., MacKenzie, C., Marteniuk, R., & Jeannerod, M. (1991). Selective perturbation of visual input during prehension movements. 1. The effects of changing object position. *Experimental Brain Research*, *83*, 502–512.

Piaget, J. (1969). *The mechanisms of perception*. London: Routledge & Kegan Paul.

Rizzolatti, G., & Craighero, L. (2004). The mirror neuron system. *Annual Review of Neuroscience*, *27*, 169–192.

Riek, S., Tresilian, J. R., Mon-Williams, M., Coppard, V. L., & Carson, R. G. (2003). Bimanual aiming and overt attention: One law for two hands. *Experimental Brain Research*, *153*, 59–75.

Rosenbaum, D. A. (1980). Human movement initiation: Specification of arm, direction, and extent. *Journal of Experimental Psychology General*, *109*, 444–474.

Saltzman, E. (1979). Levels of sensorimotor representation. *Journal of Mathematical Psychology*, *19*, 91–163.

Saltzman, E., & Kelso, S. J. A. (1987). Skilled actions: A task-dynamic approach. *Psychological Review*, *94*(1), 84–106.

Schmidt, R. A., & Lee, T. D. (1999). Motor control and learning: A behavioral emphasis (3rd ed.). Champaign, IL: *Human Kinetics*.

Schneider, W., & Fisk, A. D. (1983). Attentional theory and mechanisms for skilled performance. In R. A. Magill (Ed.), *Memory and control of action* (pp. 119–143). Amsterdam: North-Holland.

Senju, A., Tojo, Y., Dairoku, H., & Hasegawa, T. (2004). Reflexive orienting in response to eye gaze and an arrow in children with and without autism. *Journal of Child Psychology and Psychiatry and Allied Disciplines*, *45*(3), 445–458.

Sergeant, J. A., Geurts, H., & Oosterlaan, J. (2002). How specific is a deficit of executive functioning for attention-deficit/hyperactivity disorder? *Behavioural Brain Research*, *130*, 3–28.

Sugden, D. A., & Sugden, L. G. (1992). The assessment of movement skill problems in 7- and 9-year-old children. *British Journal of Developmental Psychology*, *61*, 329–345.

Tipper, S. P., Howard, L. A., & Houghton, G. (1998). Action-based mechanisms of attention. *Philosophical Transactions of the Royal Society of London, B*, *353*, 1385–1393.

Tresilian, J. R., Stelmach, G. E., & Adler, C. H. (1997). Stability of reach-to-grasp movement patterns in Parkinson's disease. *Brain*, *120*, 2093–2111.

Wallace, S. A., & Weeks, D. L. (1988). Temporal constraints in the control of prehensile movement. *Journal of Motor Behavior*, *20*, 81–105.

Weir, P. L., MacKenzie, C. L., Marteniuk, R. G., & Cargoe, S. L. (1991). Is object texture a constraint on human prehension?: Kinematic evidence. *Journal of Motor Behavior*, *23*, 205–210.

Weir, P. L., MacKenzie, C. L., Marteniuk, R. G., Cargoe, S. L., & Frazer, M. B. (1991). The effects of object weight on the kinematics of prehension. *Journal of Motor Behavior*, *23*, 192–204.

Whiten, A., & Ham, R. (1992). On the nature and evolution of imitation in the animal kingdom: Reappraisal of a century of research. *Advances in the Study of Behavior*, *21*, 239—283.

Wing, A. M., Turton, A., & Fraser, C. (1986). Grasp size and accuracy of approach in reaching. *Journal of Motor Behavior*, *3*, 245–260.

Wing, L. (1981). Asperger's syndrome: A clinical account. *Psychological Medicine*, *11*, 115–129.

Wolpert, D. M., Ghahramani, Z., & Jordan, M. I. (1994). Perceptual distortion contributes to the curvature of human reaching movements. *Experimental Brain Research*, *98*, 153–156.

Wolpert, D. M., Ghahramani, Z.. & Flanagan, J. R. (2001). Perspectives and problems in motor learning. *Trends in Cognitive Sciences*, *5*, 487–494.

Wolpert, D. M., Miall, R. C., & Kawato, M. (1998). Internal models in the cerebellum. *Trends in Cognitive Sciences, 2*, 338–347.

Woodworth, R. S. (1898). The accuracy of voluntary movement. *Psychological Review*, *3*(2, Whole No. 13).

World Health Organization. (1992). *The ICD-10 classification of mental and behavioral disorder: Diagnostic criteria for research*. Geneva: Author.

CHAPTER 15

Neuroimaging Self–Other Mapping in Autism

JUSTIN H. G. WILLIAMS
GORDON D. WAITER

One of the more elegant aspects of the self–other mapping hypothesis of autism comes from its capacity for testability and the potential for such tests to generate new and exciting leads that increase our understanding of autism. Imitation is both highly accessible to measurement and amenable to experimental manipulation. In addition, imitation can be such a simple enough process that we may have the potential to identify its neural substrate across the age range. Through exploring the neural substrate of imitation and self–other mapping in autism, we have the opportunity not only to test the self–other hypothesis but to develop tools that serve to map both across developmental levels and between the anatomical, physiological, and behavioral abnormalities characteristic of autism spectrum disorders (ASD).

At the time of the paper by Rogers and Pennington (1991), the technological capacity to test their hypothesis was fairly limited. The last 15 years has seen an explosion in our ability to image the human brain with respect to fine structure and function. Along with developments in other areas of neurosicence we are now able to clarify the Rogers and Pennington hypothesis, as well as to make predictions that we can test with the new technology. At the core of the paper by Rogers and Pennington lays a proposal that autism is characterized by a deficit in the neural substrate for *self–other mapping*. The meaning of this term is discussed elsewhere in the book and thus we do not give it much coverage here. For the purposes of this chapter we are concerned with the integration of sensory information originating from visual sources, with that which exists as part of the "self" in the form of body schemas.

Williams, Whiten, Suddendorf, and Perrett (2001) reviewed the Rogers and Pennington hypothesis alongside some of the relevant, more recent advances in psychology and neuroscience, and some of the arguments that simple "mindreading" mechanisms might commonly serve imitation, pretense "theory of mind," and joint attention. They suggested that all these forms of action are dependent on recognizing the equivalence of an observed action to an action already existing in the behavioral repertoire. Once such connectivity has been established, a person can understand the actions of another by drawing on their own knowledge of that action—its causal relationships, consequences, associations with emotions, and beliefs. In other words, once intersubjectivity is established, one person can understand another by "stepping into his shoes." As a mechanism for understanding the mental states of others, this is known as the "simulation theory of mind" (Carruthers & Smith, 1996). They considered that a mechanism for self–other mapping might be based on "mirror neurons," and that a dysfunction of this system at early stages of development could trigger a cascade of psychopathology manifesting as excessive copying combined with a social cognitive deficit. This led to the suggestion that development of mirror neurons might be somehow dysfunctional in autism. Over the past few years we and others have been bringing neuroimaging technology to bear on this hypothesis. Other developments in autism neuroimaging research are also proving informative. In this chapter we review some of these studies and consider how the hypothesis may benefit from clarification and refinement.

THE "MIRROR NEURON" SYSTEM

First, a brief overview of mirror neurons (MNs) is warranted. MNs have been described in monkeys using single-cell recording methods (di Pellegrino, Fadiga, Fogassi, Gallese, & Rizzolatti, 1992; Gallese, Fadiga, Fogassi, & Rizzolatti, 1996; Rizzolatti, Fadiga, Gallese, & Fogassi, 1996; Rizzolatti, Fogassi, & Gallese, 2001). The property that makes them unique is that they fire in response to specific actions, both when these same actions are observed and when they are performed. They have been identified in two main brain areas. In the ventral premotor cortex, including Broca's area, neural codings exist for goal-directed actions involving hand or mouth and objects. A number of studies have now shown that these neurons can also be activated in both monkeys and humans by the sight of the same actions. Methods used to demonstrate this include magnetic electroencaphalography (Hari et al., 1998), transcranial magnetic stimulation (Fadiga et al., 1999), and functional magnetic resonance imaging (Hamzei et al., 2003). The evidence that they are involved in reaching and grasping actions and orofacial actions in humans appears unequivocal. Arbib (2005) presents the strong case that the MN system also lies at the core of a language function. Important questions are whether MNs play an additional role in imitation (see also Grezes, Armony, Rowe, & Passingham, 2003; Decety, Chapter 11, this volume) and what other roles Broca's area performs.

MNs have also been identified in somatosensory cortex in anterior parietal sulcus. These are neurons that are active during execution of an action because they receive input from proprioceptive sensory feedback following the execution of an action, as well as from visual cortex during observation of actions. This appears to be an important area where visual information about observed actions can be analyzed in relation to preexisting knowledge of action achieved through proprioceptive feedback. Recently, MNs have been described in monkey inferior parietal cortex that code for the same action goals or intentions (Fogassi et al., 2005). Therefore, while previous MNs coded for the action type such as pincer grip or grasp, these neurons code for the action intention, such as whether an object is being picked up to be eaten or placed elsewhere. For further discussion of the MN system, see Decety (Chapter 11, this volume).

FUNCTIONAL IMAGING OF IMITATION

We have recently performed a functional magnetic resonance imaging (fMRI) study with a view to comparing MN-related activity during imitation in individuals with ASD, (described fully in Williams, Waiter, Gilchrist, et al., 2006). We utilized a protocol developed by Iacoboni and colleagues (1999, 2001), who carried out a study of imitation using fMRI to test the hypothesis that MNs play a role in human imitation. Iacoboni and colleagues' task involved the imitation of a finger movement during brain scanning and five control conditions. The finger movement shown was an animation of five still pictures shown successively for 0.6 seconds each, of either the index or middle finger being extended. There were five control conditions consisting of two other execution and three other observation-only conditions. In one execution control, execution was carried out in response to observing a cross marking either finger on a still photograph of the hand (symbolic cue condition). In the second it was in response to a cross on one side of the screen (spatial cue condition). In the observation controls, the three types of visual stimuli were simply observed. Brain activity during imitation could then be compared to observation only and also two execution conditions. We therefore sought to utilize this protocol to compare brain activity during imitation in participants with ASD to normal controls.

Participants with ASD were all right-handed males ages 13–20 years with normal IQ, recruited from our clinical population and through voluntary agencies. All had an unequivocal clinical diagnosis of ASD and all met full diagnostic criteria for autism on the Autism Diagnostic Interview—Revised (ADI-R, 2000) (Lord, Rutter, & Le Couteur, 1994). All but one met diagnostic criteria for ASD on the Autism Diagnostic Observation Schedule (Lord et al., 2000). He was retained because the validity of his diagnosis was in no doubt from high scores on the ADI-R and clinical knowledge. All had IQ assessed on the Wechsler Adult Intelligence Scale-IV or the Wechsler Intelligence Scale for Children. Participants were then matched to controls of similar age and IQ. All participants underwent fMRI scanning using the paradigm described by Iacoboni and colleagues (1999, 2001), using the same stimuli kindly provided by these authors. We carried out all analyses using statistical parametric mapping and a random-effects approach.

Task performance during scans was very close to 100%, with just two subjects making minor errors on two occasions. This means that group differences were not due to performance differences but, rather, because the groups are using their brain differently during imitation. Of 124 scan blocks processed (4 per subject), 54 from controls and 52 from subjects with ASD were free from movement artifact and therefore suitable for analysis.

The results may be examined with respect to two questions. One question concerns how the neural substrate of imitation more generally differs in its functioning between the two groups. Another question is how MNs function differently in the two groups. First, though, some discussion of fMRI may be helpful.

Functional Magnetic Resonance Imaging and Maps of Brain Activation

To obtain the SPM maps shown in Plate 15.1 is a complex, multistage process that may benefit from some explanation for readers unfamiliar with the details. The first stage of fMRI data collection involves a structural brain scan that can divide up the brain to fit a large three-dimensional grid of small cubes about 2 mm × 2 mm, known as voxels (a three-dimensional equivalent of the pixel). As everyone has a different-shaped brain, a standard warping algorithm is required to transform each brain scan in a standard way to make it conform to a standard shape. The functional imaging process measures fluctuations in the amount of oxygenated blood (the "BOLD signal" stands for blood oxygen level dependent signal) over the time course of the scan at each voxel. Another algorithm, taking into account the hemodynamic delay between activity and the BOLD signal change, then ascribes a level of activity, related to oxygen consumption, to each condition.

In this study we then compared these measures across conditions and groups using random-effects models. These models differ from fixed-effects models in that fixed-effects models effectively just compare the group means and so do not differentiate between within-subject and within-group variation. While the fixed-effect findings only make a statement about group differences in the subjects studied, the findings of random-effects models can be generalized to the wider population. The downside of the random-effects approach is that effect sizes are reduced and studies are less sensitive to more subtle findings. To generate the maps shown, a threshold must be set so that areas can be identified where effects sizes are above that threshold. If the threshold is too low, type 1 errors and chance findings occur. This is a particular problem because of the many thousands of comparisons being carried out, in view of the number of voxels. If it is too high, important group differences are missed. In our studies we have chosen to use a threshold of $p < 0.001$ uncorrected for multiple comparisons. Examining more limited areas of the brain, and having *a priori* hypotheses about areas where differences might be found, reduces the prospect of making chance findings.

Functioning of Mirror Neurons

Therefore, to determine whether mirror neurons functioned differently between the two groups, we sought to repeat the analytic approach taken by Iacoboni and colleagues (1999), though within the framework of statistical parametric mapping (SPM). This involved contrasting activity in the imitative condition with the average of the two other execution conditions. The area examined was narrowed to include only frontal and parietal regions. This was partly because the established MN areas are located in these regions, and also because the conditions contained very different visual content, and by reducing our area of comparison, we could increase the study's sensitivity. The results can be considered for parietal and premotor areas separately.

Parietal Activations

In the maps shown in Plate 15.1, voxels are identified where the difference in activity between imitation and execution rose above the $p < 0.001$ threshold, uncorrected for multiple comparisons. It can be seen that this activation is more extensive for the control group than the ASD group in somatosensory cortex. We then took these results forward to a second analysis where we examined the interaction of this contrast with group status. Curiously, this did not confirm group differences in anterior parietal cortex. The reasons for this became apparent when we did more localized studies. For the areas where peaks of activity were identified in the ASD and control groups, we selected 27 voxels (about 1 cm^3) and examined the mean activity in this region for each of the six conditions (27 voxels × 4 measures for each condition × 15 subjects per group = 1,500 measures per condition per group). The results are shown in Figure 15.1a and 15.1b. It can be seen that activity during imitation was not as extensive in the ASD group, not reaching the second location. However, it was also less during action execution, so that the contrast of imitation versus execution did not reveal an interaction at the $p < 0.001$ threshold.

As mentioned previously, this area in the inferior parietal lobe is at the anterior of the intraparietal sulcus in somatosensory cortex where activity is increased by proprioceptive input as well as visual input. These findings seem to suggest diminished proprioceptive input into these areas during action–execution as well as during imitation. Could it be that individuals with autism suffer from diminished proprioceptive input to parietal cortex? Tsatsanis and colleagues (2003) have suggested poor connectivity between

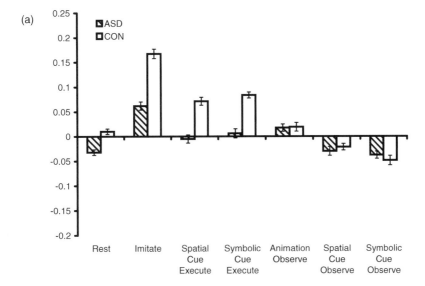

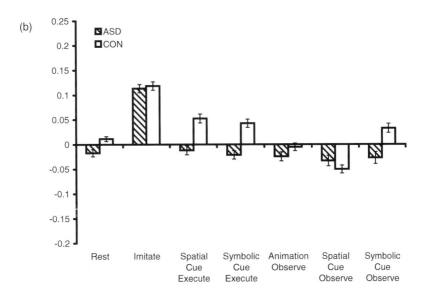

FIGURE 15.1. Parameter estimates determined from SPM fit of model to time course data for two areas in anterior parietal lobe close to anterior parietal sulcus showing relative contributions of experimental conditions to BOLD signal. Area (a) was a peak of activity in controls (x = 59, y = –26, z = 27)and area (b) was a peak of activity in participants with ASD (x = 61, y = –18, z = 38).

thalamus and cortex in ASD, which could mean that proprioceptive feed-back could also be adversely affected as a consequence. These findings raise the possibility that self–other mapping is impaired in ASD in parietal cortex, because actions performed by the "self" are poorly represented in the form of neural codings in anterior parietal cortex. This is consistent with the MN hypothesis of autism (Williams et al., 2001). It is also consistent with the suggestion made elsewhere in this volume (Dewey & Bottos, Chapter 17; Rogers & Williams, Chapter 12) that autism is associated with a kinaes-thetic deficit.

Broca's Area

We did not find any cluster in Broca's area in our contrasts that were at odds with the findings by Iacoboni and colleagues (1999). This is puzzling as we had attempted a close replication of their experiment. One possible cause of differences was verbal rehearsal. We took care to ensure participants did not use this, but this was not reported by Iacoboni's group. Other researchers (Grezes et al., 2003; Jackson, Meltzoff, & Decety, in press; Makuuchi, 2005) have also failed to find imitation-specific activity in Broca's area during hand-related tasks, and have suggested that it is required for converting instruction into action. This in itself may be an important component of imitation even if it is not specific to it. Similarly, it has been suggested that Broca's area may be involved in the preparation and/or the selection of motor action (Jackson et al., in press; Zhang, Feng, Fox, Gao, & Tan, 20040, which was integral to both control and imitative tasks in our study.

Functioning of the Neural Substrate of Imitation
Amygdala

The second aim of this study was to identify differences between groups relat-ing to the neural substrate of imitation more generally. To address this ques-tion we first examined the areas in which there was an interaction of group status with the contrast of imitation versus rest. First, this revealed a differ-ence in the left amygdala. Figure 15.2 shows the average time course of activa-tion in the two groups and the derived parameter estimates that were used to construct the SPMs. This shows clearly that the amygdala becomes deacti-vated during task performance in controls and especially so during imitation. No such deactivation occurs among the ASD group. It has been suggested that a circuit involving orbitofrontal cortex and the amygdala is concerned with associating memories with an emotional valence, and impairment of this func-tion lies at the core of the autistic syndrome (Baron-Cohen et al., 2000). Our finding raises the possibility that the amygdala is closely connected with imitation-related action processing systems. This would be expected if the amygdala is a key regulator of social-cognitive function, and amygdaloid

(a)

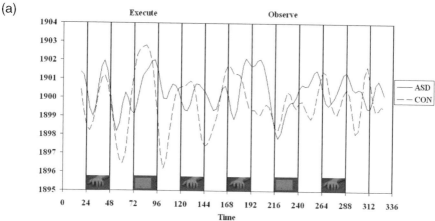

(b)

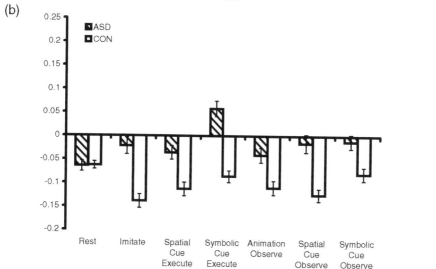

FIGURE 15.2. (a) Mean time course of activity in left amygdala during task performance showing clear activity-induced modulation during task performance that is greatest during imitation. (b) Bar graph shows parameter estimates determined from SPM fit of model to time course data showing relative contributions of experimental conditions to BOLD signal.

involvement in action–perception connectivity forms the foundations of social cognitive neural systems. Other chapters of this book have considered whether a lack of motivation may account for the imitative impairment in autism. An alternative possibility is that processes of attaching emotional valence during imitation is impaired in ASD. Therefore, the children may be equally willing and motivated to engage with imitation tasks, but they do not have similar emotional experiences when they do imitate. If children do not experience the imitation of certain types of behavior as pleasurable or otherwise, this may influence whether they imitate selectively or not, and whether imitation is experienced in a self-reinforcing manner. At the same time, they may still learn through nonimitative conditioning mechanisms such as stimulus-enhanced learning normally.

Posterior Temporal Cortex

We next examined a contrast between imitation and observation to find out what brain areas were more active during imitation compared to observation in these regions. This time we masked our data to include only the visual and temporal cortex. We then subjected this output to a further analysis to identify areas in which this contrast interacted with group status. First, we found activity in the control groups that was greater during imitation than observation alone. This involved ventral temporal cortex, areas of occipital cortex, bilateral lingual gyrus, and the motion processing areas at the temporoparietal junction. No such additional activity was found in the ASD group. This suggests that while for the control group posterior cortex was more active during imitation than observation; it functioned no differently whether individuals with ASD were either imitating or just observing. Then, of even greater interest was the group interaction with this contrast that identified an important group difference in an area of posterior temporal cortex. A region of interest analysis of this cluster is illustrated in Figure 15.3b, showing that this area was active during imitation but not action observation in controls, while the converse was true for the ASD group. This area is associated with the observation of meaningful biological movements (Puce & Perrett, 2003) and theory of mind (Castelli, Happé, Frith, & Frith, 2000; Frith & Frith, 2000; Saxe & Kanwisher, 2003; Saxe, Xiao, Kovacs, Perrett, & Kanwisher, 2004; Vogeley et al., 2001), and activity here is diminished in ASD during theory of mind (ToM) tasks (Castelli, Frith, Happé, & Frith, 2002). It seems unlikely that our imitation task required any sort of mentalizing function. However, if imitation plays a role in ToM development, then a brain area used for imitation during development, may also come to serve ToM. Our findings suggest that normally, motor activity during imitation increases activity in this region, perhaps influencing perception. Supporting this suggestion, Astafiev, Stanley, Shulman, and Corbetta (2004) also found that motor activity was associated with increased activity in occipitotemporal cortex and in the lingual gyrus. Alternatively, during imitation, visual processing areas may receive input from parietal areas serving action representation as discussed earlier, or from frontal areas associated with executive function (Decety et al., 1997). Whichever, in normal individuals this area of cortex serves a ToM function, and in this experiment only became active when motor activity and visual activity were concurrent. In the ASD group, which was likely to have poor mentalizing abilities, this area was only active during observation. Taken all together, we would suggest that early in development, imitation is associated with input

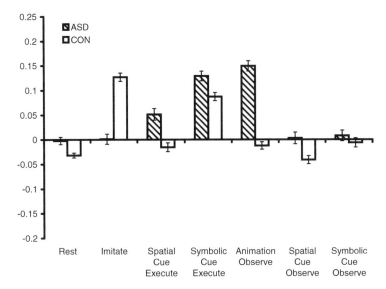

FIGURE 15.3. Parameter estimates determined from SPM fit of model to time course data for posterior temporal cortex showing relative contributions of experimental conditions to BOLD signal.

into the temporoparietal areas secondary to action execution, which leads it to serve a function of integration between action execution and matching observed actions. Consequently, only imitation activates this area, and observation of actions alone is insufficient to activate it. However, if actions are observed and the observer tries to understand them by imagining performing these same actions, this would activate this area and it would serve a ToM function. In individuals with ASD, because the integration function has failed to develop, a lack of connectivity between frontal and visual areas means that observation of actions is unaffected by such interference or methods of understanding observed action, resulting in different patterns of visual attention but poor ToM skills. This is all in keeping with the self–other mapping hypothesis and the idea that self–other mapping contributes to ToM development.

The Subcortical Route

Another brain area that was more active among the autism group than among controls was the dorsal premotor cortex. This is an area active during visuomotor association learning which uses subcortical routes including the thalamus to associate specific visual stimuli with specific actions (Toni & Passingham, 1999). This suggests that the group with ASD were using associative actions to perform the tasks. Just as one learns different motor responses to a one-way sign and a no-entry sign, it appears that the individuals in the

ASD group may have used a similar cognitive strategy, performing the tasks by executing specific learned actions that they associated with specific visual stimuli, rather than imitating by matching their action to the one they observed.

Summary of the Williams and Colleagues Study

In summary, we found evidence for diminished activation of parietal mirror neurons in autism, which we suggest is secondary to more fundamental problems with proprioceptive feedback to cortical structures. However, deficits in imitation in autism also lie "beyond the mirror" (to borrow a phrase from Arbib, 2005) in neural structures in which the MN system is embedded, serving action imagery, amygdaloid modulation, and ToM. A deficit in self–other mapping at the temporoparietal junction may have important negative consequences for the development of action understanding and ToM development. The ASD group used the dorsal premotor cortex more, suggesting greater use of visuomotor association processes in imitation. Neuroanatomical evidence that this picture resulted from neurodevelopmental failure of gray matter maturational processes and white matter connectivity is discussed further below.

OTHER NEUROIMAGING STUDIES OF IMITATION IN AUTISM

Very recently, powerful support for the MN hypothesis of autism has come from Dapretto and colleagues (2006). They compared brain activity in controls and young people with autism during facial imitation. This is a task much more likely to affect activity in Broca's region than imitation of finger movements. They found clear group differences in Broca's area as the control group activated this area much more than controls. To our knowledge, only one other neuroimaging study has examined imitation in individuals with ASD, using orofacial imitation which is more likely to activate the MN region. Nishitani, Avikainen, and Hari (2004) used magnetoencephalography to study a mixed-sex group of adults ages 19–45 years with Asperger syndrome. They projected still images of orofacial gestures for 551 milliseconds (msec) every 4 seconds onto a screen and subjects were asked to imitate them. Lip movements were recorded with electromyograms. There was no difference in the delay before which mouth movement started in each group (about 400 msec after stimulus onset), but curiously electromyographics lasted almost twice as long for the ASD group. In the control group this paradigm was associated with activation in occipital, inferior parietal, superior temporal, and Broca's areas bilaterally. Activation was diminished in Broca's area in the ASD group in that only three individuals of eight activated it on the right, and six of eight activated it on the left. Furthermore, activation of Broca's area was weaker on the left-hand side and there was delay to its activation of

Broca's area on the left. This study shows that Broca's area is less active in adults with Asperger syndrome during imitation. Interestingly, there was no difference in involvement of superior temporal sulcus in this condition, supporting the notion that the abnormality in processing occurs at the level of interaction with the motor system, rather than simply at the level of action observation.

NEUROIMAGING OF VISUOMOTOR ABILITY

One drawback of the study by Nishitani and colleagues (2004) is that it lacked a control condition. This may be required for two reasons. The first reason is to show that both groups were equally engaged in the task, as it is often a concern with studies of individuals with ASD that participants were simply not attending to the stimuli. In this case, however, the electromyographic measure and the equal activation of occipital areas in this study puts any such doubts firmly to rest. The second type of control would be a nonimitative task, because it is not clear whether the activation identified in this study is specific to imitation. As we found in our study, it is unclear exactly what activates Broca's area, and we remain unsure as to whether the deficit identified in this study was specific to imitation, or whether the circuit that was activated would have been equally active if an incongruent action was performed in response to a visual instruction.

But, while imitation may be a potent activator of the MN system, this does not necessarily mean that it is the only activator, or that imitation is the only type of motor activity in which we would expect to find abnormalities. Müller and colleagues (2003) raise the question whether even studies of simple imitation in autism are premature, as we are still unsure as to whether simple motor learning systems are functioning abnormally in autism at an even more fundamental level. They noted the literature reporting abnormalities in the functioning of the motor system in autism (see also Dewey & Bottos, Chapter 17; Mon-Williams & Tresilian, Chapter 14, this volume) and tested a group of individuals with autism, all males ages 15–43 years, all with IQ scores in the normal range, on a simple motor sequence learning task using fMRI. They found significant differences between the group of eight individuals with autism and the controls. They found that areas of activation during motor learning were much more scattered in the autism group and point to similar findings in studies of facial perception. They suggest that variability of neurofunctional organization could be a defining feature of autism. They go on to suggest that thalamocortical afferents play an important role in differentiation and that the neurofunctional disturbance in autism could reflect developmental consequences of pathways between cerebellum, thalamus, and cortex that function abnormally in autism. A further study (Müller, Cauich, Rubio, Mizuno, & Courchesne, 2004) examined differences in the time course of learning patterns between the two groups. They found that participants with autism, unlike the control participants, tended to maintain activation of sensorimotor and premotor cortex at the later stages even when learning was evident. Therefore, they do not appear to alter their strategy of approach to the task as it proceeds. The individuals in these studies come from a broad age range, are quite small in number, have varied handedness, and have a lower-than-average IQ. One possibility to consider is that poor neurofunctional organization could reflect general developmental delay, rather than a phenomenon specific to autism. We examined distribution of activation foci in our data and did not find that those related to the ASD group were any more scattered than in the control group. Nevertheless (see discussion of limitations), the finding of different time courses of learning should alert us to be cautious in the way that we interpret fMRI data in motor learning paradigms autism.

OTHER TESTS OF THE MIRROR NEURON HYPOTHESIS

Very recently, a few other studies have reported evidence in support of the MN hypothesis of autism. Using fMRI, Villalobos, Mizuno, Dahl, Kemmotsu, and Muller (2005) have shown that group differences in functional connectivity between visual cortex and Broca's area in individuals with autism. Using electroencephalography (EEG), Oberon and colleagues (2005) have shown a failure of mu-wave suppression during action observation in ASD that occurs in normal individuals when watching orofacial actions. Theoret and colleagues (2005) used the method described earlier, pioneered by Fadiga and colleagues (1995), to investigate whether action observation increased muscular-evoked potentials induced by transcaranial magnetic stimulation (TMS) administered over the premotor cortex in groups with ASD and controls. They found that when the action observed involved a to-or-away perspective, action observation failed to increase TMS-induced activity in hand muscles in the ASD group, whereas it did for controls. Finally, Hadjikhani, Joseph, Syder, Harris, and Tager-Flusberg (2005) used novel processing techniques to compare cortical thickness between groups on brain images collected using structural MRI from an ASD and a carefully matched control group. They found decreased cortical thickness in MN areas in the ASD group.

FUNCTIONAL NEUROIMAGING OF JOINT ATTENTION

Williams and colleagues (2001) suggested that joint attention would be served by an MN function because it involves relating the perception of gaze direction to executed gaze direction. Importantly, as in imitation, it is not simply a matter of mapping the executed eye direction so that it is directed to the same object as the model. It requires frequent shifts of visual attention between the object and the model (as in imitation) and also results in an effect of shared experience. We recently performed an experiment to investigate this (Williams, Waiter, Perra, Perrett, & Whiten, 2005). We made two types of video clip: The first involved the model's head in the top half of the screen whose gaze and head movements could be seen to be following a moving dot in the lower half of the screen. In the second video clip, the person was not following the dot and though he moved his head and gaze equally he did not look at the dot. Twelve individuals underwent fMRI scanning as they followed the instruction to "watch the moving dot." As they watched the dot they either experienced joint attention or they did not. Some of the results are shown in Plate 15.2. This shows that in both the nonshared and shared attention condition, both observed and executed eye movements are processed in the right side in the superior temporal sulcus (STS) and frontal eye fields, respectively. There is also activity in the superior parietal lobes on the right-hand side.

At the more robust but less sensitive condition comparison, foci of activity were present in medial frontal cortex and particularly the superior left frontal lobe in the shared condition but not the nonshared condition. This left frontal lobe activation is important because it overlaps with an area of increased gray matter volume that we identified in the ASD group that took part in our imitation experiment (Waiter et al., 2004; Plates 15.3 and 15.4). Furthermore, this area has some particularly interesting characteristics. According to Ramnani and Owen (2004), it is likely to serve an information integration function, particularly when this involves integrating a self-monitoring function with a motor output. Second, it has a characteristic cytoarchitecture of high dendritic density and low cell body density (Jacobs et al., 2001) that is reflective of both an integration function and the outcome of developmental processes such as programmed cell death and dendritic spine formation that could be impaired in autism.

We concluded that joint attention is another form of self–other matching that is associated with widespread activations of cortex and subcortical structures. However, this self–other matching was not evident through the activation of mirror neurons or through greater activation of eye movement regions, but rather, the very simple behavior of looking at the same thing as another person led specifically to the activation of left frontal cortex and anteromedial frontal cortex that is strongly associated with mentalizing activities. In this case, therefore, self–other matching appears to be dependent on frontal lobe orchestration.

FUNCTIONAL CONNECTIVITY

Just, Cherkassky, Keller, and Minshew (2004) have recently published an fMRI study showing "underconnectivity" in ASD. They used fMRI to measure changes in the time course of brain activation while reading active or passive sentences. They then calculated the correlation between the fluctuations of BOLD signal in one part of the brain with fluctuations in another part.

They reasoned that a high correlation would reflect close connectivity whereas poor correlation reflected low connectivity. They found much lower correlations across 10 pairs of regions of interest. This appears to reflect uniformly diminished cortical connectivity in ASD and would suggest that those functions most dependent on cortical connectivity would be most affected. Imitation and joint attention may well be such processes, and in this sense these authors present a hypothesis not very dissimilar to the MN hypothesis. Both hypotheses advocate a general lack of synchrony between cooperating brain centers. The MN hypothesis proposes that autism is a developmental consequence of poor connectivity between neurons serving action and perception, while the underconnectivity hypothesis advocates a more general deficit.

Furthermore, just as Williams and colleagues (2001) hypothesized that ASD would be characterized by dysfunction of mirror neurons in Broca's area in terms of disconnectivity between what is perceived and what is executed, so these authors have shown diminished synchrony between a brain area serving auditory perception and Broca's area serving speech execution. One concern with the study by Just and colleagues (2004), is that it is not clear from the study description whether participants were matched on Verbal IQ, and whether the findings are simply a general reflection of nonspecific, Verbal IQ differences. The participants in the study are described as having high-functioning autism, implying that they have all suffered impairment of language development. As they were matched on Full Scale IQ, it seems likely that they did have poorer language skills than controls. This argument may antagonize those who consider a Verbal–Performance IQ discrepancy to be an intrinsic feature of autism. We would suggest that such a tangle of arguments will always be a problem unless we are clear about the questions we are asking and the generalizability of our findings. If one is asking whether a group of people with autism who also have language delay have impaired connectivity between areas serving a language function, the answer would appear to be in the affirmative. However, if we are asking whether such impaired connectivity is core to developing the set of behavioral characteristics that define ASD (which does not necessarily require impaired language abilities), then while this study generates this hypothesis, it does not provide the evidence in support of it. Rather, diminished connectivity needs to be demonstrated in areas serving social cognitive function, as described previously.

To this end, we applied the method used by Just and colleagues (2004) to our own data. We selected 33 regions of interest and selected the BOLD signal measures for the period of imitation. A correlation matrix between the 33 pairs generated 527 correlative tests for each individual. We then calculated a mean correlation for each group for each of the 527 pairs. Our null hypothesis was that functional connectivity would be similar for any matrix pair between the two groups. We found that the mean correlation for the ASD group was 0.383, whereas it was 0.399 in the control group. This was actually a significant difference (χ^2 test, $p = 0.007$) but is clearly a very small one. We suggest that autism is not characterized by a process of generally impaired functional connectivity, and this is further discussed below.

STRUCTURAL STUDIES

A necessary step that is required to test the self–other mapping and MN hypotheses of autism is to look at structural neuroimaging studies of children with autism. It is much easier to do a structural than a functional neuroimaging study of autism because it requires that the participant spend a shorter amount of time in the scanner and it can even be done under sedation if the participant has difficulty remaining still. We do not attempt a complete review of this literature but attempt to discuss some of that which is relevant.

Perhaps the most consistent finding to have emerged not only from structural imaging studies but also from head measurements in general and post-mortem studies (Bailey et al., 1998; Woodhouse et al., 1996) is that of megencephaly in autism. A recent review by Courchesne (2004) looked at current evidence that head growth at birth below normal progresses rapidly during the first year before growth is arrested. This means that growth during the first year is overrapid and then too slow. Overgrowth is most marked in frontal, temporal, and parietal regions serving higher cognitive functions, language, and social information processing. Courchesne suggests that despite early overgrowth, development of neuronal systems is curtailed. He suggests that greatest effects may be on large pyramidal neurons, especially in frontal regions that play a key role in integrating information from multiple functional domains, and in exerting "top-down" influences on lower-level systems. He also suggests that this will lead to reduced long-distance cortical connectivity. Within Courchesne's (2004) model, "autism may be an unusual disconnection disorder with sparing (or perhaps even enhancement) of lower-level basic processing, but also with an impaired capacity to fully integrate lower-level detailed information into higher level contexts" (p. 109).

Therefore, Just and colleagues' (2004) suggestion that autism may result from disconnectivity is not a novel one. As pointed out by Frith (2004), disconnectivity has long been a concept used to explain psychiatric disorders, at least since Wernicke in 1906. It has also been evoked as an explanation for dyslexia and schizophrenia. As well as Courchesne (2004) and Muller, Kleinhans, Kemmotsu, Pierce, and Courchesne (2003), Hill and Frith (2003) also speculated that autism results from a failure of feedback connectivity, and the findings by Castelli and colleagues (2002) that are consistent with this idea have been discussed earlier. Ellis and Gunter (1999) also related Asperger syndrome to nonverbal learning disability and suggested both disorders might arise from a white matter disorder, particularly affecting the right brain. In Courchesne's model, disconnectivity is primarily between frontal cortex and the autistic syndrome arises from the lack of its influence on the rest of the cortex. The Hill and Frith model is similar. In Muller and colleagues' (2004) paper, disconnectivity arises secondary to poor connections between thalamus and cortex and the consequent failure of these areas to differentiate. Muller and colleagues' findings also raise the possibility that poor synchronicity between areas is not due to poor connectivity but to different patterns of cellular response to input. For Just and colleagues, underconnectivity is proposed as a general feature of autism though they concede that this may arise from poor orchestration by prefrontal executive function.

The MN hypothesis by Williams and colleagues (2001) comes from an evolutionary position with the view that specific adaptations that have modified primate brain function for it to serve imitation, joint attention, and ToM, and it is these adaptations that are specifically affected in autism. We hope that by identifying commonalities of affected processes in autism, we will be able to hone the specificity of the biological adaptation that is affected to result in the characteristic pattern of clinical features and experimental findings that constitute the autistic syndrome. We also suggested that connectivity would be impaired, but that adaptations specifically serving self–other connectivity will be most affected. Our findings of essentially normal functional connectivity suggests that we should focus our efforts on brain areas that serve integratory functions, such as frontal lobe, mirror neurons, and temporoparietal cortex, as opposed to looking at the connectivity between the brain areas. However, autism is a developmental disorder and the development of connectivity will affect local regional development and vice versa.

Voxel-Based Morphometry

It is important to look at the distribution of white matter connectivity in autism. If one was attempting to frame the self–other matching hypothesis of autism in terms of a hypothesis amenable to testing with structural imaging, one might well propose poor white matter connectivity between brain areas serving observation and action. In fact, white matter deficits have been reported in autism mainly in the corpus callosum. Hardan, Minshew, and Keshavan (2000) and Piven, Bailey, Ranson, and Arndt (1997) demonstrated reductions in the size of the corpus callosum, though McAlonan and colleagues (2002) described white matter deficits in the brainstem, inferior longitudinal and occipitofrontal fasciculi, and corticospinal tracts in adults with Asperger syndrome.

A limitation of studies that depend on measurements of regions of interest is that they miss differences in unexpected areas or where the delineation of the area is difficult. Voxel-based morphometry (VBM) takes a whole-brain analysis approach. Again, structural brain images of participants are all subjected to a warping algorithm to make them fit a standard template. Then the relative volumes of gray and white matter in each voxel can be compared between groups. We carried out a VBM study of gray and white matter differences in ASD (Waiter et al., 2004, 2005; see Plates 15.4 and 15.5), making our template from the brain images of our participants, so that the amount of warping necessary was minimized. We found gray matter volume increases in the right fusiform gyrus, the right temporo-occipital region, the left frontal pole, and the medial frontal cortex. These areas are all implicated in imitation. As mentioned previously, we suggested that maturation of an area involves neural pruning processes which reduce gray matter volume. As the areas were heavily used for imitation in controls compared to participants with ASD, so they showed greater maturity of this region. The only area of decreased gray matter density was in the thalamus, again consistent with the idea that this region is used more by participants with ASD than controls, because of greater learning by direct associative learning than through imitation or other more abstract approaches.

White matter differences were even more statistically significant than gray matter differences. We found widespread white matter differences— particularly in the corpus callosum and right-sided cortical white matter. These findings are consistent with the disconnectivity/underconnectivity hypotheses proposed earlier, but it is also evident that connectivity between areas serving ToM, imitation, and joint attention were especially affected, with white matter deficits being more right-sided and specifically affecting temporoparietal cortex and left orbitofrontal cortex (Plate 15.2). The MN regions in themselves did not show abnormal volumes of gray matter, suggesting that these regions have developed normally, and it is more likely to be their control or anatomical connectivity that is functionally impaired.

Other studies using VBM have also been published by Boddaert and colleagues (2004) and by McAlonan and colleagues (2005). Boddaert found many fewer differences than those in our study, with only small differences bilaterally in STS. More important though, both studies found gray matter volumes to be less in their study groups compared to ours, which found increased gray matter levels. One explanation might be that participants in the McAlonan and Boddaert study were younger (mean age = 12.0 and 9.3 years, respectively), were much more developmentally impaired in the case of the Boddaert study (mean IQ = 55), and, in contrast to ours, neither study had ASD participants matched on IQ with controls. However, the IQ differences between groups were not great in the McAlonan study and they covaried for IQ, which did not make a difference. The mean age of our participants was only 3.4 years greater than those in McAlonan's study, and thus it seems unlikely that this would explain the differences. One possible explanation may lie in methods of analysis. As mentioned, the comparison requires "warping" each image to fit a standard brain. We were concerned about problems with these procedures, when the images of young, autistic brains have to be more extensively "warped" to fit standard adult templates. We therefore constructed a group-specific template to minimize this, and generated a quite different pattern of results to those we generated previously (unpublished) using an adult template. One possibility is, therefore, that the findings of the McAlonan and Boddaert have been unduly influenced by "warping" effects rather than real gray and white matter differences. Our study is more consistent with the first VBM study of adults with ASD by Abell and colleagues (1999), supporting this explanation.

Diffusion Tensor Imaging

In recent years a new technique, diffusion tensor imaging, is showing promise. Fiber tracts mean that water molecules in the brain are forced to diffuse more in the directions along which these paths travel than in other directions. This provides a measure of "fractional anisotropy" that reflects microstructural characteristics of white matter such as fiber density and fiber diameter. Barnea-Goraly and colleagues (2004) identified tract abnormalities in bilateral ventromedial frontal cortex and bilaterally in the region of the temporo-parietal junctions in autism, in a small group of seven children and adolescents with high-functioning autism.

The Thalamus

As mentioned, our VBM study found an increase rather than a decrease in gray matter volume in ASD, consistent with Abell and colleagues (1999). Thalamic abnormalities have also been reported by Tsatsanis and colleagues (2003). They found that while thalamic volume correlated with cortical volume in controls, no such relationship existed for the ASD group. They wondered about aberrant patterns of connectivity between the thalamus and cortex. We investigated thalamus activation during imitation in our study and found it to be greater in the ASD group than in the participants. Another possible explanation then for Tsatsanis's findings is that individuals with ASD use thalamocortical learning mechanisms in preference to corticocortical learning mechanisms, perhaps irrespective of the nature of the stimulus. Looked at from an evolutionary perspective, we might suggest that while activities involving mirror neurons and social cognition are under predominantly subcortical control in nonhuman primates, social-cognitive evolution has led to greater cortical control of such activities. In the absence of social cognitive development, perhaps through the failure of connectivity development, imitation reverts to a more subcortical activity. Lewis (2004) has explored greater activation of thalamic and other limbic system learning mechanisms in his animal model of autism, suggesting that this could also explain the repetitive behaviors associated with autism.

LIMITATIONS AND THE FUTURE OF IMAGING RESEARCH IN AUTISM

Brain imaging techniques appear to have much to offer the study of ASD. However, their limitations need to be appreciated if their benefits are to be reaped appropriately. Functional imaging studies for example, reflect brain function and not anatomy. If activity levels in an area of brain are reduced, it does not mean that the anatomy is abnormal. Furthermore, they show that function is abnormal for the tasks that are part of the particular experiment. Similarly, brain activity in an area may appear normal when its function is impaired. This may be because the experimental task has not put it under the conditions that would induce abnormal function. Hence, our imitation task did not find abnormalities in Broca's area whereas Just and colleagues (2004) found poor synchrony between Broca's area and Wernicke's area. Also, fMRI does not measure function directly but uses a measure of changing blood oxygenation. Research suggests (Logothetis, 2002; Logothetis, Pauls, Augath, Trinath, & Oeltermann, 2001) that this depends on local metabolic rates which are most affected when a cellular area is processing inputs, although there is also evidence that it might be strongly affected by changes in neuroglial cell metabolism. Also, if neural cell densities differ (as we suggested occurs with gray matter difference in autism), this could also presumably affect the way the BOLD signal changes when an area becomes involved in an activity. Therefore, we need to be aware that BOLD signal change in an area may be influenced by a number of local factors that might differ between groups. Finally, there is the finding by Müller and colleagues (2004) that a brain area may continue to be activated in autism, even though activation has stopped in the controls once the task has been learned. If this is a general feature, then, in repetitive tasks averaged over a number of blocks, persistent activation will appear as increased activation. Another important concern to be raised about functional neuroimaging studies in autism is that they are usually performed in adults (adolescents in our study). However, autism is a developmental condition, and functional abnormalities in physically mature individuals with normal intelligence cannot necessarily be generalized to the whole population of people with autism. Ideally, as we increase our ability to design tasks that children can perform in the scanning environment, we will be able to ascertain a developmental picture of the neural substrate of social cognition and examine how this changes with age and social functioning. In addition, new methods may be developed that enable the measurement of function directly.

Just as functional studies on their own say nothing about anatomical structure, so structural studies do not tell us about function. However, they are essential for us to develop an understanding of the neuroanatomical abnormality of autism and what may be called its endophenotype. Nevertheless, we need to remain cautious. First, we need to be cautious in our statistical and image manipulative procedures. Apparent group differences may emerge from groups responding differently to these processing steps. Once we have the evidence of differences in white or gray matter structure, we need to ascertain which are the direct products of genetic expression and which are secondary to the effect of experience on brain structure. Here, we have suggested that increasing use of an area leads to neural pruning and greater organization. Greater use of two brain areas may also conceivably lead to changes in white matter connectivity between them. Structural studies are more straightforward in children and already prospective longitudinal studies of brain development in autism are being conducted. These will be essential in disentangling primary from secondary neuroanatomical abnormalities.

CONCLUSIONS

Our hypothesis was that people with autism would show impaired function of those neural systems that serve self–other mapping and which lie at the heart of imitation, joint attention, and ToM. These neural systems would include but would not be confined to areas in which an MN function has been established. Frontal and posterior temporal integratory functions may be especially important. Our functional neuroimaging studies of imitation in autism and joint attention largely supported this hypothesis, finding less extensive activity in the parietal MN system during imitation and a very different pattern of activity in posterior temporal cortex where we found evidence that a self–other mapping function could be central to the development of ToM. These findings have recently been complemented by a study conducted by Dapretto and colleagues (2006) providing strong evidence for low activation of Broca's area during facial imitation in young people with autism.

In addition, we found impairment in amygdaloid involvement in the action processing system. Our joint attention study showed the importance of the left superior frontal gyrus and anteromedial cortex in self–other mapping, demonstrating that it remains a much more complex process in the mature brain, than being solely dependent on the MN system. Other studies are providing evidence for more general brain impairment associated with ASD such as diminished "connectivity" and global white matter deficits. We have found gray and white matter deficits in autism to be a little more specifically associated with areas serving social cognitive function, occurring especially in areas that we have also associated with imitation or joint attention. Therefore, structural imaging studies of individuals with autistic disorder also find impairment of white and gray matter structures that serve a self–other mapping function. A simple white matter deficit seems to offer a straightforward explanation, but its specific distribution suggests that it could arise secondary to deficits in synaptic functioning.

These are promising initial steps that begin to find some congruence between the simple behavioral functions of imitation and joint attention, the more complex cognitive function of ToM, and the functional and structural abnormalities associated with autism.

As our ability to image the brain increases we will be able to study children at younger ages and map the course of the brain changes associated with social development. This offers the promise of understanding the effects of experience on brain development and identifying the key developmental processes that can be upset to result in autism.

ACKNOWLEDGMENTS

Our work is supported by grants awarded by Chief Scientist's Office of the Scottish executive, the National Alliance for Autism Research and the Health Foundation. We are very grateful to our collaborators Andrew Whiten, David Perrett, Anne Gilchrist and Alison Murray, as well as the volunteers who participated in our studies.

REFERENCES

Abell, F., Krams, M., Ashburner, J., Passingham, R., Friston, K., Frackowiak, R., et al. (1999). The neuroanatomy of autism: A voxel-based whole brain analysis of structural scans. *Neuroreport, 10*(8), 1647–1651.

Arbib, M. A. (2005). From monkey-like action recognition to human language: An evolutionary framework for neurolinguistics. *Behavioral and Brain Sciences, 28,* 105–124.

Astafiev, S. V., Stanley, C. M., Shulman, G. L., & Corbetta, M. (2004). Extrastriate body area in human occipital cortex responds to the performance of motor actions. *Nature Neuroscience, 7*(5), 542–548.

Bailey, A., Luthert, P., Dean, A., Harding, B., Janota, I., Montgomery, M., et al. (1998). A clinicopathological study of autism. *Brain, 121*(Pt. 5), 889–905.

Barnea-Goraly, N., Kwon, H., Menon, V., Eliez, S., Lotspeich, L., & Reiss, A. L. (2004). White matter structure in autism: Preliminary evidence from diffusion tensor imaging. *Biological Psychiatry, 55*(3), 323–326.

Baron-Cohen, S., Ring, H. A., Bullmore, E. T., Wheelwright, S., Ashwin, C., & Williams, S. C. (2000). The amygdala theory of autism. *Neuroscience and Biobehavioral Reviews, 24*(3), 355–364.

Boddaert, N., Chabane, N., Gervais, H., Good, C. D., Bourgeois, M., Plumet, M. H., et al. (2004). Superior temporal sulcus anatomical abnormalities in childhood autism: A voxel-based morphometry MRI study. *NeuroImage, 23*(1), 364–369.

Carruthers, P., & Smith, P. K. (1996). Introduction. In P. Carruthers & P. K. Smith (Eds.), *Theories of theories of mind* (pp. 1–8). Cambridge, UK: Cambridge University Press. 1996.

Castelli, F., Frith, C., Happé, F., & Frith, U. (2002). Autism, Asperger syndrome and brain mechanisms for the attribution of mental states to animated shapes. *Brain, 125*(Pt. 8), 1839–1849.

Castelli, F., Happé, F., Frith, U., & Frith, C. (2000). Movement and mind: A functional imaging study of perception and interpretation of complex intentional movement patterns. *NeuroImage, 12*(3), 314–325.

Courchesne, E. (2004). Brain development in autism: Early overgrowth followed by premature arrest of growth. *Mental Retardation and Developmental Disabilities Research Reviews, 10*(2), 106–111.

Decety, J., Grezes, J., Costes, N., Perani, D., Jeannerod, M., Procyk, E., et al. (1997). Brain activity during observation of actions. Influence of action content and subject's strategy. *Brain, 120*(Pt. 10), 1763–1777.

di Pellegrino, G., Fadiga, L., Fogassi, L., Gallese, V., & Rizzolatti, G. (1992). Understanding motor events: A neurophysiological study. *Experimental Brain Research, 91*(1), 176–180.

Ellis, H. D., & Gunter, H. L. (1999). Asperger syndrome: A simple matter of white matter? *Trends in Cognitive Sciences, 3*(5), 192–200.

Fadiga, L., Buccino, G., Craighero, L., Fogassi, L., Gallese, V., & Pavesi, G. (1999).

Corticospinal excitability is specifically modulated by motor imagery: A magnetic stimulation study. *Neuropsychologia, 37*(2), 147–158.

Fogassi, L., Ferrari, P. F., Gesierich, B., Rozzi, S., Chersi, F., & Rizzolatti, G. (2005). Parietal lobe: From action organization to intention understanding. *Science, 308,* 662–667.

Frith, C. (2004). Is autism a disconnection disorder? *Lancet Neurology, 3*(10), 577.

Frith, C. D., & Frith, U. (2000). In S. Baron-Cohen, H. Tager-Flusberg, & D. J. Cohen (Eds.), *The physiological basis of theory of mind: Functional neuroimaging studies* (pp. 334–356). Oxford, UK: Oxford University Press.

Gallese, V., Fadiga, L., Fogassi, L., & Rizzolatti, G. (1996). Action recognition in the premotor cortex. *Brain, 119*(Pt. 2), 593–609.

Grezes, J., Armony, J. L., Rowe, J., & Passingham, R. E. (2003). Activations related to "mirror" and "canonical" neurons in the human brain: An fMRI study. *NeuroImage, 18*(4), 928–937.

Hadjikhani, N., Joseph, R., Syder, J., Harris, G., & Tager-Flusberg, H. (2005, May 5–7). *Regional differences in the cortical thickness of the mirror neuron network in autistic spectrum disorder.* Poster presented at the meeting of International Society for Autism Research, Boston.

Hamzei, F., Rijntjes, M., Dettmers, C., Glauche, V., Weiller, C., & Büchel, C. (2003). The human action recognition system and its relationship to Broca's area: An fMRI study. *NeuroImage, 19,* 637–644.

Hardan, A. Y., Minshew, N. J., & Keshavan, M. S. (2000). Corpus callosum size in autism. *Neurology, 55*(7), 1033–1036.

Hill, E. L., & Frith, U. (2003). Understanding autism: Insights from mind and brain. *Philosophical Transactions of the Royal Society of London, B, 358,* 281–289.

Iacoboni, M., Koski, L. M., Brass, M., Bekkering, H., Woods, R. P., Dubeau, M. C., et al. (2001). Reafferent copies of imitated actions in the right superior temporal cortex. *Proceedings of the National Academy of Sciences of the USA, 98,* 13995–13999.

Iacoboni, M., Woods, R. P., Brass, M., Bekkering, H., Mazziotta, J. C., & Rizzolatti, G. (1999). Cortical mechanisms of human imitation. *Science, 286,* 2526–2528.

Jackson, P. L., Meltzoff, A. N., & Decety, J. (in press). Neural circuits involved in imitation and perspective-taking. *NeuroImage.*

Jacobs, B., Schall, M., Prather, M., Kapler, E., Driscoll, L., Baca, S., et al. (2001). Regional dendritic and spine variation in human cerebral cortex: A quantitative Golgi study. *Cerebral Cortex, 11,* 558–571.

Just, M. A., Cherkassky, V. L., Keller, T. A., & Minshew, N. J. (2004). Cortical activation and synchronization during sentence comprehension in high-functioning autism: Evidence of underconnectivity. *Brain, 127*(Pt. 8), 1811–1821.

Lewis, M. (2004, May). *Repetitive behavior in autism.* Presentation delivered at the annual meeting of the International Society for Autism Research, Sacramento.

Logothetis, N. K. (2002). The neural basis of the blood-oxygen-level-dependent functional magnetic resonance imaging signal. *Philosophical Transactions of the Royal Society of London, B, Biological Sciences, 357,* 1003–1037.

Logothetis, N. K., Pauls, J., Augath, M., Trinath, T., & Oeltermann, A. (2001). Neurophysiological investigation of the basis of the fMRI signal. *Nature, 412,* 150–157.

Lord, C., Rutter, M., & Le Couteur, A. (1994). Autism Diagnostic Interview—Revised: A revised version of a diagnostic interview for caregivers of individuals with possible pervasive developmental disorders. *Journal of Autism and Developmental Disorders, 24*(5), 659–685.

Makuuchi, M. (in press). Is Broca's area crucial for imitation? *Cerebral Cortex, 15*(5), 563–570

McAlonan, G. M., Cheung, V., Cheung, C., Suckling, J., Lam, G. Y., Tai, K. S., et al. (2005). Mapping the brain in autism. A voxel-based MRI study of volumetric differences and intercorrelations in autism. *Brain*, *128*, 268–276.

McAlonan, G. M., Daly, E., Kumari, V., Critchley, H. D., van Amelsvoort, T., Suckling, J., et al. (2002). Brain anatomy and sensorimotor gating in Asperger's syndrome. *Brain*, *125*(Pt. 7), 1594–1606.

Muller, R. A., Cauich, C., Rubio, M. A., Mizuno, A., & Courchesne, E. (2004). Abnormal activity patterns in premotor cortex during sequence learning in autistic patients. *Biological Psychiatry*, *56*(5), 323–332.

Muller, R. A., Kleinhans, N., Kemmotsu, N., Pierce, K., & Courchesne, E. (2003). Abnormal variability and distribution of functional maps in autism: An FMRI study of visuomotor learning. *American Journal of Psychiatry*, *160*(10), 1847–1862.

Nishitani, N., Avikainen, S., & Hari, R. (2004). Abnormal imitation-related cortical activation sequences in Asperger's syndrome. *Annals of Neurology*, *55*, 558–562.

Piven, J., Bailey, J., Ranson, B. J., & Arndt, S. (1997). An MRI study of the corpus callosum in autism. *American Journal of Psychiatry*, *154*(8), 1051–1056.

Ramnani, N., & Owen, A. M. (2004). Anterior prefrontal cortex: Insights into function from anatomy and neuroimaging. *Nature Reviews Neuroscience*, *5*, 184–194.

Rizzolatti, G., Fadiga, L., Gallese, V., & Fogassi, L. (1996). Premotor cortex and the recognition of motor actions. *Brain Research Cognitive Brain Research*, *3*(2), 131–141.

Rizzolatti, G., Fogassi, L., & Gallese, V. (2001). Neurophysiological mechanisms underlying the understanding and imitation of action. *Nature Reviews Neuroscience*, *2*(9), 661–670.

Rogers, S. J., & Pennington, B. F. (1991). A theoretical approach to the deficits in infantile autism. *Development and Psychopathology*, *3*, 137–162.

Saxe, R., & Kanwisher, N. (2003). People thinking about thinking people. The role of the temporo-parietal junction in "theory of mind." *NeuroImage*, *19*(4), 1835–1842.

Saxe, R., Xiao, D. K., Kovacs, G., Perrett, D. I., & Kanwisher, N. (2004). A region of right posterior superior temporal sulcus responds to observed intentional actions. *Neuropsychologia*, *42*(11), 1435–1446.

Theoret, H., Halligan, E., Kobayashi, M., Fregni, F., Tager-Flusberg, H., & Pascual-Leone, A. (2005). Impaired motor facilitation during action observation in individuals with autism spectrum disorder. *Current Biology*, *15*(3), R84–R85.

Toni, I., & Passingham, R. E. (1999). Prefrontal–basal ganglia pathways are involved in the learning of arbitrary visuomotor associations: A PET study. *Experimental Brain Research*, *127*(1), 19–32.

Tsatsanis, K. D., Rourke, B. P., Klin, A., Volkmar, F. R., Cicchetti, D., & Schultz, R. T. (2003). Reduced thalamic volume in high-functioning individuals with autism. *Biological Psychiatry*, *53*(2), 121–129.

Villalobos, M. E., Mizuno, A., Dahl, B. C., Kemmotsu, N., & Muller, R. A. (2005). Reduced functional connectivity between V1 and inferior frontal cortex associated with visuomotor performance in autism. *NeuroImage*, *25*, 916–925.

Vogeley, K., Bussfeld, P., Newen, A., Herrmann, S., Happe, F., Falkai, P., et al. (2001). Mind reading: Neural mechanisms of theory of mind and self-perspective. *NeuroImage*, *14*, 170–181.

Waiter, G. D., Williams, J. H., Murray, A. D., Gilchrist, A., Perrett, D. I., & Whiten, A. (2004). A voxel-based investigation of brain structure in male adolescents with autistic spectrum disorder. *NeuroImage*, *22*(2), 619–625.

Waiter, G. D., Williams, J. H., Murray, A. D., Gilchrist, A., Perrett, D. I., & Whiten, A. (2005). Structural white matter deficits in high-functioning individuals with autistic spectrum disorder: A voxel-based investigation. *NeuroImage*, *24*(2), 455–461.

Williams, J. H. G., Waiter, G. D., Gilchrist A., Perrett, D. I., Murray A. D., & Whiten, A. (2006). Neural mechanisms of imitation and "Mirror Neuron" functioning in autistic spectrum disorder. *Neuropsychologia*, *44*(4), 610–621.

Williams, J. H. G., Waiter, G. D., Perra, O., Perrett, D. I., & Whiten, A. (2005). An fMRI study of joint attention experience. *NeuroImage*, *25*, 133–140.

Williams, J. H., Whiten, A., Suddendorf, T., & Perrett, D. I. (2001). Imitation, mirror neurons and autism. *Neuroscience and Biobehavioral Reviews*, *25*(4), 287–295.

Woodhouse, W., Bailey, A., Rutter, M., Bolton, P., Baird, G., & Le Couteur, A. (1996). Head circumference in autism and other pervasive developmental disorders. *Journal of Child Psychology and Psychiatry, and Allied Disciplines*, *37*(6), 665–671.

Zhang, J. X., Feng, C. M., Fox, P. T., Gao, J. H., & Tan, L. H. (2004). Is left inferior frontal gyrus a general mechanism for selection? *NeuroImage*, *23*, 596–603.

CHAPTER 16

Assessment of Imitation Abilities in Autism
Conceptual and Methodological Issues

ISABEL M. SMITH
CRYSTAL LOWE-PEARCE
SHANA L. NICHOLS

The dramatic growth in research on imitation in autism over the past decade is surveyed in depth by the authors of other chapters in this volume. They discuss, from a variety of perspectives, the rationale and results of this rich literature. This chapter provides an opportunity for reflection on some of the methodological issues that arise in the rapidly expanding area of research on imitation. Our approach is first to highlight briefly some of the conceptual issues that determine or limit methodological choices. Most important, of course, are the questions of how one has defined imitation and for what purpose one is measuring it. These are weighty issues that the reader will no doubt have in mind throughout this volume; here we highlight only a few pertinent aspects. For the purpose of this chapter, we draw specifically on the literature on imitation of body movements (gestures, and other actions with and without objects). There is a small literature on imitation of facial–oral gestures in autism (e.g., Loveland et al., 1994; Rogers, Bennetto, McEvoy, & Pennington, 1996; Rogers, Hepburn, Stackhouse, & Wehner, 2003.). Vocal–verbal imitation is, of course, also slow to develop in children with autism; the relatively few studies are found largely, but not exclusively, in the behavioral intervention literature (e.g., Drash, High, & Tudor, 1999). Many of the same concerns with experimental design and control arise in studies of these classes of imitation. Our main purpose here, however, is to discuss the methodological considerations that pertain to the measurement of action imitation in autism spectrum disorders (ASD) and to address these issues as they are found in both experimental and clinical contexts.

DEFINITION OF IMITATION

It is obvious that the choice of measurement determines in part what can be measured. The question of what we mean by measuring imitation has become increasingly complex. Developments in theoretical approaches to imitation have been rapid over the last several years, fueled in part by the research on imitation in comparative psychology, the discovery of the mirror neurons as a possible neural basis for imitation (Rizzolatti, Fadiga, Gallese, & Fogassi, 1996), and burgeoning interest in the development of intentionality and how it is reflected in imitative behavior (e.g., Tomasello & Carpenter, 2005). Want and Harris (2002) made a particularly influential contribution, highlighting the various forms of imitative behavior and their different cognitive underpinnings. The literature on "imitation" in autism reveals a wide spectrum of behaviors of interest. Studies cover the gamut, for example, from Nadel and Pezé (1993), who examined the frequency of reciprocal imitation of peers by preschoolers, to magnetoencephalographic investigations of imitation of oral movements in response to picture cues (Nishitani, Avikainen, & Hari, 2004).

A number of different research interests are served by the study of imitation in autism. One fundamental distinction is whether the primary focus is on what autism reveals about the mechanisms of imitation (e.g., Heyes, 2001) or on what imitation reveals about autism (e.g., Dawson et al., 2002). Some, perhaps many, investigators have both objectives. For developmental researchers, imitation may also be an experimental tool, for example, as an assay for social–cognitive ability (Meltzoff & Decety, 2003), notably the development of intentional understanding (e.g., Tomasello & Carpenter, 2005). Findings from imitation tasks may also provide evidence of the neuropsychological basis of autism (e.g., Dawson, Meltzoff, Osterling, & Rinaldi, 1998).

The neural basis of imitation, especially as embodied in the mirror neuron system, is receiving much attention (e.g., Iacoboni, 2005; Rizzolatti, Fadiga, Fogassi, & Gallese, 2002), including within autism research (Williams et al., 2006; Williams, Whiten, Suddendorf, & Perrett, 2001). Methodological issues in this area are beyond our scope. However, we note in passing both the technical and ethical challenges inherent in obtaining images of the brains of young children with autism, in whom the imitation impairment is perhaps most evident and most informative. Moreover, despite the ingenuity of researchers in this area, there are considerable pragmatic challenges associated with imaging during imitation of ecologically meaningful actions.

Imitation in autism may also be investigated for its own sake, as, for example, in studies that seek to develop more effective ways of teaching young children with autism. These studies may converge with research that is directed toward the discovery of mechanisms that underlie imitative impairments. The assumption of such studies is that better understanding of the deficient processes may lead to interventions that more effectively remediate, compensate for, or bypass these difficulties. An excellent example of this convergence is research by Schreibman and her colleagues that provides rigorous tests of intervention methods that target specific skills such as imitation. The effects of treatment are measured on both the targeted skill and on theoretically related skills such as joint attention (Ingersoll & Schreibman, in press). Such studies contribute to the understanding of relationships among these critical skills, as well as to the development of effective interventions.

We focus first on issues related to measurement of imitation for the primary purpose of describing the imitative problem in autism and revealing the underlying mechanisms. Following this, we consider measurement issues that arise in more clinically oriented contexts.

IMPAIRED IMITATION IN AUTISM: EXPERIMENTAL STUDIES

Historically, there have been two basic approaches to the study of imitation in autism (see Smith & Bryson, 1994, for more detailed discussion). One tradition emphasized the symbolic function of imitation and considered imitative deficits an early indicator of impaired language development. An alternative perspective has emphasized imitation as an aspect of praxis, or the control of learned movements. These two lines of research are no longer as distinct, but they continue to influence the conceptualization and, hence, the measurement, of imitation in individuals with autism. Some issues that arise in the measurement of imitation in experimental studies, including the use of controls, are addressed below. The reader is referred to a special issue of the *Journal of Autism and Developmental Disorders* (Burack, 2004) for in-depth discussions of issues regarding appropriate controls for autism research in general. In our more specific but briefer discussion, we make a somewhat arbitrary distinction between (1) "control" conditions or groups, in the sense of tasks (e.g., of motor skill) administered or groups matched on a particular variable (e.g., language level) to rule out an expected influence, and (2) tasks or conditions that are designed to test possible underlying mechanisms, the effects of which are not yet determined (e.g., body schema).

Control Groups and Conditions

A major implication of the merging of early perspectives on imitation in autism (i.e., symbolic vs. praxic deficits) was recognition of the need to control for level of language functioning in experimental work in imitation (Smith & Bryson, 1994). Such controls were considered necessary because imitation and language skills are correlated in normal development (Bates, Benigni, Bretherton, Camaioni, & Volterra, 1979). Prior to the work conducted in the 1990s, lack of such controls in many studies left the question open as to whether imitation was more deficient in individuals with autism than would be predicted based on their level of language development. Subsequent studies have addressed this issue, and most have confirmed that imitation is disproportionately impaired in autism. Imitation deficits are observed for both representational and nonrepresentational gestures and do not appear to be simply a consequence of a general impairment in symbol use. As studies have been conducted with younger and younger children with autism, one challenge that has become apparent is that matching to typically developing children for language level would result in dramatically mismatched motor skills. Rogers has addressed this by matching developmentally delayed controls to the children with autism on language level, and young typically developing controls on motor skills (Rogers et al., 2003).

Another of the advances that accompanied more analytic approaches to studying imitation deficits was the introduction of control conditions to address the perceptual, memory, and motor demands imposed by elicited imitation tasks (Smith & Bryson, 1994). For example, in studies by Rogers (Rogers et al., 1996) and Smith (1996; Smith & Bryson, 1998) control conditions were used to verify that participants with autism were as able as controls to identify the gestures that they were required to imitate. These studies used picture identification control tasks in which the participants indicated the one gesture, from among foils, that was modeled (cf. pantomime recognition tasks of Bartak, Rutter, & Cox, 1975), thus ruling out problems with attention or memory as explanations of imitation deficits. Nonetheless, it should be noted that these are fairly gross measures (using static stimuli). It may still be the case that more subtle features, perhaps especially dynamic features, of gestures or movements are not processed in the same way by individuals with autism. This may occur in the context of general difficulty in processing biologically relevant motion (Blake, Turner, Smoski, Pozdol, & Stone, 2003).

In contrast to the similarity of the strategies used in the aforementioned studies to control attentional/perceptual and memory factors, different approaches were taken to account for the role of motor skills in imitation performance. Rogers and colleagues (1996) administered an additional motor control trial for each imitation item, in order to ascertain that participants were physically capable of the movements. Participants were prompted to perform the action simultaneously as the experimenter demonstrated, and both verbal and physical feedback was used to correct the posture or movement. Therefore, the control was for the ability to perform the specific movements required for each item, as each participant demonstrated his or her physical competence, with maximal support.

To account for motor skill effects on imitation, Smith and Bryson (1998) instead administered a standard test of manual dexterity, the Grooved Pegboard. Participants with autism obtained a significantly lower group mean score than did either the language-impaired control group or younger, typically developing controls (both matched to the autism group for receptive language level). Regression analyses indicated that differences in motor skills accounted for 37% of the variance in gesture imitation scores (beyond the 11% accounted for by language level). Imitation scores remained significantly low for the autism group when both the language and motor skill measures were covaried. These results demonstrated that motor skills in general do influence imitation ability, in that good motor skills provide a necessary but not sufficient condition for accurate imitation (presumably especially of more complex gestures).

This approach of testing motor skills independent of the specific gesture tasks is now common. However, not all studies with younger participants have confirmed associations between motor and imitation skills (Rogers et al., 2003). Differing statistical associations among the same skills at different points in development is a known phenomenon. One cannot conclude that because two skills are uncorrelated at one point in development, a relationship between the two might not be apparent at another developmental stage (Bates et al., 1979).

Clearly, the relationships between various aspects of motor and imitation abilities in autistic spectrum disorders have not yet been resolved (Dewey & Bottos, Chapter 17, this volume; Green et al., 2002; Rogers et al., 2003; Smith, 2000, 2004). The specific nature and strength of these relationships may depend not only on the particular actions involved but also on the age/developmental level of participants. However, given the prevalence of motor problems in autism (Smith, 2000, 2004), it is also clear that the motor demands of the tasks should be considered in any study of action imitation. In particular, investigators need to be mindful of the physical demands of imitation tasks when children with autism are compared to language-matched but much younger typically developing children. Rogers and colleagues (2003) addressed this concern by matching developmentally delayed controls to their group of children with autism on both nonverbal and verbal mental age, as well as on fine motor skill levels (and chronological age), whereas the typically developing group was matched only on the nonverbal and fine motor measures.

Nature of the Imitation Tasks

Lessons learned from research on the typical development of imitation have been relatively slow to infiltrate studies of imitation in autism. In particular, work on differences between elicited and spontaneous imitation, and on factors influencing individual differences in imitation, might inform the study of imitative phenomena in autism. There are few studies of spontaneous imitation in autism, one major constraint being, of course, the rarity of the phenomenon. Rising to this challenge, Brown and Whiten (2000) undertook a study of spontaneous imitation by both children and adults with autism. Using a time-sampling procedure (1-minute samples over 90 minutes of videotaped observations), they observed few imitative acts in any of five categories. Indeed, in both school/residential and play contexts, only 3- to 4-year-old typically developing children showed much spontaneous imitative behavior; children and adults with autism, older typical children, and children with intellectual disabilities imitated far less often. Due to the descriptive nature of the study, lack of constancy in the environments in which participants were observed, and lack of mental age controls, interpretation of these findings is difficult. This represents another instance in which the spontaneous performance of people with autism obscures competencies that can be demonstrated in more structured situations. It has long been observed that individuals with autism possess many abilities that nonetheless are rarely seen in their spontaneous repertoires. Volkmar, Lord, Bailey, Schultz, and Klin (2004) have commented recently on the need for research to address this issue more directly by taking care not to lose the phenomenon under study in the pursuit of experimental rigor.

Examining the effects of varying demands may be a more efficient research strategy than attempting to tap the limited imitative behavior of people with autism in completely natural environments. Nadel's (2002) work has been exemplary in this regard, by capitalizing on situations in which young children with autism may show *some* spontaneous imitation (i.e., in dyadic free play with peers). Any increase in structure and reduction of distractions under these more controlled conditions may account for the higher levels of spontaneous imitation observed in her study, in contrast to that of Brown and Whiten (2000). Stone and her colleagues have also explored the effects of the amount of structure provided by an adult examiner on the imitation performance of young children with autism (Stone, Ulman, Swanson, McMahon, & Turner, 2004). In addition to the expected differences in levels of imitation performance revealed by the two conditions (i.e., greater structure leading to better performance), different patterns of correlation were obtained with other skills (such as motor and visual attention skills), important information both for understanding the nature of the deficit and potentially for intervention.

The upper limits of imitative competence in individuals with autism are generally revealed in research on elicited imitation, which constitutes the vast majority of published studies. In typically developing infants and children, a number of parameters have been demonstrated to influence performance in elicited imitation paradigms. Many of these could reasonably be assumed also to affect imitation in children with autism, and additional factors may be involved. For the present purpose, the effects of several variables will be considered: the characteristics of the model, the motivational state of the child, and the methods of stimulus presentation. Substantial attention has been paid to manipulations of the types of actions in previous reviews (e.g., Smith & Bryson, 1994; Williams, Whiten, & Singh, 2004). Interestingly, comparisons of imitation of different action types by children with autism and children with other developmental disorders, or indeed with typically developing children, have been conducted on a between-groups basis. This has led to debates on issues such as whether, as a group, children with autism have more difficulty with symbolic versus nonsymbolic actions, or with body movements alone versus actions with objects. The reader is referred to several recent discussions of issues related to this aspect of imitation research, notably those by Rogers (1999; Rogers & Bennetto, 2000; Rogers et al., 2003; Stone, Ousley, & Littleford, 1997; Williams et al., 2004). For additional discussion of issues specific to the imitation of symbolic gestures and, in particular, the difficulty of disentangling the effects of meaning and familiarity/novelty, see Smith and Bryson (2005).

In the context of this methodological discussion, however, we wish to draw attention to one major issue regarding action types. Longitudinal designs have not been used to address a key question: whether, in autism, the developmental order in which actions of different types are imitated differs from what is seen in controls. This is somewhat surprising, given that Carpenter, Pennington, and Rogers (2002) found a different place for imitative learning of instrumental actions in the sequence of emergence of social–cognitive functions for children with autism than was found for typically developing children in their earlier study (Carpenter, Nagell, & Tomasello, 1998). Specifically, imitation (of arbitrary and instrumental actions) preceded joint attention in children with autism, whereas in typically developing children and those with developmental delays, joint attention preceded imitation. These data (see also Turner, Pozdol, Ulman, & Stone, 2003) invite speculation that imitation without joint attention has significant consequences for the development of language and other social–cognitive skills in children with autism. However, because cross-sectional, rather than longitudinal, data were used to infer developmental sequences for the children with autism, strong conclusions cannot be drawn from this study. Moreover, the typical developmental sequence proposed by Carpenter and colleagues (1998) has not been replicated (Slaughter & McConnell, 2003). Thus, it remains unknown whether there is a reliable typical sequence, and, if so, whether children with autism follow this in their ability to imitate different kinds of actions. A different sequence might be expected if the relationships among the functions associated with imitation (e.g., joint attention) are atypical. Additional longitudinal data are sorely needed to address these issues. Such data would supplement and clarify the findings of a considerable body of cross-sectional literature that has produced contradictory conclusions.

Methods of Eliciting Imitation

Familiarity/Characteristics of the Model

Most studies of elicited imitation in autism assess the ability of participants to respond on demand to the demonstrations of an unfamiliar experimenter, usually in a laboratory setting. Although a few might vary the setting by conducting the study in a home, preschool, or school, we are not aware of any experimental studies that have varied the familiarity of the model. Research

with typically developing infants reveals no differences when imitation is elicited by unfamiliar versus familiar partners in infants ranging from 8 to 22
months (Devouche, 2004; McCabe & Užgiris, 1983). However, given the negative response to novelty of most individuals with autism, the lack of attention
to this variable is somewhat remarkable. Our own work with typically developing infants suggests that temperamental differences among infants are
reflected in differing elicited imitative responses to their parents and an experimenter (Nichols, 2005). We are currently pursuing the relevance of these findings for autism (e.g., Nichols, Hepburn, Smith, & Rogers, 2005). Nadel's
work speaks powerfully to the social aspects of imitation for children with
autism as well as other children (see Nadel, Chapter 6, this volume).

Motivational State

Most investigators explicitly acknowledge the need to engage children in imitation tasks, so that a failure to perform cannot be attributed either to inatten-
tion or to lack of motivation. Although some authors (e.g., Trevarthen &
Aitken, 2001) have attributed imitation deficits in autism to lack of motivation, this argument is inconsistent with the data (Williams et al., 2004).
Typically in imitation research with children, the experimenter promotes a
game-like atmosphere (e.g., Stone, Ousley, & Littleford, 1997); ideally evidence that one has been successful in drawing children into the game should
be presented. For example, Rogers and colleagues (2003) presented details of
participation through analyses of the probability of producing any response
(vs. no response) across groups. They also compared the number of demonstrations required to elicit a response across groups; results of both analyses
show no differences for young children with autism and increase confidence in
the conclusions.

   With older and more able individuals with autism, the "game" approach
may be less appropriate. However, at a minimum, investigators should look
for evidence that participants' attention was engaged and that they attempted
to act contingently in response to the model's demonstration.[1] Verbal instructions are typically minimal in elicited imitation paradigms, "Do what I do"
and "Now you do it" being common prompts. Libby, Powell, Messer, and
Jordan (1997) pointed out in their study of imitation of pretend play actions
(e.g., moving an empty hand to mouth as if drinking from a cup) that only the
verbal prompts ("Look, it's a cup") identified the movement as symbolic. This
reinforces the necessity of at least ensuring that language comprehension levels of participants with autism are equivalent to those of controls in imitation
studies. The possibility of reduced attention to auditory/verbal information
should also be considered. Most clinicians and educators would share the
experience that the more "verbal" a task is perceived to be, the less appealing
to many individuals with autism.

   The use of reinforcement is an accepted method of increasing motivation
to accomplish a task. Most experimental studies of elicited imitation report

the use of noncontingent verbal praise and encouragement for effort. A few (e.g., Rogers et al., 2003) have indicated that tangible rewards were used for some children, likely a more common practice than is reported. Because immediate imitation rather than observational learning across trials is the focus of these studies, the use of reinforcement for general attempts to imitate (vs. reinforcing the imitation of any specific action) does not appear to be a problem. An interesting question, however, is the extent to which imitation performance is affected by systematic reinforcement and other operant procedures (e.g., shaping). These issues are raised again later with reference to clinical assessment and remediation of imitation impairments. Of note, however, is that Rogers and colleagues (2003) employed a teaching procedure with children who did not imitate an action after three trials. This consisted of physically prompting the child through the movement and providing a reward. These teaching trials did not contribute toward children's imitation scores but may have increased the likelihood of imitative responses in this sample (who nonetheless scored well below controls). Ingersoll, Schreibman, and Tran (2003) demonstrated that the imitation of actions with objects by children with autism was improved when correct imitation produced sensory feedback (in the form of light and/or noise), whereas this manipulation had no effect on typically developing children's performance.

Presentation of Stimuli/Models

Repetition of demonstrations is usual in elicited imitation paradigms, commonly for a total of two to three opportunities. Studies differ as to whether the child is cued to imitate after the first demonstration or whether repeated demonstrations are administered routinely before a response is expected from the child. Use of multiple demonstrations of the action in "bursts" has been adopted from studies of normal infant imitative development. Roeyers, Van Oost, and Bothuyne (1998), for example, presented gestures three times in rapid succession, with each demonstration lasting about 5 seconds. Rogers and colleagues (2003) adopted Meltzoff and Moore's (1977) procedure: Each action was repeated three times rapidly in bursts of three, for a total of nine rapid presentations for each action in each trial. Each item was then demonstrated for up to three such trials, if trials one and two elicited no response. Thus, these very young children with autism were given many opportunities to demonstrate imitation, yet performance remained at very low levels.

In some elicited imitation studies, the model is only presented once, but the gesture is held in view during the child's imitation attempt. Such simultaneous matching methods are uncommon in studies of children with autism. They clearly involve different representational demands than do conditions requiring either immediate imitation of a model from memory, or imitation following a delay (deferred imitation). Smith and Bryson (1998) manipulated model present/model absent conditions as an experimental variable; no differential effects were seen on imitation by participants with autism. However, it is curious that this issue has received little attention, given the long history of discussion of the symbolic/representational demands of imitation tasks. Also curious, given the interest in deferred imitation in typically developing infants (e.g., Barr, Dowden, & Hayne, 1996; Meltzoff, 1988), is that few investigators have studied deferred imitation in autism (Brown, 1996, cited in Dawson et al., 1998; Williams et al., 2004). In deferred imitation paradigms, the action is demonstrated, an interval is imposed, and the child has an opportunity to imitate. For obvious reasons, this paradigm is suited to actions with objects in that the presentation of the object becomes the cue to perform the action. Perhaps deferred imitation has not been studied because deficits are so apparent in most studies of immediate imitation. However, deferred imitation paradigms offer opportunities to manipulate representational demands and may be informative particularly with respect to the nature of the relationship between imitation and other symbolic activity, such as language.

Scoring Imitation Performance

Differences in approaches to scoring may influence the conclusions of imitation studies. One challenge is to develop scoring systems that reflect both the parameters that change with the normal development of imitation and the possible errors that might accompany atypical performance. Criticisms of the early literature on imitation in autism included the use of all-or-nothing approaches to scoring, which perpetuated a false impression that individuals with autism could not or did not imitate, rather than that their imitation performance was flawed. Nonetheless, pass–fail scores may be useful in studies in which the focus is on a particular measure of imitation ability as an indicator of a specific social–cognitive competency, as in Carpenter and colleagues' (2002) study of developmental sequencing of social–communication abilities.

In the few studies of spontaneous imitation in autism, presence/absence, or frequency counts are the most common forms of measurement. In Brown and Whiten's (2000) previously mentioned study, time-sampled actions were categorized as, for example, instances of a nonsymbolic action with an object. These instances were then summed over observation periods, resulting in very few observations for most individuals in their study. An additional challenge for the Brown and Whiten study was the relatively low agreement between raters on some action categories. Reliability data are essential for scoring of imitation performance, and perhaps especially when imitation attempts are atypical, as in autism. Most studies are able to demonstrate strong agreement across raters, using either correlational methods or kappa values, as appropriate to the type of measurement (Bakeman & Gottman, 1986). For practical reasons, videorecording of imitation performance is employed in most instances in order to provide evidence of scoring reliability.

Commonly, in studies of elicited imitation, ratings of imitation quality have replaced pass–fail scores. Usually, only responses that occur within a specified interval following the demonstration are scored (e.g., 20–30 seconds;

Aldridge, Stone, Sweeney, & Bower, 2000; Roeyers et al., 1998), although this information may often be lacking in published reports. In most studies coders (ideally blind to participants' diagnostic status) rate the quality of imitation performance on an ordinal scale, frequently with 3 or 4 points. Usually, scores of 0 indicate no response and/or an unrecognizable attempt, although we would argue that no response is different from a contingent behavior, however little it may resemble the target action. In most coding schemes, one or two levels encompass partial/incomplete or poorer-quality responses, and the highest ratings designate accurate reproductions of the modeled action. Total scores across multiple items, average scores per item, first scores, and best scores have all been used as dependent variables. Multiple demonstrations also create opportunities to examine finer gradations in imitation performance. Such differences in types of scores do not appear to affect conclusions. Rogers and colleagues (2003) reported that "first" and "best" scores did not differ in the context of their procedure (described previously) that provided generously for repeated attempts at imitation. It may be that multiple opportunities do not necessarily improve performance in children with autism. This question may be worth some attention, however, given that the quality of imitative responses by typically developing infants does improve over trials (Kaye & Marcus, 1978; Nichols, 2005), perhaps suggesting their differential use of self-feedback.

One potential complication arising from the use of scores summed across trials is that children may obtain the same total score for different reasons. Consider, for example, a child who imitates, but poorly, on each of six trials, obtaining scores of 2 on a 4-point scale on every trial. That child's total score (12) is indistinguishable from the same score obtained by a child whose perfect score of 4 on the first two trials is followed by scores of 1 on the other four trials. This suggests that supplementary descriptive information (such as error data) would assist in efforts to identify different patterns of performance.

Error Scoring

In studies of gesture use and imitation that stem from a neuropsychological orientation, it is common to conduct error analyses. The types of errors that are often observed in acquired (adult) apraxia are not so clearly seen in developmental dyspraxia (Dewey, 1993). Systematic attention to error types may yet be useful in distinguishing the praxic difficulties of children with ASD from those with other conditions (e.g., Hill, Bishop, & Nimmo-Smith, 1998), but presently the evidence for increased frequency of specific imitation errors in children with autism is mixed. Smith and Bryson (1998) reported an increased frequency of reversal errors (failure to take viewer's perspective into account) by children with autism, as did Whiten and Brown (1999). This unique error is consistent with other significant aspects of autism, such as reversal of I–you pronouns and impaired social understanding. However,

Green and colleagues (2002) found no differences in error patterns between children with Asperger syndrome (an ASD) and children with developmental coordination disorder. Moreover, Brown now describes the reversal error as indicative of developmental delay, rather than deviance, in children with autism (Beadle-Brown, 2004). Other types of errors, for example, in the precision of postures versus the dynamic aspects of movements, are considered to have different neuropsychological implications (Leiguarda & Marsden, 2000). Evidence of specific types of errors may be useful in addressing such questions as the relationships among gesture imitation, sensorimotor integration, and motor functions more generally. What is needed is additional evidence of error patterns from larger samples of individuals with autism at differing age and ability levels, as well as longitudinal data on the acquisition of imitation skills in children with autism.

Approximations

An alternative to classifying inaccurate imitation attempts as errors is to think of them as approximations to accurate responses. One question for longitudinal study is, therefore: As children with autism begin to imitate, do they produce the same kinds of attempts as do other beginning imitators? In our lab, Nichols (2005) has studied typically developing 9-month-old infants, who are in the early stages of copying others' actions. The aim was to provide a detailed analysis of the characteristics of early imitative responses, and of predictors and correlates of typical early imitation, with a view to refining the study of early imitation by children with autism. The study incorporates methods and scoring derived from a thorough review of the literature and provides data on a large sample of 9-month-olds as they begin to imitate. Two promising directions have emerged from this rich source of data. These pertain to the relationships between individual differences in temperament and imitation previously mentioned, and to the detailed scoring of approximate responses and changes in performance over trials. We are pursuing each of these avenues in our work with children with autism.

Levels of Imitation: Scoring Associated Behaviors

In studies with typically developing infants, Meltzoff (1990) described how, by 14 months, infants "test" an adult who mimics their actions by repeating an action, pausing, and gazing expectantly at the adult. Nadel (2002) discussed testing and other social responses to being imitated in children with autism, outlining a hierarchy of social behaviors that she proposes are associated with different levels of awareness of imitative exchanges. For example, smiling at the experimenter is considered a lower-level response than testing the mimicking experimenter by doing something unusual with an object.

A few other investigators have exploited such nonverbal cues to further distinguish among levels of children's imitative responses. In their study of the emergence of social–cognitive behaviors, Carpenter and colleagues (2002) coded as "passing" only instrumental imitation of an action on an object that was accompanied by an expectant look toward the object, indicating that the child was anticipating the effect of the action. In a similar vein, Ingersoll and colleagues (2003) measured smiling, gaze, and other responses during imitation tasks. They coded children's behavior that was directed either to the experimenter or to the objects used in the tasks and found that children with autism directed fewer social behaviors toward the experimenter while engaged in imitation. Libby and colleagues (1997) reported that whereas typically developing children and children with other developmental difficulties commented or were amused when asked to imitate counterfunctional actions with objects, children with autism tended not to do so. Similar anecdotal observations by Smith (1996) add to the evidence that children with autism may copy some acts accurately without appreciation of their intent or meaning, important for distinguishing among levels of imitative behavior such as mimicry, emulation, and true imitation (Want & Harris, 2002). Future studies should make greater use of the verbal and nonverbal clues that children provide as to their awareness of the social nature of imitation and their understanding of the actions that they imitate. These behavioral indicators may help us to identify levels of imitative responding, supplementing features of experimental designs that may constrain the types of imitation that children display.

CLINICAL ASSESSMENT AND REMEDIATION OF IMPAIRED IMITATION IN AUTISM

There are several clinical contexts in which the imitation skills of a child with autism might be assessed. These include screening and diagnosis, standardized cognitive/developmental assessment, and behavioral curriculum-based assessment.

Screening/Diagnosis

Of the recently reported screening measures for autism, most include at least one item related to imitation. The Modified Checklist for Autism in Toddlers (M-CHAT; Robins, Fein, Barton, & Green, 2001) is an example of a parent report form that asks only one imitation question, "Does your child imitate? (e.g., You make a face, will your child imitate it?)." Although imitation of facial gestures and expressions may be particularly atypical in children with autism (Loveland et al., 1994), it is a curious single example to provide, as other, manual gestures may be more frequently modeled for young children (e.g., waving and clapping). The Screening Test for Autism in Two-Year-Olds (STAT; Stone, Coonrod, & Ousley, 2000; Stone, Coonrod, Turner, & Pozdol, 2004) is a direct screening measure. Building on Stone's experimental work with the Motor Imitation Scale (Stone, Ousley & Littleford, 1997), the STAT includes four imitation items. The Autism Observation Scale for Infants (AOSI) has shown promise in prospective studies of infants with an older sibling with autism (Bryson, McDermott, Rombough, Brian, & Zwaigenbaum, in press). Failure to imitate simple motor acts (such as shaking a rattle) by 12 months is among the predictors of a later diagnosis of autism in these high-risk infants (Zwaigenbaum et al., 2005). The usefulness of imitation ability in screening for ASD will no doubt depend on the age at which screening takes place, the specific form of imitation skill, and the ability of the respondent/observer to identify the target skill (or lack thereof) reliably.

Current gold standard research diagnostic measures, the Autism Diagnostic Observation Schedule (ADOS, a direct assessment; Lord, Rutter, DiLavore, & Risi, 2001) and the Autism Diagnostic Interview—Revised (ADI-R, a parent interview; Rutter, LeCouteur, & Lord, 2003), both include aspects of imitation. In the ADOS, imitation of a pretend action is included as a task only in the developmentally lowest-level module, which is administered to children who are nonverbal, or at the single-word stage. In order to obtain a normal score on this item, the child must imitate an action performed with a "placeholder" object; for example, "flying" a wooden block as though it was an airplane. Imitation of pretence is a relatively high-level function that few young children with autism will pass (cf. Libby et al., 1997). It is possible to mimic the movement without any understanding of the symbolic nature of the action; however, this is a challenging distinction on which to make reliable judgments.

The ADI-R evaluates parent reports of imitative behavior with a particular focus on copying the behavior and actions of an individual, including mimicry of personal characteristics such as voice, gestures, or walk. Coding is based on data that suggest that individuals with a diagnosis of autism may imitate familiar routines or use of objects, but rarely an individual's manner of walking, talking, and so on. Interestingly, imitation of TV or video characters is excluded, as children with autism may show uncanny mimicry under these circumstances. The ability to imitate actions from video has been used to therapeutic advantage by several investigators to teach skills such as speech (e.g., Charlop-Christy, Le, & Freeman, 2000).

Cognitive/Developmental Assessment

Imitation is frequently assessed in the context of standardized cognitive developmental testing. Imitation skills may be implicitly important, in that tests of early skills such as the Bayley Scales of Infant Development II (Bayley, 1993), Mullen Scales of Early Learning (Mullen, 1995), and the new Merrill-Palmer—Revised Scales of Development (Roid & Sampers, 2004) have many items that require demonstration by an examiner in addition to, or in lieu of, verbal instructions. This is especially true of all tests that assess cognitive abilities for children who are functioning at lower mental ages, in the infant–toddler range. Again an issue for many young children with autism is the difficulty with performance "on demand," or in unfamiliar contexts. Examiners must be cautious in concluding a lack of competence for a child with autism if a test is heavily dependent on imitation, just as they must be aware of the verbal demands of tests. Of course, tests may also explicitly measure imitation in recognition of its importance as a substrate for social and cognitive development. The tradition of directly assessing imitation as an aspect of cognitive development owes much to Užgiris and Hunt (1975). Their ordinal scales based on Piagetian principles were very influential on early research on imitation in autism (e.g., Abrahamsen & Mitchell, 1990; Sigman & Ungerer, 1984). This research did not, however, examine whether the sequence in which imitation of various kinds of actions was accomplished differed in children with autism. Indeed, this question does not appear ever to have been addressed. The normative acquisition of imitation skills has been translated into scales by the Piaget-inspired work of Užgiris and Hunt, on one hand, and the neuropsychologically oriented approach of Bergès and Lézine (1965) on the other. However, despite the plethora of experimental studies of imitation in infants, toddlers, and young children in the past three decades, this enhanced understanding of levels of imitation has not been translated into any new normative measure. Three existing measures of imitation in autism deserve notice here. The Motor Imitation Scale (MIS; Stone, Ousley, & Littleford, 1997) is a 16-item scale developed for the study of imitation with young children with autism. Items were selected based on Piaget's developmental sequence, and the MIS demonstrates good split-half and test–retest reliability. The MIS has been used by other investigators (e.g., Ingersoll & Schreibman, in press) and appears to provide a robust general measure of impaired imitation in young children with autism. However, differential associations between MIS subscores and other developmental functions (e.g., vocal imitation with language development and object imitation with play skills) have not been replicated (Rogers et al., 2003). One difficulty may lie with the designations of items within the subscales. For example, both symbolic and nonsymbolic actions are included in the body movements category, and the characterization of actions such as "shake noisemaker" as meaningful and "bang spoon on table" as nonmeaningful is not compelling.

The Imitation Disorders Evaluation scale (IDE; Malvy et al., 1999) was intended as a measure of *abnormal* imitation in autism rather than a typical reference. The scale is scored from all clinical data on the child, including a parent interview; developmental, pediatric, and genetic assessments; and a videotaped psychiatric examination. The psychiatric examination reportedly entails "presses" for imitative behavior, as well as opportunities for observation of spontaneous imitation. Malvy and colleagues (1999) demonstrated that performance on the IDE differentiated children with autism from young typical children, and that the IDE scores of children with autism improved following 9 months of treatment. However, a weakness of the measure is the lack of standardization of the situations that are scored. Insufficient information is provided both about these contexts and about the scoring of specific behaviors. Despite this, the IDE has recently been applied in a retrospective study of young children with autism, examining behavior revealed in video-taped interactions both at home (prediagnosis) and in a clinic following diagnosis (Receveur et al., 2005). Good reliability was reported for these IDE ratings, and differences in imitative behavior emerged between lower- and higher-functioning groups of children with autism. This suggests that the measure, at least as used by its developers, is sensitive to developmental variability.

A battery of imitation tasks was also developed by Beadle-Brown (2004) for her research with children and adults with autism, consisting of 93 actions spanning the range of distinctions suggested by Smith and Bryson's (1994) review. Although the battery is admirable for its breadth, standardized procedures for administering the items were not described, limiting its general usefulness. Having been designed for use in between-subjects experimental designs, none of the scales by Stone, Ousley, and Littleford (1997), Malvy and colleagues (1999), or Beadle-Brown (2004) provide comparative normative information, other than from matched control groups. To provide a comprehensive measure for our work with children with autism, we are developing the Multidimensional Imitation Assessment (MIA; Lowe-Pearce & Smith, 2005). Our first step, which is in progress, is to confirm the sequence in which typically developing children succeed at the MIA tasks before employing it in studies with children with autism. Another unique aspect of the MIA is a parent-report component, intended to complement information from the elicited imitation paradigm with observations from familiar settings. This parent-report measure is derived from our work with typically developing infants and may hold promise for improving our understanding of both competence and performance aspects of imitation in autism (cf. Nichols, 2005).

Behavioral Assessment for Intervention Planning

An obvious application for the measurement of imitation skills is in behavioral intervention program planning and monitoring. In recognition of the crucial importance of imitation in young children's learning, and its impairment in children with autism, imitation is a major intervention target in many programs (e.g., Lovaas, 1981; Partington & Sundberg, 1998; Taylor & McDonough, 1996). In the tradition of applied behavioral analysis (ABA), the general approach to assessment is individualized and curriculum-based, rather than normative or standardized. That is, assessment is directly tied to the specific skills to be taught.

Of the widely known curricula, whereas all include imitation as a key area of focus, the sequence in which imitation of various sorts of actions is taught varies. For example, *The ME Book* (Lovaas, 1981) and the *Bridges* curriculum (Romanczyk, Lockshin, & Matey, 1996) suggest teaching of arbitrary gross motor movements (e.g., standing up, raising arms) as a first step in discrete trial imitation training. Leaf and McEachin (1999) instead suggest imitation of object manipulation as the initial phase, preceding gross motor imitation. The placement of oral–vocal–verbal imitations in relation to various aspects of motor imitation is particularly variable across curricula. Whether these different sequences reflect differing views of (or lack of data on) the typical sequence of acquisition of these skills, or merely different clinical opinions as to the relative difficulty of teaching these skills to children with autism, is unclear. This issue has, surprisingly, received little attention in either the clinical or the experimental literature, highlighting the dearth of research on oral–vocal imitation. More developmentally oriented curricula include the early work of Schopler, Lansing, and Waters (1981), whose imitation teaching activities follow a sequence based on typical developmental patterns. Rogers and Schreibman are among those who have promoted more naturalistic behavioral teaching of imitation skills (Ingersoll & Schreibman, in press; Rogers, Hall, Osaki, Reaven, & Herbison, 2001). Their approaches have built on the evidence that in typical development imitation emerges in the context of joint attention and other social–communicative behaviors. Intervention that is guided by developmental principles is perhaps influenced less by predetermined sequences than by the child's interests and existing repertoire of actions. Ingersoll and Schreibman (in press) discuss some of the limitations of more traditional behavioral approaches to the teaching of imitation, and provide a formal demonstration of the application of naturalistic behavioral teaching of imitation skills to young children with autism. This is an extremely promising area for further clinical-developmental research that has the potential to provide information about the typical and atypical development of imitation, and to maximize developmental gains for children with autism.

CONCLUSIONS

The central questions for the study of imitation in autism—why is imitation difficult for people with autism, and how can we most effectively facilitate the acquisition of imitation skills?—remain to be answered. Our intention in writing this chapter was to highlight some of the many methodological factors that must be considered when assessing imitation in the service of either of these questions. There has been an enormous amount of progress as a result of researchers bringing both new conceptual and methodological perspectives to the study of imitation in autism. Given what is now generally accepted about the different forms that copying actions may take, and the parameters that do (and do not) influence various aspects of imitation performance in people with autism, there is real promise that studies can be generated that will address our pressing questions in more sophisticated ways. In so doing, we will increase our understanding of the elusive process of imitation. Moreover, we stand to learn more about the origins of autism and about effective means for giving children with autism the powerful learning tool that imitative behavior represents.

NOTE

1. Of course, how the participants construe the nature of the task leads one back to the initial points raised in this chapter: What is imitation and how does one measure it? One has no control over the participant's *interpretation* of the task—for example, whether the goal is to imitate the form of the movement versus its goal or even its "style" (Hobson & Lee, 1999; Meyer & Hobson, 2004)—and perhaps herein lie some of the most essential issues for the study of imitation in autism.

REFERENCES

Abrahamsen, E. P., & Mitchell, J. R. (1990). Communication and sensorimotor functioning in children with autism. *Journal of Autism and Developmental Disorders, 20,* 75–86.

Aldridge, M. A., Stone, K. R., Sweeney, M. H., & Bower, T. G. R. (2000). Preverbal children with autism understanding the intentions of others. *Developmental Science, 3*(3), 294–301.

Bakeman, R., & Gottman, J. M. (1986). *Observing interaction: An introduction to sequential analysis.* Cambridge, UK: Cambridge University Press.

Barr, R., Dowden, A., & Hayne, H. (1996). Developmental changes in deferred imitation by 6-to-24-month-old infants. *Infant Behavior and Development, 19,* 159–170.

Bartak, L., Rutter, M., & Cox, A. (1975). A comparative study of infantile autism and specific developmental receptive language disorder. I. The children. *British Journal of Psychiatry, 126,* 127–145.

Bates, E., Benigni, L., Bretherton, I., Camaioni, L., & Volterra, V. (1979). *The emergence of symbols: Cognition and communication in infancy.* New York: Academic Press.

Bayley, N. (1993). *Bayley Scales of Infant Development* (2nd ed.). San Antonio, TX: Psychological Corporation.

Beadle-Brown, J. (2004). Elicited imitation in children and adults with autism: The effect of different types of actions. *Journal of Applied Research in Intellectual Disabilities, 17,* 37–48.

Bergès, J., & Lézine, I. (1965). *The imitation of gestures.* London: The Spastics Society Medical Education and Information Unit with William Heinemann Books Ltd.

Blake, R., Turner, L. M., Smoski, M. J., Pozdol, S. L., & Stone, W. L. (2003). Visual recognition of biological motion is impaired in children with autism. *Psychological Science, 14,* 151–157.

Brown, J., & Whiten, A. (2000). Imitation, theory of mind, and related activities in autism: An observational study of spontaneous behavior in everyday contexts. *Autism, 4,* 185–204.

Bryson, S. E., McDermott, C., Rombough, V., Brian, J., & Zwaigenbaum, L. (in press). The Autism Observation Scale for Infants: Scale development and reliability data. *Journal of Autism and Developmental Disorders.*

Burack, J. A. (Ed.). (2004). Research methodology—Matching [Special issue]. *Journal of Autism and Developmental Disorders, 34*(1).

Carpenter, M., Nagell, K., & Tomasello, M. (1998). Social Cognition, joint attention, and communicative competence from 9 to 15 months of age. *Monographs of the Society for Research in Child Development, 63*(4), 1–176.

Carpenter, M., Pennington, B. F., & Rogers, S. J. (2002). Interrelations among social–cognitive skills in young children with autism. *Journal of Autism and Developmental Disorders, 32*(2), 91–106.

Charlop-Christy, M. H., Le, L., & Freeman, K. A. (2000). A comparison of video modeling with in vivo modeling for teaching children with autism. *Journal of Autism and Developmental Disorders, 30*(6), 537–52.

Dawson, G., Meltzoff, A. N., Osterling, J., & Rinaldi, J. (1998). Neuropsychological correlates of early symptoms of autism. *Child Development, 69*(5), 1276–1285.

Dawson, G., Webb, S., Schellenberg, G. D., Dager, S., Friedman, S., Aylward, E., et al. (2002). Defining the broader phenotype of autism: Genetic, brain, and behavioral perspectives. *Development and Psychopathology, 14*(3), 581–611.

Devouche, E. (2004). Mother versus stranger: A triadic situation of imitation at the end of the first year of life. *Infant and Child Development, 13*(1), 35–48.

Dewey, D. (1993). Error analysis of limb and orofacial praxis in children with developmental motor deficits. *Brain and Cognition, 23*, 203–221.

Drash, P. W., High, R. L., & Tudor, R. M. (1999). Using mand training to establish an echoic repertoire in young children with autism. *Analysis of Verbal Behavior, 16*, 29–44.

Green, D., Baird, G., Barnett, A. L., Henderson, L., Huber, J., & Henderson, S. (2002). The severity and nature of motor impairment in Asperger's syndrome: A comparison with specific developmental disorder of motor function. *Journal of Child Psychology and Psychiatry, 43*, 655–668.

Heyes, C. (2001). Causes and consequences of imitation. *Trends in Cognitive Sciences, 5*(6), 253–261.

Hill, E. L., Bishop, D. V. M., & Nimmo-Smith, I. (1998). Representational gestures in developmental coordination disorder and specific language impairment: Error types and the reliability of ratings. *Human Movement Science, 17*, 655–678.

Hobson, P., & Lee, A. (1999). Imitation and identification in autism. *Journal of Child Psychology and Psychiatry, 40*(4), 649–659.

Iacoboni, M. (2005). Neural mechanisms of imitation. *Current Opinion in Neurobiology, 15*(6), 632–637.

Ingersoll, B., & Schreibman, L. (in press). Teaching reciprocal imitation skills to young children with autism using a naturalistic behavioral approach: Effects on language, pretend play, and joint attention. *Journal of Autism and Developmental Disorders.*

Ingersoll, B., Schreibman, L., & Tran, Q. H. (2003). Effect of sensory feedback on immediate object imitation in children with autism. *Journal of Autism and Developmental Disorders, 33*(6), 673–683.

Kaye, K., & Marcus, J. (1978). Imitation over a series of trials without feedback: Age six months. *Infant Behavior and Development, 1*, 141–155.

Leaf, R., & McEachin, J. (Eds.). (1999). *A work in progress.* New York: DRL Books.

Leiguarda, R. C., & Marsden, C. D. (2000). Limb apraxias: Higher-order disorders of sensorimotor integration. *Brain, 123*(5), 860–879.

Libby, S., Powell, S., Messer, D., & Jordan, R. (1997). Imitation of pretend play acts by children with autism and Down syndrome. *Journal of Autism and Developmental Disorders, 27*, 365–383.

Lord, C., Rutter, M., DiLavore, P. C., & Risi, S. (2001). *Autism Diagnostic Observation Schedule—WPS (WPS edition).* Los Angeles: Western Psychological Services.

Lovaas, O. I. (1981). *Teaching developmentally disabled children.* Austin, TX: Pro-Ed.

Loveland, K., Tunali-Kotoski, B., Pearson, D., Brelsford, K., Ortegon, J., & Chen, R. (1994). Imitation and expression of facial affect in autism. *Development and Psychopathology, 6*, 433–444.

Lowe-Pearce, C., & Smith, I. M. (2005, June). *Multidimensional Imitation Assessment (MIA): Development of a comprehensive imitation measure for young children.* Poster presented at the annual meeting of the Canadian Psychological Association, Montreal.

Malvy, J., Roux, S., Zakian, A., Debuly, S., Sauvage, D., & Barthélémy, C. (1999). A brief clinical scale for the early evaluation of imitation disorders in autism. *Autism*, *3*(4), 357–369.

McCabe, M. A., & Užgiris, I. C. (1983). Effects of model and action on imitation in infancy. *Merrill-Palmer Quarterly*, *29*(1), 69–82.

Meltzoff, A. N. (1990). Foundations for developing a concept of self: The role of imitation in relating self to other and the value of social modeling and self practice in infancy. In D. Cicchetti & M. Beeghly (Eds.), *The self in transition* (pp. 139–164). Chicago: University of Chicago Press.

Meltzoff, A. N., & Decety, J. (2003). What imitation tells us about social cognition: A rapprochement between developmental psychology and cognitive neuroscience. *Philosophical Transactions of the Royal Society of London, B, Biological Science*, *358*, 491–500.

Meltzoff, A. N., & Moore, M. K. (1977). Imitation of facial and manual gestures by human neonates. *Science*, *198*, 75–78.

Meyer, J. A., & Hobson, R. P. (2004). Orientation in relation to self and other: The case of autism. *Interaction Studies*, *5*, 221–244.

Mullen, E. M. (1995). *Mullen Scales of Early Learning*. Circle Pines, MN: American Guidance Service.

Nadel, J. (2002). Imitation and imitation recognition: Functional use in preverbal infants and nonverbal children with autism. In A. N. Meltzoff & W. Prinz (Eds.), *The imitative mind* (pp. 42–73). Cambridge, UK: Cambridge University Press.

Nadel, J., & Pezé, A. (1993). What makes immediate imitation communicative in toddlers and autistic children? In J. Nadel & L. Camaioni (Eds.), *New perspectives in early communicative development* (pp. 139–156). London: Routledge.

Nichols, S. L. (2005). *Information processing abilities and parent–child interaction: Prediction of imitative ability in the first year*. Unpublished doctoral dissertation, Dalhousie University, Halifax, NS, Canada.

Nichols, S., Hepburn, S. L., Smith, I. M., & Rogers, S. (2005, May). *Temperament matters: Imitative abilities of young children with autism, fragile X, and developmental delay*. Poster presented at the annual meeting of the International Meeting for Autism Research, Boston.

Nishitani, N., Avikainen, S., & Hari, R. (2004). Abnormal imitation-related cortical activation sequences in Asperger's syndrome. *Annals of Neurology*, *55*, 558–562.

Partington, J. W., & Sundberg, M. L. (1998). *The assessment of basic language and learning skills: An assessment, curriculum guide, and tracking system for children with autism or other developmental disabilities*. Danville, CA: Behavior Analysts.

Receveur, C., Lenoir, P., Désombre, H., Roux, S., Barthélémy, C., & Malvy, J. (2005). Interaction and imitation deficits from infancy to 4 years of age in children with autism: A pilot study based on videotapes. *Autism*, *9*, 69–82.

Rizzolatti, G., Fadiga, L., Gallese, V., & Fogassi, L. (1996). Premotor cortex and the recognition of motor actions. *Brain Research: Cognitive Brain Research*, (2),131–41.

Rizzolatti, G., Fadiga, L., Fogassi, L., & Gallese, V. (2002). From mirror neurons to imitation: Facts and speculations. In A. N. Meltzoff & W. Prinz (Eds.), *The imitative mind* (pp. 247–266). Cambridge, UK: Cambridge University Press.

Robins, D., Fein, D., Barton, M., & Green, J. (2001). The Modified Checklist for Autism in Toddlers: An initial study investigating the early detection of autism and pervasive developmental disorders. *Journal of Autism and Developmental Disorders*, *31*, 131–144.

Roeyers, H., Van Oost, P., & Bothuyne, S. (1998). Immediate imitation and joint attention in young children with autism. *Development and Psychopathology*, *10*(3), 441–450.

Rogers, S. J. (1999). An examination of the imitation deficit in autism. In J. Nadel & G. Butterworth (Eds.), *Imitation in infancy* (pp. 254–283). New York: Cambridge University Press.

Rogers, S. J., & Bennetto, L. (2000). Intersubjectivity in autism: The roles of imitation and executive function. In A. M. Wetherby & B. M. Prizant (Eds.), *Autism spectrum disorders: A transactional developmental perspective* (pp. 79–107). Baltimore: Brookes.

Rogers, S. J., Bennetto, L., McEvoy, R., & Pennington, B. F. (1996). Imitation and pantomime in high-functioning adolescents with autism spectrum disorders. *Child Development*, 67(5), 2060–2073.

Rogers, S. J., Hall, T., Osaki, D., Reaven, J., & Herbison, J. (2001). The Denver Model: A comprehensive, integrated educational approach to young children with autism and their families. In J. S. Handleman & S. L. Harris (Eds.), *Preschool education programs for children with autism* (pp. 95–133). Austin, TX: Pro-Ed.

Rogers, S. J., Hepburn, S. L., Stackhouse, T., & Wehner, E. (2003). Imitation performance in toddlers with autism and those with other developmental disorders. *Journal of Child Psychology and Psychiatry*, 44(5), 763–781.

Roid, G., & Sampers, J. (2004). *Merrill-Palmer Revised Scales of Development*. Wood Dale, IL: Stoelting.

Romanczyk, R. G., Lockshin, S., & Matey, L. (1996). *The individualized goal selection curriculum*. (Available from: Clinical Behavior Therapy Associates. Suite 5, 3 Tioga Boulevard, Apalachin, NY 13732)

Rutter, M., Le Couteur, A., & Lord, C. (2003). *Autism Diagnostic Interview—Revised*. Los Angeles: Western Psychological Services.

Schopler, E., Lansing, M., & Waters, L. (1981). *Individualized assessment and treatment for autistic and developmentally disabled children. Vol. III: Teaching activities for autistic children*. Austin, TX: Pro-Ed.

Sigman, M., & Ungerer, J. (1984). Cognitive and language skills in autistic, mentally retarded and normal children. *Developmental Psychology*, 20(2), 293–302.

Slaughter, V., & McConnell, D. (2003). Emergence of joint attention: Relationships between gaze following, social referencing, imitation, and naming in infancy. *Journal of Genetic Psychology*, 164, 54–71.

Smith, I. M. (1996). *Imitation and gesture representation in autism*. Unpublished doctoral dissertation, Dalhousie University, Halifax, NS, Canada.

Smith, I. M. (2000). Motor functioning in Asperger syndrome. In A. Klin, F. R. Volkmar, & S. S. Sparrow (Eds.), *Asperger syndrome* (pp. 97–124). New York: Guilford Press.

Smith, I. M. (2004). Motor problems in children with autistic spectrum disorders. In D. Dewey & D. E. Tupper (Eds.), *Developmental motor disorders* (pp. 152–168). New York: Guilford Press.

Smith, I. M., & Bryson, S. (1994). Imitation and action in autism: A critical review. *Psychological Bulletin*, 116(2), 259–273.

Smith, I. M., & Bryson, S. (1998). Gesture imitation in autism I: Nonsymbolic postures and sequences. *Cognitive Neuropsychology*, 15(6), 747–770.

Smith, I. M., & Bryson, S. E. (2005). *Symbolic imitation and the representation of actions and objects in autism*. Manuscript in review.

Stone, W. L., Coonrod, E. E., & Ousley, O. Y. (2000). Screening Tool for Autism in Two-Year-Olds (STAT): Development and preliminary data. *Journal of Autism and Developmental Disorders*, 30(6), 607–612.

Stone, W. L., Coonrod, E. E., Turner, L. M., & Pozdol, S. L. (2004). Psychometric properties of the STAT for early autism screening. *Journal of Autism and Developmental Disorders*, 34(6), 691–702.

Stone, W. L., Ousley, O., & Littleford, C. D. (1997). Motor imitation in young children with autism: What's the object? *Journal of Abnormal Child Psychology*, 25(6), 475–485.

Stone, W. L., Ousley, O.Y., Yoder, P. J., Hogan, K. L., & Hepburn, S. L. (1997). Nonverbal communication in two- and three-year-old children with autism. *Journal of Autism and Developmental Disorders*, 27(6), 677–696.

Stone, W. L., Ulman, T. C., Swanson, A., McMahon, C., & Turner, L. (2004, May). *Structured vs. naturalistic object imitation in young children with ASD*. Poster presented at the International Meeting for Autism Research, Sacramento CA.

Taylor, B. A., & McDonough, K. A. (1996). Selecting teaching programs. In C. Maurice (Ed.), *Behavioral intervention for young children with autism: A manual for parents and professionals* (pp. 63–177). Austin TX: Pro-Ed.

Tomasello, M., & Carpenter, M. (2005). Intention-reading and imitative learning. In S. Hurley & N. Chater (Eds.), *Perspectives on imitation: From neuroscience to social science: Vol. 2. Imitation, human development, and culture* (pp. 133–148). Cambridge, MA: MIT Press.

Trevarthen, C., & Aitken, K. J. (2001). Infant intersubjectivity: Research, theory, and clinical applications. *Journal of Child Psychology and Psychiatry*, 42(1), 3–48.

Turner, L., Pozdol, S., Ulman, T. C., & Stone, W. L. (2003, April). *The relation between social-communication skills and language development in young children with autism*. Paper presented at the biennial meeting of the Society for Research in Child Development, Tampa, FL.

Užgiris, I. C., & Hunt, J. (1975). *Assessment in infancy*. Chicago: University of Illinois Press.

Volkmar, F. R., Lord, C., Bailey, A., Schultz, R. T., & Klin, A. (2004). Autism and pervasive developmental disorders. *Journal of Child Psychology and Psychiatry*, 45(1), 135–70.

Want, S. C., & Harris, P. L. (2002). How do children ape? Applying concepts from the study of non-human primates to the developmental study of "imitation" in children. *Developmental Science*, 5(1), 1–13.

Whiten, A., & Brown, J. D. (1999). Imitation and the reading of other minds: Perspectives from the study of autism, normal children and non-human primates. In S. Bråten (Ed.), *Intersubjective communication and emotion in ontogeny: A sourcebook* (pp. 260–280). Cambridge, UK: Cambridge University Press.

Williams, J. H., Whiten, A., & Singh, T. (2004). A systematic review of action imitation in autistic spectrum disorder. *Journal of Autism and Developmental Disorders*, 34(3), 285–299.

Williams, J. H., Whiten, A., Suddendorf, T., & Perrett, D. I. (2001). Imitation, mirror neurons and autism. *Neuroscience Behavioral Review*, 25, 287–95.

Williams, J. H. G., Waiter, G. D., Gilchrist, A., Perrett, D. I., Murray, A. D., & Whiten, A. (2006). Neural mechanisms of imitation and "mirror neuron" functioning in autistic spectrum disorder. *Neuropsychologia*, 44(4), 610–621.

Zwaigenbaum, L., Bryson, S., Rogers, T., Roberts, W., Brian, J., & Szatmari, P. (2005). Behavioral manifestations of autism in the first year of life. *International Journal of Developmental Neuroscience*, 23, 143–152.

CHAPTER 17

The Effect of Motor Disorders on Imitation in Children

DEBORAH DEWEY
SHAUNA BOTTOS

According to *Webster's New Collegiate Dictionary* (1979), imitation is defined as "the execution of an act supposedly as a direct response to the perception of another person performing the act" (p. 567). When one individual imitates another, he or she copies or reproduces the actions of that person. Imitation is one of the basic processes that individuals use to learn and to develop skills, including motor skills, and it is through imitation and practice that children develop proficiency in the performance of movement. Through imitation, sensory and motor activity become consolidated into representative thought, which in turn allows the children to develop the symbolism necessary for the accurate performance of gestures in specific situations (Berges & Lezine, 1965).

Although most children display normal development of motor skills, there is a significant minority of children that have difficulty with the acquisition of these skills. These children are referred to as displaying developmental coordination disorder (American Psychiatric Association, 1994) or specific developmental disorder of motor function (World Health Organization, 1989, 1992). Deficits in the performance of motor skills have also been noted in many children with autism spectrum disorders (Smith, 2004). This chapter discusses the motor and gestural/imitation deficits displayed by children with developmental motor deficits and autism spectrum disorders. The motor dysfunction and gestural deficits evidenced in children with developmental motor disorders and children with autism spectrum disorders are examined and compared. Finally, we explore processes that could underlie impairments in gestural performance and imitation in children with developmental coordination disorder and autism spectrum disorders.

DESCRIPTIONS AND DEFINITIONS
OF DEVELOPMENTAL MOTOR PROBLEMS

Developmental motor disorders have been discussed in the research literature
for almost 100 years (Cermak, 1985; Orton, 1937). They have been treated as
a single disorder; however, there is increasing evidence that there are different types of developmental motor disorders (Cermak, 1985; Denckla &
Roeltgen, 1992; Dewey, 2002). Many different terms have been used to refer
to children whose coordination difficulties and physical awkwardness are
sufficiently severe to interfere with everyday activities, including minimal
brain dysfunction (Gillberg, 1985), perceptual–motor dysfunction (Laszlo,
Bairstow, Bartrip, & Rolfe, 1988), clumsy child syndrome (Cratty, 1994;
Gubbay, 1975), developmental dyspraxia (Ayres, Mailloux, & Wendler,
1987; Cermak, 1985), and more recently specific developmental disorder of
motor function (World Health Organization, 1989, 1992) and developmental
coordination disorder (American Psychiatric Association, 1994). Investigators
and clinicians agree that these children are distinguished from their typically
developing peers by a pervasive slowness in the easy acquisition of motor
skills in spite of normal intelligence and freedom from diagnosed neurological
disorders (Hall, 1988; Polatajko, Fox, & Missiuna, 1995). The prevalence of
developmental motor disorders is estimated to be about 5–10% in school-age
children (American Psychiatric Association, 1994; Henderson & Hall, 1982).
Furthermore, although it was once believed that children outgrew their difficulties in motor functioning, research over the past 20 years has demonstrated
that in many of these children, the motor deficits persist into adolescence and
adulthood (Blondis, Snow, Roizen, Opacich, & Accordo, 1993; Cantell,
1998; Cantell, Smyth, & Ahonen, 2003; Losse et al., 1991).

Apraxia

In the adult literature many types of apraxia (i.e., motor disorders) have been
proposed: ideational, ideomotor, frontal, premotor, and limb-kinetic (Brown,
1972; Hecaen & Alberta, 1978; Luria, 1966). The two major types of adult
acquired apraxia described in the literature are, however, ideational and
ideomotor apraxia. Ideational apraxia is characterized by defective performance of a sequence of gestures. The individual elements of the sequence are
performed correctly; however, there is a disruption in the logical sequence of
the separate elements. Thus, a person is unable to plan actions to accomplish
an intended goal (e.g., make a cup of coffee). In ideomotor apraxia, the performance of isolated gestures is disturbed but the general plan of the action is
preserved. Individuals with this type of apraxia show better performance of
gestures to imitation and when using the actual objects compared to verbal
command. They can often tell how to execute a task, but they cannot perform
the individual actions required (Hecaen, 1981; Roy, 1978). Ideational and
ideomotor apraxia are most frequently associated with left-hemisphere dam-

age to the parietal–occipital areas of the cerebral cortex; however, the damage in ideational apraxia is usually greater and often bilateral (Roy, 1978).

Roy (1978) suggested that adult acquired apraxia could be better conceptualized as either planning or execution. He identified two types of planning apraxias, primary and secondary. In primary planning apraxia, the individual has lost the ability to sequence or plan any activity, whether or not it has a discernible motor component. This type of apraxia is believed to result from damage to the frontal area. Secondary planning apraxia results in a disturbance in the sequencing of actions. This disorder, however, is not due to an inability to plan. Rather, the spatial information sent to the area (frontal) responsible for planning is disordered. The frontal area depends on sensory information from the parietal–occipital area to plan movements successfully. Therefore, damage to parietal–occipital regions, which is associated with spatial problems, results in an inability to plan motor behavior. The second type of apraxia, executive apraxia, results from damage to the premotor area. In executive apraxia, the individual can plan the movement sequences necessary for accurate performance but is unable to execute the action in a coherent movement pattern.

Both Cermak (1985) and Dewey (Dewey, 2002; Dewey, Kaplan, Wilson, & Crawford, 1999) have applied Roy's (1978) conceptualization of adult apraxia to developmental motor disorders. In the pediatric population, execution disorders would be characterized by poorly coordinated performance in children who know what to do; disorders of planning would be characterized by uncertainties surrounding what to do and how to move. The utility of this view in pediatrics populations, however, is open to question and more research is needed. Investigations that adequately control for variables that could have an impact on children's ability to successfully execute motor acts (e.g., visual–spatial deficits), and variables that are relevant to the ability to successfully plan and carry out motor sequences (e.g., memory), are necessary to further our understanding of the developmental motor deficits displayed by pediatric populations.

Developmental Motor Disorders

In the motor development area, clinicians typically use the terms *developmental coordination disorder (DCD), specific developmental disorder of motor function (SDDMF), and developmental dyspraxia* interchangeably. Among researchers, however, they are rarely used synonymously, and there is much debate surrounding their exact definitions. Table 17.1 provides the DSM-IV and ICD-10 definitions for DCD and SDDMF, respectively, and various definitions of developmental dyspraxia found in the literature.

Because of the differences among the definitions and diagnostic criteria proposed for DCD, SDDMF, and developmental dyspraxia, a question that must be asked is whether these different diagnoses identify children with the same disorder (Cantell, Kooistra, & Larkin, 2001). The descriptions of the

TABLE 17.1. Definitions of DCD, SDDMF, and Developmental Dyspraxia

Developmental coordination disorder[a]	Specific developmental disorder of motor function[b]	Developmental dyspraxia
1. A disorder in which the main feature is a serious impairment in the development of motor coordination that is not solely explicable in terms of general intellectual retardation or of any specific congenital or acquired neurological disorder. Performance of daily activities that require motor coordination is substantially below that expected given the person's chronological age and measured intelligence (Criterion A). 2. The disturbance in Criterion A interferes with academic achievement or activities of daily living (Criterion B). 3. The diagnosis is made if the coordination difficulties are not due to a general medical condition and the criteria are not met for pervasive developmental disorder (Criterion C). 4. If mental retardation is present, the motor difficulties exceed those usually associated with it (Criterion D).	1. The child's motor coordination, on fine or gross motor tasks, should be significantly below the level expected on the basis of his or her age and general intelligence. This is best assessed on the basis of an individually administered, standardized tests. 2. The difficulties in coordination should have been present since early in development (i.e., they should not constitute an acquired deficit). (It is usual for the motor clumsiness to be associated with some degree of impaired performance on visual–spatial cognitive tasks.)	1. A disorder in planning and carrying out skilled, nonhabitual motor acts in the correct sequence.[c] 2. A disorder in movement planning; no deficits in movement execution.[d] 3. A disorder in the performance of representational gestures, nonrepresentational gestures, and movement sequences.[e]

a DSM-IV (American Psychiatric Association).
b ICD-10 (World Health Organization, 1992).
c Ayres (1972, 1985).
d Sugden and Keogh (1990); Cermak (1985).
e Denckla and Roeltgen (1992); Dewey (1995).

specific motor problems experienced by children with DCD, SDDMF, and developmental dyspraxia are often very similar. Children identified with these disorders are described as having difficulty with goal-directed actions that could be due to problems in movement execution such as balance and coordination and problems in movement planning (Henderson & Barnett, 1998). The definitions of DCD and SDDMF both emphasize that the child must display a significant impairment in motor coordination on various tasks. The definitions of developmental dyspraxia, however, do not focus on the issue of motor coordination. Rather, they emphasize that dyspraxia is a disorder in movement planning and gestural performance (Cermak, 1985, 1991; Denckla & Roeltgen, 1992; Dewey, 1995; Sugden & Keogh, 1990).

In the developmental literature, the word *gesture* is used to connote the ability to perform skilled motor acts or sequences of purposeful motor movements and the ability to use tools (Dewey, 1995; Hill, 1998; Kaplan, 1968). The term *praxis* has been used in a similar way (Cermak, 1985; Dewey & Kaplan, 1992; Dewey, Roy, Square-Storer, & Hayden, 1988). Children with developmental dyspraxia display impairments when performing meaningful gestures (i.e., gestures related to meaningful or familiar acts such as waving good-bye), nonmeaningful gestures (i.e., gestures related to nonmeaningful acts such as imitating postures), and gesture sequences (i.e., a series of gestures that result in the appropriate completion of an action) (Dewey, 1995). Thus, compared to DCD and SDDMF, developmental dyspraxia is a much more circumscribed disorder and could be viewed as a specific subtype or subcategory of DCD or SDDMF. It is noteworthy that ICD-10 specifically mentions that children with dyspraxic deficits would be included in the diagnostic category of SDDMF.

Although many of the same diagnostic criteria are used to make a diagnosis of DCD or SDDMF, there are some clear differences, the most notable being that children with mental retardation (MR) can be diagnosed with DCD if the motor problems exceed those usually associated with MR, but not with SDDMF (the definition of SDDMF excludes children with MR). A second difference that is particularly relevant to focus of this book is the fact that DSM-IV states that diagnosis (of DCD) is made if the criteria are not met for pervasive developmental disorder. Therefore, children who meet criteria for autism spectrum disorders (ASD) cannot be diagnosed with DCD. The definition of SDDMF does not specifically exclude children with a diagnosis of ASD; however, because it excludes children with MR, many children with ASD could not be diagnosed with SDDMF. It would be possible, however, for high-functioning children with ASD to receive a diagnosis of SDDMF.

This discussion highlights the fact that there is no universally agreed-on set of characteristics to describe and diagnose children with developmental motor disorders. The field, however, does agree that these children are extremely slow in their development of motor skills and that this results in functional motor performance deficits. Many, if not most, children with ASD also display deficits in the performance of motor skills (Smith, 2004). The question then is whether the motor deficits displayed by children with ASD differ from those displayed by children with developmental motor disorders. Please note that throughout the rest of this chapter, the term *DCD* is used to refer to developmental motor deficits in children, except when giving details of specific studies that identified their participants as specifically displaying SDDMF.

MOTOR DEFICITS IN CHILDREN WITH DEVELOPMENTAL COORDINATION DISORDER

Basic Visual–Motor Skills

Children with DCD have been reported to manifest motor deficits in virtually every motor domain. They tend to work more slowly than their typically developing peers and trade speed for accuracy (Missiuna & Pollock, 1995; Schoemaker et al., 2001). Performance on tasks that require rapid or accurate goal-directed movements is often impaired (Huh, Williams, & Burke, 1998; Johnston, Burns, Brauer, & Richardson, 2002; Schoemaker et al., 2001). Slowness of reaction time is particularly apparent for bimanual, compared to unimanual, reaching movements, and this is true for both symmetrical (i.e., both hands moved to targets located at the same distance) and asymmetrical (i.e., both hands moved to targets situated at different distances) reaching (Williams, Huh, & Burke, 1998). Movement time, a measure of the speed of movement execution (Williams, 2002), is also considerably slower in many children with DCD (Henderson, Rose, & Henderson, 1992; Huh et al., 1998). Poor rhythmic coordination or timing of movement, evident on finger-tapping tests, and deviant force control capabilities (e.g., too much, too little, or variability in the amount of force applied in a given task) are commonly observed in these children (Lundy-Ekman, Ivry, Keele, & Woollacott, 1991; Piek & Skinner, 1999; Volman & Geuze, 1998a, 1998b; Williams, 2002; Williams, Woollacott, & Ivry, 1992). In addition to general slowness, and timing and force control deficits, children with DCD often display fine motor (Smits-Engelsman, Niemeijer, & Van Galen, 2001) and handwriting difficulties (Denckla & Roeltgen, 1992). Unusual pencil grasps and immature prehension of scissors have also been noted in this population (Missiuna & Pollock, 1995; Rodger et al., 2003). They have also been found to display abnormalities in postural control (Johnston et al., 2002; Wann, Mon-Williams, & Rushton, 1998). Wann and colleagues (1998) reported that the postural control of children with DCD was similar to that observed in younger children (i.e., a greater reliance on visual information for balance control and less on proprioceptive cues). This suggests that at least for some children with DCD, there may be a developmental lag in the acquisition of the skills necessary for adequate postural control. There is also some suggestion that a developmental lag may affect the acquisition of other motor skills (Cantell et al., 2003; Hill, 1998; Hill, Bishop, & Nimmo-Smith, 1998). In addition to basic motor skills deficits, children with DCD have been reported to display impairments in kin-esthetic perception (i.e., the ability to apprehend the position in space of body parts and the force, timing, amplitude and direction of movement using proprioceptive and vestibular input) (Laszlo & Bairstow, 1983; Piek & Coleman-Carman, 1995) and visual–motor integration (Wilson & McKenzie, 1998), both of which could result in impaired motor performance.

Most studies that have examined motor functioning in children with DCD and other neurodevelopmental disorders have focused on the *product* dimension of motor performance. The product dimension reflects the level of performance on a task, such as the accuracy of performance or the time taken to perform the task relative to some expected level of performance (i.e., test norms). Children with various neurodevelopmental disorders could, however, display the same level of performance on the product dimension for different reasons. To better understand the nature of motor impairments in children, investigators need to focus on the *process* dimension of motor performance. The process dimension refers to how the child achieves the product (i.e., level of motor performance). Analyses of the factors that underlie the performance of motor skills and the presence of certain types of errors are ways in which the process dimension of motor performance can be assessed.

Gesture/Imitation

When we use the term *gesture*, we are typically referring to nonverbal commu-nicative actions (e.g., waving good-bye and pointing). In neuropsychology, however, *gesture* has come to connote a wider range of *actions* from the imita-tion of meaningless movements to the demonstration of how an object should be used (e.g., show me how you comb your hair). Furthermore, in the neuro-psychology literature, deficits in gestural performance are often associated with deficits in motor function and are labeled *apraxia* or *dyspraxia*. A spe-cific impairment in the performance of communicative gestures has not been noted in children with DCD; however, empirical studies have reported that the motor performance of gestures is much poorer in children with DCD com-pared to control children (Dewey, 1993; Hill, 1998).

To better understand the gestural deficits displayed by children with DCD, researchers have examined the effects of different input modalities and response conditions on gestural performance. Children's performance on ges-tures to verbal command versus imitation, meaningful versus nonmeaningful gestures, transitive gestures (those *requiring the use* of an object, e.g., comb your hair with a comb) versus intransitive gestures (those that *do not require an object*, e.g., salute), and single gestures versus complex gestures (e.g., those involving a sequence of gestures) have been examined (Dewey, 1995; Dewey & Kaplan, 1992; Hill, 1998). In a comprehensive study by Dewey and Kaplan (1992), the gestural performance of children with developmental motor prob-lems was compared to that of similar-age typically developing children. Results indicated that the children with DCD performed more poorly than typically developing peers on meaningful and nonmeaningful gestures. Furthermore, these impairments were evident across movement systems (i.e., orofacial and limb). Closer examination of the task demands indicated that the children with motor deficits had particular difficulty with the performance of complex gesture sequences compared to single gestures, more problems with transitive compared to intransitive gestures, and more difficulties performing gestures to verbal command than to imitation. Furthermore, for meaningful gestures (i.e., limb and orofacial) children with DCD showed significant improvements when performing gestures to imitation compared to verbal command.

Hill (1998) also compared the performance of children with DCD to that of age-matched controls on both meaningful and nonmeaningful gesture tasks. She included two additional comparison groups, children with specific language impairment (SLI) and a younger, motor-matched control group. Consistent with Dewey and Kaplan (1992), Hill found that children with DCD performed more poorly on tests of transitive gestures and intransitive gestures compared to the age-matched normally developing controls. Results also revealed that the children with DCD, the children with SLI, and the younger motor-matched control children all displayed similar levels of difficulty with tasks requiring the production of meaningful gestures. Furthermore, performance of each group of children improved significantly when performing meaningful gestures to imitation compared to verbal command. On tasks that required the production of nonmeaningful hand postures or sequences of hand postures, few errors were noted and no group differences were found. This finding is counterintuitive as one would expect that familiarity would aid in the accurate performance of gestures. Hill suggests, however, that familiarity with a gesture might lead to less reliance on visual monitoring of the gesture and hence less accurate execution. This lack of visual monitoring could result in the children relying on kinesthetic information to perform the gesture. As kinesthetic difficulties have been implicated in the motor deficits manifest by children with DCD (Laszlo et al., 1988; Wilson & McKenzie, 1998), problems in this area could have contributed to the poorer performance of the children with DCD on the tasks that involved familiar gestures. Also intriguing was Hill's finding that the children with DCD produced a similar number of errors as the younger motor-matched control group. This is consistent with the view that children with DCD display a general delay in the development of gesture.

In a more recent study, Zoia, Pelamatti, Cuttini, Casotto, and Scabar (2002) investigated the impact of input modality on the gestural performance of children with and without DCD in three age bands (i.e., 5–6 years, 7–8 years, and 9–10 years). Transitive gestures were examined using four input modalities: (1) imitation, which involved the reproduction of the gesture performed by the investigator; (2) visual plus tactile, for which a real object or tool was used; (3) visual, which required the child to mime the use of a seen object; and (4) verbal command, in which the child performed the gesture requested by the experimenter. Results revealed that the limb gesture skills of normally developing children followed a progressive maturation pattern with the imitation, visual plus tactile, and visual modalities maturing before the verbal modality. Children with DCD performed more poorly than their peers without motor deficits on every input modality. With the exception of the verbal command condition, differences between children with DCD and the control children became less marked with increasing age and for the oldest age band (i.e., 9–10-year-olds) no differences were found between the children with DCD and control children in the imitation and the visual conditions. For each age band, the imitation and visual plus tactile conditions resulted in significantly better gestural performance than the verbal condition. Zoia and colleagues suggest that difficulties in integrating information obtained from these different sensory systems (i.e., visual, tactile, and kinesthetic) and in using verbal information could account for the inaccurate or clumsy performance of skilled motor movements by children with DCD. Zoia and colleagues also noted that the ability to effectively use these different types of information was age dependent with the imitation and visual plus tactile facilitating gestural performance in children under 6 years of age, visual information facilitating gestural performance by around 7–8 years of age, and verbal information facilitating gestural performance only around 9 years of age. The improved performance with age on all input modalities and the catchup with the typical control children on the visual and imitation modalities at 9–10 years of age provides further support for the contention that children with DCD display a general maturational delay in gestural development and that this delay could be the result of delays in the development of visual–verbal–perceptual integration.

In conclusion, the literature on gestural and particularly imitative deficits in children with DCD suggests that impairments in gestural performance are characterized by a maturational delay in normal development and are not the result of a specific deficit. Examination of the types of errors that these children display could, however, provide us with insight into the specific *processes* that contribute to these delays.

Error Analyses of Gestures

Dewey (1993) examined the types of errors made by children with DCD and their normally developing peers when producing gestures. She found that the children with DCD demonstrated significantly more *action errors* (i.e., alterations in the typical timing, force, and amplitude required to complete the movement) and *movement errors* (i.e., the palm of the hand is incorrectly rotated relative to the child's arm or position, or the plane through which the movement typically occurs is not used) for both transitive and intransitive limb gestures relative to normally developing children. Inaccurate judgments in the timing, force, and amplitude necessary to perform gestures accurately has also been observed in other samples of children with DCD (Lundy-Ekman et al., 1991; Piek & Skinner, 1999; Williams, 2002). Dewey (1993) also noted that the children with DCD displayed significantly more *posture errors* (i.e., incorrect position or shape of the limb) when performing transitive limb gestures, but not when performing intransitive gestures compared to the typically developing children. This latter result is consistent with the findings of other researchers that suggest children with DCD display deficits in postural control (Johnston et al., 2002; Wann et al., 1998).

Hill, Bishop, and Smith (1998) undertook a similar qualitative analysis of the error patterns displayed by children with DCD, age-matched controls, a younger motor-matched control group, and an SLI group. Several results from this study are noteworthy. First, Hill and colleagues reported that all the gestures performed by the children in all four groups were correct conceptually. In other words, they resembled the correct action. Second, the children in the DCD, SLI, and the control groups produced similar types of errors. Third, there was a trend for children in the DCD, SLI, and younger control group to produce more of each of these errors than the age-matched controls and to perform similarly to one another (suggesting an immaturity in the development of gestures for children with DCD and SLI). Finally, performance to imitation tended to reduce error production; however, it did not eliminate it. Examination of the specific types of errors revealed that children in the DCD, SLI, and younger motor-matched control groups demonstrated significantly more errors related to *spatial orientation* (i.e., hand deviating from the appropriate spatial position), *external configuration* (i.e., correctly gripping an object, but failing to take into account the length of the object when performing the action), and *internal configuration* (i.e., correctly using an object, but showing an incorrect orientation of the object) relative to the older control children. Therefore, the children in these three groups were more likely to place their hand too close to their mouth when miming using a toothbrush (external configuration), or their hand grip would not allow a comb to come into contact with their hair when demonstrating the use of a comb (internal configuration). The children in the DCD, SLI, and younger motor-matched groups also displayed more *body-part-as-object errors* (i.e., used part of the anatomy to represent the object such as using one's finger to represent a toothbrush when miming brushing one's teeth) than the older controls. The authors concluded that the gestural errors displayed by the children with DCD, SLI, and the younger motor-matched controls were indicative of imprecise implementation of the sequence of movements, as opposed to an inability to conceptualize the action.

MOTOR DEFICITS IN CHILDREN
WITH AUTISM SPECTRUM DISORDERS
Basic Visual–Motor Skills

ASD include a range of conditions with similar phenotypes (autistic disorder, Asperger's disorder, and pervasive developmental disorder not otherwise specified) (American Psychiatric Association, 1994). Whether these DSM-IV subgroups reflect clinical or theoretically meaningful distinctions remains contro-versial (Fein et al., 1999). For the purposes of this chapter, we use the term *ASD* to refer to these conditions, except when presenting details of specific study criteria or when otherwise required for clarity.

Research has reported that children with ASD display a variety of motor skills deficits (Ghaziuddin & Butler, 1998; Ghaziuddin, Butler, Tsai, & Ghaziuddin, 1994; Gillberg, 1989; Green et al., 2002; Hauck & Dewey, 2001; Hughes, 1996; Manjiviona & Prior, 1995; Miyahara et al., 1997; Page & Boucher, 1998) similar to those displayed by children with DCD, including deficits in motor planning (Hughes, 1996), motor coordination (Ghaziuddin & Butler, 1998; Ghaziuddin et al., 1994), fine motor skills (Szatmari, Tuff, Finlayson, & Bartolucci, 1990), and gross motor and oromotor skills (Page & Boucher, 1998). In addition, children with ASD display stereotyped and repet-itive behaviors (e.g., hand flapping, finger flicking, and complex whole-body movement). These repetitive behaviors, which are specific to ASD and not seen in children with DCD, have a substantial motor component. From a motor development perspective, however, they do not represent impairments in motor execution or motor planning but rather deviant motor behavior. For more detailed discussions of repetitive motor behavior in children with ASD consult Lewis and Bodfish (1998) and Turner (1999).

Differential motor skill patterns have been associated with the different subtypes of ASD. In Kanner's (1943/1973) initial description of autism, motor skills were described not only as unimpaired but a strength of children with autism. In contrast, Asperger (Asperger, 1944/1991) and Wing (1981) reported that motor clumsiness was associated with Asperger syndrome (AS). Recent studies that have compared the motor skills of children with AS and children with high-functioning autism (HFA; children with prototypical autism who present without mental retardation) suggest that impaired motor performance does not distinguish these two groups, and that no particular motor difficulties are specific to children with AS (Ghaziuddin & Butler, 1998; Iwanaga, Kawasaki, & Tscuchida, 2000; Miller & Ozonoff, 2000). More detailed reviews of this issue are provided by Smith (2000, 2004) and Ghaziuddin, Tsai, and Ghaziuddin (1992).

A recent study by Rinehart, Bradshaw, Brereton, and Tonge (2001) sug-gests, however, that some subtle differences in motor functioning may exist between children with different subtypes of ASD. Rinehart and colleagues (2001) investigated whether the motor dysfunction in HFA and AS was due to deficits in movement preparation or movement execution and whether there were any differences between children with HFA and AS in terms of their movement planning and movement execution abilities. Based on the work of Hughes (1996), they hypothesized that children with HFA and AS would dis-play deficits in motor preparation. Diagnoses were made according to the DSM-IV criteria and each child was matched to a typically developing child on the basis of age, sex and Full Scale IQ. A simple motor reprogramming task was used to examine separately the preparation and the execution of movements. Children were required to depress a target button as quickly as possible in response to its illumination. Once this target button was pressed, the next target was illuminated and the children were required to press it. The task involved alternating repeatedly, as quickly as possible between these two target buttons. On each trial the children were cued one time to move in an unexpected direction (i.e., "oddball" movement). Results indicated that speed of motor execution on this task was similar for the typically developing group, the HFA group, and the AS group. However, both the HFA and AS groups differed from the typically developing group in movement preparation, but in different ways. The typically developing children displayed slower movement preparation prior to the oddball movements but responded faster on the trials immediately following the oddball movement. In contrast, children with HFA displayed fast movement preparation times for all movements and were unaffected by the oddball movements, whereas children with AS showed slower movement preparation following the oddball trials. The authors concluded that children with HFA and AS showed deficits in movement preparation, with intact movement execution ability, and that "poorly planned movement" may be a more accurate description of the motor impairment displayed by children with ASD. The differences in movement preparation between children with HFA and AS suggested that children with HFA showed a lack of anticipation (for oddball movements) when preparing movements and individuals with AS showed a deficit in motor programming after an unexpected movement. Rinehart and colleagues suggested that these differences in impaired movement preparation could be attributed to differential impairment in the frontalstriatal area. They also acknowledged that attentional processing could be a confounding factor. Research suggests that both children with HFA and AS display deficits in spatial attention (Bryson, Landry, & Wainwright, 1997; Burback, Enns, Stauder, Mottron, & Randolph, 1997). It is important then for future research to attempt to tease out the contribution of impaired attentional processes to motor functioning in children with ASD. Studies using comparison groups of children with DCD and attention-deficit/hyperactivity disorder (ADHD) could assist us in learning more about the interaction of motor, attentional, and sensory–perceptual processes and their influence on motor performance in children with ASD and related conditions.

Gesture/Imitation

In the clinical literature, the difficulties in gestural performance noted in children with ASD typically refer to impairments in communicative gesture (Attwood, 1998; Gillberg, 1991) and not deficits in motor function. Many empirical studies, however, have employed tasks involving imitation of gestures and object use. The findings of these studies indicate that children with ASD display impairments on various tasks associated with gesture production, including imitation of manual and oral gestures and imitation of tool use (Green et al., 2002; Rogers, Hepburn, Stackhouse, & Wehner, 2003; Stone, Ousley, &

Littleford, 1997; Williams, Whiten, & Singh, 2004). See Rogers and Williams (Chapter 12, this volume) for a detailed discussion of imitation deficits in children with ASD.

COMPARISON OF THE MOTOR DEFICITS IN DEVELOPMENTAL COORDINATION DISORDER VERSUS AUTISM SPECTRUM DISORDERS

When investigating motor impairments in children, it is important to consider what might be the most appropriate control group(s). Most of the research to date has compared the motor performance of children with DCD or ASD to typically developing children. It is essential, however, that the motor performance of children with various developmental disorders be compared. Such investigations would allow us to determine if the profile of motor skills differs among children with various developmental disorders.

In a recent study, Green and colleagues (2002) examined the extent and severity of the motor impairment of 11 children with AS compared to 9 children with SDDMF. Children's motor skills were assessed on the Movement Assessment Battery for Children (MABC; Henderson & Sugden, 1992). Results indicated that all the children with AS had significant motor impairments and that they did not differ from the SDDMF group in terms of their overall performance on the motor assessment measure. Dewey and Crawford (2005) examined the motor skills of children with DCD (n = 38) and compared them to those of children with ASD (n = 49) and children with no evidence of problems in motor coordination (n = 78). The ASD group included 22 children who had been diagnosed with autism, 12 who had been diagnosed with AS, and 15 who had been diagnosed with pervasive developmental disorder not otherwise specified (PDDNOS) based on DSM-IV criteria (American Psychiatric Association, 1994). Children's motor skills were assessed using the Bruininks–Oseretsky Test of Motor Performance—Short Form (BOTMP-SF). Results indicated that the children with DCD and the children with ASD scored significantly lower than the normal comparison children on the BOTMP-SF when age and IQ were controlled (see Table 17.2). The children with DCD and the children with ASD did not differ from each other in terms of their overall level of performance. The findings of these two studies suggest that the severity of the motor difficulties displayed by children with developmental motor disorders and ASD are similar. It is possible, however, that the nature of the motor impairment evidenced by these two groups of children differs.

Gesture/Imitation

Both children with DCD and ASD display deficits in the performance of gestures. Do these two groups of children, however, display different types of gestural deficits and are these gestural deficits due to motor impairment? It

TABLE 17.2. Motor and Gesture Test Scores for Children with ASD, Children with DCD, and Normal Controls

	ASD (n = 49)		DCD (n = 38)		Normal controls (n = 78)	
	M	SD	M	SD	M	SD
Males/females	43/6		26/12		59/19	
Chronological age (years)	10.2	3.4	11.3	1.7	11.3	2.4
IQ	88.2	20.8	97.2	14.5	111.2	12.6
BOTMP	33.78	13.02	39.70	9.15	73.90	7.74
Transitive gesture—command	8.17	3.42	13.16	2.11	13.91	2.54
Transitive gestures—imitation	8.86	3.11	14.53	1.70	15.31	2.04
Intransitive gestures—command	8.57	4.55	15.67	1.31	15.31	2.04
Intransitive gestures—imitation	11.11	3.76	16.81	1.49	16.19	1.75

has been suggested that the difficulties in gestural performance seen in children with ASD may be due to a deficits in motor functioning (DeMeyer et al., 1972; Smith & Bryson, 1994). Jones and Prior (1985) and Smith and Bryson (1994, 1998) reported that children with ASD were significantly less accurate than control children on various tests that demanded the performance of gestures such as the imitation of static postures, imitation of dynamic sequences, and the use of objects. Smith and Bryson also reported that manual dexterity accounted for 37% of the variance in posture imitation in children with ASD. In contrast, a recent study by Rogers and colleagues (2003) found that motor functioning did not account for a significant amount of variance on imitation scores in children with ASD when overall developmental level was controlled for. These studies, however, did not directly address the question whether the imitative deficit noted in children with ASD was due to an impairment in motor functioning. Recent studies by Green and colleagues (2002) and Dewey and Crawford (2005), however, provide some insight.

Green and colleagues (2002) examined the performance of children with SDDMF and AS on the Gesture Test (Cermak, Costers, & Drake, 1980). This test included two components. The first required the children to demonstrate 10 meaningful gestures to verbal command and the second required the imitation of 10 nonmeaningful actions. Results revealed that the children with AS had significantly more difficulty performing the meaningful gestures to command and imitating gestures than did the children with SDDMF. Dewey and Crawford (2005) compared the gestural performance of children with DCD, ASD, and typically developing children on six meaningful transitive limb gestures (e.g., show me how you brush your teeth with a toothbrush) and six meaningful intransitive limb gestures (e.g., show me how you wave good-bye) performed to verbal command and to imitation. This praxis test was similar to that used by Dewey and Kaplan (1992). The testing was completed in one session and the children's performance of the gestures was videotaped for later scoring. Videotapes were scored for level of gestural development using a system based on Kaplan's (1968) hierarchy of gestural development (Dewey & Kaplan, 1992) by a rater who was blind to the diagnoses of the children. Previous research has demonstrated that this method of scoring has a high degree of reliability (Dewey & Kaplan, 1992). Results revealed significant group differences in the performance of transitive gestures to command, and intransitive gestures to command when age and IQ were controlled (see Table 17.2). The ASD group scored significantly lower than the children with DCD and the typically developing children on both types of gestures. Significant differences also emerged for transitive and intransitive gestures to imitation with the ASD group scoring significantly lower than the other groups. The children with DCD did not differ significantly from the typically developing group on any of the measures of gestural performance. Furthermore, all groups showed better performance of gestures to imitation compared to command. Thus, providing a visual model resulted in improved performance of gestures for all children, including children with ASD. Of note is the fact that although the children with ASD and DCD showed similar deficits in motor skills relative to normal controls, only the children with ASD showed a significant deficit in gestural performance. Thus, the deficits in gestural performance displayed by children with ASD could not be attributed solely to a motor deficit.

Error Analysis

The studies by Green and colleagues (2002) and Dewey and Crawford (2005) also examined errors in gestural production. Green and colleagues reported that the children with AS made marginally more spatiotemporal errors than children with SDDMF but that this differences was not statistically significant. They also reported that there was no difference between the groups in the pattern of errors. In contrast, Dewey and Crawford, using an error analyses system similar to that used by Dewey (1993), found that children with ASD displayed significantly more incorrect actions, extension errors, distortion errors, body-part-as-object errors, orientation errors, and location errors when performing gestures to command and imitation than children with DCD and normal control children when IQ and age were controlled (see Table 17.3 for definition of errors). Were there certain types of errors, however, that accounted for a significantly greater percentage of total errors in children with ASD compared to children with DCD and typically developing children? Examination of group differences in the distribution of errors (% contribution of a particular error type to the total errors made) revealed that for gestures to command, children with ASD displayed a significantly higher proportion of orientation, distortion, and incorrect action errors than children with DCD and typically developing controls (see Table 17.4). Of note, however, was the fact that the children with ASD showed a significantly lower proportion of posture errors than children in the other two groups. For gestures to imitation, a similar pat-

TABLE 17.3. Limb Praxis Errors

Level of gestural development	Error	Definition
3	Correct	Action correctly performed.
2	Extension	An over- or underextension of the movement (e.g., when combing hair, the hand holding the comb touches the head; when brushing teeth, the child extends the brush so it appears he or she is brushing the sides of the cheeks as well).
2	Delay	A 3-second delay between the end of the instructions and the beginning of the movement.
2	Other	A movement error not otherwise specified (e.g., not opening the lips when brushing the teeth; keeping eyes closed when hammering).
2	Helper	Subject uses another part of the body to help with the movement (e.g., crossing the fingers of one hand with the help of the other; using the left hand to tuck the thumb of the right hand in when making a fist).
1	Distortion	A change in the amplitude, force, or timing of a movement; the typical force, timing, or amplitude required to perform the movement is altered and may include abnormally increased, decreased, or irregular rates of production (e.g., overly vigorous hammering; writing in 2-foot-tall letters).
1	Posture	An incorrect position of the hand (e.g., putting the thumb inside the fist; not holding the hammer or toothbrush correctly).
1	Orientation	Incorrect rotation of the palm of the hand relative to the arm, or the plane through which the movement normally occurs is not used; most common in the salute.
1	Location	Action performed at the wrong location; most common in the salute, when the hand goes over the midline of the face.
1	Body part	Body part used as an object rather than an imitation of the use of that object (e.g., using fingers as scissors; using fingers as a comb).
0	Absence of action	No action performed.
0	Incorrect action	Action performed but it is incorrect (e.g., the child snaps fingers when he or she is supposed to salute).

TABLE 17.4. Proportion of Error (%) for Gestures to Command in Children with ASD, Children with DCD, and Normal Controls

Errors	ASD (n = 49)	DCD (n = 38)	Normal controls (n = 78)
Extension	29.4	37.7	34.4
Delay	5.7	2.9	2.0
Other	2.1	6.7	5.2
Helper	0.4	1.4	1.0
Distortion*	16.1	7.2	5.2
Posture**	13.3	22.3	37.2
Orientation***	5.7	2.4	0.3
Location	4.2	7.5	3.9
Body part	15.1	10.0	9.1
Absence of action	1.4	1.2	4.7
Incorrect action****	6.7	0.8	1.6

Note. Significant group differences in the proportion of error: * $p < .001$; ** $p = .003$; *** $p = .002$; **** $p = .001$.

tern emerged for orientation, distortion, and postural errors; children with ASD also displayed significantly more other errors than the children with DCD and the typically developing controls (see Table 17.5). These findings reveal that the distribution of error types in children with ASD differed from that of children with DCD and normal controls. Furthermore, they provide some suggestions regarding the processes that could be influencing gestural performance in children with ASD, which is discussed in more detail in a later section of this chapter.

Delay or Deficit in Gesture/Imitation

In children with DCD and ASD, are the impairments in gestural/imitation skills due to a delay in the development of these skills or an actual deficit? The findings of Dewey and colleagues (Dewey, 1991, 1993; Dewey & Kaplan, 1992, 1994), as well as those of Hill (1998) and Zoia and colleagues (2002), are consistent with the view that children with DCD display a general maturational delay in the acquisition of gestural skills. Williams and colleagues (2004) in their review on action imitation in children with autism suggest that the literature provides support for the view that autism is characterized by a delay in the normal development of imitative skills rather than an absolute deficit. This conclusion is based research that has reported no differences in action imitation between children with autism and controls groups matched on verbal mental age (Libby, Powell, Messer, & Jordan, 1997; Morgan, Cutrer, Coplin, & Rodrigue, 1989) and studies that have found that

TABLE 17.5. Proportion of Error (%) for Gestures to Imitation in Children with ASD, Children with DCD, and Normal Controls

Errors	ASD (n = 49)	DCD (n = 38)	Normal controls (n = 78)
Extension	34.1	45.6	44.3
Delay	0.6	0.03	0.10
Other*	5.2	0.9	0.8
Helper	0.5	0.3	0.04
Distortion**	22.0	6.	10.1
Posture***	13.7	32.4	28.3
Orientation****	5.8	0.7	0.6
Location	8.6	9.4	8.6
Body part	8.7	4.4	4.3
Absence of action	0.5	0.04	0.2
Incorrect action	0.7	0.04	1.2

Note. Significant group differences in the proportion of error: * $p = .002$; ** $p = .002$; *** $p = .027$; **** $p < .001$.

group differences in imitative skills diminished in older populations (Royeurs, Van Oost, & Bothuyne, 1998). Thus, for both children with DCD and ASD, the general consensus is that problems in gestural performance are the result of a delay in the normal development of gestural/imitative skills; however, prospective longitudinal studies are needed to confirm this.

Neural Correlates

Neuroimaging studies provide some insight in the neural correlates of motor functioning in children with ASD, DCD, and other developmental disorders (i.e., ADHD and dyslexia). Until recently, the cerebellum and the prefrontal cortex were not thought to be involved in the same functions. The cerebellum was thought to be critical for motor skills, while the dorsolateral prefrontal cortex was considered essential for complex cognitive abilities (Diamond, 2000). Evidence from neuroimaging studies suggests, however, that there is a close relationship between these two brain regions (Berman et al., 1995; Desmond, Gabrieli, Wagner, Ginier, & Glover, 1997; deZubicaray et al., 1998; Flament, Ellermann, Ugurbil, & Ebmer, 1994; Schlosser et al., 1998; Van Mier et al., 1994).

Numerous studies of children with ASD have found evidence of pathology in the cerebellum (Bailey et al., 1998; Courchesne, 1991, 1997; Gaffney, Tsai, Kuperman, & Minchin, 1987; Guerin et al., 1996). Recent neuropathological and neuroimaging studies have also found evidence that individuals with ASD have frontal lobe damage. Carper and Courchesne (2000) found that frontal lobe volume was increased in some patients with autism and that this increase correlated with the degree of cerebellar abnormality. Although neuroimaging studies have not specifically examined children with DCD, studies of children with ADHD and dyslexia, both of which are associated with motor problems (Fawcett & Nicolson, 1995; Piek, Pitcher, & Hay, 1999), have reported cerebellar and frontal abnormalities (Berquin et al., 1998; Castellanos, 1997; Castellanos et al., 1996; Mostofsky, Reiss, Lockhart, & Denckla, 1998). Examinations of the motor behaviors of children with ADHD and dyslexia also provide support for the neural bases of the motor impairments seen in these populations. Investigations of the motor behavior of children with ADHD suggest that their motor impairments are associated with cerebellar dysfunction (problems in balance, rapid alternating movements and consistently producing movements of the correct distance or correct timing) (Diamond, 2000). Problems in timing precision on bimanual tasks, a cerebellar function (Ivry & Keele, 1989; Keele & Ivry, 1990), have also been reported in children with dyslexia (Wolff, Michel, Ovrut, & Drake, 1990). Thus, children with these developmental disorders display concomitant motor problems that appear to be associated with cerebellar dysfunction.

Research also suggests a close link between cerebellar and frontal lobe functions and that the cerebellum and the frontal cortex are parts of an interconnected neural system in which the dysfunction at one site can cause maldevelopment of other brain sites (Carper & Courchesne, 2000; Diamond, 2000). Investigators have shown that abnormal neural activity can affect the development of the cerebral cortex (Killackey, 1990; Quartz & Sejnowski, 1997). Therefore, abnormal neural activity in the cerebellar projections to the frontal cortex could cause maldevelopment of the frontal lobes and any other brain region receiving this input (Carper & Courchesne, 2000; Diamond, 2000). Diamond (2000) suggests that another reason why abnormalities of the neocerebellum and the prefrontal cortex occur in the same disorder may be because both regions "have extended periods of maturation; insults too late in development to affect the maturation of other neural structures can have profound consequences for both prefrontal and cerebellar development" (p. 49). Thus, the coexistence of frontal and cerebellar abnormalities helps in explaining the co-occurrence of motor and cognitive impairments in children with various developmental disorders.

Research has also suggested that the basal ganglia and specifically the caudate nucleus are important for movement control such as selecting the proper movement, the appropriate muscles to perform the movement, and the appropriate force to execute the movement (Groves, 1983; Stelmach & Worringham, 1988). The caudate is also a major output structure of dorsolateral prefrontal cortex (Selemon & Goldman-Rakic, 1988). Studies of children with ADHD have reported size reductions and reduced left–right asymmetry in the caudate nucleus (Filipek et al., 1997; Hynd et al., 1993). Neuroimaging studies have also found reduced activity in the caudate in children with ADHD during the performance of cognitive tasks (Lou, Henriksen,

Bruhn, Borner, & Nielsen, 1989; Teicher, Ito, Glod, & Barber, 1996; Vaidya et al., 1998).

Many children with developmental disorders display not only motor problems but also problems in visual–motor integration. In fact, problems in visual–motor integration and visual perception have been found to be areas of particular difficulty for children with DCD and ASD (Smith, 2004; Wilson & McKenzie, 1998). Studies of adult patients with brain damage suggest that both cerebral hemispheres are involved in visual–motor integration, but that the right hemisphere plays a more important role given the greater frequency of visual–motor problems associated with right-hemisphere lesions (Damasio, 1985). Lesions of the parietal cortex, particularly when the injury is on the right, have been found to result in deficits in visual perception and deficits in fine motor coordination associated with visual guidance (Andersen, 1987). Neuroimaging studies of preterm children with spastic diplegia have reported that lesions in the parietal and/or occipital white matter are associated with visual–spatial deficits (Goto, Ota, Iai, Sugita, & Tanabe, 1994). Rourke (1995) has hypothesized that nonverbal learning disabilities, which are found in children with DCD and AS, and have visual–spatial deficits as a major feature, are the result of lesions in the white matter of the right hemisphere. Thus, the nondominant (i.e., right) hemisphere, and particularly the right parietal lobe, appears to be involved in visual–spatial processes that contribute to visual–motor integration. Visual–motor integration also requires, however, that information be exchanged between the parietal region and the motor areas of the frontal cortex (Quintana & Fuster, 1993) with the subcortical areas providing an integrative function (Alexander, Delong, & Strick, 1986). As a result, deficits in visual–motor integration could arise from frontal and subcortical, as well as parietal, lobe lesions (Marshall et al., 1994).

In summary, the foregoing discussion emphasizes the close interconnections of the various brain regions that are involved in motor and cognitive functioning. Because of these interconnections, abnormalities in one area of the brain could have a detrimental effect on the development and functioning of another region. These bidirectional influences may account for the "comorbidities" in motor impairment displayed by children with various neurodevelopmental disorders.

PROCESSES THAT CONTRIBUTE TO GESTURAL IMPAIRMENTS

There is a general consensus that difficulty with motor learning is a key feature of DCD. Although children with DCD learn motor skills, they typically require more practice than average, and the quality of movement may be compromised considerably (Cermak, Gubbay, & Larkin, 2002). Beyond this, however, there is little agreement regarding the processes that contribute to the deficits in gestural performance and specifically imitation manifest by children with DCD. A number of hypotheses, however, have been advanced to account for the imitative deficit seen in children with ASD. Williams and colleagues (2004) provide a detailed discussion of these various hypotheses and conclude that the specific imitative deficit in children with ASD reflects a deficit in self–other mapping (Rogers & Pennington, 1991). This hypothesis is supported by the fact that a number of studies have reported the presence of reversal errors on imitation (i.e., the basic components of the imitation are correct but the children are unable to alter their perspective accordingly) (Hobson & Lee, 1999; Ohta, 1987; Whiten & Brown, 1999). Dewey and Crawford (2005) also found that children with ASD displayed significantly more reversal errors (i.e., orientation error) than children with DCD and normal controls when performing gestures to command and imitation and that these errors accounted for approximately 6% of the total error, in both conditions. Other research, however, brings into question Williams and colleagues' conclusion that self–other mapping problems offer the most parsimonious explanation for imitation deficits in children with ASD.

Previous research has suggested that children with DCD and ASD have deficits in proprioception, sensory integration, and visual processing (Ayres, 1985; Dewey & Kaplan, 1992; Sellers, 1995; Smith, 2004; Smyth & Mason, 1997, 1998; Zoia et al., 2002). Such deficits could account for difficulties in postural control and balance, as well as the deficits in gestural skills. Deviant timing of postural muscle activity, which results in inadequate postural control and poor execution of skilled movements, has been postulated to be a contributor to the upper-limb coordination difficulties manifest by children with DCD (Johnston et al., 2002). Inaccuracies in force, timing, and amplitude due to sensory deficits could also result in gestures executed to verbal command or imitation being performed in a distorted manner and are possible mechanisms underlying praxis (i.e., gestural) deficits in children (Dewey, 1993; Dewey & Crawford, 2005). Further research is needed, however, to clarify the influence of sensory functioning on the performance of gestures.

Although most research has focused on the difficulties with motor output displayed by children with DCD, some researchers have suggested that the dyspraxic deficits seen in some children with DCD may result from an impairment in the internal representation of gesture (Ayres, 1985; Denckla & Roeltgen, 1992). A study by Wilson, Maruff, Ives, and Currie (2001) supports the idea that children with DCD have an impaired ability to generate internal representations of movements. A visually guided pointing task (VGPT) was used to measure movement duration for real and imagined movements in 20 children with DCD at 8 and 12 years of age, and normally developing controls matched on age and Verbal IQ. The task required that the children make a series of real or imagined alternating movements between two target locations on a table using a pencil held in the preferred hand. For the imagined trials, the children's eyes were open and their hands remained fixed at the starting location (while holding the pencil) while they imagined their hand moving between the two target locations. The distance between the two target locations remained constant, while the width of the targets varied between 1.9 and

30 millimeters. The movements were performed under two load conditions: with or without the addition of a 200-gram weight attached to the top of the pencil. The time the children took to perform the real and imagined movement sequences was recorded. Results revealed that the normally developing children's performance conformed to Fitts's law (i.e., an inverse relationship between speed and accuracy: Smaller targets require more accurate movements, and result in slower movement duration relative to larger targets where accuracy demands are less) when executing real movements and imagined movements. In contrast, for children with DCD, only their real movements conformed to this trade-off between speed and accuracy. Movements simulated in their imagination did not. Furthermore, the effect of load differed between groups. For real movements, movement duration did not differ between the load and no-load conditions for either group, whereas for imagined movements, movement duration increased under the load condition for the normally developing controls but *not* for the children with DCD. This weight-related slowing of imagined movements in the normally developing controls was hypothesized to occur because the children were required to program a greater muscle force in order to overcome the additional weight when moving the pencil. When actually performing the pointing movements, this additional force allowed the children to move at the same speed as when no weight was attached. Thus, when required only to imagine the movement while carrying the load, the normally developing children interpret the increased force as an increased duration, which consequently resulted in the imagined movements being performed more slowly. Similar findings have been reported in normal adults under similar conditions (Decety, Jeannerod, & Prablanc, 1989). The children with motor deficits, however, fail to take into account the implication of this increased force on the duration of their movement. This pattern of performance suggests that children with DCD are impaired in their ability to mentally represent volitional movements, and that an impaired ability to program both relative force and timing appears to underlie this difficulty (Wilson et al., 2001). Smith and Bryson (1994) have suggested that deficits in the internal representation of movement could underlie the deficits in imitation seen in children with ASD. Further research with children with DCD and ASD is needed, however, before any definitive conclusions can be made concerning the contribution of impairments in internal representation to imitation performance.

Dewey (1995) suggested that the gestural disturbances seen in children with DCD are the result of a conceptual linguistic disturbance. The finding that children with ASD displayed significantly more incorrect actions when performing representational gestures is consistent with the idea that a conceptual linguistic disturbance underlies imitation deficits in children with ASD (Dewey & Crawford, 2005). According to this hypothesis, both language and gestures rely on a common underlying capacity for communication (Bates, Benigni, Bretherton, Camaioni, & Volterra, 1979). Kaplan (1977) concurred with this view, suggesting that gestural representation and language both involve symbolic behavior. Consequently, if the ability to "symbolize" is impaired, the development of language and gestural skills would be delayed. Conversely, as language skills develop so would gestural skills. Support for a linguistic conceptual disturbance is evident in the finding that children who are unable to provide a name for a particular object are often unable to provide a gesture for that object (Kaplan, 1977), as well as the finding that children with language impairments frequently display deficits in gestural performance (Dewey & Wall, 1997; Hill, 1998; Hill et al., 1998; Thal, Tobais, & Morrison, 1991). Research with individuals with ASD also suggests a link between language and gestural development. Stone and colleagues (1997) reported that motor imitation skills in children with autism improved from 2 to 3 years of age and that imitation of body movements was associated with expressive language. Rogers and colleagues (2003) also found that the verbal development quotient on the Mullen Scales of Early Learning was a significant predictor of imitative ability in young children with autism. Although research with children with DCD, ASD, and language impairments suggests a significant relationship between gestural impairments and conceptual linguistic disturbance, longitudinal research is needed to determine if there is a causal relationship between gestural and language impairments, the direction of such a relationship, or whether the cause of these deficits is due to some other common factor.

The research literature also suggests that neurodevelopmental delay plays a significant role in gestural performance. Studies of children with developmental motor problems and children with ASD have found that deficits in gestural performance are associated with poorer cognitive functioning (Dewey & Kaplan, 1994; Rogers et al., 2003). Furthermore, Dewey and Crawford (2005) found that the cognitive level was highly associated with performance of transitive, $r = .53$, $p < .01$, and intransitive, $r = .52$, $p < .01$, limb gestures to command and transitive, $r = .58$, $p < .01$, and intransitive, $r = .44$, $p < .01$, limb gestures to imitation in children with ASD, those with DCD, and typically developing children. Thus, studies that examine imitation ability in children need to take cognitive level into account.

CONCLUSION

Research that has investigated the motor skills of children with ASD and children with DCD suggests that they display similar problems in motor skills and that the severity of the motor deficit is similar (Dewey & Crawford, 2005; Green et al., 2002). When the gestural/imitation performance of these two groups of children was compared, however, the children with ASD were more impaired than children with DCD (Dewey & Crawford, 2005). Thus, although both groups display similar levels of motor dysfunction, children with

ASD are more impaired in the performance of gestures. For both children with DCD and ASD, problems in gestural performance appear to be associated with a delay in normal imitative development rather then a specific deficit. Longitudinal studies of gestural development in children with DCD and ASD are needed, however, to clearly chart the developmental profile and to identify the various processes that contribute to this delay.

Williams and colleagues (2004) stated that imitation deficits are specific to children with autism, as long as perceptual and motor capacities are intact. This statement suggests that the imitation deficits found in children with other developmental disorders such as DCD could only be due to motor and perceptual problems, and that the processes that contribute to the imitation deficits in children with ASD are different from the processes associated with imitation problems in other pediatric populations. This conclusion is somewhat premature as some of the hypotheses that have been advanced regarding the processes that contribute to imitation deficits in children with DCD suggest that they may not be due to motor–perceptual deficits. Furthermore, imitation performance in clinical conditions such as ADHD and dyslexia in comparison to children with ASD still needs to be examined. Finally, the research evidence to date on children with DCD and ASD does not provide definitive support for any particular hypothesis concerning the basis for imitative deficits in these populations.

Imitation is a learned skill that requires the child to generate an idea about the action and then plan how that action will be performed. The normal development of imitation is dependent on the normal development of many other abilities (e.g., cognitive, language, and motor). Therefore, problems in various areas of development could have an impact on the development of imitation. Future research investigating the processes that underlie imitation deficits in children with DCD and ASD should take into account not only motor functioning but also cognitive and language functioning, and in the case of children with ASD, the severity of the autism deficit. Such investigations must also consider the fact that these are developmental disorders and that they are constantly evolving. As a result, processes that may be associated with imitation deficits in young children with ASD may not be associated with imitation deficits in older children. Furthermore, as various abilities (e.g., language and motor) improve with age and with intervention, certain processes that may not have been associated with imitation ability may now be found to be correlates.

The heterogeneity of children with DCD and ASD make these youngsters compelling yet complex to study. The precise processes that underlie the disturbances in gesture/imitation remain poorly understood and need to be investigated further. A more comprehensive understanding of the gestural and particularly the imitation deficits manifest by these children and greater knowledge of the processes implicated in such deficits could be of crucial importance in facilitating the development of appropriate interventions that target the specific areas of deficiency in these children.

ACKNOWLEDGMENTS

This research was supported by grants from the Scottish Rite Charitable Foundation of Canada, the Alberta Children's Hospital Foundation and the Canadian Institutes of Health Research.

REFERENCES

Alexander, G. E., Delong, M. R., & Strick, P. L. (1986). Parallel organization of functionally segregated circuits linking basal ganglia and cortex. *Annual Review of Neuroscience, 9,* 357–381.

American Psychiatric Association. (1994). *Diagnostic and statistical manual of mental disorders* (4th ed.). Washington, DC: Author.

Andersen, R. A. (1987). Inferior parietal lobule function in spatial perception and visuomotor integration. In F. Plum, V. B. Mountcastle, & S. R. Geiger (Eds.), *The handbook of physiology: Section 1: The nervous system. Vol. 5. Higher functions of the brain* (pp. 483–518). Bethesda, MD: American Physiological Society.

Asperger, H. (1991). "Autistic psychopathy" in childhood. In U. Frith (Ed.), *Autism and Asperger syndrome* (pp. 37–92). Cambridge, UK: Cambridge University Press. (Original work published 1944)

Attwood, T. (1998). *Asperger's syndrome: A guide for parents and professionals.* London: Jessica Kingsley.

Ayres, A. J. (1972). *Southern California sensory integration tests.* Los Angeles: Western Psychological Services.

Ayres, A. J. (1985). *Developmental apraxia and adult onset apraxia.* Torrance, CA: Sensory Integration International.

Ayres, A. J., Mailloux, Z. K., & Wendler, C. L. (1987). Developmental dyspraxia: Is it a unitary function? *Occupational Therapy Journal of Research, 7,* 93–110.

Bailey, A., Luthert, P., Dean, A., Harding, B., Janota, I., Montgomer, M., et al. (1998). A clinicopathological study of autism. *Brain, 121,* 889–905.

Bates, E., Benigni, L., Bretherton, I., Camaioni, L., & Volterra, V. (1979). *The emergence of cognition and communication in infancy.* New York: Academic Books.

Berges, J., & Lezine, I. (1965). *The imitation of gestures.* London: William Heinemann Medical Books.

Berman, K. F., Ostrem, J. L., Randoulph, C., Gold, J., Goldberg, T. E., Coppola, R., et al. (1995). Physiological activation of a cortical network during performance of the Wisconsin Card Sorting Test: A positron emission tomography study. *Neuropsychologia, 33,* 1027–1046.

Berquin, P. C., Gidd, J. N., Jacobsen, L. K., Burger, S. D., Krain, A. L., Rapiport, J. L., et al. (1998). Cerebellum in attention-deficit hyperactivity disorder. A morphometric MRI study. *Neurology, 50,* 1087–1093.

Blondis, T. A., Snow, J. H., Roizen, N. J., Opacich, K. J., & Accordo, P. J. (1993). Early maturation of motor-delayed children at school age. *Journal of Child Neurology, 8,* 323–329.

Brown, J. (1972). *Aphasia, apraxia, and agnosia: Clinical and theoretical aspects.* Springfield, IL: Thomas.

Bryson, S. E., Landry, R., & Wainwright, J. A. (1997). A componential view of executive dysfunction in autism: Review of recent evidence. In J. A. Burack & J. T. Enns (Eds.), *Attention, development, and psychopathology* (pp. 232–262). New York: Guilford Press.

Burback, J. A., Enns, J. T., Stauder, J. E. A., Mottron, L., & Randolph, B. (1997). Attention and autism: Behavioral and electrophysiological evidence. In D. J. Cohen & F. R. Volkmar (Eds.), *Handbook of autism and pervasive developmental disorders* (2nd ed., pp. 226–247). New York: Wiley.

Cantell, M. (1998). Developmental coordination disorder in adolescence: Perceptual–motor, academic and social outcomes of early motor delay. *LIKES—Research Report on Sport and Health, 112.*

Cantell, M., Kooistra, L., & Larkin, D. (2001). Approaches to intervention for children with developmental coordination disorder. *New Zealand Journal of Disability Studies, 9,* 106–119.

Cantell, M. H., Smyth, M. M., & Ahonen, T. K. (2003). Two distinct pathways for developmental coordination disorder: Persistence and resolution. *Human Movement Science, 22,* 413–431.

Carper, R. A., & Courchesne, E. (2000). Inverse correlation between frontal lobe and cerebellum sizes in children with autism. *Brain, 123,* 836–844.

Castellanos, F. X. (1997). Toward a pathophysiology of attention-deficit/hyperactivity disorder. *Clinical Pediatrics, 36,* 381–393.

Castellanos, F. X., Giedd, J. N., Marsh, W. L., Hamburger, S. D., Vaituzis, A. C., Dickstein, D. P., et al. (1996). Quantitative brain magnetic resonance imaging in attention-deficit hyperactivity disorder. *Archives of General Psychiatry, 53,* 607–616.

Cermak, S. A. (1985). Developmental dyspraxia. In E. A. Roy (Ed.), *Neuropsychological studies of apraxia and related disorders* (pp. 225–248). Amsterdam: North-Holland.

Cermak, S. A. (1991). Somatodyspraxia. In A. G. Fisher, E. A. Murray, & A. C. Bundy (Eds.), *Sensory integration: Theory and practice* (pp. 137–170). Philadelphia: Davis.

Cermak, S. A., Costers, W., & Drake, C. (1980). Representational and non-representational gestures in boys with learning disabilities. *American Journal of Occupational Therapy, 34,* 19–26.

Cermak, S. A., Gubbay, S. S., & Larkin, D. (2002). What is developmental coordination disorder? In S. A. Cermak & D. Larkin (Eds.), *Developmental coordination disorder* (pp. 2–22). Albany, NY: Delmar Thomson Learning.

Courchesne, E. (1991). Neuroanatomical imaging in autism. *Pediatrics, 87,* 781–790.

Courchesne, E. (1997). Brainstem, cerebellar and limbic neuroanatomical abnormalities in autism. *Current Opinions in Neurobiology, 7,* 269–278.

Cratty, B. J. (1994). *Clumsy child syndromes: Descriptions, evaluation and remediation.* Chur, Switzerland: Harwood Academic.

Damasio, A. R. (1985). Disorders of complex visual processing: Agnosias, achromatopsia, Balint's syndrome and related difficulties of orientation and construction. In M. M. Mesulam (Ed.), *Principles of behavioral neurology* (pp. 259–288). Philadelphia: Davis.

Decety, J., Jeannerod, M., & Prablanc, C. (1989). The timing of mentally represented actions. *Behavioural Brain Research, 34,* 35–42.

DeMeyer, M. K., Alpern, G. D., Barton, S., DeMeyer, W. E., Churchhill, D. W., Hington, J. N., et al. (1972). Imitation in autistic, early schizophrenic, and non-psychotic subnormal children. *Journal of Autism and Childhood Schizophrenia, 2,* 264–287.

Denckla, M. B., & Roeltgen, D. P. (1992). Disorders of motor function and control. In I. Rapin & S. J. Segalowitz (Eds.), *Handbook of neuropsychology, Vol. 6: Child neuropsychology* (pp. 455–476). Amsterdam: Elsevier Science.

Desmond, J. E., Gabrieli, J. D. E., Wagner, A. D., Ginier, B. I., & Glover, G. H. (1997). Lobular patterns of cerebellar activation in verbal working memory and finger tapping tasks as revealed by functional MRI. *Journal of Neuroscience, 17,* 9675–9685.

Dewey, D. (1991). Praxis and sequencing skills in children with sensorimotor dysfunction. *Developmental Neuropsychology, 7,* 197–206.

Dewey, D. (1993). Error analysis of limb and orofacial praxis in children with developmental motor deficits. *Brain and Cognition, 23*, 203–221.

Dewey, D. (1995). What is developmental dyspraxia? *Brain and Cognition, 29*, 254–274.

Dewey, D. (2002). Subtypes of developmental coordination disorder. In S. A. Cermak & G. D. Larkin (Eds.), *Developmental coordination disorder* (pp. 40–68). Albany, New York: Delmar Thomson Learning.

Dewey, D., & Crawford, S. G. (2005). Motor and praxis skills in children with autism spectrum disorder: A comparison with developmental coordination disorder. *Journal of the International Neuropsychological Society, 11*, 108.

Dewey, D., & Kaplan, B. J. (1992). Analysis of praxis task demands in the assessment of children with developmental motor deficits. *Developmental Neuropsychology, 8*, 367–379.

Dewey, D., & Kaplan, B. J. (1994). Subtyping of developmental motor deficits. *Developmental Neuropsychology, 10*, 265–284.

Dewey, D., Kaplan, B. J., Wilson, B. N., & Crawford, S. G. (1999). *Developmental coordination disorder and developmental dyspraxia: Are we talking about the same thing?* Paper presented at the 27th annual meeting of the International Neuropsychology Society, Boston.

Dewey, D., Roy, E. A., Square-Storer, P. A., & Hayden, D. (1988). Limb and oral praxic abilities of children with verbal sequencing deficits. *Developmental Medicine and Child Neurology, 30*, 743–751.

Dewey, D., & Wall, K. (1997). Praxis and memory deficits in language impaired children. *Developmental Neuropsychology, 13*, 507–512.

deZubicaray, G. I., Williams, S. C., Wilson, S. J., Rose, S. E., Brammer, M. J., Bullmore, E. T., et al. (1998). Prefrontal cortex involvement in selective letter generation: A functional magnetic resonance imaging study. *Cortex, 34*, 389–401.

Diamond, A. (2000). Close interrelation of motor development and cognitive development and the cerebellum and prefrontal cortex. *Child Development, 71*, 44–56.

Fawcett, A. J., & Nicolson, R. I. (1995). Persistent deficits in motor skill of children with dyslexia. *Journal of Motor Behavior, 27*, 235–240.

Fein, D., Stevens, M. C., Dunn, M., Waterhouse, L., Allen, D., Rapin, T., et al. (1999). Subtypes of pervasive developmental disorder: Clinical characteristics. *Child Neurology, 5*, 1–23.

Filipek, P. A., Semrud-Clikeman, M., Steingard, R. J., Renshaw, P. F., Kennedy, D. N., & Biederman, J. (1997). Volumetric MRI analysis comparing subjects having attention-deficit hyperactivity disorder with normal controls. *Neurology, 48*, 589–601.

Flament, D., Ellermann, J., Ugurbil, K., & Ebner, T. J. (1994). Functional magnetic resonance imaging (fMRI) of cerebellar activation while learning to correct for visuo-motor errors. *Society for Neuroscience Abstracts, 20*, 20.

Gaffney, G. R., Tsai, L. Y., Kuperman, S., & Minchin, S. (1987). Cerebellar structure in autism. *American Journal of Diseases in Children, 141*, 1330–1332.

Ghaziuddin, M., & Butler, E. (1998). Clumsiness in autism and Asperger syndrome: A further report. *Journal of Intellectual Disabilities Research, 42*, 43–48.

Ghaziuddin, M., Butler, E., Tsai, L., & Ghaziuddin, N. (1994). Is clumsiness a marker for Asperger syndrome? *Journal of Intellectual Disabilities Research, 38*, 519–527.

Ghaziuddin, M., Tsai, L. Y., & Ghaziuddin, N. (1992). A reappraisal of clumsiness as a diagnostic feature of Asperger syndrome. *Journal of Autism and Developmental Disorders, 22*, 651–656.

Gillberg, C. (1989). Asperger syndrome in 23 Swedish children. *Developmental Medicine Child Neurology, 31*, 520–531.

Gillberg, C. (1991). Clinical and neurobiological aspects of Asperger's syndrome in six families. In U. Frith (Ed.), *Autism and Asperger syndrome*. Cambridge, UK: Cambridge University Press.

Gillberg, L. C. (1985). Children with minor neurodevelopmental disorders III: Neurological and neurodevelopmental problems at age 10. *Developmental Medicine and Child Neurology, 27,* 3–16.

Goto, M., Ota, R., Iai, M., Sugita, K., & Tanabe, Y. (1994). MRI changes and deficits of higher brain functions in preterm diplegia. *Acta Paediatrica, 83,* 506–511.

Green, D., Baird, G., Barnett, A. L., Henderson, L., Huber, J., & Henderson, S. E. (2002). The severity and nature of motor impairment in Asperger's syndrome: A comparison with specific developmental disorder of motor function. *Journal of Child Psychology and Psychiatry, 43,* 655–668.

Groves, P. M. (1983). A theory of the functional organization of the neostriatum and the neostriatal control of voluntary movement. *Brain Research Reviews, 286,* 109–132.

Gubbay, S. S. (1975). *The clumsy child: A study of developmental apraxic and agnosic ataxia*. Philadelphia: Saunders.

Guerin, P., Lyon, G., Barthelemy, C., Sostak, E., Chevrollier, V., Garreau, B., et al. (1996). Neuropathological study of a case of autistic syndrome with severe mental retardation. *Developmental Medicine and Child Neurology, 38,* 203–211.

Hall, D. M. B. (1988). The children with DCD. *British Medical Journal, 296,* 375–376.

Hauck, J. A., & Dewey, D. (2001). Hand preference and motor functioning in children with autism. *Journal of Autism and Developmental Disorders, 31,* 265–277.

Hecaen, H. (1981). Apraxia. In S. Filskov & T. Boll (Eds.), *Handbook of clinical neuropsychology* (pp. 257–286). New York: Wiley.

Hecaen, H., & Alberta, M. L. (1978). *Human neuropsychology*. New York: Wiley.

Henderson, L., Rose, P., & Henderson, S. (1992). Reaction time and movement time in children with a developmental coordination disorder. *Journal of Child Psychology and Psychiatry, 33,* 895–905.

Henderson, S., & Barnett, A. (1998). The classification of specific motor coordination disorders in children: Some problems to be solved. *Human Movement Science, 17,* 449–469.

Henderson, S. E., & Hall, D. (1982). Concomitants of clumsiness in young school children. *Developmental Medicine and Child Neurology, 24,* 448–460.

Henderson, S. E., & Sugden, D. A. (1992). *Movement Assessment Battery for Children*. London: Psychological Corporation.

Hill, E. L. (1998). A dyspraxic deficit in specific language impairment and developmental coordination disorder? Evidence from hand and arm movements. *Developmental Medicine and Child Neurology, 40,* 388–395.

Hill, E. L., Bishop, D. V. M., & Nimmo-Smith, I. (1998). Representational gestures in developmental coordination disorder and specific language impairment: Error-types and the reliability of ratings. *Human Movement Science, 17,* 655–678.

Hobson, R. P., & Lee, A. (1999). Imitation and identification in autism. *Journal of Child Psychology and Psychiatry, 40,* 649–659.

Hughes, C. (1996). Planning problems in autism at the level of motor control. *Journal of Autism and Developmental Disorders, 26,* 99–107.

Huh, J., Williams, H. G., & Burke, J. R. (1998). Developmental of bilateral motor control in children with developmental coordination disorders. *Developmental Medicine and Child Neurology, 40,* 474–484.

Hynd, G. W., Herm, K. L., Novey, E. S., Eliopulos, D., Marshall, R., Gonzalez, J. J., et al. (1993). Attention-deficit hyperactivity disorder and asymmetry of the caudate nucleus. *Journal of Child Neurology, 8,* 339–347.

Ivry, R. B., & Keele, S. W. (1989). Timing functions of the cerebellum. *Journal of Cognitive Neuroscience, 1,* 136–152.

Iwanaga, R., Kawasaki, C., & Tscuchida, R. (2000). Brief report: Comparison of sensory-motor and cognitive function between autism and Asperger syndrome in preschool children. *Journal of Autism and Developmental Disorders, 30*, 169–174.

Johnston, L. M., Burns, Y. R., Brauer, S. G., & Richardson, C. A. (2002). Differences in postural control and movement performance during goal directed reaching in children with developmental coordination disorder. *Human Movement Science, 21*, 583–601.

Jones, V., & Prior, M. (1985). Motor imitation and neurological signs in autistic children. *Journal of Autism and Developmental Disorders, 15*, 37–46.

Kanner, L. (1973). *Childhood psychosis: Initial studies and new insight*. Washington, DC: V. H. Winston. (Original work published 1943)

Kaplan, E. (1968). *The development of gesture*. Unpublished doctoral dissertation, Clark University, Worchester, MA.

Kaplan, E. (1977). Praxis: Development. In B. Wolman (Ed.), *International encyclopedia of psychiatry, psychology, psychoanalysis, and neurology* (pp. 26–29). New York: Van Nostrand.

Keele, S. W., & Ivry, R. (1990). Does the cerebellum provide a common computation for diverse tasks? A timing hypothesis. *Annals of the New York Academy of Sciences, 608*, 179–207.

Killackey, H. A. (1990). Neocortical expansion: An attempt toward relating phylogeny and ontogeny. *Journal of Cognitive Neuroscience, 2*, 1–17.

Laszlo, J. I., & Bairstow, P. J. (1983). Kinaesthesis: Its measurement training and relationship to motor control. *Quarterly Journal of Experimental Psychology, 35*, 411–421.

Laszlo, J. I., Bairstow, P. J., Bartrip, J., & Rolfe, U. T. (Eds.). (1988). *Clumsiness or perceptuo-motor dysfunction?* Amsterdam: Elsevier Science.

Lewis, M. H., & Bodfish, J. W. (1998). Repetitive behavior disorders in autism. *Mental Retardation and Developmental Disabilities, 4*, 80–89.

Libby, S., Powell, S., Messer, D., & Jordan, R. (1997). Imitation of pretend play acts by children with autism and Down syndrome. *Journal of Autism and Developmental Disorders, 27*, 365–383.

Losse, A., Henderson, S. A., Elliman, D., Hall, D., Knight, E., & Jongmans, M. (1991). Clumsiness in children: Do they grow out of it? A 10-year follow-up study. *Developmental Medicine and Child Neurology, 33*, 55–68.

Lou, H. C., Henriksen, L., Bruhn, P., Borner, H., & Nielsen, J. B. (1989). Striatal dysfunction in attention deficit and hyperkinetic disorder. *Archives of Neurology, 46*, 48–52.

Lundy-Ekman, L., Ivry, R., Keele, S. W., & Woollacott, M. (1991). Timing and force control deficits in clumsy children. *Journal of Cognitive Neuroscience, 3*, 367–376.

Luria, A. R. (1966). *Higher cortical functions in man*. New York: Basic Books.

Manjiviona, J., & Prior, M. (1995). Comparison of Asperger syndrome and high-functioning autistic children on a test of motor impairment. *Journal of Autism and Developmental Disorders, 25*, 23–39.

Marshall, R. S., Lazar, R. M., Binder, J. R., Desmond, D. W., Drucker, P. M., & Mohr, J. P. (1994). Intrahemispheric localization of drawing dysfunction. *Neuropsychologia, 32*(4), 493–502.

Miller, J. N., & Ozonoff, S. (2000). The external validity of Asperger disorder: Lack of evidence from the domain of neuropsychology. *Journal of Abnormal Psychology, 109*(2), 227–238.

Missiuna, C., & Pollock, N. (1995). Beyond the norms: Need for multiple sources of data in the assessment of children. *Physical and Occupational Therapy in Pediatrics, 15*(4), 57–71.

Miyahara, A., Tsujii, M., Hori, M., Nakanishi, K., Kageyama, H., & Sugiyama, T. (1997). Brief report: Motor incoordination in children with Asperger's syndrome and learning disabilities. *Journal of Autism and Developmental Disorders, 27*, 597–603.

Morgan, S. B., Cutrer, P. S., Coplin, J. W., & Rodrigue, J. R. (1989). Do autistic children differ from retarded and normal children in Piagetian sensorimotor functioning? *Journal of Child Psychology and Psychiatry, 30,* 857–864.

Mostofsky, S. H., Reiss, A. L., Lockhart, P., & Denckla, M. B. (1998). Evaluation of cerebellar size in attention-deficit hyperactivity disorder. *Journal of Child Neurology, 13*(9), 434–439.

Ohta, M. (1987). Cognitive disorders of infantile autism: A study employing the WISC, spatial relationship conceptualization, and gesture imitation. *Journal of Autism and Developmental Disorders, 17,* 45–62.

Orton, S. T. (1937). *Reading, writing and speech problems in children.* New York: Norton.

Page, J., & Boucher, J. (1998). Motor impairments in children with autistic disorder. *Child Language Teaching and Therapy, 14,* 233–259.

Piek, J. P., & Coleman-Carman, R. (1995). Kinaesthetic sensitivity and motor performance of children with developmental co-ordination disorder. *Developmental Medicine and Child Neurology, 37,* 976–984.

Piek, J. P., Pitcher, T. M., & Hay, D. A. (1999). Motor coordination and kinaesthesis in boys with attention deficit-hyperactivity disorder. *Developmental Medicine and Child Neurology, 41,* 159–165.

Piek, J. P., & Skinner, R. A. (1999). Timing and force control during a sequential tapping task in children with and without motor coordination problems. *Journal of the International Neuropsychological Society, 5,* 320–329.

Polatajko, H. J., Fox, A. M., & Missiuna, C. (1995). An international consensus on children with developmental coordination disorder. *Canadian Journal of Occupational Therapy, 62,* 3–6.

Quartz, S. R., & Sejnowski, T. J. (1997). The neural basis of cognitive development: A constructivist manifesto. *Behavioural Brain Science, 20,* 537–556.

Quintana, J., & Fuster, J. M. (1993). Spatial and temporal factors in the role of prefrontal and parietal cortex in visuomotor integration. *Cerebral Cortex, 3,* 122–132.

Rinehart, N. J., Bradshaw, J. L., Brereton, A. V., & Tonge, B. J. (2001). Movement preparation in high-functioning autism and Asperger disorder: A serial choice reaction time task involving motor reprogramming. *Journal Autism and Developmental Disorders, 31,* 79–88.

Rodger, S. J., Ziviani, J., Watter, P., Ozanne, A., Woodyatt, G., & Springfield, E. (2003). Motor and functional skills of children with developmental coordination disorder: A pilot investigation of measurement issues. *Human Movement Science, 22,* 461–478.

Rogers, S. J., Hepburn, S. L., Stackhouse, T., & Wehner, E. (2003). Imitation performance in toddlers with autism and those with other developmental disorders. *Journal of Child Psychology and Psychiatry, 44,* 763–781.

Rogers, S. J., & Pennington, B. F. (1991). A theoretical approach to the deficits in infantile autism. *Developmental Psychopathology, 3,* 137–162.

Rourke, B. P. (1995). *Syndrome of nonverbal learning disabilities: Neurodevelopmental manifestations.* New York: Guilford Press.

Roy, E. (1978). Apraxia: A new look at an old syndrome. *Journal of Human Movement Studies, 4,* 191–210.

Royeurs, H., Van Oost, P., & Bothuyne, S. (1998). Immediate imitation and joint attention in young children with autism. *Developmental Psychopathology, 10,* 441–450.

Schlosser, R., Hutchinson, M., Joseffer, S., Rusinek, H., Saarimaki, A., Stevenson, J., et al. (1998). Functional magnetic resonance imaging of human brain activity in a verbal fluency task. *Journal of Neurology Neurosurgery, and Psychiatry, 64,* 492–498.

Schoemaker, M. M., van der Wees, M., Flapper, B., Verheij-Jansen, N., Scholten-Jaegers, S.,

& Geuze, R. H. (2001). Perceptual skills of children with developmental coordination disorder. *Human Movement Science, 20*, 111–133.

Selemon, L. D., & Goldman-Rakic, P. S. (1988). Common cortical and subcortical targets of the dorsolateral prefrontal and posterior parietal cortices in the rhesus monkey: Evidence for a distributed neural network subserving spatially guided behavior. *Journal of Neuroscience, 8*(11), 4049–4068.

Sellers, J. S. (1995). Clumsiness: Review of causes, treatments, and outlook. *Physical and Occupational Therapy in Pediatrics, 15*, 39–55.

Smith, I. M. (2000). Motor functioning in Asperger syndrome. In A. Klin, F. R. Volkmar, & S. S. Sparrow (Eds.), *Asperger syndrome* (pp. 97–124). New York: Guilford Press.

Smith, I. M. (2004). Motor problems in children with autistic spectrum disorders. In D. Dewey & D. E. Tupper (Eds.), *Developmental motor disorders: A neuropsychological perspective* (pp. 152–168). New York: Guilford Press.

Smith, I. M., & Bryson, S. E. (1994). Imitation and action in autism: A critical review. *Psychological Bulletin, 116*, 259–273.

Smith, I. M., & Bryson, S. E. (1998). Gesture imitation in autism I: Nonsymbolic postures and sequences. *Cognitive Neuropsychology, 15*, 747–770.

Smits-Engelsman, B. C. M., Niemeijer, A. S., & Van Galen, G. P. (2001). Fine motor deficiencies in children diagnosed as DCD based on poor grapho-motor ability. *Human Movement Science, 20*, 161–182.

Smyth, M. M., & Mason, U. C. (1997). Planning and execution of action in children with and without developmental coordination disorder. *Journal of Child Psychology and Psychiatry, 38*, 1023–1037.

Smyth, M. M., & Mason, U. C. (1998). Use of proprioception in normal and clumsy children. *Developmental Medicine and Child Neurology, 40*, 672–681.

Stelmach, G. E., & Worringham, C. J. (1988). The preparation and production of isometric force in Parkinson's disease. *Neuropsychologia, 26*, 93–103.

Stone, W. L., Ousley, O. Y., & Littleford, C. D. (1997). Motor imitation in young children with autism: What's the object? *Journal of Abnormal Child Psychology, 25*, 475–485.

Sugden, D., & Keogh, J. (1990). *Problems in movement skill development.* Columbia: University of South Carolina Press.

Szatmari, P., Tuff, L., Finlayson, M. A., & Bartolucci, G. (1990). Asperger's syndrome and autism: Neurocognitive aspects. *Journal of the American Academy of Child Adolescent Psychiatry, 29*, 130–136.

Teicher, M. H., Ito, Y., Glod, C. A., & Barber, N. I. (1996). Objective measurement of hyperactivity and attentional problems in ADHD. *Journal of American Academy of Child and Adolescent Psychiatry, 35*, 334–342.

Thal, D., Tobais, S., & Morrison, D. (1991). Language and gesture in late talkers: A 1-year follow-up. *Journal of Speech and Hearing Research, 34*, 604–612.

Turner, M. (1999). Annotation: Repetitive behaviour in autism: A review of psychological research. *Journal of Child Psychology and Psychiatry, 40*, 839–849.

Vaidya, C. J., Austin, G., Kirkorian, G., Ridlehuber, H. W., Desmond, J. E., Glover, G. H., et al. (1998). Selective effects of methylphenidate in attention deficit hyperactivity disorder: A functional magnetic resonance study. *Proceedings of the National Academy of Sciences, USA, 95*, 14494–14499.

Van Mier, H., Petersen, S. E., Tempel, L. W., Perlmutter, J. S., Snyder, A. Z., & Raichle, M. E. (1994). Practice related changes in a continuous motor task measured by PET. *Society for Neuroscience Abstracts, 20*, 361.

Volman, M. J. M., & Geuze, R. H. (1998a). Relative phase stability of bimanual and visuomanual rhythmic coordination patterns in children with a developmental coordination disorder. *Human Movement Science, 17*, 541–572.

Volman, M. J. M., & Geuze, R. H. (1998b). Stability of rhythmic finger movement in children with a developmental coordination disorder. *Motor Control, 2*, 34–60.

Wann, J. P., Mon-Williams, M., & Rushton, K. (1998). Postural control and coordination disorders: The swinging room revisited. *Human Movement Science, 17*, 491–513.

Webster's new collegiate dictionary (H. Bosley, Ed.). (1979). Springfield, MA: Merriam.

Whiten, A., & Brown, J. (1999). Imitation and the reading of other minds: Perspectives from the study of autism, normal children and non-human primates. In S. Bråten (Ed.), *Intersubjective communication and emotion in early ontogeny* (pp. 260–280). Cambridge, UK: Cambridge University Press.

Williams, H. (2002). Motor control in children with developmental coordination disorder. In S. A. Cermak & D. Larkin (Eds.), *Developmental coordination disorder: Theory and practice* (pp. 117–137). Albany, NY: Delmar Thomson Learning.

Williams, H., Huh, J., & Burke, J. (1998). *Planning of unimanual and bimanual responses in children with developmental coordination disorder: A reaction time analysis.* Unpublished data, Motor Development and Control Laboratory, University of South Carolina, Columbia.

Williams, H. G., Whiten, A., & Singh, T. (2004). A systematic review of action imitation in autistic spectrum disorder. *Journal of Autism and Developmental Disorders, 34*, 285–299.

Williams, H. G., Woollacott, M. H., & Ivry, R. (1992). Timing and motor control in clumsy children. *Journal of Motor Behavior, 24*, 165–172.

Wilson, P., Maruff, P., Ives, S., & Currie, J. (2001). Abnormalities of motor and praxis imagery in children with DCD. *Human Movement Science, 17*, 491–513.

Wilson, P. H., & McKenzie, B. E. (1998). Information processing deficits associated with developmental coordination disorder: A meta-analysis of research findings. *Journal of Child Psychology and Psychiatry, 39*, 829–840.

Wing, L. (1981). Asperger's syndrome: A clinical account. *Psychological Medicine, 11*(1), 115–129.

Wolff, P. H., Michel, G. F., Ovrut, M., & Drake, C. (1990). Rate and timing precision of motor coordination in developmental dyslexia. *Developmental Psychology, 26*, 349–359.

World Health Organization. (1989). *The ICD-9 classification of mental and behavioural disorders: Clinical descriptions and diagnostic guidelines.* Geneva, Switzerland: Author.

World Health Organization. (1992). *The ICD-10 classification of mental and behavioural disorders: Clinical descriptions and diagnostic guidelines.* Geneva, Switzerland: Author.

Zoia, S., Pelamatti, G., Cuttini, M., Casotto, V., & Scabar, A. (2002). Performance of gesture in children with and without DCD: Effects of sensory input modalities. *Developmental Medicine and Child Neurology, 44*, 699–705.

CHAPTER 18

Conclusions

BRUCE F. PENNINGTON
JUSTIN H. G. WILLIAMS
SALLY J. ROGERS

In this final chapter, we offer our broad conclusions about the material presented in the preceding chapters and present some new theoretical ideas that were stimulated by reading those chapters.

BROAD CONCLUSIONS

The chapters in this text describe efforts to examine imitative behavior through many different lenses—typical and atypical developmental patterns, various types of imitative behavior, imitation as it occurs in newborn infants and mirroring adults. Chapters consider the (probably bidirectional) effects of imitative behavior on language development, peer relations, parent–child interaction patterns, and instrumental learning. Also examined is imitative behavior at many levels of analysis, from microanalytic behavior analysis of movement patterns involved in gestural and facial imitation to brain activation patterns that occur when imitating others.

Integration of the contributions of these chapters leads one to consider the main topic areas that are addressed by the authors in this volume: imitation in typical development, the brain bases of imitation, and imitation in atypical development, with autism as a particular focus of interest.

Imitation in Typical Development

Several integrative conclusions can be drawn from the chapters that address imitative behavior in typical development. One is struck by the pervasiveness of imitation (defined more loosely in this chapter as copying of another's behavior) in human social encounters. Experiences of volitional and non-volitional imitation, of imitating and being imitated, appear to occur from the first interactive hour of life, occur at high rates of frequency in positive interpersonal interactions, and occur across sensory modalities (these cross-modality imitations were described by Stern, 1985, as "attunements"). Given that observing an action (which also may activate automatic mimicry) and doing an action activate some common neural circuitry, and that some of these "mirror neurons" fire to multimodal stimuli and would thus register an attunement as an imitation, then truly our interpersonal moments from birth on are filled with countless episodes of the experience of mirrored exchanges between partners, both actual (behavior matching, whether intentional or unintentional) and virtual (implicit matches involving activation of one's own action circuitry in response to a partner's familiar actions).

Furthermore, the occurrence of imitative behavior in interpersonal exchanges influences the nature of the relationship between partners. We respond to being imitated, whether intentionally or unintentionally, with positive emotions. We like people better, feel closer to them, and have more sustained, organized, and cooperative interactions with them during reciprocal imitation, and this is apparent in infancy and in adulthood. This ongoing multimodal matching and the emotional tone it engenders may be the social glue or reinforcement system of dyadic exchanges—the social function of imitation that Užgiris (1981) defined so many years ago.

Imitation is foundational for culture, the means by which behavior is transmitted from person to person, both behavior involving instrumental acts—skills, tools, language, and traditions—and much more personal and less visible behaviors—the use of eye contact and touch in interactions, tone and pitch of voice, postures and gait, gestures, and facial displays.

Intentional imitation of vocal and gestural acts precedes acquisition of language and tool use in ontogeny and appears to influence skills acquisition in each of these areas. Given the evolutionary evidence from other species, as well as humans, it appears likely that ontogeny recapitulates phylogeny in this area. The fact that the mirror neuron system is activated by imitation, by meaningful use of objects and by language, adds additional weight to the arguments for the importance of imitation to human evolution, as developed particularly by Donald (1991). Our growing knowledge of the activation of the mirror neuron system during imitation also supports Donald's thesis that imitative capacities in humans developed along with neural specialization for that skill. Hypotheses about the importance of imitation for development of other early social-communicative skills are beginning to be supported by longitudinal data from infant development. There is a growing body of data supporting the role of imitation, both behavioral and vocal, in language acquisition in the second year of life, thoroughly reviewed by Charman (Chapter 5). Developmental, as opposed to modular, accounts of theory of mind have also stressed the importance of imitation as the foundation for the understanding of others' psychological experiences. In infancy, this hypothesized relationship is best tested by examining relations between imitative skills and development of intentionality and joint attention behavior. Unfortunately, there is thus far relatively little longitudinal data from typically developing infants that we can use to test this hypothesis. The same is true of the relations between imitation and symbolic play. While Piagetian theory makes very strong claims for continuity between the two, we have too little data to either substantiate or refute the hypothesis, even though more than 50 years have elapsed since the hypothesis was made. Similarly, we have little information about the continuity of imitative abilities over time, or the contributions of imitative ability in the first few hours, weeks, and months of life to these developments during the toddler period.

Neural Correlates of Imitation and Being Imitated

Chapters by Decety (Chapter 11) and Williams and Waiter (Chapter 15) highlight the findings of the rapidly expanding neuroscience of imitation. One must step way from the current tendency to discuss mirror neurons as if they represented a brain structure dedicated to imitation. Imitation is not the result of a structure but, rather, of a large network involving many different loci. Imitation appears to involve an orchestra of parietal, temporal, and frontal circuitry. The network is activated in response to behavior that is meaningful, intentional, and imitable at a personal level, and it is activated in response to watching or doing. Imitation resembles language in this way—a receptive and an expressive vocabulary, with learning in one mode contributing to learning in the other.

Work on mirror neurons has reminded us that behavioral distinctions do not always map neatly onto brain distinctions, as mirror neurons respond similarly to both observing and executing a meaningful action. This key finding opens up the broader question of how similar and different various social learning behaviors are at the level of brain circuits. For instance, how distinct are mimicry and intentional imitation at the neural level? In Chapter 10, Whiten has very nicely reviewed a more differentiated taxonomy of social learning that has emerged from comparative studies. Claims that nonhuman primates could imitate may be explained by simpler mechanisms, and thus, as with claims for neonatal imitation, the debate has given rise to a tighter definition of imitation along with increasingly sophisticated experiments. Types of social learning have been identified that are not imitation in this strict sense (learning how to perform an action through seeing how it is done) but, rather, arise through alternative simpler mechanisms such as enhancement (from watching a conspecific act on the environment), observational conditioning (which is similar to the phenomenon of social referencing in human development, whereby infants use a caretaker's emotion to assign a valence to a novel object or event), affordance learning, end-state emulation, and object movement reenactment. Furthermore, the emphasis of the classification process has also been on those cognitive processes unique to primates, as opposed to those that are more ubiquitous among social animals such as social mimicry. A more refined taxonomy is beginning to be applied to the development of imitation in humans (Want & Harris, 2002), but already it is becoming apparent that in humans, different emphases may warrant alternative approaches. In humans the value of the social-bonding role of imitation is a much more salient issue than whether or not infants can imitate. For example, Nielsen, Suddendorf, and Dissanayake (Chapter 7) trace a normal developmental transition in the second year of human life from emulation to synchronic imitation, which serves a specifically social purpose. The dramatic increase of synchronic imitation in the second year and beyond is seen in the imitative protoconversations documented by Nadel, Guérini, Pezé, and Rivet (1999) and the increase in both vocal and action imitation between mothers and children documented by Masur and Ritz (1984).

Therefore, while the comparative psychologists have been required to go to great lengths to discriminate between matching behavior that serves to learn and acquire novel actions in the behavioral repertoire and that which serves a social function of facilitating group or other coordinated social behavior, for humans it may be more important to see the commonalities, particularly with respect to mechanisms. For example, given that the observation of orofacial action is a potent activator of the mirror neuron system, and given the likely role of the mirror neuron system in imitation, it seems likely that mimicry and imitation both utilize similar cross-modal action–perception coupling processes, though the role of executive function probably differs.

Thus, as discussed in Chapter 11 (Decety), the various types of matching responses that comparative psychologists discuss—stimulus enhancement, goal emulation, mimicry—appear to activate many of the same neural circuits in humans and should probably not be considered independent or unrelated behaviors.

Finally, although the idea of similar reverberating neural circuits during experiences of observation and execution of familiar movements may raise concerns about self–other boundaries and the locus of a sense of agency, especially in early development, the neuroimaging studies reviewed (and conducted) by Decety have addressed this clearly. While many neural circuits activate to both observing and executing a meaningful act, the right inferior parietal lobe appears to have a specific role in assigning self or other agency to acts. These findings support Stern's (1985) suggestion from 20 years ago that there is no evidence of self–other confusion or merging in infant experiences, including imitation.

Imitation in Atypical Development

To the extent that imitation is one of the fundamental processes underlying development of language, tool use, and social behavior, we should expect that significant developmental differences in many areas would also involve imitative differences, and so it is. Children with delayed learning—or mental retardation—also show delayed acquisition of imitative skills. Children with specific motor difficulties have specific difficulties imitating others' movements, as is reviewed by Dewey and Bottos (Chapter 17). Children with specific language impairments have difficulties with motor imitation that very closely resemble difficulties of children with primary problems in motor coordination, both at the level of performance and also in the individual error level (Hill, 1998; Hill, Bishop, & Nimmo-Smith, 1998).

In addition, there is recent evidence of unusual strengths in imitative behavior. A set of papers from Hepburn, Fidler, Rogers, and colleagues documents such strengths in young children with Williams syndrome. A group of 23 preschoolers with Williams syndrome showed unusually strong imitative responses, involving both facial expression and intentional motor acts, during empathy probes, compared to a group of 30 clinical comparison children matched for chronological and mental age (Fidler, Hepburn, Most, Philofsky, & Rogers, in review). In addition, the children with Williams syndrome were as socially responsive in dyadic exchanges as those with typical development matched for mental age. Surprisingly, however, they showed abnormally low levels of initiating joint attention, and their responses in this domain did not differ from a comparison group of children with autism, matched for chronological and mental age, and were significantly reduced compared to the typical comparison group (Hepburn, Philofsky, Fidler, & Rogers, in review). These studies are demonstrating strong relations between imitative behavior and social relatedness in this Williams syndrome sample but a lack of relation between imitation and joint attention initiation in this group. This suggests some degree of independence between imitation and joint attention development.

Finally, the role of imitation in atypical development as a therapeutic tool deserves mentioning. Teaching children through modeling and imitation is a crucial aspect of human pedagogy and requires far more awareness of the pragmatic aspects of the pedagogical relationship than is often considered (Csibra & Gergely, 2005). Yet, the capacity for most children, including those with a variety of disabilities, to understand and participate in the pedagogical process is seen in the therapies that have evolved for treatment of children with motor impairments, language impairments, and learning problems of various types. Procedures for teaching speech to deaf children (and a second language to hearing children) rely particularly on the teacher's ability to teach the pragmatics of the language through imitation and simulation of social-communicative processes evoked in the children.

Imitation and Autism

That imitation is particularly affected in autism was demonstrated as early as 1972, by the first comparative study of imitation by Marian DeMyer and colleagues. Continuing evidence led two groups to develop strong theories about the primary nature of an imitative deficit in autism and hypothesized neural underpinnings. In 1991, Rogers and Pennington were the first to suggest imitation as a primary neuropsychological deficit in autism. They hypothesized that the imitative problem in autism reflected difficulties in the coordination of representations of self and other. They hypothesized an early imitative impairment in autism occurring during infancy and directly affecting development of dyadic relations. They further suggested that imitative development would contribute substantially (though not fully) to impairments in joint attention, language, symbolic play, and theory of mind, both in autism and in typical development. Furthermore, they suggested that the imitative impairment in autism reflected impairments at a functional neural level but did not specify a precise locus for the neural abnormalities, though they implicated dysfunctional limbic-frontal circuitry very early in life.

The second major conceptual leap concerning imitation in autism was provided by Williams, Whiten, Suddendorf, and Perrett (2001), who tied together the autism-specific problems of self–other mapping seen in imitation, the presence of repetitive behavior including abnormal imitation involving echolalia and sometimes echopraxia in autism, and recent findings concerning the prefrontal cortex and mirror neuron systems to hypothesize a specific neural mechanism for autism. Building from the cascade model suggested by Rogers and Pennington (1991), Williams and colleagues sketched out a model in which abnormalities in the mirror neuron system underlay the developmental impairments specific to autism, interfering with imitation and with the formation and coordination of self–other representations, and underlying problems with reciprocal exchange of affect, attention, pragmatics of language, empathy, and theory of mind laid out in Rogers and Pennington's cascade model of autism. They also hypothesized that abnormal repetitive behavior in autism represented a failure of frontal lobe executive processes, which could also be due to mirror neuron deficits leading to a lack of socially acquired executive abilities. Finally, they suggested significant evolutionary development from apes to humans in the development of the mirror neuron system as a foundation for social cognition in humans via simulation processes.

Both of these papers made specific predictions, many of which have been tested and reported on in this volume. We now review the five hypotheses made in the original two papers and examine whether subsequent empirical data have supported them. After that, we consider how well theoretical notions from Rogers and Pennington (1991) have stood the test of time.

Hypotheses of Rogers and Pennington (1991) and Williams and Colleagues (2001)

1. *Deficits in imitation, affect sharing, and joint attention in the first year of life, at the earliest points at which symptoms occur, including the sensitivity of imitation as a screener for autism risk.* Examination of symptoms in the first year of life has been occurring using parental report and retrospective video analysis for the last decade. In addition, this year marks the first publi-

cation of a new paradigm for answering this question, prospective studies of infant siblings of children with autism, who have increased risk for developing autism. One study has been published and two are in press at this time. Zwaigenbaum and colleagues (2005) reported on 65 infant siblings examined repeatedly from ages 6 to 24 months of life, compared to a typically developing longitudinal sample of 23 infants. Seven of the 65 high-risk infants were positive for autism at 24 months of age, whereas none of the comparison infants were positive. Measures taken at 6 months did not predict outcomes of the infants who would develop autism as a group, though individual children did show atypical responses at that age. Infants who would later develop autism were temperamentally less active than others. At age 12 months, overall scores on an infant screener identified six of the seven children, and imitation, social smiling, and language development were three of the (many) behaviors that distinguished them. Reports by Yirmiya and colleagues (in press; Yirimiya, Gamliel, Shaked, & Sigman, in press) examined 4-month-old infant sibs in the still-face paradigm and reported differences in infant synchrony and affective sharing, though imitation was not examined. Although science in this area is just beginning to be reported, there is positive preliminary evidence of abnormalities in imitation and affect sharing in infants who will later be diagnosed with autism. Thus, support for this hypothesis is beginning to accumulate.

2. *Relationships will exist among imitation, emotion sharing, joint attention, symbolic play, and language in typical development and autism.* Cross-sectional studies of imitation in autism have begun to support this hypothesis. Rogers, Hepburn, and Stackhouse (2003) demonstrated concurrent relations among imitation skills, joint attention, and social responsivity but not play or language development in a group of 2-year-olds with autism. Scambler, Hepburn, Rutherford, Wehner, and Rogers (in press) have reported concurrent relations between emotional responsivity and joint attention behavior (but not imitation) in the same sample.

Longitudinal studies of the interrelations of the five target skills have begun to appear. Perhaps the first study of this type was reported by Mundy, Sigman, and Kasari (1990), who demonstrated that joint attention behavior predicted later language acquisition in children with autism. Charman (2003) has made the first report on a group of infants with autism identified at 18 months and followed to age 42 months. Imitation skill and gaze alternation (joint attention to share interest) at 20 months (but not play skills or eye contact during the blocking-teasing tasks) were both significantly related to language development at 42 months, even with IQ effects partialed out. Rutherford, Hepburn, Young, and Rogers (in press) have reported both concurrent and longitudinal relations between joint attention behavior at age 2 and symbolic play abilities at age 4 in a group of children with autism, but imitation was not related to play skills either concurrently or longitudinally. Stone, Ousley, and Littleford (1997) reported that gestural imitation was predictive of language development, and object imitation was predictive of play development in 2-year-olds with autism. In a longitudinal study concerning typical development, Charman and colleagues (2000) reported that imitation skills at 20 months predicted language development at 44 months, while alternating gaze at 20 months predicted theory of mind abilities at 44 months.

To summarize the aforementioned evidence, relations among these key variables have been demonstrated, both concurrently and longitudinally, but the evidence is rather spotty at this time. No studies have reported longitudinal data on all five variables across time in the same sample. The hypothesis has some support, but at this point almost all studies involve only correlations, either simple or partial. While it is evident that these constructs are not independent of each other, understanding the causal and predictive relations among them requires much more rigor in both measurement and analysis. A longitudinal study that is large enough to lend itself to robust statistical analysis that can tease out both construct dependence and causal relations would serve this purpose.

3. *A pattern of profile differences involving related deficits in imitation, joint attention, affect sharing, and symbolic play will differentiate young children with autism from appropriate comparison groups.* This hypothesis is very well supported at this point. Several different groups studying young children with autism from 18 months to 3 years of age have described significant group differences in all four of these areas in comparison to both typically developing children and clinical groups, carefully matched developmentally. (Charman et al., 1997; Rogers et al., 2003; Rutherford & Rogers, 2003; Scambler et al., in press; Stone, Ousley, & Littleford, 1997; Stone, Ousley, Yoder, Hogan, & Hepburn, 1997).

4. *Electrophysiological studies will demonstrate autism-specific deficits in mimicry.* In the past decade, several different papers have reported deficits in facial responsiveness or mimicry to affective stimuli social mimicry deficits in children with autism (Corona, Dissanayake, Arbelle, Wellington, & Sigman, 1998; McIntosh, Reichmann-Decker, Winkielman, & Wilbarger, in press; Scambler et al., in press; Sigman, Dissanayake, Corona, & Espinosa, 2003; Sigman, Kasari, Kwon, & Yirmiya, 1992). While most of these papers used microanalytic coding from videotapes to examine facial expressions, McIntosh and colleagues (in press) used electromyography recordings to demonstrate an absence of rapid automatic response and perseveration of an intentional imitation response, ruling out a lack of normal motor capacity. Moody and McIntosh (Chapter 4) document a social mimicry deficit in older individuals with autism and distinguish social mimicry from intentional imitation. Social mimicry is rapid, automatic, and unintentional. Both Chapter 4 and Chapter 1 (by Rogers) argue that neonatal imitation may not be separable from the development of social mimicry and may facilitate emotional correspondence between two interacting partners. We continue to hypothesize that a starting-state impairment in facial imitation/mimicry could undermine early affective exchanges and lead to the various knock-on effects postulated by the original theory. We need to test whether a social mimicry deficit is found in prospective studies of infants at risk for autism, and such experiments are cur-

rently underway with high-risk samples involving infant siblings of children with autism. Thus, this hypothesis concerning an autism-specific deficit in automatic imitation, or mimicry, has initial support in the first reported study of electromyography and autism (McIntosh et al., in press), but this area is clearly in need of much more work.

5. *Imaging studies will indicate altered activation of mirror neuron regions during imitation (and other mental state) tasks in subjects with autism.* Several studies using neuroimaging methods to examine response to imitation tasks and mirror neuron system activation in participants with autism have been published within the last year. These studies uniformly report brain function differences of persons with autism during imitation tasks, many of which involve mirror neuron systems, as well as limbic differences particularly involving amygdala activation, as reviewed by Williams and Waiter (Chapter 15). Nishitani, Avikainen, and Hari (2004) demonstrated reduced mirror neuron system activation in Broca's area using magneto-encephalography in a group of adults with Asperger syndrome during a facial observation–imitation paradigm. Oberman and colleagues (2005) showed a failure of mu wave suppression, which they stated reflected impaired mirror neuron system activation during action observation in a group of subjects with autism. Theoret and colleagues (2005) used transcranial magnetic stimulation (TNS) during action observation and execution tasks involving meaningless finger movements. They report an autism-specific lack of normal activation of mirror neuron systems during the observation condition in motor cortex, and furthermore, an abnormal response to difference in self versus other directed movements. Williams and colleagues (2006) report a functional magnetic resonance imaging (fMRI) study using Iacoboni's paradigm, which found autism-specific abnormalities in parietal mirror neurons and amygdala activation during observation and execution tasks. A recent paper by Dapretto and colleagues (2005) reported autism-specific mirror neuron system deficits in Broca's area, among others, during observation–execution of facial movements. Moreover, this study used eye-tracking technology to ensure that all subjects were looking at the stimuli, and a separate imitation task in which it was demonstrated that the subjects with autism were capable of intentional imitation of the target movements.

Finally, a study by Hadjikhani, Joseph, Snyder, and Tager-Flusberg (in press) reported decreased cortical thickness in mirror neurons in a group with autism compared to controls using structural MRI technology. Thus, evidence supportive of this hypothesis is accumulating concerning abnormal mirror neuron activation during observing and imitating other people's actions.

Theoretical Ideas in the 1991 Paper

Rogers and Pennington (1991) proposed that self–other correspondences were the key to the normal development of social cognition and that the development of social cognition began at birth, was continuous, and was rooted in early imitative and affective exchanges. Although our paper did not use these terms, this view of development was emergentist or constructivist and contrasted with a maturational, modular view in which certain cognitive operations necessary for understanding others (e.g., metarepresentation) somewhat abruptly "came on line" at much later ages. The emergentist view of the development of social cognition (e.g., Johnson & Morton's, 1991, account of infant face processing) holds that some minimal initial biases favoring social stimuli are present at birth (i.e., innate), but that more detailed social representations are then learned through extensive practice with those favored inputs. In the Rogers and Pennington model, the key initial biases were neonatal imitation and the salience of affect. Through imitative and affective exchanges, young infants began learning about their own and others' bodily and emotional states, thus setting the stage for later learning about the cognitive mental states of attention, intention, and, eventually, belief. Although our 1991 paper did not refer to the concept of *embodiment* (e.g., Barsalou, 1999; Lakoff & Johnson, 1999) per se, the construct was central to the paper's hypotheses concerning the development of early social cognition. In our 1991 paper, shared experiences at higher levels of abstractness (like belief) were considered to be rooted in early-shared bodily experiences (see also Meltzoff & Gopnik, 1993). As Bruner once said in his commentary on a theory-of-mind symposium, "To get to the propositional attitudes, one must climb the ladder of praxis." In other words, epistemic attitudes grow out of affective and bodily attitudes. Both bodily postures and facial affect convey a preparedness to act in a certain way (i.e., a motivational state). Eventually, the young child learns that another's attention, intention, and belief are also informative about how they will act. To simulate and predict another's behavior, the child must learn about their motivational and epistemic attitudes.

Correspondingly, our 1991 model of atypical development of early social communication and cognition in autism was a cascade model in which a problem (such as an imitation deficit) that prevented a child from participating in early imitative and affective exchanges would undermine the learning of more detailed social representations, including the later acquired ones involving the cognitive mental states of attention, intention, and belief. The 1991 paper also provided a model of social development in the case of blindness, where a sensory impairment limits access to imitative and affective exchanges, thus producing a phenocopy of autism due to a form of environmental deprivation. Such a phenocopy of autism is also observed in orphans with minimal early social input (e.g., Rutter et al., 1999). Later publications (Mundy & Neal, 2000; Pennington, 2002) have discussed how many of the associated features of autism (such as mental retardation and language deficits) can be thought of as secondary to the deprivation that would result from being "unhooked" from social interactions. Thus, a seemingly small initial problem could have devastating knock-on effects because it would prevent a child from acquiring most socially transmitted knowledge, as well as the deep enculturation of various attentional and executive skills (Donald, 1991, 2001). As Nelson (1996) pointed out, imitation "furnishes" the mind. These furnishings include not only cultural contents, like a particular language, set of social rules, or various event scripts (see Loth & Gómez, Chapter 8), but also a deeper set of domain general cognitive procedures, like temporally extended working memory. Enculturation teaches us not only what to think but also *how* to think. A child growing up outside a social culture would think in a very different way than a child inside one. Such a child would focus on different phenomena in the world, and would acquire different types of knowledge (e.g., specialized interests) and different cognitive procedures. If the human brain is a flexible, powerful computer, how it operates and what it learns depends crucially on how it is initially programmed.

Summary

We would argue that these theoretical aspects of our 1991 model—the continuous role of imitation in the development of normal social cognition, which is rooted in early imitative and affective exchanges, and a cascade model of the development of autism—have stood the test of time.

Next we turn to new ideas stimulated by the reading of this volume. These new ideas include ones about (1) the evolution of imitation, (2) the motor equivalence problems in gestural understanding, (3) the indeterminacy problem in autism, (4) whether imitation is an elemental or molar function, and (5) how self–other mapping relates to other aspects of development.

NEW IDEAS

Evolution of Imitation

Evolutionary developmental biology (e.g., Carroll, 2005) teaches us that the genetic changes that lead to the evolution of differences *between* species will be ones that alter development *within* a species. In other words, evolution acts mainly by regulating when genes that are shared by many animals are turned on and off in development. So, the evolution of human imitation, language, and social cognition will likely be attributable mainly to changes in gene regulation instead of the evolution of wholly new genes. Thus, one can ask what is distinct about the genetic bases of human development that lead to neonatal imitation and permit the development of other later emerging forms of imitation documented in these chapters. We do not yet know the answer to this question, but we are beginning to discover which genes evolved rapidly to support human oral language (such as the FOXP2 gene (Fisher, Vargha-Khadem, Watkins, Monaco, & Pembrey, 1998) and genes implicated in dyslexia (McGrath, Smith, & Pennington, in press; Pennington & Olson, 2005). Moreover, there could well be some overlap between genes that evolved for human language and genes that evolved for human imitation because both require precise motor control, mapping intrinsically variable motor tokens onto invariant units (types) of meaning, and, of course, intermodal mapping.

We also know that the evolution of the human brain greatly increased its size relative to body size, with a disproportionate increase in the size of the neocortex (Finlay & Darlington, 1995) and a disproportionate increase in the length of the developmental period. It would not take too many genetic changes to support these two changes because they are both changes in the *regulation* of brain development. We have recent evidence (Evans, et al., 2005; Mekel-Bobrov et al., 2005) that some of the genetic mutations supporting a larger human brain are relatively recent, having occurred only in the past 5,000–60,000 years or so, which means they would coincide with significant changes in the development of human culture. So, the human brain and human culture co-evolved, leading to an infant who was biologically prepared to be a partner in the long process of cultural transmission from elders to children.

The genetic changes in autism will undoubtedly be ones that alter brain development to interfere with the ability to be such an infant partner. Whether the genetic changes in autism do so in a specific (e.g., no innate preference for voices of faces) or general way (e.g., failure to prune long-distance connections leading to a failure of integration) remains to be discovered.

Specifically, we can ask how the patterning of human development fits with the goal of cultural transmission. Obviously, imitation and a protracted developmental period are prerequisites, as is a brain large enough to support powerful statistical learning and storage of a wealth of culturally transmitted information. But beyond those things, it seems that the particular profile of human motor development may play a role. Young infants' motor control of their eyes and face are much more advanced than their control of locomotion. Their prolonged period of locomotor helplessness means they will have an extended period of learning from face-to-face interactions, which establish an interpersonal reference frame and the understanding that gestures refer to both external events and internal states and can communicate shared (or not shared) attitudes.

Thus an early ability via neonatal imitation to mirror facial movements and a prolonged opportunity for face-to-face learning both seem distinctively human, but such copying of facial expressions must have evolved out of matching behaviors found in other primates, which leads us to a discussion of the motor equivalence problem.

The Motor-Equivalence Problem for Gestural Understanding

One could integrate these domains of development (imitation, language, and social cognition) by focusing on what is common about the different gestural "languages" the infant masters in the first 18 months of life. Before mainly relying on oral language, an infant acquires many intentional communicative functions through a variety of what Trevarthen (2001) calls protoconversations. (Nadel also applies this term to synchronic imitative exchanges in the second and third years of life.) These early protoconversations include affective "conversations" in the first 6 months of life and protodeclarative conversations about objects in the second 6 months. Both of these early forms of conversation involve (1) directed communicative gestures, (2) learning the mapping between gestures and meaning (i.e., solving the problem of reference), (3) turn taking, and (4) understanding that self and other can both share and not share an experience. Children both create gestures through meaning-imbued movement patterns and learn to interpret the meaning of others' gestures via the common code of perception–action couplings. But for gestural development to proceed from procedural to declarative, and from dynamic to symbolic, more than perception–action couplings are needed. Intentional communication involves the directed transmission of meanings. Communicative gestures must be tied to common meaning for both giver and receiver, and be differentiated from those with a different meaning.

What is the reference frame for the meaning of the earliest communicative gestures, facial expressions, and body postures and movements? Clearly, that reference frame is affect. Different expressions and gestures display different affects or fundamental motivations (reasons for the action). We can define affective states as rudimentary "plans"; each motivational state is a preparedness to act in a certain way (e.g., engage, aggress, avoid, and withdraw). Thus, the "common code" for communicative acts must have at least three components: perception, action, and shared affect or motivation.

One can relate these three components to the three components of the familiar "triangle" connectionist models used to explain aspects of speech (Joanisse, 2000) and reading development (Harm & Seidenberg, 1999). In Joanisse's model of speech acquisition, the infant learns to map acoustic features (perception) onto articulatory gestures (action) under the influence of shared meaning (which is related to motivation). One can imagine a similar model for learning about facial or manual gestures. In each case, visual features of a model's gesture (perception) are mapped onto a child's motor plans (action) under the influence of meaning (motivation).

For each kind of gestural language, we can ask what innate biases, if any, including what kind of innate intermodal mapping, what kind of experiential input, and what kind of learning algorithms, are needed. We can also ask what the developmental relations are, if any, among the three domains: learning about facial, vocal, and manual gestures. Does motivation provide the first "semantic field"—one that is later added to and differentiated into many other axes of meaning? Or, is learning the semantics of the nonaffective world an entirely different affair? A continuous theory of early social cognition says "no."

Infants develop an early repertoire of gestures that emerge in a seemingly maturational fashion (such as vocal, manual, or facial babbling). The particular cultural context selects from these universal gestures and tunes these to the repertoire of gestures used in that culture. This process has been well described for speech sounds; a similar process likely operates for both facial and manual features.

In mastering this repertoire of communicative gestures, the infant must solve the motor equivalence problem: Which of the intrinsically variable gestural tokens belong to the same type? Solving the mapping between tokens and types can probably be accomplished by both statistical learning and semantics. The latter, while dependent on understanding of reference and underlying intent, is a much more efficient and rapid process. Just as a phoneme is defined as the minimal difference in sound that makes a difference in meaning, a "faceme" or a "mimeme" would be a minimal difference in a facial or manual gesture that makes a difference in meaning. Solving the token/type problem in any gestural domain would appear to require imitation of gestures made by caretakers in a communicative exchange with the infant, and the shaping effects of contingent responses from the partner responding to infants' self-generated gestures. Although infants appear to practice on their own, matching would mainly occur in protoconversations with a caretaker. One would expect the quantity and quality of these protoconversations to affect how quickly the infant learns the relevant set of gestures and their referents. Anything in the infant–caretaking interactive loop that severely restricted the quantity and quality of these protoconversations would deprive the infant of the input necessary for learning and generating these gestural communicative symbols. Thus we postulate that the cause of autism is something that disrupts this interactive loop, such as an early imitation deficit. But nailing down exactly what causes this disruption in autism is very difficult, as the next section explains.

The Indeterminacy Problem in Autism

Our ability to provide a psychological explanation of a developmental disorder depends on several factors, including (1) the range of behaviors affected by the disorder, (2) the age of onset of the disorder, and, most important, (3) our understanding of normal development in the behavioral domain most affected by the disorder. Understanding autism is a "tall order" on all three counts. The range of behaviors affected is broad, the age of onset is early, and our theoretical understanding of the normal development of early social cognition is still developing. A telling contrast is provided by developmental dyslexia, where the range of affected behaviors is much narrower, the onset is later, and a much more mature theory of normal reading development is available (including connectionist models).

A difficult problem in science generally, and the behavioral sciences in particular, is that there are potentially an infinite number of theoretical models consistent with the data. This problem is the *indeterminacy* problem. We would argue that the indeterminacy problem is particularly acute in the case of autism. So, the frustration for the autism researcher is that just about any candidate primary deficit for autism could be either a cause or a result of other competing candidate deficits, especially when these deficits are studied later in the development of people with autism. For instance, the prosopagnosia that is observed in a subset of people with autism could be either a cause or a result of problems relating with others. And the same is true for postulated primary deficits in social orienting, joint attention, imitation, or executive functions.

Autism presents us with a Gordian knot in which many key strands of social, cognitive, and linguistic development are intertwined. Until we deconstruct the normal development of early social cognition and have good *prospective* data on which elements of early social cognition are impaired and intact in children who are later diagnosed with autism, it will be hard to untie this Gordian knot.

We would like to know what counts as an explanatory primitive, an elemental component of early social cognition, and which social behaviors represent combinations of these elements. Is neonatal orienting too top-heavy (and therefore face-like) configurations a single element? Is the neonatal preference for the human (and mother's) voice? Is neonatal mimicry? the social smile? contagious crying? Are any of these elemental components or are they combinations of other elements? If so, are they impaired in autism and related to later social cognitive milestones in normal development? For our cascade model to work, we need to fulfill both requirements: (1) impairment in an early elemental component and (2) that elemental component must be required for later social development to proceed normally. Some possible early deficits, like diminished orientation to faces or voices or directed social smile, do not seem consequential enough to undermine later social development in a major way, because infants with various peripheral handicaps can also miss these experiences and still can develop normal reciprocal social relations. A more fundamental early deficit is needed to explain the development of autism. Of the various elements of early social cognition, deficits in which ones are consequential enough to produce autism?

Retrospective and comparative studies have succeeded in rejecting some candidate neuropsychological deficits as primary, such as a deficit in cognitive theory of mind, executive dysfunction, and sensory modulation. The executive deficit appears to increase with the development of autism and thus may be secondary rather than primary. If we move beyond single cognitive deficit models and consider the possibility of multiple interacting deficits (Pennington, in press), then some of these rejected primary deficits could return as risk factors that interact with other deficits. Although the possibility of single neuropsychological deficit subtypes of autism has been considered, the possibility of a multiple deficit model of autism has received less attention.

It is possible that the current group of infant sibling prospective studies will not identify any single element of very early social cognition that is impaired in infants who will later develop autism. Autism may emerge as a failure to integrate these elementary components, as Charman has discussed (Chapter 5). A failure of integration fits with some of what we have learned about aberrant brain development in autism. There is macrocephaly in a sub-set of children with autism and a failure at the functional level to demonstrate the level of coherence found in typical brain development (Bailey, Phillips, & Rutter, 1996). Coherence is the correlation of activity between widely sepa-rated parts of the cortex, such as posterior and frontal sites. An integrative failure could manifest somewhat abruptly at the behavioral level as deficits in joint attention, affect sharing, understanding reference, and synchronic imita-tion, rather than being the cascading effects of an earlier deficit, like a failure in neonatal imitation. If this proves to be the case, we can reject the cascade model proposed by Rogers and Pennington (1991). A failure in integration could also impair the capacity for identification, which Hobson has proposed as a core psychological deficit in autism, while preserving many of its compo-nents.

The original Gordian knot proved to be an intractable problem that would only be solved by the man who became Alexander the Great. The prob-lem with it was that there were no loose ends and it was difficult to find a place to begin. A solution to our problem may be to examine our knot more closely for some loose or common threads, perhaps in deeper levels of analy-sis. In contrast to a focus on elemental developmental or neuropsychological impairments in autism, it may be more fruitful to move to commonalities in terms of the neural substrate. After all, autism is a syndrome, a cluster of symptoms that come together more often than by chance alone. Therefore, it is likely that different symptoms share a common core neural deficit.

Imitation: An Elemental or Molar Function?

The foregoing discussion as to whether the primary precursors of autism relate to specific or integrational functions bears strong parallels to similar controversies concerning models of imitation. Is imitation a specific and autonomous capacity, or is it constructed from simpler parts? This discussion seeks to complement and expand on the Brass and Heyes (2005) contrast between specialist and generalist models of solutions to the correspondence problem.

Specialist Models

Imitation requires translating the perception of an action from one sensory modality into an executed motor action. If this can be achieved, that action can be copied by any number of individuals with the requisite motor skills and cultural transmission is possible. Computational neuroscientists (Dautenhahn & Nehaniv, 2002) have appreciated the technical difficulties of such a process and who have termed this *the correspondence problem* (see also Heyes, 2001). One view of imitation within cognitive neuroscience is that the correspon-dence problem makes imitation into something special and unique as a cogni-tive process, such that it requires a very specific mechanism for it to function.

A well-known specialist theory is the active intermodal matching (AIM) model of Meltzoff and Moore (1997) that proposes an innate supramodal representation containing information about organ relations.

Generalist Theories

Generalist theories suggest that those brain areas that serve imitation serve other functions as well. Therefore, although mirror neurons contribute to the imitation process, they are neither necessary nor sufficient for it. Heyes (2001), as reviewed by Rogers (Chapter 1), has offered the associative sequence learning theory and ideomotor theory, which purport that imitation is mediated by general learning and motor control mechanisms. Nevertheless, even within this model, imitation is still considered a type of motor learning.

A more radical molar or generalist perspective on imitation would be to consider that imitation is dependent on a broad range of cognitive functions, including language, motor planning, attentional skills, causal understanding, and so on. Development of these functions may be variably dependent on imitation, but the development of imitation also depends on the functioning of these other capacities. Normal development is therefore characterized by parallel development of a range of cognitive and affective processes that all contribute to imitation. Impairment of any of these functions will result in impaired or abnormal development of imitation and could perhaps result in clinical presentations that resemble autistic disorder. The level of interdependence may be variable for the different processes. Interdependence with affective (motivational) processes may be crucially important for imitation to become a meaningful, self-reinforcing activity whereby it becomes a productive force in self-development. For example, in the absence of affective reinforcement for useful imitation, imitation may also end up being driven by factors such as the sensory salience of observed behaviors, resulting in the symptoms of echolalia and echopraxia that we commonly observe in autism. In contrast, isolated impairments of symbolic thought or language, movement skill, or visual attentional regulation may simply affect the profile of imitative skill development. Nevertheless, as with the integrationist model of autism, imitation is still just one of many social functions that could be affected in autism like other social functions, by such factors as poor social interest.

Self–Other Mapping as a Property of Elemental Functions

Considering imitation in a radically generalist light begs the question of how elemental processes develop and how the correspondence problem is solved. We predict that the mechanism required for imitation is required for more capacities than just imitation. We argue that mirror neurons are not confined to a particular region, just as they are not confined to any modality. Rather, it is a property of some neurons that serve representations in one modality to form connections with other neurons that serve matching representations in other modalities. Furthermore we postulate that some sort of "marker" system enables the brain to know the difference between actions and perceptions that tend to occur together but are different to actions and perceptions that are matched. Models put forward by Keysers and Perrett (2004), Brass and Heyes (2005), and Heyes (2001) argue how they could come into being.

Our modified hypothesis and our solution to our Gordian knot is to consider that higher-level human cognitive capacities can be engaged by both nonsocial and social contexts, and that basic human cognitive operations require some additional property to make them appropriate for use within an interpersonal context. We would predict that all the cognitive functions outlined in Figure 18.1 can exist without this additional property such that they can operate in their own way in an asocial context. This "add-on" property occurs in two parts. First is a self–other matching function that can label those perceptions that match the existing repertoire as such. The second is the capacity to use that self–other matching function to compare representations associated with perceived actions to those within the existing behavioral repertoire. This allows for perceptions to be interpreted, to be seen as something more than they are when taken literally or at their face value. This occurs for the perception of actions, whether gestural, functional, irrelevant, or instructive, and for linguistic material, whether spoken or written.

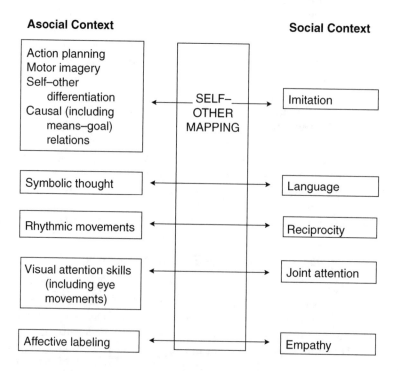

FIGURE 18.1. Basic cognitive operations in social and asocial contexts.

This interpretive, creative exploration of perceived action is associated with emotional and imaginative activity as well as the observer experimenting with the generation of novel action responses that vary in their fidelity to the perceived action patterns. The issue of novelty is essential for it is this that enables the cognitive function to develop. Rather than self–other matching being something that happens in a spatially isolated part of the brain, it is a novel and specifically human feature of cognitive processing that is integral to its underlying cognitive functions including imitation and joint attention, as well as motor skills and executive function and symbolic functions such as language. Successful concurrent development of self–other matching with the other processes results in the development of imitation, empathy, joint attention, language, and reciprocity. Self–other mapping is both the cognitive precursor and the integrational function.

Autism is characterized by poor development of the self–other function, reflected in variably poor development of other dependent cognitive functions. The word development is crucial, referring to a process not just of expansion of the behavioral repertoire but also expansion of an increasingly complex and sophisticated response set through the incorporation of an ever-expanding experience of novel situations and creative problem solving. Autism may be framed as a deficit in a core problem of self–other mapping, or in the integration of a number of otherwise disparate cognitive functions through the self–other mapping function.

CONCLUSION

In closing, the thinking and the data reflected in the chapters in this volume assert the strong role that imitation plays in the early development of a wide range of social-communicative skills in human development, and this is as true for children with developmental disorders as it is for children with typical development. That imitative deficits could be an important aspect in the development and symptomatology in autism, first suggested by DeMyer and colleagues (1972) and again by Rogers and Pennington (1991), has certainly been supported by a host of studies carried out over the past decade or more. Hypothesized developmental ties among imitation, dyadic reciprocal engagement and affect sharing, and joint attention, suggested by Stern (1985) in terms of typical development, and by Rogers and Pennington (1991) in terms of autism, are beginning to be supported by data from studies of both typical and atypical early development. Furthermore, the suggestion by Williams and colleagues (2001) that in autism, disturbances in activation of the mirror neuron system may be associated with core difficulties in coordination of self–other representations as seen in imitation and other aspects of social cognition, has also begun to be supported.

However, the support has thus far been piecemeal and the hypotheses not yet rigorously tested. Major questions to be answered include (1) the neural bases of autism and the extent to which brain differences in autism involve general as opposed to specific capacities; (2) the extent to which core differences in autism involve general information processing as opposed to specifically social stimuli; (3) the extent to which social differences in autism have to do with deficits in small initial starting-state biases as opposed to failure of later integrations; (4) the extent to which any of the "core" social phenomena (imitation, joint attention, affect reading, or sharing) are elemental; (5) the neural mechanisms at work in each; and (6) the nature of the relations among these core social phenomena. Until these questions are answered, for both typical development and autism, the indeterminacy problem remains, the hypotheses laid out in the theory papers cannot be rigorously tested, and the causal roles of social imitation in typical development remain unclear.

REFERENCES

Bailey, A. Phillips, W., & Rutter, M. (1996). Autism: Towards an integration of clinical, genetic, neuropsychological, and neurobiological perspectives. *Journal of Psychology and Psychiatry, 37,* 89–126.

Barsalou, L. W. (1999). Perceptural symbol systems. *Behavioral and Brain Sciences, 22,* 577–609.

Brass, M., & Heyes, C. (2005). Imitation: Is cognitive neuroscience solving the correspondence problem? *Trends in Cognitive Science, 9,* 489–495.

Carroll, S. B. (2005). *Endless forms most beautiful.* New York: Norton.

Charman, T. (2003). Why is joint attention a pivotal skill in autism? *Philosophical Transactions of the Royal Society, B, 358,* 315–324.

Charman, T., Baron-Cohen, S., Swettenham, J., Baird, G., Cox, A., & Drew, A. (2000). Testing joint attention, imitation and play as infancy precursors to language and theory of mind. *Cognitive Development, 15*(4), 481–498.

Charman, T., Swettenham, J., Baron-Cohen, S., Cox, A., Baird, G., & Drew, A. (1997). Infants with autism: An investigation of empathy, pretend play, joint attention, and imitation. *Developmental Psychology, 33,* 781–789.

Corona, R., Dissanayake, C., Arbelle, S., Wellington, P., & Sigman, M. (1998). Is affect aversive to young children with autism? Behavioral and cardiac responses to experimenter distress. *Child Development, 69,* 1494–1502.

Csibra, G., & Gergely, G. (2005). Social learning and social cognition: The case for pedagogy. In M. H. Johnson & Y. Munakata (Eds.), *Processes of change in brain and cognitive development. Attention and performance*(pp. 249–274). Oxford, UK: Oxford Press.

Dapretto, M., Davies, M. S., Pfeifer, J. H., Scott, A. A., Sigman, M., Bookheimer, S. Y., et al. (2005). Understanding emotions in others: mirror neuron dysfunction in children with autism spectrum disorders. *Nature Neuroscience, 9,* 28–30.

Dautenhahn, K., & Nehaniv, C. L. (2002). *Imitation in animals and artifacts.* Cambridge, MA: MIT Press.

DeMyer, M. K., Alpern, G. D., Barton, S., DeMyer, W. E., Churchill, D.W., Hingtgen, J. N., et al. (1972). Imitation in autistic, early schizophrenic, and nonpsychotic subnormal children. *Journal of Autism and Childhood Schizophrenia, 2,* 264–287.

Donald, M. (1991). *Origins of the modern mind.* Cambridge, MA: Harvard University Press.

Donald, M. (2001). *A mind so rare: The evolution of human consciousness.* New York: Norton.

Evans, P. D., Gilbert, S. L., Mekel-Bobrov, N., Vallender, E. J., Anderson, J. R., Vaez-Azizi, L. M., et al. (2005). Microcephalin, a gene regulating brain size, continues to evolve adaptively in humans. *Science, 309,* 1717–1720.

Fidler, D. J., Hepburn, S. L., Most, D. E., Philofsky, A., & Rogers, S. J. (in review). *Emotional responsivity in young children with Williams syndrome.*

Finlay, B. L., & Darlington, R. B. (1995). Linked regularities in the development and evolution of mammalian brains. *Science, 268,* 1578–1584.

Fisher, S. E., Vargha-Khadem, F., Watkins, K. E., Monaco, A. P., & Pembrey, M. E. (1998). Localization of a gene implicated in a severe speech and language disorder. *Nature Genetics, 18,* 168–170.

Hadjikhani, N., Joseph, R. M., Snyder, J., & Tager-Flusberg, H. (in press). Anatomical differences in the mirror neuron system and social cognition network in autism. *Cerebral Cortex.*

Harm, M. W., & Seidenberg, M. S. (1999). Phonology, reading acquisition, and dyslexia: Insights from connectionist models. *Psychological Review, 106,* 491–528.

Hepburn, S. L., Philofsky, A., Fidler, D., & Rogers, S. J. (in review). *Social–perceptual and cognitive skills in young children with Williams syndrome.*

Heyes, C. (2001). Causes and consequences of imitation. *Trends in Cognitive Science, 5,* 253–261.

Hill, E. L. (1998). A dyspraxic deficit in specific language impairment and developmental coordination disorder? Evidence from hand and arm movements. *Developmental Medicine and Child Neurology, 40,* 388–395.

Hill, E. L., Bishop, D.V. M., & Nimmo-Smith, I. (1998). Representational gestures in developmental coordination disorder and specific language impairment: Error-types and the reliability of ratings. *Human Movement Science, 17,* 655–678.

Joanisse, M. F. (2000). *Connectionist phonology.* Unpublished doctoral dissertation, University of Southern California.

Johnson, M., & Morton, J. (1991). *Biology and cognitive development: The case of face recognition.* Oxford, UK: Blackwell.

Keysers, C., & Perrett, D. I. (2004). Demystifying social cognition: A Hebbian perspective. *Trends in Cognitive Sciences, 8,* 501–507.

Lakoff, G., & Johnson, M. (1999). *Philosophy in the flesh: The embodied mind and its challenge to western thought.* New York: Basic Books.

Masur, E. F., & Ritz, E. G. (1984). Patterns of gestural, vocal, and verbal imitation performance in infancy. *Merrill-Palmer Quarterly, 30,* 369–392.

McGrath, L., Smith, S. D., & Pennington, B. F. (in press). Breakthroughs in the search for dyslexia candidate genes. *Trends in Molecular Medicine.*

McIntosh, D. N., Reichmann-Decker, A., Winkielman, P., & Wilbarger, J. L. (in press). When the social mirror breaks: Deficits in automatic, but not voluntary mimicry of emotional facial expressions in autism. *Developmental Science, 5*(3).

Mekel-Bobrov, N., Gilbert, S. L., Evans, P. D., Vallender, E. J., Anderson, J. R., Hudson, R. R., et al. (2005). Ongoing adaptive evolution of ASPM, a brain size determinant in Homo sapiens. *Science, 309,* 1720–1722.

Meltzoff, A., & Gopnik, A. (1993). The role of imitation in understanding persons and developing a theory of mind. In S. Baron-Cohen, H. Tager-Flusberg, & D. J. Cohen (Eds.), *Understanding other minds* (pp. 335–366). Oxford, UK: Oxford University Press.

Meltzoff, A. N., & Moore, K. M. (1997). Explaining facial imitation: A theoretical model. *Early Development and Parenting, 6,* 179–192.

Mundy, P., & Neal, R. (2000). Neural plasticity, joint attention, and a transactional social-orienting model of autism. *International Review of Research in Mental Retardation*, 20, 139–1687.

Mundy, P., Sigman, M., & Kasari, C. (1990). A longitudinal study of joint attention and language development in autistic children. *Journal of Autism and Developmental Disorders*, 20, 115–128.

Nadel, J., Guérini, C., Pezé, A., & Rivet, C. (1999). The evolving nature of imitation as a format for communication. In J. Nadel & G. Butterworth (Eds.), *Imitation in infancy* (pp. 209–234). Cambridge, UK: Cambridge University Press.

Nelson, K. (1996). *Language in cognitive development: Emergence of the mediated mind.* Cambridge, UK: Cambridge University Press.

Nishitani, N., Avikainen, S., & Hari, R. (2004). Abnormal imitation-related cortical activation sequences in Asperger's syndrome. *Annals of Neurology*, 55, 558–562.

Oberman, L. M., Hubbard, E. M., McCleery, J. P., Altschuler, E. L., Ramachandran, V. S., & Pineda, J. A. (2005). EEG evidence for mirror neuron dysfunction in autism spectrum disorders. *Brain Research: Cognitive Brain Research*, 24, 190–198.

Pennington, B. F. (2002). *The development of psychopathology: Nature and nurture.* New York: Guilford Press.

Pennington, B. F. (in press). A multiple-deficit model for understanding developmental disorders. *Cognition.*

Pennington, B. F., & Olson, R. (2005). Genetics of dyslexia. In M. Snowling & C. Hulme (Eds.), *The science of reading: A handbook* (pp. 453–472). Oxford, UK: Blackwell.

Rizzolatti, G., Fogassi, L., & Gallese, V. (2001). Neurophysiological mechanisms underlying the understanding and imitation of action. *National Review of Neuroscience*, 2, 661–670.

Rogers, S. J., Hepburn, S. L., & Stackhouse, T. (2003). Imitation performance in toddlers with autism and those with other developmental disorders. *Journal of Child Psychology and Psychiatry and Allied Disciplines*, 44, 763–781.

Rogers, S. J., & Pennington, B. F. (1991). A theoretical approach to the deficits in infantile autism. *Development and Psychopathology*, 3, 137–162.

Rutherford, M. D., Hepburn, S., Young, G. S., & Rogers, S. J. (in press). A longitudinal study of pretend play in autism. *Journal of Autism and Developmental Disorders.*

Rutherford, M. D., & Rogers, S. J. (2003). Cognitive underpinnings of pretend play. *Journal of Autism and Developmental Disorders*, 33, 289–302.

Rutter, M., Andersen-Wood, L., Beckett, C., Bredenkamp, D., Castle, J., Groothues, C., et. al. (1999). Quasi-autistic patterns following severe early global privation. *Journal of Child Psychology and Psychiatry*, 40, 537–549.

Scambler, D., Hepburn, S., Rutherford, M. D., Wehner, E., & Rogers, S. J. (in press). Emotional responsivity in children with autism, children with other developmental disabilities, and children with typical development. *Journal of Autism and Developmental Disorders.*

Sigman, M., Dissanayake, C., Corona, R., & Espinosa, M. (2003). Social and cardiac responses of young children with autism. *Autism*, 7, 205–216.

Sigman, M. D., Kasari, C., Kwon, J. H., & Yirmiya, N. (1992). Responses to the negative emotions of others by autistic, mentally retarded, and normal children. *Child Development*, 63, 796–807.

Stern, D. N. (1985). *The interpersonal world of the human infant.* New York: Basic Books.

Stone, W. L., Ousley, O. Y., & Littleford, C. D. (1997). Motor imitation in young children with autism: What's the object? *Journal of Abnormal Child Psychology*, 25, 475–485.

Stone, W. L., Ousley, O. Y., Yoder, P. J., Hogan, K. L., & Hepburn, S. L. (1997). Nonverbal communication in two and three-year-old children with autism. *Journal of Autism and Developmental Disorders, 27*, 677–696.

Theoret, H., Halligan, E., Kobayashi, M., Fregni, F., Tager-Flusberg, H., & Pascual-Leone, A. (2005). Impaired motor facilitation during action observation in individuals with autism spectrum disorder. *Current Biology, 15*, R84–R85.

Trevarthen, C. (2001). Infant intersubjectivity: Research, theory, and clinical applications. *Journal of Child Psychology and Child Psychiatry, 42*, 3–28.

Užgiris, I. C. (1981). Two functions of imitation during infancy. *International Journal of Behavioral Development, 4*, 1–12.

Want, S. C., & Harris, P. L. (2002). How do children ape? Applying concepts from the study of non-human primates to the developmental study of "imitation" in children. *Developmental Science, 5*, 1–41.

Williams, J. H., Waiter, G. D., Gilchrist, A., Perrett, D. I., Murray, A. D., & Whiten A. (2006). Neural mechanisms of imitation and "mirror neuron" functioning in autistic spectrum disorder. *Neuropsychologia, 44*(4), 610–621.

Williams, J. H. G., Whiten, A., Suddendorf, T., & Perrett, D. I. (2001). Imitation, mirror neurons and autism. *Neuroscience and Biobehavioral Reviews, 25*, 287–295.

Yirmiya, N., Gamliel, I., Pilowsky, T., Feldman, R., Baron-Cohen, S., & Sigman, M. (in press). The development of siblings of children with autism at 4 and 14 months: Social engagement, communication, and cognition. *Journal of Child Psychology and Psychiatry*.

Yirmiya, N., Gamliel, I., Shaked, M., & Sigman, M. (in press). Cognitive and verbal abilities of 24- to 36-month-old siblings of children with autism. *Journal of Autism and Developmental Disorders*.

Zwaigenbaum, L., Bryson, S., Rogers, T., Roberts, W., Brian, J., & Szatmari, P. (2005). Behavioral manifestations of autism in the first year of life. *International Journal of Developmental Neuroscience, 23*, 143–152.

Index

Asperger syndrome, 110, 177, 186, 345–346
  MEG study of, 295
  motor skills and, 409–410
  neuroimaging studies of orofacial gestures, 362–363
  object imitation study of, 280
  white matter and, 367, 368
Assessments
  behavioral, 392–393
  cognitive/developmental, 390–392
  experimental studies, 378–389
  of movement, 340–341
  screening measures, 389–390
Assessors, for autism, 436–437
Associative sequence learning (ASL), 11–12, 253
Attention deficit-hyperactivity disorder (ADHD), 417
Attentional flexibility, 285–286
Autism Diagnostic Interview—Revised (ADI-R), 390
Autism Diagnostic Observation Schedule (ADOS), 390
Autism Diagnostic Observation Schedule—Generic, 208
Autism Observation Scale for Infants (AOSI), 390
Autism spectrum disorders (ASD)
  cascade model, 440–441
  clinical perspectives, 199–202
  cognitive functioning and, 421
  deficits characterizing, 72
  deficits in cultural knowledge and, 177–189
  deficits in mapping action, goal, and intention, 103–104
  echolalia, 78, 96–97, 207, 303, 447
  echopraxia, 303, 447
  end-state emulation and, 236–237
  eye contact and eye tracking, 58–59, 177–178, 287, 339–340
  genetic changes and, 442
  gestural impairments and, 419–421
  identification problems and, 218–219
  in imitation, identification, and self-other relations, 202–210
  in imitation and language development, 106–107, 110
  indeterminacy problem in, 444–446
  linguistic processing deficits and, 108
  megencephaly in, 367
  mirror neuron system and, 11, 296–297, 353. See also Mirror neuron system
  molar theories of imitation and, 447
  motor deficits in developmental coordination disorder and, 411–418, 421–422

neuroimaging
  of functional connectivity, 365–367
  of imitation activity, 354–363
  structural studies, 367–370
  of visuomotor ability, 363–364
phenocopies, 440
prehension in, 345–348
responses to being imitated and, 210, 302–303
risk assessors, 436–437
screening measures, 389–390
self–other mapping and, 210, 284, 285, 352–353, 419, 449
social cognition and, 440–441
thalamus and, 370
theory of mind deficit and, 166–169, 177–187
white matter connectivity and, 368–370
See also Children with autism; Imitation in autism; Mimicry and autism
Automatic imitation, 282, 289. See also Mimicry
Autonomic nervous system, facial expressions and, 264–265

Basal ganglia, 417
Bayley Scales of Infant Development II, 390
Behavioral assessment, 392–393
Behavioral reenactment paradigm, 203
Belief systems, 169
Bilateral dorsal premotor area, 265
Bilateral lingual gyrus, 360
Birds, imitation and, 243
Blindness, 440
Blood oxygen level dependent signal. See BOLD signal
"Body babbling," 10
Body-level imitation, 292–293
BOLD (blood oxygen level dependent) signal, 355, 371
Brain evolution, 293–294, 442
Brain imaging. See Functional magnetic resonance imaging; Neuroimaging studies
Brainstem, 368
Broca's area, 260, 261, 262, 265
  Asperger syndrome and, 295, 439
  language development and, 109
  mirror neurons and, 108, 109, 294, 353, 366
  neuroimaging studies, 358, 362–363, 371
Brodmann's area 46, 264

Capuchin monkeys, 233
CAST. See Childhood Asperger Syndrome Test
Caudate nucleus, 417